Catheter-Related Infections

INFECTIOUS DISEASE AND THERAPY

Series Editors

Brian E. Scully, M.B., B.Ch.
Harold C. Neu, M.D.

College of Physicians & Surgeons
Columbia University
New York, New York

Catheter-Related Infections

edited by
Harald Seifert
Institute of Medical Microbiology
University of Cologne
Cologne, Germany

Bernd Jansen
Johannes Gutenberg University
Mainz, Germany

Barry M. Farr
University of Virginia Health Sciences Center
Charlottesville, Virginia

MARCEL DEKKER, INC.   NEW YORK · BASEL · HONG KONG

Library of Congress Cataloging-in-Publication Data

Catheter-related infections / edited by Harald Seifert, Bernd Jansen,
    Barry M. Farr
        p. cm. — (Infectious disease and therapy; v. 20)
    Includes index.
    ISBN 0-8247-9848-1 (hardcover: alk. paper)
    1. Nosocomial infections. 2. Catheterization—Complications.
    I. Seifert, Harald, Dr. II. Jansen, Bernd. III. Farr, Barry M. IV. Series.
        [DNLM: 1. Cross Infection—etiology. 2. Catheterization—adverse
    effects. W1 IN406HMN v.20 1997 / WC 195 C363 1997]
    RC112.C38   1997
    616.9—dc21
    DNLM/DLC
    for Library of Congress   97-2630
                                                                                              CIP

The publisher offers discounts on this book when ordered in bulk quantities. For more information, write to Special Sales/Professional Marketing at the address below.

This book is printed on acid-free paper.

MARCEL DEKKER, INC.
270 Madison Avenue, New York, New York 10016
http://www.dekker.com

Current printing (last digit):
10 9 8 7 6 5 4 3 2 1

PRINTED IN THE UNITED STATES OF AMERICA

Series Introduction

Marcel Dekker, Inc., has for many years specialized in the publication of high-quality monographs in tightly focused areas in a variety of medical disciplines. These have been of great value to both the practicing physician and the research scientist as sources of detailed and up-to-date information presented in an attractive format. During the last decade, there has been a veritable explosion in knowledge in the various fields related to infectious diseases and clinical microbiology. Antimicrobial resistance, antibacterial and antiviral agents, AIDS, Lyme disease, infections in immunocompromised patients, and parasitic diseases are but a few of the areas in which an enormous amount of significant work has been published. The Infectious Disease and Therapy series covers carefully chosen topics that should be of interest and value to the practicing physician, the clinical microbiologist, and the research scientist.

Brian E. Scully, M.B., B.Ch.
Harold C. Neu, M.D.

Preface

The past several decades have witnessed major progress in many fields of medicine, such as the treatment of the critically ill in intensive care units, management of patients with hematologic malignancy, dialysis for end-stage renal disease, and transplantation for organ failure.

Many of these advances have involved an increasing reliance on intravascular catheters for the administration of medications, fluids, total parenteral nutrition, and blood products, as well as for hemodynamic monitoring. Catheters have been placed within the central nervous system for a variety of clinical indications, including the management of patients with hydrocephalus, intracranial pressure monitoring, and the administration of intraventricular antibiotics. Catheters have been employed for the management of patients on hemodialysis and continuous ambulatory peritoneal dialysis (CAPD).

Catheterization using an initially sterile catheter, however, may quickly be complicated by infection. A variety of microorganisms have been implicated, some originating from the hospital environment or the hands of hospital personnel, and others coming from the patient's own skin flora. It is clear that the density of cutaneous flora varies with different parts of the body, and that these skin organisms are the ones most likely to cause an endogenous infection. When a catheter is inserted into the neck or beneath the clavicle, higher microbial densities at these sites may lead to a greater risk of infection than for catheters inserted into the arm. Occasionally these infections come from other sources, such as contaminated infusate or hematogenous spread from a distant infection (e.g., urinary tract infection). Although remarkable improvements have been made in catheter design and composition, vascular catheters continue to be a major source of nosocomial infection that extends hospital stay and increases hospital costs.

Although most cases of catheter-related infections are resolved with catheter removal and antibiotic therapy, serious complications may result, including septic thrombophlebitis, endocarditis, and metastatic infection of distant sites. Prevention of these infections would have an important impact on patient mortality and the cost-effectiveness of hospital care.

In this book, experts from several countries have contributed their knowledge of various aspects of catheter-related infections. The pathogenesis and epidemiology of catheter-related infections are addressed in detail, with special focus on the types of catheters and the etiological agents involved. This book provides the clinician with current information about diagnosis, major complications, and management of catheter-related infections. Situations in which removal of the indwelling catheter is essential for cure are contrasted with those in which the device may be preserved. Finally, various approaches to the prevention of catheter-related infections are emphasized.

Harald Seifert
Bernd Jansen
Barry M. Farr

Contents

Contributors

Roger Bayston, M.Med.Sci., M.Sc., Ph.D., F.R.C.Path. University Research Fellow (S/L), Clinical Microbiologist, University Department of Microbiology and Infectious Diseases, City Hospital, Nottingham, England

Verena A. Briner, M.D. Head, Department of Medicine, Hospital of Lucerne, Lucerne, Switzerland

Arnaldo Colombo, M.D., Ph.D. Director, Special Mycology Laboratory, Division of Infectious Diseases, São Paulo Federal Medical School, São Paulo, Brazil

Barry M. Farr, M.D., M.Sc. Hospital Epidemiologist, University of Virginia Health Sciences Center, and the William S. Jordan Jr. Professor of Medicine and Epidemiology, Department of Internal Medicine, University of Virginia, Charlottesville, Virginia

André Fleer, M.D., Ph.D. Medical Microbiologist, Department of Medical Microbiology, University Hospital for Children and Youth "Het Wilhelmina Kinderziekenhuis," Utrecht, The Netherlands

Leo J. Gerards, M.D., Ph.D.   Pediatrician-Neonatologist, Department of Neonatology, University Hospital for Children and Youth "Het Wilhelmina Kinderziekenhuis," Utrecht, The Netherlands

Mathias Herrmann, M.D.   Associate Physician, Department of Medical Microbiology, University of Münster, Münster, Germany

Bernd Jansen, M.D., Ph.D.   Professor and Head, Department of Hygiene and Environmental Medicine, Johannes Gutenberg University, Mainz, Germany

Tannette G. Krediet, M.D.   Pediatrician-Neonatologist, Department of Neonatology, University Hospital for Children and Youth "Het Wilhelmina Kinderziekenhuis," Utrecht, The Netherlands

Karl G. Kristinsson, M.D., Ph.D., F.R.C.Path.   Associate Professor, Department of Clinical Microbiology, National University Hospital, Reykjavik, Iceland

Dennis G. Maki, M.D.   Ovid O. Meyer Professor of Medicine and Head, Section of Infectious Diseases, Department of Medicine, University of Wisconsin Hospital and Clinics, Madison, Wisconsin

C. Glen Mayhall, M.D.   Professor of Internal Medicine and Hospital Epidemiologist, Departments of Internal Medicine and Healthcare Epidemiology, University of Texas Medical Branch at Galveston, Galveston, Texas

Leonard A. Mermel, D.O., Sc.M.   Assistant Professor of Medicine, Brown University School of Medicine, and Medical Director, Department of Epidemiology and Infection Control, Rhode Island Hospital, Providence, Rhode Island

Georg Peters, M.D.   Professor of Medical Microbiology and Chairman, Institute of Medical Microbiology, University of Münster, Münster, Germany

Issam I. Raad, M.D., F.A.C.P.   Associate Professor of Medicine and Chief, Section of Infection Control, Department of Infectious Diseases, University of Texas M.D. Anderson Cancer Center, Houston, Texas

John J. Roord, M.D., Ph.D.   Pediatrician-Infectiologist, Department of Pediatrics, University Hospital for Children and Youth "Het Wilhelmina Kinderziekenhuis," Utrecht, The Netherlands

Hossam Safar, M.D.*   Fellow in Infectious Diseases, Department of Internal Medicine, University of Texas M.D. Anderson Cancer Center, Houston, Texas

Current affiliation: University of Texas Health Science Center.

Harald Seifert, M.D.   Associate Professor of Medical Microbiology, Institute of Medical Microbiology and Hygiene, University of Cologne, Cologne, Germany

Robert J. Sherertz, M.D.   Professor of Medicine and Hospital Epidemiologist, Division of Infectious Diseases/Internal Medicine, Bowman Gray School of Medicine, Winston-Salem, North Carolina

Henri Alexander Verbrugh, M.D., Ph.D.   Professor of Clinical Microbiology, Department of Medical Microbiology and Infectious Diseases, Erasmus University Hospital Rotterdam, Rotterdam, The Netherlands

Andreas Voss, M.D., Ph.D.   Hospital Epidemiologist, Department of Medical Microbiology, University Hospital St. Radboud, Nijmegen, The Netherlands

Sergio B. Wey, M.D., Ph.D.   Associate Professor, Division of Infectious Diseases, São Paulo Federal Medical School, São Paulo, Brazil

Andreas F. Widmer, M.S., M.D.   Director, Division of Clinical Epidemiology, University Hospital Basel, Basel, Switzerland

Pathogenesis of Vascular Catheter-Related Infections

Robert J. Sherertz
Bowman Gray School of Medicine, Winston-Salem, North Carolina

I. INTRODUCTION

Vascular catheter infections can develop for many reasons, but they must begin with catheter colonization by microorganisms through either one or both of two routes: (1) colonization of the outside of the catheter, or (2) colonization of the inside of the catheter. Colonization of the outside of the catheter can occur owing to skin microorganisms, direct extension of a contiguous infectious process, or hematogenous seeding of the catheter from a distant site (Fig. 1). In all three of these circumstances, the microorganisms must have been able to evade or overwhelm the immune system. Colonization of the inside of the catheter can happen by either the introduction of microorganisms through the catheter hub or contamination of infusion fluid (Fig. 1). These locations inside the catheter are not accessible to the immune system and therefore may require a much lower number of microorganisms to produce infection. Colonization of a catheter by either route can then progress to clinical manifestations—i.e., infection. This chapter will attempt to provide an understanding of the mechanisms by which catheter colonization/infection develops, identify factors that modify these mechanisms, and suggest areas for future research.

II. CATHETER COLONIZATION VS. CATHETER INFECTION

The diagnosis of catheter-related infection is a complex subject that is covered in detail elsewhere in the book. Using a variety of quantitative culture methods it has been possible to show an association between greater numbers of microorganisms on the catheter and inflammation or catheter-related bacteremia. With the roll-plate culture method 13% of catheters with <15 cfu had associated inflammation vs. 64% of catheters with ≥ 15 cfu (1). Similarly, the risk of catheter-related bacteremia varied with the number of organisms quantitated: 0/225 catheters with <15 cfu, 4/25 with ≥15 cfu, and 4/13 with ≥1000 cfu (1). Similar findings from other studies using different quantitative culture methods (2–5) suggest that clinical manifestations; i.e., fever, purulence, bacteremia, "sepsis," etc. may be directly related to the number of organisms on the catheter.

Strong support for a quantitative relationship between the number of microorganisms on a catheter and clinical manifestations has been provided by the sonication catheter culture method (6,7). In a study of 1681 consecutive catheters cultured in a clinical microbiology laboratory there was a high correlation ($r = 0.93$) between the number of organisms removed by sonication and the percent of catheters associated with positive blood cultures growing the same organism (6). Using this same culture method in a rabbit model of subcutaneous *Staphylococcus aureus* infection, it has been possible to show a very high correlation between the number of cfu of *S. aureus* removed from the catheters and the percent of catheters with associated purulence ($r = 0.99$; Fig. 2) (7). Thus, the more organisms on a catheter in vivo, the more likely there will be clinical signs and symptoms of infection.

One significant question that remains to be answered in relation to catheter colonization/infection is why some catheters have visible biofilm containing microorganisms by scanning and transmission electron microscopy and yet have negative cultures. Raad et al. (8) found in a group of cancer patients that biofilms were present on the internal and external surfaces of all central catheters within several days of catheter insertion. Even in culture-negative catheters, more than 30% of the internal surface of the catheter and nearly 10% of the external surface was covered by biofilm containing microorganisms. Similar findings with culture negative catheters were found by Tenney et al. in the same patient population (9) and by Passerini et al. with Swan-Ganz catheters (10). This suggests either that the biofilm is nonviable or that it must be cultured using a different method in order to recover the organisms. A better understanding of this phenomenon may help in the prevention of vascular catheter infection.

Sources of Infecting Organisms

Studies have been done in recent years attempting to identify the source of microorganisms that cause vascular catheter infection. These studies have used

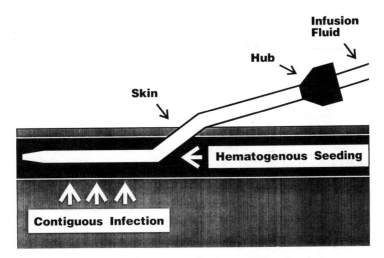

Figure 1 Sources of vascular catheter infection. Vascular catheter infection develops most commonly from organisms originating at the skin surface followed by the catheter hub, and then much less frequently from infusion fluid, hematogenous seeding, or continuous infection.

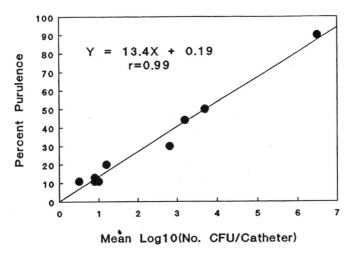

Figure 2 Relationship of the number of organisms removed from vascular catheters by sonication and the likelihood of these catheters being associated with purulent infection. Each symbol represents a mean taken from five to 10 catheters implanted in a rabbit model of subcutaneous *Staphylococcus aureus* infection.

quantitative culture methods to culture the skin around the catheter, the catheter hub or lumen, and the infusate, as well as attempting to identify other sites of infection that may have seeded the catheter through the bloodstream. With short-term catheters (average duration ≤ 8 days) studies have found that catheter colonization comes predominantly from the skin (75–90%), followed by the hub/lumen (10–50%), the bloodstream (3–10%), and infusate (2–3%) (11–13). For catheters in place for longer durations (>8 days), the relative frequencies of different sources of catheter colonization are not as well known, because many long-term catheters are not routinely removed related to questions of infection. Data are available for both short-term and longer-term catheters comparing the catheter hub versus the skin as sources of catheter-related bacteremia (Table 1). For short-term catheters the skin is more likely than the hub/lumen to be the source of catheter-related bacteremia (92% vs. 42%), whereas with longer-term catheters the hub/lumen is more likely the source (66% vs. 26%) (11–17). Additional evidence supporting these conclusions has been provided by Raad et al., who found that the quantity of biofilm on the internal surface of the catheter was less than the external surface during the first 10 days of catheterization, but increased steadily thereafter until it equaled or exceded the biofilm on the external surface (8).

1. Skin

The best evidence that the skin is the most common source of microorganisms for infections involving short-term catheters has been provided by Maki et al., who

Table 1 Relative Contribution of the Skin Entry Site vs. the Catheter Hub/Lumen to Catheter-Related Bacteremia

Study	Catheter type	Average duration	No. CRB	Skin	Hub/lumen
Mermel et al. (13)	Swan-Ganz	3 d	2	2	1
Flowers et al. (12)	CVC	5 d	4	3	2
Maki et al. (11)	CVC	8 d	6	6	2
		≤ 8 d		11/12	5/12
				92%	42%
Almirall et al. (15)	Hemodialysis	20 d	9	6	3
Linares et al. (14)	CVC/TPN	22 d	20	2	14
Cheesbrough et al. (16)	Hemodialysis	26 d	12	4	12
Weightman et al. (17)	Cancer Rx	115 d	11	0/6	8/10
		> 8 d		12/47	34/51
				26%	66%

looked at multiple risk factors for catheter-related infection and then performed multivariate analysis (18–21). In four studies, involving peripheral catheters (18), arterial catheters (19), Swan-Ganz catheters (13), and central catheters (20), colonization of the catheter insertion site with $>10^2$ cfu was the strongest risk factor (three studies) (13,18,19) or second-strongest risk factor (one study) (20) for catheter-related infection. Molecular typing of skin microorganisms and catheter microorganisms has substantiated the link demonstrated epidemiologically (13). By comparing data from quantitative skin cultures of the exit sites of central versus peripheral catheters, Maki has also found that peripheral catheters have fewer microorganisms on the skin at the exit site than central catheters and suggested that this could explain the lower risk of infection associated with peripheral catheters (21). A possible explanation for this observation could be the lower skin temperatures found on the skin of the extremities in comparison to the skin of the trunk. This hypothesis is interesting and disserves further investigation.

Additional evidence that the skin is the source of the majority of early catheter infections has been provided by a number of studies in both animal models and patients aimed at reducing the number of microorganisms on the skin surface or in the subcutaneous space next to the catheter (Table 2). These studies have shown that sterile technique (22), maximum sterile barriers (23,24), better skin antisepsis (25–27), topical ointments (28,29), catheter cuffs (11,12,30), and

Table 2 Interventions That Reduce the Risk of Infections Associated With Short-Term (≤ 8 days) Vascular Catheters by Decreasing the Number of Microorganisms on the Skin or in the Subcutaneous Space Next to the Catheter

Sterile technique
    Sterile technique is better than nonsterile technique—rats (22)
    Maximum sterile drapes—patients (23,24)
Better skin antisepsis
    Povidone iodine scrub followed by alcohol/tincture of iodine wipe—dogs (25)
    Chlorhexidine—patients (26,27)
Topical ointment
    Povidone iodine ointment—hemodialysis patients (28)
    Mupirocin—patients (29)
Catheter cuffs
    4 different types were effective—dogs (30)
    Ag-coated collagen cuffs—patients (11,12)
Anti-infective coatings
    Dicloxacillin, clindamycin, fusidic acid, chlorhexidine, penicillin, Ag-sulfadiazine, Ag-sulfadiazine plus chlorhexidine, silver wire—animals (7,31–36)
    Ag-sulfadiazine plus chlorhexidine, TDMAC-cefazolin, minocycline-rifampin-patients (37–44)

anti-infective coatings (7,31–44) have all been effective at reducing the risk of infection associated with short-term catheters. Conversely, contamination of the skin with antiseptic skin preparation solutions containing microorganisms has been shown to increase the risk of catheter-related infection (45–48).

2. Hub

In addition to the culture localization studies that suggest that the hub is the source of the majority of long-term (>8 days), catheter-related infections, there are a number of investigations in both animal models and patients that support this contention. Luminal disinfection with vancomycin/heparin, chlorine dioxide, gentamicin/chymotrypsin, and vancomycin/ciprofloxacin/heparin have all been shown to be effective at decreasing the risk of catheter-related infection (Table 3) (49–53). There have also been studies done with several new devices designed to reduce the risk of contaminating the catheter hub which have been shown to reduce the risk of catheter-related infection (54–57). Conversely, interventions that are designed to decrease the risk of infections by targeting skin microorganisms should not have much effect on decreasing the risk of infections associated with long-term catheters. In two studies of cancer patients with catheters in place longer than 20 days, silver-coated collagen cuffs were not effective at decreasing the risk of catheter-related infection (58,59). One additional study by Goldschmidt et al. (60), demonstrated that the precise cut-off of short term versus long term catheters is not clear. They found that in cancer patients with catheters inserted into the internal jugular for an average of 12 to 13 days that silver-coated catheters decreased the risk of catheter-related colonization/infection. Most long-term catheters in cancer patients are inserted in the operating room with maximum barrier sterile drapes. If the internal jugular catheters in this study were inserted with less than maximum sterile drapes, the efficacy of the anti-infective coating may be explainable by the greater risk of infection associated with this method of insertion (23,24).

Table 3 Interventions That Reduce the Risk of Infections Associated With Long-Term (> 8 days) Vascular Catheters by Decreasing the Number of Microorganisms in the Lumen of the Catheter

---

Luminal disinfection
  Chymotrypsin/gentamicin, chlorine dioxide—animals (49,50)
  Vancomycin/heparin, minocycline/EDTA, vancomycin/ciprofloxacin/heparin—
    patients (51–53)
Engineering controls
  Antibiotic lock—animals (54)
  Betadine connection shield, I-system, antibiotic lock—patients (55–57)

---

3. Bloodstream

Hematogenous seeding of vascular catheters has been shown to occur infrequently (1–3), but it is still an important source of catheter-related infection. In a recent study by Maki and Will of risk factors for central venous catheter-related infection in ICU patients, exposure to an unrelated bacteremia was the strongest risk factor for infection (20). Hematogenous seeding has been documented to occur almost exclusively in ICU patient populations (20,61–63). This probably means that this patient population is the most likely to experience an unrelated bloodstream infection while having a catheter in place; it does not mean that hematogenous seeding of vascular catheters will not occur outside of an ICU setting.

4. Intravenous Fluids

Like hematogenous seeding, contamination of intravenous fluids is an infrequent source of vascular catheter infection. However, it is an extremely important source because of the potential for outbreaks to occur associated with contamination of intravenous fluids. This source of infection as well as how to investigate a possibly contaminated product has been reviewed in detail by Maki (64–66). A summary of the major causes of this type of infection is shown in Table 4. Intrinsic contamination (during the manufacturing process) occurs less commonly than extrinsic contamination (in use).

Table 4 Major Causes of Infusion-Related Catheter Infection

Extrinsic contamination
    Arterial pressure monitoring infusate
    Blood products
    Heart lung machine
    Hemodialysis-related
    Hyperalimentation solutions
    Intra-aortic balloon pumps
    Lipid emulsions, including propafol
    Medication vials, especially multidose vials
    Parenteral crystaloids, especially those containing dextrose
    Skin antiseptics
    Warming baths
Intrinsic contamination (during manufacturing)
    Blood products
    Commercial crystaloid solutions, especially those containing dextrose
    IV drugs

Source: Modified from Ref. 65.

Table 5 Unique Abilities of Certain Bacteria to Grow in Different Solutions

---

Distilled water
 Acinetobacter
 Pseudomonas
 Serratia
Lactated Ringer's
 Enterobacter
 Ps. aeruginosa
 Serratia
Normal saline
 Bacteria, not yeast
5% dextrose
 Citrobacter
 Enterobacter
 Klebsiella
 Pseudomonas cepacia
 Serratia
25% dextrose/TPN
 Candida
Lipid emulsions
 Almost any bacteria; yeasts
 Malassezia furfur

Source: From Refs. 64–67.

Many studies have demonstrated that different fluids favor the growth of different microorganisms. Table 5 summarizes the most important associations in this regard. A particularly unique example of the differential growth of microorganisms was provided by a nationwide outbreak of Enterobacteriacae infections in the United States involving 5% dextrose solutions. As part of the investigation it was demonstrated that this IV solution favored the growth of *Klebsiella, Enterobacter, Citrobacter,* and *Pseudomonas cepacia* (67,68). These organisms were capable of reaching concentrations of 10^5 cfu/ml within 24 hours at room temperature. The outbreak actually developed secondary to intrinsic contamination of the fluid bottle—screw-cap closure associated with a change in the cap liner from one material (gilsonite) to another (elastomer) (69,70). Unbeknownst to the manufacturer the original gilsonite material had antibacterial properties which the replacement elastomer material did not have (70) and thus allowed the growth of microorganisms after contamination occurred during the manufacturing process.

The growth characteristics of different solutions can be used to help focus an outbreak investigation. In an outbreak of *Candida* bloodstream infections in a neonatal intensive care unit the unique ability of *Candida* to grow in hyperalimentation fluid suggested the most obvious location for contamination to be occurring in a complex system of fluid delivery (71). In other outbreaks, such as the recent report of extrinsic contamination of the anesthetic propafol, the ability of lipid emulsions to support the growth of a wide range of microorganisms forced the consideration of a broad range of outbreak mechanisms (72). A detailed summary of the mechanisms of a wide variety of infusion-related blood-stream infection has been provided by Pittet (73).

5. Contiguous Infection

Direct extension of microorganisms from adjacent infected tissue to a vascular catheter is uncommon except in burn patients. In patients with large burns it is frequently necessary to insert a vascular catheter through burned skin. Because of the high frequency of heavy colonization/infection of burned skin, burn patients have a high frequency of catheter-related infection (63,74,75).

III. MICROORGANISMS

The microbiology of catheter-related infections has been carefully investigated in a number of studies. In one large study of 1681 consecutive vascular catheters sent to a microbiology laboratory for culture by sonication, there was a predictable spectrum of culture results with sterile catheters being most common (53.9%), followed by colonized catheters ($<10^2$ cfu; 33.8%), infected catheters ($\geq 10^2$ cfu with no associated positive blood culture growing the same organism; 7.6%), and finally by infected catheters with associated bloodstream infection (4.7%) (6). Thus, colonized catheters were much more common than infected catheters.

Coagulase-negative staphylococci (*Staphylococcus epidermidis* > other CNS) were the most common organisms growing $\geq 10^2$ cfu, followed by *Pseudomonas aeruginosa*, yeasts (*C. albicans* > other yeasts), enterococci, *Staphylococcus aureus*, and *Enterobacter* (Table 6) (6). This ranking by quantitative culture is very similar to a composite ranking calculated by pooling the results of different studies of vascular catheter infections that employed quantitative culture methods (76). The high frequency of *Ps. aeruginosa* isolates most likely represented the large number of catheters removed from burn patients (26%). The ranking of organisms by frequency of catheter-related bloodstream infection is quite different: coagulase-negative staphylococci, followed by *S. aureus*, *C. albicans*, enterococci, *Ps. aeruginosa*, and *E. cloacae* (Table 7). This ranking closely parallels pooled data from prospective studies looking for catheter-related bacteremias using quantitative culture methods (77). Polymicrobial catheter-related bloodstream infection was uncommon (9%).

Focusing on the three most common causes of catheter-related bloodstream infection—*S. epidermidis*, *S. aureus*, and *C. albicans*—there are clinical data demonstrating a hierarchy of virulence. Again looking at data from the same

Table 6 Frequency of Microorganisms Isolated From Sonicated Catheter Cultures With $\geq 10^2$ cfu

Organism	Frequency	%
Coagulase-negative staphylococci	189	36.5
Pseudomonas aeruginosa	75	14.5
Yeasts	43	8.3
Enterococci	41	7.9
Staphylococcus aureus	40	7.7
Enterobacter species	22	4.2
Corynebacterium species	21	4.1
Escherichia coli	20	3.9
Alpha-hemolytic streptococci	16	3.1
Klebsiella species	10	1.9
Proteus species	7	1.4
Bacillus species	5	1.0
Serratia species	4	0.8
Acinetobacter species	4	0.8
Other	21	4.1
Total	518	

Table 7 Risk of Positive Blood Cultures Within 48 hours Prior to Catheter Removal Associated With Positive Catheter Cultures ($\geq 10^2$ cfu) for the Six Most Common Organisms Causing Vascular Catheter Infections

Organism	Catheters (N)	Positive blood cultures			
		N	Rank	%	Rank
C. albicans	20	15	3	75	1
S. aureus	26	18	2	69	2
E. cloacae	12	6	6	50	3
E. faecalis	30	10	4	33	4
Ps. aeruginosa	32	10	4	31	5
Coagulase-negative staphylococci	99	29	1	29	6

study of vascular catheters cited above (6), the most remarkable difference was the much higher frequency of associated bloodstream infection with *C. albicans* and *S. aureus* catheter infections than with coagulase-negative staphylococcal (CNS) infections (15/20 and 18/26 vs. 29/99, respectively; $P \le 0.0004$; χ^2). This suggests greater virulence for *S. aureus* and *C. albicans* than CNS. *S. aureus* was more likely to have more than one positive blood culture prior to catheter removal (*S. aureus* 1.7 ± 0.8 vs. *C. albicans* 1.2 ± 0.8; CNS – 1.2 ± 0.4; $P \le 0.02$, Mann-Whitney). The titer of *S. aureus* cfu removed by sonication (*S. aureus*: $N = 60$, mean $= 3.74 \pm 1.83$) was higher than for the other two organisms (*C. albicans*: $N = 65$, mean $= 3.05 \pm 1.78$; *S. epidermidis*: $N = 77$, mean $= 2.64 \pm 1.14$; $P \le 0.03$, Mann-Whitney). *S. aureus* was also more likely to have purulence documented by the clinicians at the catheter exit site than the other two organisms ($P < 0.05$) (6). Collectively, these findings suggest that *S. aureus* is more virulent than *C. albicans*, which is more virulent than *S. epidermidis* at causing vascular catheter infection.

A. *Staphylococcus epidermidis*

It is striking that although *S. epidermidis* is less virulent at causing vascular catheter infections than *S. aureus*, *C. albicans*, and other organisms as well (see above) (6), it is the most common cause of catheter infection and catheter-related bacteremia, as well as the most common cause of infection associated with most other implantable medical devices (78). Equally notable, *S. epidermidis* is an uncommon cause of infection in the absence of medical devices (79). Thus, while it is tempting to conclude that the overall greater frequency of *S. epidermidis* causing catheter-related infection is due to the much greater frequency of isolating these organisms from the skin than other organisms that cause catheter infection (80), the link between *S. epidermidis* infections and foreign bodies suggests that the pathogenesis of *S. epidermidis* infections must be related to its ability to survive in vivo in the presence of a foreign body.

The first step toward producing catheter infection must be adherence of the organism to the catheter. Hydrophobic strains of CNS are more likely to colonize naked medical devices in vitro than are hydrophilic strains (81–84). There are some recent in vitro data that suggest that pili-like structures may be involved in the adherence of *S. epidermidis* to naked medical devices (85). There are also data that suggest that *S. epidermidis* has an adhesin that is important for adherence to naked plastic (86). The data on in vitro adherence to uncoated polymers should be quite relevant to adherence to catheter hubs or lumina, but it is not clear whether it will have relevance in vivo where the external surface of catheters becomes coated with a wide range of proteins, including fibrinogen, fibronectin, and albumin. There are studies demonstrating that *S. epidermidis* binds to fibronectin and collagen (87,88) and that it has an adhesin that is important in the pathogenesis of hematogenous catheter infection and endocarditis (89,90).

However, to date there is no clear consensus that adherence to any of the proteins that coat medical devices is absolutely necessary to the pathogenesis of CNS infections of catheters or other medical devices (78). Further work is necessary to understand the events required for initial attachment of *S. epidermidis* and other CNS to medical devices.

The best-studied potential virulence factor for *S. epidermidis* is capsular "slime." Using a tube assay it has been demonstrated by Christensen et al. that 63% of pathogenic strains of *S. epidermidis* produce slime vs. 37% of nonpathogenic strains (91,92). They have further shown that *S. epidermidis* strains associated with vascular catheter infection produce thicker bacterial films than blood culture contaminants (93). Similar studies have been performed by many different investigators all over the world with similar findings (78). Some evidence exists that slime may impede phagocytosis by neutrophils (94). More significant evidence that slime production might be a virulence factor was provided when it was shown that a slime producing strain of *S. epidermidis* was more virulent in animal models than a daughter strain that did not produce slime (95,96). Unfortunately, the slime-negative mutant used in these studies has also been shown to have differences in antibiotic resistance, and both changes have been thought to occur secondary to phase variation (95). While this does not disprove that slime is a virulence factor, it makes the question more difficult to answer. One interesting speculation that might explain the presence of slime made by CNS is that they may be marine organisms and their ability to form slime may have evolved as a mechanism for maintaining attachment to rocks and other underwater surfaces (78,97). The ultimate solutions to these questions will require slime-negative mutants that do not have other associated phenotypic changes.

B. Staphylococcus aureus

Localization studies have shown that the majority of *S. aureus* infections originate at the skin surface (11/16; 69%) (3,14–16). These data suggest that *S. aureus* must be present on the skin surface where the catheter is inserted. Colonization of the skin with *S. aureus* is felt to be a function of *S. aureus* nasal colonization (98). Nasal carriage of *S. aureus* has been linked in general to an increased risk of *S. aureus* infection (99–104) and to an increased risk of vascular access infection (105–110). In chronic hemodialysis patients, interventions that decrease the rate of *S. aureus* nasal carriage decrease the risk of *S. aureus* vascular access infection (105,106).

For a vascular catheter infection to develop, *S. aureus* must then be able to extend from the skin surface and survive and multiply in the subcutaneous space. This involves evading being killed by neutrophils, the principal defense against *S. aureus* (98). Patient populations who have neutrophil defects that affect their being able to kill *S. aureus* have been shown to have an increased risk of *S. aureus* vascular catheter infection (107–109,111–114). *S. aureus* makes a number of potential virulence factors including a wide array of enzymes (catalase, hyaluronidase, nuclease, β-lactamase, coagulase, staphylokinase) and toxins (α-toxin, β-toxin, γ-toxin, δ-toxin, leukocidin, epidermolytic toxins, enterotoxins, toxic shock syndrome toxin, staphylococcal superantigens) (98). However, except for catalase production with its ability to interfere with neutrophil killing (115), the relative contribution of each to evading neutrophils has been difficult to sort out (98).

S. aureus has been clearly demonstrated to have enhanced virulence in the presence of a foreign body. This finding was first shown in humans with silk sutures by Elek and Conen (116). We have recently found that the same thing was true in rabbits using polyurethane vascular catheters implanted in the subcutaneous space (7). Characteristics of *S. aureus* that may increase its virulence in association with a foreign body include surface receptors for proteins that will allow it to adhere to foreign bodies and the ability to form a glycocalyx. *S. aureus* has been shown to adhere to at least six proteins that may facilitate its attachment to foreign bodies: fibrinogen (117), fibronectin (118), laminin (119), thrombospondin (120), collagen IV (121), and von Willebrand factor (122). Studies using coverslips removed from subcutaneous chambers in guinea pigs (123), vascular catheters removed from patients (124,125), and ex vivo canine artiovenous shunts (126) suggest that fibrinogen is the protein that mediates early adherence and that fibronectin is the protein that mediates adherence after the foreign body has been in place for a while. Adherence to these proteins is also the likely explanation for hematogenous seeding of vascular catheters by *S. aureus*. After adherence, some strains of *S. aureus* have the ability to form a glycocalyx, which may help them evade phagocytes (127). Since many *S. aureus* strains do not have this characteristic, it may not have great importance in the pathogenesis of foreign body infections.

An interesting question is whether the ability of *S. aureus* to interact with the coagulation system has any importance relative to its virulence with vascular catheter infections. *S. aureus* makes a coagulase that can clot blood (128); a staphylokinase that can lyse clots by activating plasminogen to plasmin (129); and surface receptors that can bind plasmin (130), fibrinogen, and fibrin (117). This combination of traits is unique among microorganisms and suggests some adaptive response to interactions with the coagulation system. Patient studies have suggested a possible link between infection and catheter-related thrombosis. Press et al. found that five of six thrombosed, central venous silicone catheters were associated with infection compared with 10 of 123 catheters without thrombosis (131). In a similar study, Raad et al. demonstrated that catheter-related blood stream infections were associated with venous mural wall thrombosis (seven of 27 episodes vs. zero of 45 without thrombosis), and *S. aureus* was four times more likely to cause the infection than any other organism (132). While these two studies do not provide information that helps distinguish whether the infection comes before or after the clot, the former is clearly one possibility. With

S. aureus this raises the possibility of coagulase being a virulence factor. Studies in mouse (133) and rabbit (134) using coagulase-deficient mutants produced by allele-replacement mutagenesis have not been able to demonstrate this possibility. The significance of such animal model results is difficult to interpret because most animals have differences in their coagulation systems related to *S. aureus* compared to humans. For example, staphylocoagulase does not coagulate mouse blood (135), and staphylokinase is a poor activator of rabbit plasminogen (136). Further studies will be necessary before the true importance of the ability of *S. aureus* to interact with the coagulations system in humans is known.

C.   Yeast (*Candida albicans*)

C. albicans, like *S. aureus*, has a much greater ability to cause catheter-related bloodstream infection than other microorganisms (6). Unlike *S. aureus*, relatively little is known about the pathogenesis of catheter-related candidemia. In studies of patients receiving hyperalimentation that have attempted to localize the origin of microorganisms, *C. albicans* is isolated from the skin surface only about half the time, suggesting that at least half the time the organism originated either external to the patient or elsewhere in the body and gets to the catheter hematogenously (3,14). The easiest mechanism by which *C. albicans* can reach the catheter from a source external to the body is through a line break (71). If the line break is into hyperalimentation fluid, *C. albicans* will have a selective growth advantage in comparison to gram-positive and gram-negative bacteria (71,137,138).

Evidence for hematogenous seeding of vascular catheters has been provided by a study that found that *C. albicans* vascular catheter infections were more likely to be associated with a preexisting other site of infection ($P \leq 0.05$) than other microorganisms causing catheter infections (6). In the absence of another site of infection, *C. albicans* may reach the bloodstream from the gastrointestinal tract associated with antibiotic therapy and/or immunosuppression (139,140). *C. albicans* has surface receptors for a number of proteins found on epithelial, endothelial, and foreign body surfaces including fibronectin (141), fibrinogen (142), and vitronectin (143); and animal model studies suggest that adherence to fibronectin is important related to hematogenous seeding of distant sites (144,145). It has been hypothesized that *C. albicans'* ability to disseminate hemogenously is a direct extension of its ability to bind to epithelial cells and survive on mucosal surfaces (146).

At the present time it is poorly understood when and under what circumstances *C. albicans* can extend from the skin surface and multiply in the subcutaneous space surrounding a vascular catheter. The use of anti-infective agents (polymyxin-neomycin-bacitracin, chlorhexidine) at the skin surface can lead to an overgrowth of *Candida*, which may facilitate infection (12,147). *C. albicans* makes a proteinase that is found extracellularly and that appears to be an important virulence factor in an animal model (148). The organism makes no known toxins. It is unclear whether the presence of a foreign body augments the survival of the organism in the same way that it does for staphylococci. Further investigation will be necessary to understand the pathogenic factors that facilitate catheter-related *C. albicans* infection (149).

IV. FOREIGN BODY EFFECTS ON THE HOST

While it is considered common knowledge among medical personnel that "foreign bodies" predispose to infection, relatively little is known about how foreign bodies affect their host. Immediately after insertion foreign bodies will interact with various host defense enzymatic systems including coagulation, fibrinolytic, kallikrein-kinin, and complement (150,151). These interactions facilitate cellular responses by neutrophils, platelets, lymphocytes, and macrophages. Ultimately four major categories of host responses have been described (152): (1) the material releases toxic compounds which kill the surrounding tissue; (2) the material is nontoxic but is gradually resorbed and replaced by the surrounding tissue; (3) the material is nontoxic, is biologically inactive, cannot be degraded, and is ultimately encapsulated; and (4) the material is nontoxic and highly interactive, and forms chemical bonds with the surrounding tissue, which stabilizes it. The mechanisms of the responses observed in these categories are just beginning to be elucidated. A detailed discussion of these considerations is beyond the scope of this chapter, but excellent reviews are available elsewhere (151,153). Instead, this section will focus on what is known about how foreign bodies predispose to infections.

The effect of foreign bodies on the risk of infection was first appreciated using suture material, where it was found that the presence of a silk, cotton, or Dacron suture would increase the risk of infection by up to 1000-fold (116,154,155). Similar observations have been made with other materials including sponges, cotton dust, blood, soil, hemostatic materials, and vascular catheter material (7,156–158). None of these early studies provided any clues as to why this occurred.

A great deal of the work examining mechanisms by which foreign bodies might increase the risk of infection has been done by a group of investigators in Geneva, Switzerland (151). Zimmerli et al. performed the first study of this type (159). Using a guinea pig model of foreign body implantation, they found that complement-mediated opsonic activity was substantially depleted in the fluid surrounding the foreign body, but that this was not enough in itself to predispose to infection (159). It was also found that neutrophils isolated from inside of a tissue cage had decreased bactericidal activity compared with neutrophils from peripheral blood or peritoneal exudate (159) and subsequently demonstrated that these neutrophils had defective oxidative metabolism and granulocyte enzyme content (160). Similar neutrophil functional defects have been described in association with neutrophil exposure to nonphagocytosable surfaces and referred to as "frustrated phagocytosis" (160–165). The time course of these two effects is that the neutrophil defect appears within the first 6 hours and then subsequently disappears, and that the complement depletion occurs more slowly appearing after the first 6 hours (159,160). The neutrophil defect can be partially corrected by adding tumor necrosis factor (TNF) or bacterial cell wall components that raise TNF levels (166). It is not clear whether the described neutrophil defects apply to all foreign bodies nor by what mechanism(s) they occur.

Neutrophil phagocytosis and killing on surfaces are also affected by the composition of the surface. In 1946, Wood et al. found that phagocytosis of unopsonized pneumococci occurred on filter paper, cloth, fiberglass, and fixed tissue specimens, but not on glass, paraffin, or cellophane (167). More recently it was shown that on polymethylmethacrylate (PMMA) coverslips neutrophils have difficulty killing *S. aureus* adhering spontaneously to uncoated coverslips or coverslips coated with albumin, but when PMMA coverslips were coated with fibronectin, fibrinogen, laminin, vitronectin, or type IV collagen that neutrophil killing of *S. aureus* was greatly enhanced (168,169). The mechanisms for why neutrophils can phagocytose and kill organisms on some surfaces but not on others are not known at this time. It is interesting that coating PMMA with proteins that can promote adherence of bacteria also facilitates neutrophil killing. This raises the possibility that neutrophil adherence may be important for phagocytosis and killing on foreign bodies.

Studies with vascular catheters have provided additional evidence that the foreign body defect may vary with different materials. In a rabbit model of subcutaneous *S. aureus* infection, it was shown that silicone catheters are easier to infect than catheters made of polyurethane, Teflon, or polyvinlychloride (170). Interestingly, the greater risk of infection associated with silicone catheters varied with the strain of *S. aureus* used (170). The greater risk of infection associated with silicone was present at the time of insertion but disappeared within 2 days after insertion (Fig. 3) associated with the histologic appearance of a ring of neutrophils (rabbit heterophiles) around the catheter (170). Paradoxically, even in the absence of *S. aureus* inoculation, silicone catheters have a greater pericatheter neutrophilic response than the other catheter materials. This suggested that silicone surfaces generate a greater chemotactic stimulus than other materials, but also that the neutrophils did not work as well on silicone surfaces as they do on other materials. In vitro it was shown that the same silicone catheters produced tenfold greater serum complement activation with C5a generation than polyurethane or polyvinylchloride, confirming the potential for generating a greater chemotactic gradient in vivo (171). It was further shown that neutrophil chemotaxis toward a serum stimulus was greater on silicone surfaces than on polyurethane surfaces (172). Of note, the serum complement activation on silicone surfaces was sufficient to significantly inhibit neutrophil chemotaxis toward

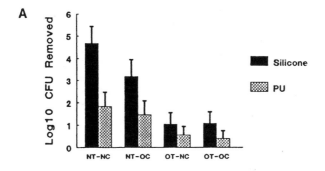

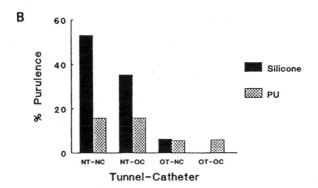

Figure 3 Effect of catheter tunnel and catheter surface on the risk of infection in the catheter shuffle experiment. NT = new tunnel (created on the day of *Staphylococcus aureus* inoculation); OT = old tunnel (created 2 days prior to *S. aureus* inoculation); NC = new catheter (inserted on the day of *S. aureus* inoculation); OC = old catheter (inserted on the day of *S. aureus* inoculation). Each catheter was inoculated with 10^2 cfu *S. aureus* and harvested 7 days later. N = 9 or 10 for each bar. (A) Quantitative catheter culture mean titers. (B) Percent of catheters with associated purulence. This figure was published with the permission of the Journal of Biomedical Materials Research (Ref. 170).

another chemotactic stimulus (formyl-methionine-leucine-phenylalanine); this did not occur on polyurethane surfaces. This raised the possibility that excessive complement activation by silicone surfaces could interfere with neutrophil chemotaxis toward bacteria. Although surface phagocytosis of bacteria does not require complement opsonization, optimal surface killing does require intact complement (173–176). Thus, excessive complement activation by silicone surfaces might also interfere with bacterial killing as well. These findings suggest that further efforts should be made to understand the importance of complement activation by silicone in the pathogenesis of foreign body infection.

Other possible explanations for the greater risk of infection associated with silicone catheters include a direct toxic effect on neutrophils (177) and greater bacterial adherence to silicone catheters (125). Lopez-Lopez et al. demonstrated that neutrophils incubated in a solution containing siliconized latex catheters had greater inhibition of superoxide formation than neutrophils incubated with PVC, Teflon, or PU catheters (177). The causative agent(s) for this effect were not identified. Vaudaux et al. have found that silicone catheters removed from patients have the greatest adherence of *S. aureus* in comparison to PU and PVC catheters (125). Although this may be a function of the greater potential for clots to form on silicone catheters than on other catheter materials (178), it still may play a role in the pathogenesis of infection.

V. CONCLUSIONS

We are just beginning to understand the pathogenesis of vascular catheter infection. Like virtually all infectious processes, there is a spectrum that ranges from asymptomatic colonization to symptomatic infection. Overall, the severity of the infection appears to be a function of the number of organisms on the catheter. However, some catheters have a demonstrable biofilm containing organisms that do not grow in culture, and this observation needs to be understood. Early catheter infections are caused primarily by skin microorganisms, and late infections by catheter hub or lumen contamination. The three most common organisms causing catheter-related bloodstream infection—*S. epidermidis*, *S. aureus*, and *C. albicans*—differ strikingly in their virulence and known mechanisms for causing infection. Significant advances have been made related to understanding how some foreign bodies interact with the immune system to produce the "foreign body effect." Localized immune defects have been identified including decreased neutrophil bactericidal activity, altered neutrophil chemotaxis, and localized complement depletion. Unfortunately, there is almost no information available about how polymer surfaces cause these defects at the molecular level. The future of improving our understanding of the pathogenesis of vascular catheter infection lies in the continued development of in vitro systems and animal models that will allow systematic investigation into how polymer surface chemistry affects host immunity.

REFERENCES

1. Maki DG, Weise CE, Sarafin HW. A semi-quantitative culture method for identifying intravenous-catheter-related infection. N Engl J Med 1977; 296:1305–1309.
2. Cleri DJ, Corrado ML, Seligman SJ. Quantitative culture of intravenous catheters and other intravascular inserts. J Infect Dis 1980; 141:781–786.

3. Bjornson HS, Colley R, Bower RH, Duty VP, Schwartz-Fulton JT, Fischer JE. Association between microorganism growth at the catheter insertion site and colonization of the catheter in patients receiving total parenteral nutrition. Surgery 1982; 92:721–727.

4. Brun-Buisson C, Abrouk F, Legrand P, Huet Y, Larabi S, Rapin M. Diagnosis of central venous catheter-related sepsis. Critical level of quantitative tip cultures. Arch Intern Med 1987; 147:873–877.

5. Heard SO, Davis RF, Sherertz RJ, et al. Influence of sterile protective sleeves on the sterility of pulmonary artery catheters. Crit Care Med 1987; 15:499–502.

6. Sherertz RJ, Raad II, Belani A, et al. Three-year experience with sonicated vascular catheter cultures in a clinical microbiology laboratory. J Clin Microbiol 1990; 28:76–82.

7. Sherertz RJ, Carruth WA, Hampton AA, Byron MP, Solomon DD. Efficacy of antibiotic-coated catheters in preventing subcutaneous *Staphylococcus aureus* infection in rabbits. J Infect Dis 1993; 167:98–106.

8. Raad I, Costerton W, Sabharwal U, Sacilowski M, Anaissie E, Bodey GP. Ultrastructural analysis of indwelling vascular catheters: a quantitative relationship between luminal colonization and curation of placement. J Infect Dis 1993; 168:400–407.

9. Tenney JH, Moody MR, Newman KA, Schimpff SC. Adherent microorganisms on lumenal surfaces of long-term intravenous catheters. Arch Intern Med 1986; 146:1949–1954.

10. Passerini L, Phang PT, Jackson FL, Lam K, Costerton JW, King EG. Biofilms on right heart flow-directed catheters. Chest 1987; 92:440–446.

11. Maki DG, Cobb L, Garman JK, Shapiro JM, Ringer M, Helgerson RB. An attachable silver-impregnated cuff for prevention of infection with central venous catheters: a prospective randomized multicenter trial. Am J Med 1988; 85:307–314.

12. Flowers RH III, Schwenzer KJ, Kopel RF, Fisch MJ, Tucker SI, Farr BM. Efficacy of an attachable subcutaneous cuff for the prevention of intravascular catheter-related infection. JAMA 1989; 261:878–883.

13. Mermel LA, McCormick RD, Springman SR. The pathogenesis and epidemiology of catheter-related infection with pulmonary artery Swan-Ganz catheters: a prospective study utilizing molecular subtyping. Am J Med 1991; 91(suppl 3B):197S–205S.

14. Linares J, Sitges-Serra A, Garau J, Perez JL, Martin R. Pathogenesis of catheter sepsis: a prospective study with quantitative and semiquantitative cultures of catheter hub and segments. J Clin Microbiol 1985; 21:357–360.

15. Almirall J, Gonzalez J, Rello J, et al. Infection of hemodialysis catheters: incidence and mechanisms. Am J Nephrol 1989; 9:454–459.

16. Cheesbrough JS, Finch RG, Burden RP. A prospective study of the mechanisms of infection associated with hemodialysis catheters. J Infect Dis 1986; 154:579–589.

17. Weightman NC, Simpson EM, Speller DCE, Mott MG, Oakhill A. Bacteraemia related to indwelling central venous catheters: prevention, diagnosis and treatment. Eur J Clin Microbiol Infect Dis 1988; 7:125–129.

18. Maki DG, Ringer M. Evaluation of dressing regimens for prevention of infection with peripheral intravenous catheters. JAMA 1987; 258:2396–2403.

19. Maki DG, Ringer M. Prospective study of arterial catheter-related infection: incidence, sources of infection and risk factors. In: Proceedings of the Twenty-ninth

Interscience Conference on Antimicrobial Agents and Chemotherapy. Houston: American Society for Microbiology, 1989. Abstract 1075.

20. Maki DG, Will L. Risk factors for central venous catheter-related infection within the ICU. A prospective study of 345 catheters. In: Proceedings of the Thirtieth Interscience Conference on Antimicrobial Agents and Chemotherapy. Atlanta: American Society for Microbiology, 1990. Abstract 715.

21. Maki DG. Marked differences in skin colonization of insertion sites for central venous, arterial and peripheral IV catheters. In: Proceedings of the Thirtieth Interscience Conference on Antimicrobial Agents and Chemotherapy. Atlanta: American Society for Microbiology, 1990. Abstract 712.

22. Popp M, Brennan MF. Long-term vascular access in the rat: importance of asepsis. Am J Physiol 1981; 241:H606–H612.

23. McCormick R, Maki DG. The importance of maximal sterile barriers during the insertion of central venous catheters: a prospective study. In: Proceedings of the Twenty-ninth Interscience Conference on Antimicrobial Agents and Chemotherapy. Houston: American Society for Microbiology, 1989. Abstract 1077.

24. Raad II, Hohn DC, Gilbreath BJ, et al. Prevention of central venous catheter-related infections by using maximal sterile barrier precautions during insertion. Infect Control Hosp Epidemiol 1994; 15:231–238.

25. Burrows CF. Inadequate skin preparation as a cause of intravenous catheter-related infection in the dog. JAVMA 1982; 180:747–749.

26. Maki DG, Alvarado CJ, Ringer MA. A prospective, randomized trial of povidone-iodine, alcohol and chlorhexidine for prevention of infection with central venous and arterial catheters. Lancet 1991; 338:339–343.

27. Mimoz O, Pieroni L, Lawrence C, Edouard A, Samii K. Prospective trial of povidone-iodine and chlorhexidine for prevention of catheter-related sepsis. In: Proceedings of the Thirty-fourth Interscience Conference on Antimicrobial Agents and Chemotherapy. Orlando: American Society for Microbiology, 1994. Abstract J56.

28. Levin A, Mason AJ, Jindal KK, Fong IW, Goldstein MB. Prevention of hemodialysis subclavian vein catheter infections by topical povidone-iodine. Kid Int 1991; 40:934–938.

29. Hill RLR, Fisher AP, Ware RJ, Wilson S, Casewell MW. Mupirocin for the reduction of colonization of internal jugular cannulae—a randomized, controlled trial. J Hosp Infect 1990; 15:311–321.

30. Knight J, Boyd SJ, van Paasschen WH, Cole JJ, Scribner BH. Use of barrier materials to prevent infection around percutaneous implants. J Surg Res 1973; 15:30–34.

31. Trooskin SZ, Donetz AP, Harvey RA, Greco RS. Prevention of catheter sepsis by antibiotic bonding. Surgery 1985; 97:547–551.

32. Sherertz RJ, Forman DM, Solomon DD. Efficacy of dicloxacillin-coated polyurethane catheters in preventing subcutaneous *Staphylococcus aureus* infection in mice. Antimicrob Agents Chemother 1989; 33:1174–1178.

33. Sherertz R, Hu Q, Clarkson L, Felton S. The chlorhexidine on Arrow catheters may be more important that Ag sulfadiazine at preventing catheter-related infection. In: Proceedings of the Thirty-third Interscience Conference on Antimicrobial Agents and Chemotherapy. New Orleans: American Society for Microbiology, 1993. Abstract 1622.

34. Greenfeld J, Sampath L, Baradarian R, Stylianos S, Modak S. In: Proceedings of the Thirty-third Interscience Conference on Antimicrobial Agents and Chemotherapy. New Orleans: American Society for Microbiology, 1993. Abstract 1620.

35. Bach A, Bohrer H, Motsch J, Martin E, Geiss HK, Sonntag HG. Prevention of bacterial colonization of intravenous catheters by antiseptic impregnation of polyurethane catheters. J Antimicrob Chemother 1994; 33:969–978.

36. Bodey GP, Zermeno A, Raad I. Novel approach for the prevention of catheter infections: iontophoretic catheter using silver wire. In: Proceedings of the Thirty-fourth Interscience Conference on Antimicrobial Agents and Chemotherapy. Orlando: American Society for Microbiology, 1994. Abstract J197.

37. Maki DG, Wheeler SJ, Stolz SM, Mermel LA. Clinical trial of a novel antiseptic central venous catheter. In: Proceedings of the Thirty-first Interscience Conference on Antimicrobial Agents and Chemotherapy. Chicago: American Society for Microbiology, 1991. Abstract 461.

38. Kamal GD, Pfaller MA, Rempe LE, Jebson PJR. Reduced intravascular catheter infection by antibiotic bonding. A prospective, randomized controlled trial. JAMA 1991; 265:2364–2368.

39. Clemence MA, Anglim AM, Jernigan JA, et al. A study of prevention of catheter related bloodstream infection with an antiseptic impregnated catheter. In: Proceedings of the Thirty-fourth Interscience Conference on Antimicrobial Agents and Chemotherapy. Orlando: American Society for Microbiology, 1994. Abstract J199.

40. Lovell RD, Corbett JB, Lowery GE. Efficacy of antiseptic impregnated central venous catheters in reducing the rate of bloodstream infections in intensive care units of a tertiary referral hospital. Presented at the Fifth Annual Meeting of the Society for Healthcare Epidemiology of America. San Diego, 1995. Abstract 51.

41. Raymond NJ, Steinberg JP. Impact of antiseptic impregnation on central venous catheter-associated bloodstream infections. Presented at the Fifth Annual Meeting of the Society for Healthcare Epidemiology of America. San Diego, 1995. Abstract 52.

42. Pfeiffer J, Bennett ME, Simpson ML. Comparison of catheter-related bacteremias using chlorhexidine/silver impregnated central venous catheters versus non-impregnated catheters. Presented at the Fifth Annual Meeting of the Society for Healthcare Epidemiology of America. San Diego, 1995. Abstract M48.

43. Cohen Y, Fosse JP, Karoubi P, et al. Prospective assessment of the value of the Arrow "Hands-off" catheter in the prevention of systemic infections associated with pulmonary artery catheters. In: Proceedings of the Thirty-fifth Interscience Conference on Antimicrobial Agents and Chemotherapy. San Francisco: American Society for Microbiology, 1995. Abstract J9.

44. Raad I, Darouiche R. Central venous catheters coated with minocycline and rifampin for the prevention of catheter-related bacteremia. In: Proceedings of the Thirty-fifth Interscience Conference on Antimicrobial Agents and Chemotherapy. San Francisco: American Society for Microbiology, 1995. Abstract J7.

45. Dixon RE, Kaslow RA, Mackel DC, Fulkerson CC, Mallison GF. Aqueous quaternary ammonium antiseptics and disinfectants. Use and misuse. JAMA 1976; 236:2415–2417.

46. Frank MJ, Schaffner W. Contaminated aqueous benzalkonium chloride. An unnecessary hospital infection hazard. JAMA 1976; 236:2418–2419.

47. Fox J, Beaucage CM, Folta CA Thornton GW. Nosocomial transmission of *Serratia marcescens* in a veterinary hospital due to contamination by benzalkonium chloride. J Clin Microbiol 1981; 14:157–60.

48. Kahan A, Phillippon A, Paul G, et al. Nosocomial infections by chlorhexidine solution contaminated with *Pseudomonas pickettii* (Biovar VA-I). J Infect 1983; 7:256–263.

49. Dennis MB, Jones DR, Tenover FC. Chlorine dioxide sterilization of implanted right atrial catheters in rabbits. Lab Anim Sci 1989; 39:51–55.

50. Palm U, Boemke W, Bayerl D, Schnoy N, Juhr N-C, Reinhardt HW. Prevention of catheter-related infections by a new, catheter-restricted antibiotic filling technique. 1991; 25:142–152.

51. Schwartz C, Henrickson KJ, Roghmann K, Powell K. Prevention of bacteremia attributed to luminal colonization of tunneled central venous catheters with vancomycin-susceptible organisms. J Clin Oncol 1990; 8:1591–1597.

52. Raad I, Hachem R, Sherertz R. Minocycline-EDTA flush solution for the prevention of vascular catheter infection. In Proceedings of the Thirty-fourth Interscience Conference on Antimicrobial Agents and Chemotherapy. Orlando: American Society for Microbiology, 1994. Abstract J57.

53. Sheth KJ, Henrickson KJ. Prevention of recurrent central venous catheter infections with a novel flush solution in a patient on long-term hemodialysis. Pediatr Nephrol 1993; 7:506.

54. Segura M, Alia C, Valverde J, Franch G, Rodriguez JMT, Sitges-Serra A. Assessment of a new hub design and the semiquantitative catheter culture method using an in vivo experimental model of catheter sepsis. J Clin Microbiol 1990; 28:2551–2554.

55. Halpin DP, O'Byrne P, McEntee G, Hennessy TP, Stephens RB. Effect of a betadine connection shield on central venous catheter sepsis. Nutrition 1991; 7:33–34.

56. Inoue Y, Nezu R, Matsuda H, et al. Prevention of catheter-related sepsis during parenteral nutrition: effect of a new connection device. JPEN 1992; 16:581–585.

57. Segura M, Lerma FA, Tellado JM, et al. Clinical trial of the effect of a new catheter hub on the prevention of central venous catheter-related sepsis. In: Proceedings of the Thirty-fifth Interscience Conference on Antimicrobial Agents and Chemotherapy. San Francisco: American Society for Microbiology, 1995. Abstract J10.

58. Clementi E, Marie O, Arlet G, et al. Usefulness of an attachable silver-impregnated cuff for prevention of catheter-related sepsis? In: Proceedings of the Thirty-first Interscience Conference on Antimicrobial Agents and Chemotherapy. Chicago: American Society for Microbiology, 1991. Abstract 460.

59. Groeger JS, Lucas AB, Coit D, et al. A prospective, randomized evaluation of the effect of silver impregnated subcutaneous cuffs for preventing tunneled chronic venous access catheter infections in cancer patients. Ann Surg 1993; 218:206–210.

60. Goldschmidt H, Hahn U, Salwender H, et al. Prevention of catheter related infections by silver coated central venous catheters in oncological patients after chemotherapy. In: Proceedings of the Thirty-fourth Interscience Conference on Antimicrobial Agents and Chemotherapy. Orlando: American Society for Microbiology, 1994. Abstract J198.

61. Band JD, Maki DG. Infections caused by indwelling arterial catheters for hemodynamic monitoring. Am J Med 1979; 67:735–741.

62. Maki DG, Hassemer CH. Endemic rate of fluid contamination and related septicemia in arterial pressure monitoring. Am J Med 1981; 70:733–738.

63. Maki DG, Jarrett F, Sarafin HW. A semiquantitative culture method for identification of catheter-related infection in the burn patient. J Surg Res 1977; 22:513–520.

64. Maki DG. Infections due to infusion therapy. In: Bennett JV, Brachman PS, eds. Hospital Infections. Boston: Little, Brown, and Company, 1992:849–898.

65. Maki DG. Infections caused by intravascular devices. In: Bisno AL, Waldvogel FA, eds. Infections Associated With Indwelling Medical Devices. Washington: ASM Press, 1994:155–212.

66. Maki DG. Epidemic nosocomial bacteremias. In: Wenzel RP, ed. CRC Handbook of Hospital Acquired Infections. Boca Raton, FL: CRC Press, 1981:371–512.

67. Maki DG, Growth properties of microorganisms in infusion fluid and methods of detection. In: Phillips I, ed. Microbiologic Hazards of Intravenous Therapy. Lancaster, England: MTP Press, 1977:13–47.

68. Maki DG, Martin WT. Nationwide epidemic of septicemia caused by contaminated infusion products. IV. Growth of microbial pathogens in fluids for intravenous infusion. J Infect Dis 1975; 131:267–272.

69. Maki DG, Rhame FS, Mackel DG, Bennett JV. Am J Med 1976; 60:471–485.

70. Mackel DC, Maki DG, Anderson RL, Rhame FS, Bennett JV. Nationwide epidemic of septicemia caused by contaminated intravenous products: mechanisms of intrinsic contamination. J Clin Microbiol 1975; 2:486–497.

71. Sherertz RJ, Gledhill KS, Hampton KD, et al. Outbreak of *Candida* bloodstream infections associated with retrograde medication administration in a neonatal intensive care unit. J Pediatr 1992; 120:455–461.

72. Bennett SN, McNeil MM, Bland LA, et al. Postoperative infections traced to contamination of an intravenous anesthetic, propofol. N Engl J Med 1995; 333:147–154.

73. Pittet D. Nosocomial bloodstream infections. In: Wenzel RP, ed. Prevention and Control of Nosocomial Infections. Baltimore: Williams & Wilkins, 1993:512–555.

74. Franceschi D, Gerding RL, Phillips G, Fratianne RB. Risk factors associated with intravascular catheter infections in burned patients: a prospective, randomized study. J Trauma 1989; 29:811–816.

75. Pruitt BA Jr, McManus WF, Kim SH, Treat RC. Diagnosis and treatment of cannula-related intravenous sepsis in burn patients. Ann Surg 1980; 191:546–554.

76. Widmer AF. IV-related infections. In: Wenzel RP, ed. Prevention and Control of Nosocomial Infections. Baltimore: Williams & Wilkins, 1993:556–579.

77. Hampton AA, Sherertz RJ. Vascular-access infections in hospitalized patients. Surg Clin North Am 1988; 68:57–71.

78. Christensen GD, Baldassarri L, Simpson WA. Colonization of medical devices by coagulase-negative staphylococci. In: Bisno AL, Waldvogel FA, eds. Infections Associated With Indwelling Medical Devices. Washington DC: American Society for Microbiology, 1994:45–78.

79. Lowy FD, Hammer SM. *Staphylococcus epidermidis* infections. Ann Intern Med 1983; 99:834–839.

80. Kloos WE, Musselwhite MS. Distribution and persistence of *Staphylococcus* and *Micrococcus* species and other aerobic bacteria on human skin. Appl Microbiol 1975; 30:381–394.
81. Hogt AH, Dankert J, de Vries JA, Feijen J. Adhesion of coagulase-negative staphylococci to biomaterials. J Gen Microbiol 1983; 129:2959–2968.
82. Pascual A, Fleer A, Westerdaal NAC, Verhoef J. Modulation of adherence of coagulase-negative staphylococci to Teflon catheters in vitro. Eur J Clin Microbiol 1986; 5:518–522.
83. Fleer A, Verhoef J, Hernandez AP. Coagulase-negative staphylococci as nosocomial pathogens inneonates: the role of host defense, artificial devices, and bacterial hydrophobicity. Am J Med 1986; 80(suppl 6B):161–165.
84. Schadow KW, Simpson WA, Christensen GD. Characteristics of adherence to plastic tissue culture plates of coagulase-negative staphylococci exposed to subinhibitory concentrations of antimicrobial agents. J Infect Dis 1988; 157:71–77.
85. Timmerman CP, Fleer A, Besnier JM, de Graaf L, Cremers F, Verhoef J. Characterization of a proteinaceous adhesin of *Staphylococcus epidermidis* which mediates attachment to polystyrene. Infect Immun 1991; 59:4187–4192.
86. Muller E, Hubner J, Gutierrez N, Takeda S, Goldmann DA, Pier GB. Isolation and characterization of transpon mutants of *Staphylococcus epidermidis* deficient in capsular polysaccharide/adhesin and slime. Infect Immun 1993; 61:551–558.
87. Switalski LM, Ryden C, Rubin K, Ljungh A, Hook M, Wadstrom T. Binding of fibronectin to *Staphylococcus* strains. Infect Immun 1983; 42:628–633.
88. Wadstrom T, Speziale P, Rozgonyi F, Ljungh A, Maxe I, Ryden C. Interactions of coagulase-negative staphylococci with fibronectin and collagen as possible first step of tissue colonization in wounds and other tissue trauma. Zentralbl Bakteriol Mikrobiol Hyg Abt 1987; 16(suppl):83–91.
89. Kojima Y, Tojo M, Goldmann DA, Tosteson TD, Pier GB. Antibody to the capsular polysaccharide/adhesin protects rabbits against catheter-related bacteremia due to coagulase-negative staphylococci. J Infect Dis 1990; 162:435–441.
90. Takeda S, Pier GB, Kojima Y, et al. Protection against endocarditis due to *Staphylococcus epidermidis* by immunization with capsular polysaccharide/adhesin. Circulation 1991; 84:2539–2546.
91. Christensen GD, Bisno AL, Parisi JT, McLaughlin B, Hester MG, Luther RW. Nosocomial septicemia due to multiply antibiotic-resistant *Staphylococcus epidermidis*. Ann Intern Med 1982; 96:1–10.
92. Christensen GD, Simpson WA, Bisno AL, Beachey EH. Adherence of slime-producing strains of *Staphylococcus epidermidis* to smooth surfaces. Infect Immun 1982; 37:318–326.
93. Christensen GD, Simpson WA, Younger JJ, et al. Adherence of coagulase-negative staphylococci to plastic tissue culture plates: a quantitative model for the adherence of staphylococci to medical devices. J Clin Microbiol 1985; 22:996–1006.
94. Johnson GM, Lee DA, Regelmann WE, Gray ED, Peters G, Quie PG. Interference with granulocyte function by *Staphylococcus epidermidis* slime. Infect Immun 1986; 54:13–20.
95. Christensen GD, Baddour LM, Simpson WA. Phenotypic variation of *Staphylococ-*

cus epidermidis slime production in vitro and in vivo. Infect Immun 1987; 55:2870–2877.

96. Christensen GD, Baddour LM, Madison BM, et al. Colonial morphology of staphylococci on Memphis agar: phase variation of slime production, resistance to β-lactam antibiotics, and virulence. J Infect Dis 1990; 161:1153–1169.

97. Gunn BA, Colwell. Numerical taxonomy of staphylococci isolated from the marine environment. Int J Syst Bacteriol 1983; 33:751–759.

98. Waldvogel FA. *Staphylococcus aureus* (including toxic shock syndrome). In: Mandell GL, Bennett JE, Dolin R, eds. Principles and Practice of Infectious Diseases. New York: Churchill Livingstone, 1995:1754–1777.

99. Tulloch LG. Nasal carriage in staphylococcal skin infections. Br Med J 1954; 2:912–913.

100. Solberg CO, A study of carriers of *Staphylococcus aureus* with special regard to quantitative bacterial estimations. Acta Med Scand [Suppl] 1965; 436:1–96.

101. White A. Increased infection rates in heavy nasal carriers of coagulase positive staphylococci. Antimicrob Agents Chemother 1963; 3:667–670.

102. Weinstein HJ. The relation between the nasal-staphylococcal-carrier state and incidence of postoperative complications. N Engl J Med 1959; 260:1303–1308.

103. Nahmias Aj, Shulman J. Epidemiology of staphylococci. In: Cohen JO, ed. The Staphylococci. New York: John Wiley, 1972:486–502.

104. Lye WC, Leong SO, van der Straaten J, Lee EJ. *Staphylococcus aureus* CAPD-related infections are associated with nasal carriage. Adv Periton Dialy 1994; 10:163–165.

105. Yu VL, Goetz A, Wagener M, et al. *Staphylococcus aureus* nasal carriage and infection in patients on hemodialysis. Efficacy of antibiotic prophylaxis. N Engl J Med 1986; 315:91–96.

106. Boelaert JR, van Landuyt HW, Godard CA, et al. Nasal mupirocin ointment decreases the incidence of *Staphylococcus aureus* bacteraemias in haemodialysis patients. Nephrol Dialy Transplant 1993; 8:235–239.

107. Jacobson MA, Gellermann H, Chambers H. *Staphylococcus aureus* bacteremia and recurrent staphylococcal infection in patients with acquired immunodeficiency syndrome and AIDS-related complex. Am J Med 1988; 85:172–176.

108. Skoutelis AT, Murphy RL, MacDonell KB, VonRoenn JH, Sterkel CD, Phair JP. Indwelling central venous catheter infections in patients with acquired immune deficiency syndrome. J Acquired Immune Deficiency Syndromes 1990; 3:335–342.

109. Mukau L, Talamini MA, Sitzmann JV, Burns RC, McGuire ME. Long-term central venous access vs other home therapies: complications in patients with acquired immunodeficiency syndrome. JPEN 1992; 16:455–459.

110. High *Staphylococcus aureus* nasal carriage rate in patients with acquired immunodeficiency syndrome or AIDS-related complex. Am J Infect Control 1990; 18:64–69.

111. Murphy PM, Lane HC, Fauci AS, Gallin JI. Impairment of neutrophil bactericidal capacity in patients with AIDS. J Infect Dis 1988; 158:627–630.

112. Ellis M, Gupta S, Galant S, et al. Impaired neutrophil function in patients with AIDS or AIDS-related complex: a comprehensive evaluation. J Infect Dis 1988; 158:1268–1276.

113. Bock SN, Lee RE, Fisher B, et al. A prospective randomized trial evaluating prophylactic antibiotics to prevent triple-lumen catheter-related sepsis in patients treated with immunotherapy. J Clin Oncol 1990; 8:161–169.

114. Klempner MS, Noring R, Mier JW, Atkins. Acquired chemotactic defect in neutrophils from patients receiving interleukin-2 immunotherapy. N Engl J Med 1990; 322:959–65.

115. Mandell GL. Catalase, superoxide dismutase, and virulence of *Staphylococcus aureus*. In vitro and in vivo studies with emphasis on staphylococcal leukocyte interaction. J Clin Invest 1975; 55:561–566.

116. Elek SD, Conen PE. The virulence of *Staphylococcus pyogenes* for man: a study of the problems of wound infection. Br J Exp Pathol 1961; 42:266–277.

117. Hawiger J, Timmons S, Strong DD, Cottrell BA, Riley M, Doolittle RF. Indentification of a region of human fibrinogen interacting with staphylococcal clumping factor. Biochemistry 1982; 21:1407–1413.

118. Kuusela P. Fibronectin binds to *Staphylococcus aureus*. Nature 1978; 276:718–720.

119. Lopes JD, Dos Reis M, Brentani RR. Presence of laminin receptors in *Staphylococcus aureus*. Science 1985; 229:275–277.

120. Hermann M, Suchard SJ, Boxer LA, Waldvogel FA, Lew PD. Thrombospondin binds to *Staphylococcus aureus* and promotes staphylococcal adherence to surfaces. Infect Immun 1991; 59:279–288.

121. Vercellotti GM, Lussenhop D, Peterson PK, et al. Bacterial adherence to fibronectin and endothelial cells: a possible mechanism for bacterial tissue tropism. J Lab Clin Med 1984; 103:34–43.

122. Herrmann M, Hartleib J, Weber S, Schiphorst M, Sixma JJ, Peters G. Interaction of *S. aureus* with Von Willebrand factor and· indentification of a putative Von Willebrand binding-protein. Presented at the 33rd Annual Meeting of the Infectious Disease Society of America, San Francisco, 1995. Abstract 8.

123. Francois P, Vaudaux P, Greene C, McDevitt D, Foster TJ. Unpublished data.

124. Vaudaux P, Pittet D, Haeberli A, et al. Host factors selectively increase staphylococcal adherence on inserted catheters: a role for fibronectin and fibrinogen or fibrin. J Infect Dis 1989; 160:865–875.

125. Vaudaux P, Pittet D, Haeberli, et al. Fibronectin is more active than fibrin or fibrinogen in promoting *Staphylococcus aureus* adherence to inserted intravascular devices. J Infect Dis 1993; 167:633–641.

126. Vaudaux PE, Francois P, Proctor RA, et al. Use of adhesion-defective mutants of *Staphylococcus aureus* to define the role of specific plasma proteins in promoting bacterial adhesion to canine arteriovenous shunts. Infect Immun 1995; 63:585–590.

127. Falcieri E, Vaudaux P, Huggler E, Lew D, Waldvogel F. Role of bacterial exopolymers and host factors on adherence and phagocytosis of *Staphylococcus aureus* in foreign body infections. J Infect Dis 1987; 155:524–531.

128. Loeb L. The influence of certain bacteria on the coagulation of blood. J Med Res 1903; 10:407–419.

129. Lack CH. Staphylokinase: an activator of plasma protease. Nature 1948; 161:559–560.

130. Sherertz RJ, Lottenberg R. Unpublished data.

131. Press OW, Ramsey PG, Larson EB, Fefer A, Hickman RO. Hickman catheter infections in patients with malignancies. Medicine 1984; 63:189–200.

132. Raad II, Luna M, Khalil S-AM, Costerton JW, Lam C, Bodey GP. The relationship between the thrombotic and infectious complications of central venous catheters. JAMA 1994; 271:1014–1016.

133. Phonimdaeng P, O'Reilly M, Nowlan P, Bramley AJ, Foster TJ. The coagulase of *Staphylococcus aureus* 8325-4. Sequence analysis and virulence of site-specific coagulase-deficient mutants. Molec Microbiol 1990; 4:393–404.

134. Sherertz RJ, Foster TJ. Unpublished data.

135. Smith W, Hale JH. The nature and mode of action of *Staphylococcus* coagulase. Br J Exp Pathol 1944; 25:101–109.

136. Devriese LA. A simplified system for biotyping *Staphylococcus aureus* strains from different animal species. J Appl Bacteriol 1984; 56:215–220.

137. Gelbart SM, Reinhardt GF, Greenlee HB. Multiplication of nosocomial pathogens in intravenous feeding solutions. Appl Microbiol 1973; 26:874–879.

138. Goldmann DA, Martin WT, Worthington JW. Growth of bacteria and fungi in total parenteral nutrition solutions. Am J Surg 1973; 126:314–318.

139. Ekenna O, Sherertz R. Factors affecting colonization and dissemination of *Candida albicans* from the gastrointestinal tract of mice. Infect Immun 1987; 55:1558–1563.

140. de Repentigny L, Phaneuf M, Mathieu LG. Gastrointestinal colonization and systemic dissemination by *Candida albicans* and *Candida tropicalis* in intact and immunocompromised mice. Infect Immun 1992; 60:4907–4914.

141. Klotz SA, Hein RC, Smith RL, Rouse JB. The fibronectin adhesin of *Candida albicans*. Infect Immun 1994; 62:4679–4681.

142. Casanova M, Lopez-Ribot JL, Monteagudo C, Llombart-Bosch A, Sentandreu R, Martinez JP. Indentification of a 58-kilodalton cell surface fibrinogen-binding mannoprotein from *Candida albicans*. Infect Immun 1992; 60:4221–4229.

143. Jakab E, Paulson M, Ascencio F, Ljungh A. Expression of vitronectin and fibronectin binding by *Candida albicans* yeast cells. APMIS 1993; 101:187–193.

144. Scheld WM, Strunk RW, Balian G, Calderone RA. Microbial adhesion to fibronectin in vitro correlates with production of endocarditis in rabbits. Proc Soc Exp Biol Med 1985; 180:474–482.

145. Klotz SA, Smith RL, Stewart BW. Effect of an arginine-glycine-aspartic acid-containing peptide on hematogenous candidal infections in rabbits. Antimicrob Agents Chemother 1992; 36:132–136.

146. Klotz SA. Plasma and extracellular matrix proteins mediate in the fate of *Candida albicans* in the human host. Med Hypotheses 1994; 42:328–334.

147. Mahayni R, Chowdri HR, McGowan H, Zervos MJ. Evaluation of risk factors and epidemiology for fungemia after introduction of a chlorhexidine Bio-patch for central venous catheter dressings. Presented at the 34th Interscience Conference on Antimicrobial Agents and Chemotherapy, Orlando, 1994. Abstract 111.

148. Kwon-Chung KJ, Lehman D, Good C, Magee PT. Genetic evidence for the role of extracellular proteinase in virulence of *Candida albicans*. Infect Immun 1985; 49:571–575.

149. Edwards JE Jr. *Candida* species. In: Mandell GL, Bennett JE, Dolin R, eds. Princi-

ples and Practice of Infectious Diseases. New York: Churchill Livingstone, 1995:2289–2306.

150. Murabayashi S, Nose Y. Biocompatability: bioengineering aspects. Artific Organs 1986; 10:114–121.

151. Vaudaux PE, Lew DP, Waldvogel FA. Host factors predisposing to and influencing therapy of foreign body infections. In: Bisno AL, Waldvogel FA, eds. Infections Associated With Indwelling Medical Devices. Washington, DC: ASM Press, 1994:1–29.

152. Hench LL, Wilson J. Surface-active biomaterials. Science 1984; 226:630–636.

153. Greco RS. Implantation Biology. The Host Response and Biomedical Devices. Boca Raton: CRC Press, 1994.

154. James RC, MacLeod CJ. Induction of staphylococcal infections in mice with small inocula introduced on sutures. Br J Exp Pathol 1961; 42:266–277.

155. Edlich RF, Panek PH, Rodeheaver GT, Kurtz LD, Edgerton MT. Surgical sutures and infection: a biomaterial evaluation. J Biomed Mater Res Symp 1974; 5:115–126.

156. Cipola AF, Narat JK. Effect of absorbable sponges on infection. Surg 1948; 24:828–831.

157. Georgiade NG, King EH, Harris WA, Tenery JH, Schlech BA. Effect of three proteinaceous foreign materials on infected and subinfected wound models. Surgery 1975; 77:569–576.

158. Noble WC. The production of subcutaneous staphylococcal skin lesions in mice. Br J Exp Pathol 1965; 46:254–262.

159. Zimmerli W, Waldvogel FA, Vaudaux P, Nydegger UE. Pathogenesis of foreign body infection: description and characteristics of an animal model. J Infect Dis 1982; 146:487–497.

160. Zimmerli W, Lew DP, Waldvogel FA. Pathogenesis of foreign body infection. Evidence of a local granulocyte defect. J Clin Invest 1984; 73:1191–1200.

161. Henson PM. The immunologic release of constituents from neutrophil leukocytes. I. The role of antibody and complement on nonphagocytosable surfaces or phagocytosable particles. J Immunol 1971; 107:1535–1546.

162. Johnston RB, Lehmeyer JE. Elaboration of toxic oxygen by-product by neutrophils in a model of immune complex disease. J Clin Invest 1976; 57:836–841.

163. Klock JC, Bainton DF. Degranulation and abnormal bactericidal function of granulocytes procured by reversible adhesion to nylon wool. Blood 1976; 48:149–161.

164. Wright DG, Gallin JI. Secretory responses of human neutrophils: exocytosis of specific (secondary) granules by human neutrophils during adherence in vitro and during exudation in vivo. J Immunol 1979; 123:258–294.

165. Yanai M, Quie PG. Chemiluminescence by polymorphonuclear leukocytes adhering to surfaces. Infect Immun 1981; 123:285–294.

166. Vaudaux P, Grau GE, Huggler E, et al. Contibution of tumor necrosis factor to host defense against staphylococci in a guinea pig model of foreign body infections. J Infect Dis 1992; 166:58–64.

167. Wood WB Jr, Smith MR, Watson B. Studies on the mechanism of recovery in pneumococcal pneumonia. IV. The mechanism of phagocytosis in the absence of antibody. J Exp Med 1946; 84:387–401.

168. Vaudaux P, Zulian G, Huggler E, Waldvogel FA. Attachment of *Staphylococcus aureus* to polymethylmethacrylate increases its resistance to phagocytosis and foreign body infection. Infect Immun 1985; 50:472–477.

169. Herrmann M, Jaconi MEE, Dahlgren C, Waldvogel FA, Stendahl O, Lew DP. Neutrophil bactericidal activity against *Staphylococcus aureus* adherent on biological surfaces. J Clin Invest 1990; 86:942–951.

170. Sherertz RJ, Carruth WA, Marosok RD, Espeland MA, Johnson RA, Solomon DD. Contribution of vascular catheter material to the pathogenesis of infection: the enhanced risk of silicone in vivo. J Biomed Mater Res 1995; 29:635–645.

171. Marosok R, Washburn R, Indorf A, Solomon D, Sherertz R. Contribution of vascular catheter material to the pathogenesis of infection: depletion of complement by silicone elastomer in vitro. J Biomed Mater Res. In press.

172. Indorf A, Clarkson L, Sherertz R. Neutrophil chemotaxis on polymer surfaces. Presented at the 33rd Interscience Conference on Antimicrobial Agents and Chemotherapy, New Orleans, 1993. Abstract 552.

173. Lee DA, Hoidal JR, Clawson CC, Quie PG, Peterson PK. Phagocytosis by polymorphonuclear leukocytes of *Staphylococcus aureus* and *Pseudomonas aeruginosa* adherent to plastic, agar, or glass. J Immunol Methods 1983; 63:103–114.

174. Gordon DL, Rice JL. Opsonin-dependent and independent surface phagocytosis of *Staphylococcus aureus* proceeds independently of complement and complement receptors. Immunology 1988; 64:709–714.

175. Gordon DL, Avery VM, Rice JL, McDonald PJ. Surface phagocytosis of *Staphylococcus epidermidis* and *Escherichia coli* by human neutrophils: serum requirements for opsonization and chemiluminescence. Fems Microbiol Immunol 1989; 1:417–423.

176. Avery VM, Gordon DL. Antibacterial properties of breast milk: requirements for surface phagocytosis and chemiluminescence. Eur J Clin Microbiol Infect Dis 1991; 10:1034–1039.

177. Lopez-Lopez G, Pascual A, Perea EJ. Effect of plastic catheters on the phagocytic activity of human polymorphonuclear leukocytes. Eur J Clin Microbiol Infect Dis 1990; 9:324–328.

178. Spilezewski KL, Anderson JM, Schaap RN, Solomon DD. In vivo biocompatability of catheter materials. Biomaterials 1988; 9:253–256.

2

Diagnosis of Catheter-Related Infections

Karl G. Kristinsson
National University Hospital, Reykjavik, Iceland

I. INTRODUCTION

Catheter-related infections, like infections associated with other foreign bodies, are usually low-grade infections caused by commensal bacteria. The symptoms and signs can therefore be subtle and go undetected, especially as vascular catheters are common in seriously ill patients, who may have many other reasons for subtle signs of infection such as low-grade pyrexia. This is unfortunate as catheters are placed directly into the vascular tree, and the infection may progress to bacteremia and sepsis, quite often without any prior signs and symptoms of local infection. It is therefore not surprising that intravascular catheters are a major source of nosocomial sepsis (1).

Early diagnosis is important, to prevent morbidity and excess length of hospital stay as well as to reduce the cost of additional treatment. Catheter-associated infections are difficult to treat and often require catheter removal. Replacement of long intravascular catheters is costly and not without risks. Delay in diagnosis may allow the microorganisms to colonize the catheter and form thick layers of organisms and extracellular materials (e.g., staphylococcal slime) (2), sometimes together with a fibrin sheath (on the outside of catheters) (3,4), which may make eradication impossible without catheter removal (5). Antibacterial treatment alone is much more likely to be successful if it is started before the organisms have established biofilms.

There have been many attempts to find simple and reliable methods to diagnose catheter-associated infections. Most require examination of a catheter segment after the catheter has been removed, and therefore only provide a retrospective diagnosis. This means that a large number of catheters will be removed unnecessarily, as they have not been colonized, and some may be removed too late. The laboratory methods available to diagnose catheter infections before catheter removal are not as accurate but are helpful together with clinical symptoms and signs.

Catheter-associated infections will be considered as local or systemic infections, where localized infection can be either an exit site infection, tunnel infection, or catheter colonization without any symptoms or signs. Systemic infections are catheter-related bloodstream infections (bacteremias or sepsis). This chapter deals with the microbiological diagnosis of infections associated with intravascular catheters; the diagnosis of infections associated with cerebrospinal fluid shunts and peritoneal catheters is covered in the respective chapters.

II. CLINICAL DIAGNOSIS

As this chapter focuses mainly on the microbiological diagnosis of catheter-related infections, the description of the clinical diagnosis is brief. For more detailed description of clinical diagnosis, see Chapter 8. Localized infections are confined to the catheter and surrounding tissues, whereas systemic infections are bloodstream infections (bacteremia or septicemia).

A. Localized Infections

Colonization of the catheter surface with microorganisms is often, but not always, associated with localizing clinical infections. Catheter colonization will be discussed in the section on microbiological diagnosis.

1. Exit Site Infections

When the exit site (insertion site) becomes infected, it is usually accompanied with the classical signs of inflammation (erythema, warmth, tenderness, and swelling). However, such inflammation can be due to mechanical and/or chemical irritation, and be sterile (6). This is especially true for peripheral catheters and peripherally placed central venous catheters. Maki and co-workers defined inflammation at the catheter site as presence of lymphangitis, purulence, or at least two of the following: erythema, tenderness, increased warmth, or a palpable thrombosed vein (7). They found that local inflammation was significantly more common when the catheters had positive semiquantitative culture than when they were negative ($P < 0.001$) (see description of the semiquantitative culture in section IIIA1b). The majority of the catheters in their study were peripheral catheters (87%). Another, more recent study looked at the clinical predictors of infection of central venous catheters used for total parenteral nutrition (8). The following insertion site variables were considered for 142 catheters: erythema (>4 mm), tenderness, swelling, and extravasation. The dependent variable was catheter infection, also defined as having a positive semiquantitative culture after removal. The only insertion site variable that was significantly ($P < 0.05$) associated with catheter infection was erythema, in both univariate analysis ($P = 0.049$) and multivariate analysis using stepwise logistic regression ($P = 0.03$). Purulence around the catheter has been considered a more reliable sign for catheter infection (1), although this was not considered as a separate variable in the aforementioned study. Exit site purulence is also easily accessible for culture, but exit site cultures will be considered in a following section.

Exit site infections can thus be defined as erythema, tenderness, induration, and/or purulence within 2 cm of the skin at the exit site of the catheter.

2.   Tunnel Infection

When the local infection extends subcutaneously along the track of tunneled long-term catheters, it is termed tunnel infection. It is characterized by erythema, swelling, and associated cellulitis along the subcutaneous track (9). This should not be confused with infusion phlebitis, which is a common complication of intravenous therapy, occurring in as many as 35% of peripheral intravenous infusions in some hospitals (6). This is mainly due to either chemical and/or mechanical irritation, and increases with the duration of cannulation. This phlebitis has been estimated to be associated with "infected catheters" (i.e., with positive semiquantitative cultures) in about 20% of catheters (10).

Tunnel infections will be defined as erythema, tenderness, and induration in the tissues overlying the catheter and >2 cm from the exit site.

3.   Suppurative Phlebitis

Suppurative phlebitis is one of the most serious complications of intravenous therapy and occurs with unusually high frequency in burn patients (4.2% of 4636 patients; 10a). It is more frequently associated with catheters inserted by cutdown techniques, and its incidence increases with prolonged duration of vein cannulation. It is a major source of sepsis and often begins very insidiously. Local inflammation is present in less than half the cases, and there may be days before the full clinical picture of fever, chills, and hypotension becomes manifest (10). In the study of burn patients by Pruitt and co-workers (10a), the most frequent presentation was that of a positive blood culture in association with clinical sepsis, and the causative organisms reflected the flora colonizing the burn wounds. Overall,

Staphylococcus aureus was the commonest cause. If suppurative thrombophlebitis is suspected, cannulated and previously cannulated veins should be thoroughly examined. If the suspected vein is accessible, it should be explored for the presence of pus, by "milking" the vein by digital pressure, beginning proximal to the estimated site of the previously resident catheter tip and proceeding distal to the site of cannulation. Extrusion of pus confirms the diagnosis. For central veins, the diagnosis may have to rely on positive blood cultures and demonstration of a thrombotic vein (using imaging techniques).

Bacteremia persisting for >48 hours after catheter removal and initiation of appropriate antimicrobial therapy may indicate intravascular infectious complications such as endocarditis or septic thrombophlebitis.

B. Systemic Infections

Systemic infections are catheter-related bloodstream infections where other sources for the organisms have been excluded. The bloodstream infection can either be bacteremia (or fungemia) without significant signs of infection or be associated with a severe toxic febrile state—sepsis. Since catheter-related bloodstream infection is usually a diagnosis of exclusion, diagnosis can be difficult. This is especially true for seriously ill patients in intensive care units and immunocompromised patients, who may have more than one focus of infection, and in addition more than one intravascular catheter. The general clinical features of catheter-related bloodstream infections are indistinguishable from bloodstream infection arising from any other site. Local infection around the catheter may implicate the catheter as a source of infection, but this lacks both specificity and sensitivity. This is because of the frequent lack of local signs of infection in sepsis associated with intravascular catheters and because of the frequency of infusion phlebitis, which may mimic catheter-related infections and thus lead to overestimation of infection (11). Retrospective clinical evidence implicating the catheter as a source of infection is the resolution of clinical sepsis after catheter removal.

Several key observations have been suggested that should alert the physician of the possibility of catheter-associated infections (12,13). They can also be of value in differentiating catheter-related bloodstream infections from other septic syndromes (see Table 1).

C. Examination After Catheter Removal

After the catheter has been removed, symptoms and signs of the infection should subside and disappear. If they do not, the results of the catheter cultures should be reviewed, and the exit site and catheter tunnel examined. In most cases the infection is probably not catheter-related, but the possibility of tunnel infection,

Table 1 Clinical Observations Suggesting Catheter-Related
Bloodstream Infection

1. The patient has received infusion therapy from the outset of
   bacteremia/sepsis.
2. Local phlebitis and/or inflammation at the catheter insertion site, especially if
   associated with expressible purulence.
3. Primary bacteremia/sepsis—i.e., no other focus can be found.
4. Sepsis occurring in a patient not otherwise at high risk for bacteremia.
5. The precipitous onset of overwhelming sepsis, often with shock (often
   indicative of massively contaminated infusate or suppurative phlebitis).
6. Localized embolic disease distal to cannulated artery.
7. Hematogenous *Candida endophthalmitis* in patients receiving total parenteral
   nutrition.
8. Sepsis apparently refractory to "appropriate" antimicrobial therapy.
9. Resolution of febrile syndrome after catheter removal.

septic thrombophlebitis, infective endocarditis, and other septic complications
has to be excluded.

III. MICROBIOLOGICAL DIAGNOSIS

Many different sites have been cultured in an attempt to predict catheter-related
bloodstream infections (Fig. 1). These are the catheter tip, the catheter hub, the
intracutaneous portion of the catheter, the exit site and surrounding skin, and
blood obtained from peripheral veins and through the catheter. Because the most

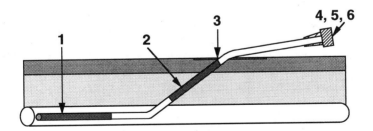

Figure 1 Diagram demonstrating the sites that have been cultured for the purpose of predicting catheter-associated infections. The sites are: (1) catheter tip, (2)
intracutaneous portion of catheter, (3) exit site and/or surrounding skin, (4) catheter
hub, (5) inside of catheter, and (6) quantitative blood cultures.

common organisms causing catheter-associated infections are the coagulase-negative staphylococci, important skin commensals, and frequent blood culture contaminants, the diagnosis by culture is not straightforward (14). The issue is further complicated by the fact that there is some disagreement on the pathogenesis of catheter-associated infections. Some authors maintain that colonization starts at the exit site and spreads along the outside of the catheters to the tip and the bloodstream (15,16); others consider hub colonization as the initial event with subsequent intraluminal progression to the tip (17). This may be because many authors have analyzed long central venous and short peripheral venous catheters together in their studies. In fact, the infection can start by either mechanism. For long intravenous tunneled catheters, hub colonization and migration of organisms along the inside of the catheters are much more important than for short peripheral intravenous lines, where exit site colonization and migration along the outside of catheters are more important. This will not be discussed further in this chapter, but it explains why more than one type of culture may be needed for diagnosis of catheter related infections.

A.   Diagnosis After Catheter Removal

1.   Culture of Catheter Segments

a.   Broth Cultures

To prove that bacteremia is caused by bacteria arising from an intravascular catheter, it is necessary to demonstrate the same organism on the catheter and in the blood.

The easiest method to demonstrate bacteria on the surface of catheter segments is just to place them in broth and incubate. However, these cultures are only qualitative as a single bacterium will give the same end result as 1000 bacteria. In addition, broth cultures can also fail to demonstrate slow-growing and fastidious pathogens in mixture with fast-growing organisms. Although these cultures may in some instances be more sensitive than semiquantitative cultures, they are much less specific and have a very low positive predictive value. When catheters are removed, they have to be pulled back through the exit site in the skin, and as a single skin microorganism can give a positive broth culture, false-positive cultures are common. Broth cultures are therefore poor predictors of catheter colonization and catheter-related infections. This method has now been replaced by semiquantitative or quantitative cultures in most places, and broth cultures should never be used as the only culture method. When broth cultures are negative, however, the probability of a catheter associated infection is low.

b.   Semiquantitative Culture of the Catheter Surface

In 1977, Maki and co-workers evaluated a semiquantitative culture technique for identifying infection due to intravascular catheters and compared it to broth culture (7). Colony counts on the semiquantitative culture plates were bimodally distributed, and local inflammation was more frequent with catheters yielding 15 or more colonies (64% as opposed to 18%); thus the presence of 15 or more colonies was considered to signify "infection."* An each of the four cases of catheter-related bacteremia detected in the study, 1000 or more colonies were found by this technique. The authors concluded that 15 colonies as the lower limit for a positive semiquantitative culture was probably too conservative, and that larger studies would be required to determine a lower limit for the best sensitivity and specificity. The method used in this study has become the standard method for culturing intravascular catheters and will therefore be described in detail. It must be noted, however, that of the 250 catheters studied, 185 (74%) were short (5.7 cm) peripheral venous catheters.

> Method: *Any antimicrobial or blood present on the skin around the catheter is first removed with an alcohol pledget. The catheter is then withdrawn with sterile forceps, while the externalized portion is being kept directed upward and away from the skin surface. For short peripheral catheters, the entire length, beginning several millimeters inside the former skin-surface catheter interface, is aseptically amputated and cultured. With longer catheters, two segments 5 to 7 cm are cultured, a proximal one beginning several millimeters inside the former skin catheter interface, and the tip. Catheter segments are transported to the laboratory in a sterile tube. In the laboratory each catheter segment is transferred to the surface of a normal (diameter 10 cm) 5% blood agar plate, and rolled back and forth across the surface at least four times, with a slight downward pressure exerted by a flamed forceps. Plates are subsequently incubated at 37°C.*

Numerous studies have used this or a similar method, but only a few of the earlier ones will be mentioned here. In a study of 114 umbilical catheters the results of the semiquantitative cultures did not correlate with local erythema, but 83% of the patients were receiving systemic antibiotics, and their use significantly reduced the number of positive cultures (18). In addition, this study failed to show a significant difference between semiquantitative cultures of tip and of intraumbilical portion of the catheter as Maki and colleagues had shown for the tip and the intracutaneous portions (7). In another study, positive semiquantitative cultures were significantly associated with bacteremia, but there was no significant association with any local symptoms except the presence of frank purulence (19). Again, there was no significant difference noted between the cultures of

---

* Today it is generally accepted that the detection of ≥15 cfu (roll plate method) in the absence of clinical symptoms is considered as "catheter colonization," whereas a catheter-related infection is probable in the case of ≥15 cfu together with accompanying symptoms.

transcutaneous segments and the tip segments. A study of 50 short peripheral venous cannulae in neonates, in which both the inside and outside of the cannulae were cultured quantitatively, showed that the outside cultures were positive in all cases, whereas four inside cultures were negative despite positive outside cultures (20). This study failed to show an association between local inflammation and positive cultures but was too small to demonstrate an association with bacteremia. Jones and co-workers evaluated the method in cancer patients, where they studied 379 catheters (all but one long IV catheters), of which 47 were positive by the semiquantitative method (21). Local signs of infection were somewhat more likely to be associated with positive cultures, but not significantly, and although positive cultures were significantly more often associated with bacteremia than negative cultures, five of 12 catheters associated with bacteremia were completely negative on the semiquantitative culture.

The following three studies have attempted to improve the sensitivity and specificity of the method by evaluating different criteria for positivity.

1. In a large study of 780 central venous catheters in an intensive care unit, Collignon and co-workers evaluated the sensitivity and predictive values of semiquantitative cultures of the catheter tips, in predicting catheter-associated bacteremia (using clinical definitions, where bacteremia was considered catheter-related if the same organism was cultured from two or more blood samples collected at different times and primary infective sites other than the catheter could not be identified) (22). When five or more colonies were taken as a positive result, the sensitivity was 92% and the specificity 83%, but the positive predictive value was only 9%. The results for a threshold of ≥15 colonies were similar, and increasing the level of test positivity to ≥100 colonies increased the positive predictive value only to 10%; however, the study population had a very low prevalence of catheter-related bacteremia (14).

2. Kristinsson et al. studied 236 unselected long central venous catheter tips, in which all the eight patients with catheter-related sepsis had >50 colonies by the semiquantitative culture, and all but one had >100 colonies (catheter-related sepsis defined as bacteremia where the same organism was isolated from the peripheral venous and also the intravascular line cultures) (23). The predictive value of a positive culture being associated with catheter related infection or probable infection was 46% for >15 colonies and 56% for ≥100 colonies, and the negative predictive values were 99% and 93%, respectively.

3. In a study of 119 long intravascular catheter tips from critically ill patients with suspected catheter-related sepsis, Rello and co-workers (24) found that thresholds of 15 and 50 colonies gave the same sensitivity, 92%, but the specificity was 78% and 86%, respectively (bacteremia

classified as catheter-related if a microorganism was cultured from a blood sample and if no primary site other than the intravascular catheter could be identified. In this study local infection was also considered to represent catheter-related sepsis). In that population the positive predictive values were 34% and 44%, respectively, and the negative predictive value 99% for both—figures very similar to those in the study of Kristinsson and co-workers (23).

c. Quantitative Culture of the Inside of the Catheters

Another approach to diagnose intravascular catheter associated infections was described by Cleri and co-workers (25). They cultured the inside of the intradermal and intravascular segments quantitatively and found that growth of >1000 colonies from the inside of a segment was significantly associated with bacteremia. Most of the catheters studied were short IV catheters (112 of 149). Catheter-associated bacteremia occurred in 13 instances, and for all of those the catheter segments grew >10^3 colonies. The likelihood of catheter-associated bacteremia increased from 29% with 10^3 to 10^4 colonies per segment to 100% with >10^6 colonies per segment. Their method is as follows:

> *The intradermal segment, the first centimeter distal to the mark on the insert, is separated from the remainder of the insert (the intravascular segment) and placed in 2 ml of trypticase soy broth. A needle is inserted into the proximal end of the intravascular segment, which is immersed in 2 ml or 10 ml broth (depending on the size of the insert) and flushed three times. The broths are serially diluted 100-fold, and 0.1 ml of each dilution is streaked onto blood agar. After incubation the number of colony-forming units is calculated by multiplying the number of colonies by 10 times the dilution factor and dividing by the volume of broth in which the insert had been immersed.*

With methods available to quantify the number of bacteria, both on the inside and on the outside of catheters, which method is better in predicting catheter-related bacteremia? Linares and co-workers used both the semiquantitative method of Maki to culture the outside and the quantitative method of Cleri to culture the inside of intravascular and subcutaneous segments of long intravascular catheters to determine the routes of infection in 20 cases of catheter-related bacteremia/fungemia (17). The intravascular tip had >15 colonies on the outside in 18 cases (90%) and >1000 colonies on the inside in 19 cases (95%), whereas the corresponding figures for the subcutaneous segment were 13 (65%) and 15 (75%), respectively. Using a slight modification of the method by Cleri and co-workers (25), Kristinsson and co-workers compared both techniques for 236 unselected long intravascular catheters (23). Results of both culture methods and sufficient clinical information were available for 193 catheters. There was a good correlation between results from both methods, but cultures from the outside of catheters produced more falsely positive results. Of the eight patients who had catheter-related bacteremia/fungemia, all cultures were positive by both methods, except for one patient where the quantitative culture from the inside showed fewer than 15 colonies. This patient had been treated with an appropriate antibiotic intravenously.

d.   Quantitative Culture After Catheter Vortexing or Ultrasonication

It may be technically difficult to roll a long segment of catheter across an agar surface in a way that dislodges most bacteria from the catheter surface onto the surface of the agar. Likewise, flushing the inside of catheters may in some cases be difficult. To avoid these problems, Brun-Buisson and colleagues (26) modified the method described by Cleri and co-workers (25); instead of flushing the inside of the catheter segments, they vortexed the catheter segment in sterile water for 1 min before diluting the solution for quantitative cultures. Most of the catheter tips growing 10^3 colony-forming units/ml (CFU/ml) or more were associated with clinical symptoms of infection. Catheters yielding less than 10^3 CFU/ml were usually either contaminated or colonized, without clinical evidence of sepsis. A cutoff concentration of 10^3 CFU/ml was 97.5% sensitive and 88% specific to diagnose catheter-related sepsis.

Bjornsson and co-workers used a slightly different technique in a study of the association between microorganism growth at the catheter insertion site and colonization of the catheter in patients receiving total parenteral nutrition (15). After placing 2 ml of sterile fluid in the tube containing the catheter segment, the tube was centrifuged vigorously for 90 sec to elute bacteria from the catheter, which were subsequently enumerated by standard dilution plate count methods. Of the 74 catheters studied, five were associated with bacteremia or fungemia, all of which had more than 10^3 CFU isolated from the intravascular catheter segment.

It has also been suggested that some microorganisms may adhere so avidly to catheter surfaces that they are not dislodged by rolling, flushing, or vortexing (27). Sonication might be a good method to remove sessile adherent organisms buried in the biofilm layer. To be able to enumerate accurately large number of bacteria adherent to the catheter, Sherertz and co-workers used sonication to dislodge the bacteria from the catheters (28). Over a 3-year period they cultured 1681 catheters by placing them in 10 ml of broth, sonicating for 1 min (55,000 Hz, 125 W), and vortexing for 15 sec before taking a 0.1-ml sample into either 0.9 ml or 9.9 ml of broth. Then 0.1 ml of these dilutions and 0.1 ml of the broth were surface-plated by a loop on blood agar. The sonication method allowed quantification of the number of CFU removed from a catheter for between 10^2 and 10^7 CFU. For catheter cultures in which $\geq 10^2$ CFU grew, a linear regression equation could be calculated ($r = 0.93$; increase in CFU associated with increase in the percentage of positive blood cultures). In a study where semiquantitative and quantitative cultures were performed together with culture after ultrasonication, the ultrasonication did not increase the sensitivity of the cultures (23). Infected catheters with insignificant growth by the semiquantitative or quantitative methods did not show significant growth on culture after ultrasonication.

e. Summary and Conclusion

The objective of all the culture methods mentioned above is to diagnose a catheter-related infection by differentiating the catheters that are associated with infection from those that are not. It is clear that culturing catheter segments in broth does not achieve this, although this is one of the most sensitive methods. Quantification of some sort is clearly necessary to differentiate contamination from colonization/infection. Direct comparison of all the quantitative and semi-quantitative methods is difficult, as these studies have variable numbers of patients, different patient/risk groups, different types of catheters, and varying definitions for infection in each study. In addition, in many studies the finding of a positive catheter culture has been a part of the definition of catheter-related bacteremia. This could overestimate the sensitivity of the methods if the catheter cultures are falsely negative (11). In fact it has been demonstrated that almost all indwelling central venous catheters have visible adherent microorganisms on their surface, but only few organisms can be cultured (27). Table 2 lists the quoted studies according to culture method, together with the number and type of catheters studied and number of bacteremias.

No one method is clearly the best. The semiquantitative culture method described by Maki and co-workers (7), using ≥15 colonies as the criterium for a positive culture, is simple and has been the method most frequently used in published studies to date. Many of the other methods appear to be just as good. In a comparison of the semiquantitative method, quantitative culture of the inside and culture after ultrasonication, in the normal routine hospital setting, a threshold of 100 CFU and culturing the inside of the catheters were the best predictors of infection (23).

By studying the ultrastructure of indwelling vascular catheters with scanning and transmission electron microscopy and comparing the results with the results of the semiquantitative roll technique and culture after ultrasonication, Raad and co-workers came up with several interesting and important findings (27). External colonization was predominant in the first 10 days of catheter placement, while luminal colonization became predominant after 30 days. This would indicate that the semiquantitative roll technique would be most useful for short-term catheters (as indeed most of the catheters were in the original study of Maki and co-workers), whereas for long-term catheters the internal surface should be cultured. Ideally both surfaces should always be cultured, but this may not be practical. In the same study, the sensitivity of the semiquantitative roll-plate technique of the catheter tips was only 42% to 45%, as opposed to 65% to 72% for culture after sonication of the tips. The authors concluded that in order to isolate sessile or

Table 2 List of Studies According to Culture Method

Study	No. studied	Long catheters	Short catheters	Bac- teremia
Semiquantitative culture of external surface				
Maki et al. (7)	250	65	185	4
Adam et al. (18)	114	114	0	?
Moyer et al. (19)	101	101	0	5
Wilkins et al. (20)	50	0	50	0
Jones et al. (21)	379	378	1	12
Collignon et al. (22)	780	780	0	14
Kristinsson et al. (23)	236	236	0	8
Rello et al. (24)	119	119	0	11
Quantitative culture of internal surface				
Cleri et al. (25)	189	> 35	> 112	13
Linares et al. (17)	20	20	0	20
Kristinsson et al. (23)	236	236	0	8
Quantitative culture after vortexing/ultrasonication				
Brun-Buisson et al. (26)	331	331	0	36
Bjornson et al. (15)	74	74	0	10
Sherertz et al. (28)	1681	?	?	?
Kristinsson et al. (23)	236	236	0	8

semisessile organisms, the more disruptive method of sonication might be necessary. These data therefore suggest that culture after ultrasonication should be the most sensitive method, and it is also easy to quantitate. However, ultrasonication may not be practical in many laboratories, and since there is no consensus as to which method should be used, the technique one chooses is not critical as long at it is a semiquantitative or quantitative method, preferably standardized for the population/catheters under study.

2. Microscopy of Catheter Segments

Microbiological cultures normally need overnight incubation before they can be examined for growth. In an attempt to reduce the time taken to decide whether removed catheters are colonized or not, several investigators have studied the possibility of using microscopy of catheter segments for diagnosis. The catheters were either stained by Gram or acridine orange stains before examination.

a. Gram Staining

Cooper and Hopkins first studied the value of Gram staining catheter segments (29). The catheter segments were Gram-stained in disposable Petri plates, which were discarded after each staining. Solutions were permitted to flow through the lumen of the catheter to stain the inside of the catheters. After they had been blotted dry on filter paper, at least 200 fields were examined under the oil immersion objective ($\times 1000$). In a study of 330 catheters, where a single organism per 20 oil immersion fields was designated as positive, the method had a 100% sensitivity and 97% specificity in predicting colonization (according to the criteria of Maki et al.; 7) with positive and negative predictive values of 84% and 100%, respectively. This study has been criticized for being time-consuming and impractical (30), and in a study of 27 catheters Kristinsson and Spencer were able to achieve a sensitivity of only 47% with this method (31). They examined only 25 to 35 oil immersion fields, and the procedure took up to 30 min to complete.

To overcome the problems of examining the cylindrical catheter surface, an alternative method has been described, where the catheter segments were rolled over the surface of a glass slide in a shallow narrow line of sterile saline solution (32). The slide was subsequently fixed and stained, and the entire length of the impression smear was examined. The sensitivity of this method was 83% and the specificity 81%, but the positive predictive value was only 44% (in predicting a positive semiquantitative culture).

b. Acridine Orange Staining

Zufferey et al. (33) have also tried to speed up the process of examining catheter segments under the microscope. They stained 710 catheter segments with the fluorochrome dye acridine orange. The catheters were examined with a fluorescence microscope, first dry at a $\times 100$ magnification, and if there was no fluorescence detected after 3 min of examination, it was considered negative. If fluorescent material was detected, the catheter was also examined with an oil immersion lens at $\times 1000$ magnification to see the morphology of the fluorescent material. This method was again compared with the semiquantitative culture (7) and showed a sensitivity of 84% and specificity of 99%.

In a study on the value of direct catheter staining in the diagnosis of intravascular-catheter related infections, both Gram staining and acridine orange staining had poor sensitivity in predicting results of semiquantitative cultures, 44% and 71%, respectively (34). The Gram staining method had higher specificity—91%, as opposed to 77% with acridine orange staining.

The main problems associated with diagnosing catheter colonization by microscopy are as follows: frequent fine focusing is necessary owing to the cylindrical shape of the catheter; opaque catheters can be difficult/impossible to examine; the technique is relatively time-consuming and seems to lack sensitivity. Not much is gained by the microscopy as the catheter has to be removed, and if the patient's pyrexia has not settled after 24 hours, an alternative cause for the fever should be searched for. At this time culture results should also be available.

B.   Diagnosis Without Catheter Removal

1.   Blood Cultures

Blood cultures are needed for the diagnosis of bacteremia. Ordinary peripheral blood cultures do not differentiate catheter-related bacteremia from bacteremia of other origin and will not be considered further. Obtaining blood through central venous catheters was first proposed as a convenient means of performing blood cultures, without the need of peripheral venipuncture (35,36). However, this has the disadvantage of false-positive cultures, caused by contamination or colonization of the catheters (37). On the other hand, obtaining blood through the central venous catheter could possibly be of help in diagnosing catheter-related infection if there is a way to differentiate between catheter-related sepsis, catheter colonization, and catheter contamination. Quantitative blood cultures have been used for this purpose since 1979 (38), when in a case report it was clearly demonstrated that the origin of a bacteremia was indeed the catheter. The method is as follows:

> Blood is drawn from a peripheral vein and through the catheter after 20 ml of saline solution has been flushed through. In addition to normal cultures, 1 ml of blood from the peripheral vein and from the catheter is added to 10 ml of molten liquid tryptic soy agar, and the mixture is plated in a Petri dish and allowed to settle. Because of high colony counts in blood from the catheter, 0.1 ml of that blood is used subsequently. Plates are examined after overnight incubation and the number of CFU is determined.

In the original study blood drawn from a peripheral vein had 25 CFU/ml, whereas blood drawn through the catheter had >10,000 CFU/ml.

Many studies have subsequently confirmed the usefulness of quantitative cultures of blood collected through the catheter and through a peripheral vein in diagnosing catheter-related bacteremia or fungemia (16,39–44), with only one exception (45). Routine quantitative blood cultures once or twice weekly have, on the other hand, not been helpful in detecting impending bacteremia (16,39). Basically three methods have been used for the quantification of blood cultures:

1. Pour plate method. An aliquot of the blood is mixed with a sterile anti-coagulant and then with molten agar (16,40,42,44). After the agar has settled and the plates have been incubated, the colonies are counted.
2. The method using the lysis centrifugation tubes (41,43,45,46) (Isolator; Du Pont Co.). The blood is inoculated into tubes containing a cell-lysing

agent, saponin, a foam-reducing agent, and sodium polyanetholesulfonate. After mixing, the tube is centrifuged, the supernatant removed, and the concentrate used to inoculate agar plates. The technique has been found to be valuable both because of early detection (47) and because it allows quantification by colony counts (48).

3. Direct inoculation of blood onto agar media (39). Pour plates may be cumbersome to use, as they require mixing the blood with molten agar. Quantitative cultures can also be made by inoculating 0.5-ml sample of blood directly onto the surface of each of two chocolate agar plates. The blood is dispersed over the agar by gentle rotation, a technique that could be mastered by the house staff on the hospital wards.

In most cases blood taken from the infected catheters had much higher colony counts than the blood taken from a peripheral vein, often 100 to 1000× times higher, although this was not invariable. Capdevila and co-workers (42) studied 107 long intravascular catheters. Using a colony count fourfold higher in blood drawn through the catheter than in simultaneously drawn peripheral blood as a cut-off value, they obtained a sensitivity of 94%, specificity of 100%, and a positive predictive value of 100%. A single bacterial count >100 CFU/ml in the quantitative culture of the catheter blood specimen in the presence of a positive qualitative peripheral blood culture of the same organism was also highly suggestive of catheter-related sepsis.

Despite the usefulness of quantitative blood cultures, there are certain practical difficulties in their use. One has either to use a separate blood culture system (Isolator, Du Pont Co.) or to transport the blood immediately to the laboratory where pour plates or surface inoculations can be performed (inoculating the agar plates on the wards is not compatible with most infection control guidelines). Laboratories using the pour plate method have to keep a stock of molten agar available at all times.

2. Culture of the Catheter Hub

Culturing the catheter hub is based on the assumption that the infection is likely to have originated from the hub and is therefore more appropriate for long intravascular catheters, especially tunneled catheters.

In a study on the pathogenesis of catheter-related sepsis, Linares et al. (17) investigated 135 subclavian catheters, where 20 catheters gave rise to catheter-related bacteremia. The catheter hub was considered the source in 14 cases, the infusate in 2, hematogenous seeding in 2, and skin/exit site in 2 (17). The hub was actually cultured after catheter removal, by flushing through the lumen with broth and subsequent quantitative culture. The authors concluded that the catheter hub was the most common site of origin of organisms causing catheter tip infection and bacteremia. This would therefore suggest that culturing the catheter hub, without removal, could be of value.

In a prospective study to investigate the potential of surveillance hub cultures before catheter removal, Fan *et al.* (49) cultured 142 catheters of which 28 were designated as infected. The hub was cultured by inserting a swab into the hub and rubbing it repeatedly against its interior surface. This could be done after cleaning the outside of the hub with a disinfectant (49). The swab was then streaked onto agar plates for semiquantitative culture. The sensitivity of the surveillance hub culture in predicting catheter-related bacteremia was 34.5% and the specificity 87.6%, as opposed to 37.9% and 71.7%, respectively, for surveillance skin/exit site cultures. Combining these culture methods yielded a sensitivity of 79.3% and a specificity of 74.3%.

Cercenado et al. (50) compared two diagnostic methods (skin and hub culture) in a prospective study of 139 intravascular catheters (95 long central vein, 44 short peripheral) to develop a simple and rapid diagnostic procedure to diagnose catheter-associated infections, obviating unnecessary catheter removal. Of the 139 catheters, 79 had clinical evidence of infection, and of these 35 were infected according to semiquantitative culture of the tip. Superficial cultures were positive ($\geq$15 CFU/plate) in 34 of those 35 (17 skin, 9 hub, 7 both, and 1 with a different organism isolated in superficial and catheter cultures). All catheters with negative superficial cultures had a negative tip culture. The sensitivity and specificity of skin and hub cultures for intravascular catheters with clinical evidence of infection were 97.1% and 68.2%, respectively. No distinction was made between short and long catheters.

Hub cultures can be useful in predicting catheter-related bacteremias, but should preferably be used together with skin/exit site cultures. Negative skin and hub cultures have a high negative predictive value.

3. Intraluminal Culture

Jakobsen and co-workers (51) evaluated an intraluminal sampling method to assess catheter colonization of 35 central venous catheters. In an attempt to find the major route of contamination, they also examined 32 of the catheters with semiquantitative culture of the tip and culture of the skin/exit site (51). The intraluminal sampling was performed by a plastic obturator (guidewire) that was inserted into the lumen along its entire length and withdrawn under rotation. The distal 3 to 4 cm of the obturator was then rolled back and forth, at least four times, across the surface of an agar plate for culture. All catheters colonized intraluminally had positive catheter tip cultures. Two patients with positive skin/exit site cultures had negative catheter tip cultures. None of the catheters that had negative tip cultures were colonized intraluminally. There was a significantly better correlation between organisms cultured from the tip and intraluminally than between the tip and the skin/exit site. None of the patients developed bacteremia during the study, so the value of the technique in predicting catheter-related bacteremia could not be assessed, but the authors concluded that the method was relatively easy and reliable.

4. Culture of Skin and Exit Site

In cases where the infection starts at the exit site and migrates along the subcutaneous tract, exit site cultures could be of value. Several investigators have cultured the skin surrounding the exit site or the exit site itself, in an attempt to predict catheter colonization or to investigate the pathogenesis of intravascular catheter-associated infections. The methods used for culture and the criteria for positive cultures have varied, and some are not described in detail. This makes a direct comparison of these studies difficult. However, to get a rough idea about the value of these cultures, the sensitivity and specificity of the methods in predicting catheter colonisation (according to the semiquantitative method described by Maki and co-workers; 7) was calculated; the results are shown in Table 3. There is a wide variation in the sensitivity of these cultures, with values as low as 11% (17) and as high as 100% (52). This difference can not be due to the difference in the methods alone, as in both studies giving these conflicting results, the exit site alone was cultured. Fan and co-workers also employed exit site cultures, with a sensitivity of 38% (49). Bjornson and co-workers (15) and Raad and co-workers (53) cultured a 24-cm^2 area around the insertion site semiquantitatively, by rubbing a premoistened swab with two sets of 10 back-and-forth strokes over the area. Armstrong and co-workers cultured a slightly smaller area (8), but Cercenado and co-workers (50) and Guidet and co-workers (52) only cultured a 9- to 10-cm^2 area with a dry swab, and still got a sensitivity of 72% and 100% respectively. The specificity of these cultures was roughly similar (71% to 100%).

Four of these studies also investigated catheter hub cultures (see Sect. IIIB2), and the investigators were able to increase the sensitivity of these methods by combining the results. In the first study (17), the sensitivity of the hub cultures increased from 80% to 90% by combining them with the results of the exit site cultures. The high colonization rate of the catheter hub in relation to the other sites was used as an argument for the importance of the hub in the pathogenesis of catheter-associated infections (54). This study is different from the others, as only patients with confirmed catheter-related bacteremia were included (i.e., 20 of 135 catheterized patients). In the second study the sensitivity of the hub culture in predicting catheter-related bacteremia (identical bacteria isolated from both the catheter tip and peripheral blood) was 34% and the skin culture 38%, but combining the results increased the sensitivity to 79% (49). The specificity did not decrease materially by combining the results. In the third study 57% of patients with infected catheters (≥15 CFU, semiquantitative culture of catheter

Table 3   Sensitivity and Specificity of Cultures of Exit Site and/or Surrounding Skin in Predicting Catheter Colonization [as Judged by Semiquantitative Cultures (Ref. 7) or Quantitative Culture (Ref. 26) of the Catheter Tip]

Study	Type of catheters studied	No. of catheters studied	Area of skin cultured	Threshold for positive skin culture	Colonized catheters (%)	Sensitivity (%)	Specificity (%)
Bjornsson et al. (15)	Subclavian	74	25 cm²	> 1000	19 (26)	68	89
Snydman et al. (16)	Tunneled subclavian	59	ES	> 0	14 (24)	95	76
Linares et al. (17)	Subclavian	20	ES	> 0	18 (90)	11	NA
Fan et al. (49)	Subclavian/ jugular	142	ES	≥15	29 (20)	38	72
Armstrong et al. (8)	Central vc	152	5 cm²	≥50	20 (13)	45	94
Cercenado et al. (50)	Central/ peripheral	139	10 cm²	≥15	53 (38)	72	71
Guidet et al. (52)	Central vc	50	9 cm²	> 15	10 (20)	100	72
Raad et al. (53)	Central vc	15	24 cm²	≥1000	3 (20)	75	100

Abbreviations: ES = catheter exit site and the skin immediately surrounding it cultured, but the area was not specified; NA = sufficient information not available, as the study included only the 20 catheters associated with catheter-related bacteremia.

tip) had a positive skin culture (≥15 CFU/plate), 23% had a positive hub culture (≥15 CFU/plate), but combining the results identified 94% of infected catheters (50). In the fourth study the sensitivity of the skin culture (>15 CFU) was already 100% in predicting catheter colonization (>1000 CFU/ml in quantitative tip culture; 26), but the specificity of combining both cultures increased from 72% to 95% (52). These results therefore show an increased benefit in combining the two culture methods, which is not surprising as organisms can colonise catheters from the exit sites, the catheter hubs, or both.

5.   Microscopy of Blood Aspirated Through Catheters

All the methods to diagnose infection before catheter removal discussed so far are based upon microbiological cultures which normally take about 1 day to become positive. Rushforth and co-workers have described a method that uses an acridine orange leukocyte cytospin to prepare a slide for ultraviolet microscopy and that takes less than 1 hour (55). In a study of 95 episodes of suspected sepsis in 51 pediatric patients receiving parenteral nutrition, catheter-related bacteremia was diagnosed in 31 cases by quantitative blood cultures. The acridine orange leukocyte cytospin test predicted catheter-related bacteremia with 87% sensitivity and 94% specificity. This may therefore be a useful test when rapid diagnosis is important, but some laboratories may not have access to both cytospin and fluorescence microscope. Further, the value of the method in adult patients has to be evaluated.

6.   Organism Characteristics

a.   Slime Production

Catheter-associated infections are most commonly caused by coagulase-negative staphylococci. Because coagulase-negative staphylococci are also important skin commensals and frequent contaminants in clinical specimens, many authors have attempted to find a laboratory test that would differentiate pathogens from contaminants.

S. epidermidis adheres and grows on the surface of synthetic polymers, develops into microcolonies, and, during the process of colonization, produces extracellular slime (2). Investigators have tried to correlate this property with the pathogenicity of coagulase-negative staphylococci. Ishak and colleagues found that slime production was significantly more common in strains causing sepsis than in contaminants and skin isolates (56). All the pathogens were identified as S. epidermidis. They concluded that differentiation to species level and the slime production test (57) predicted the clinical significance of blood isolates of coagulase-negative staphylococci with an overall accuracy of 89%.

In an investigation of 588 clinical isolates of coagulase-negative staphylococci, 81% of 59 infectious episodes associated with prosthetic devices were due to slime-producing isolates, whereas there was no significant difference in the frequency of slime-positive vs. slime-negative isolates in patients without a prosthetic device (58). Younger and colleagues studied 51 pathogens and 34 contaminants from cerebrospinal fluid shunts; 88% of the pathogens were adherent (slime producers) compared with 61% of contaminants (59). Kotilainen studied 64 strains from bacteremias, and 53% were adherent slime producers as opposed to 29% of 489 single blood culture isolates considered contaminants (60). In contrast, Kristinsson and colleagues did not find slime production to be a useful marker for significant disease, except that it was more difficult to eradicate infections caused by slime producers than those caused by non-slime producers (61). Also, Ludlam and colleagues did not find infecting strains to be more likely to produce slime than noninfecting strains (in chronic ambulatory peritoneal dialysis) (62). The aforementioned investigators, except Younger and colleagues (59), used the method described by Christensen and colleagues to detect slime production (57).

Despite some correlation between slime production and clinical significance, the likelihood of an infecting strain being a slime producer varies markedly between different studies. Thus, the test for slime production is not accurate enough to differentiate between infecting and noninfecting strains in a clinical situation. However, it may be used as one of several markers for the clinical significance of an isolate.

b.   Speciation and Typing

Culturing coagulase-negative staphylococci from the blood and the catheter tip does not necessarily imply catheter-related bacteremia. There are currently over 30 staphylococcal species, many of which can cause catheter-associated infections (14). Accurate diagnosis depends on the isolation of identical organisms from both the catheter and the blood. When coagulase-negative staphylococci are isolated, especially from different sites, identification to a species level is necessary. However, the commonest species, *S. epidermidis*, is a large and heterogenous group of organisms, which means that further typing is usually necessary. Although *S. epidermidis* is by far the commonest species involved in foreign body-associated infections, the speciation itself is of limited value in deciding clinical significance as it is also the predominant species in the normal flora of humans (14).

Numerous methods have been used for the typing of coagulase-negative staphylococci. The discussion of the advantages and disadvantages of the various typing methods are outside the scope of this chapter, but good reviews of the subject have been written (14,63). More recent methods include sodium dodecyl sulfate (SDS) polyacrylamide gel electrophoresis (PAGE) of staphylococcal extracellular products (64), SDS-PAGE and immunoblotting (65), cellular DNA restriction patterns (66), restriction polymorphism of the rRNA gene region (67), hybridization patterns obtained with three probes (68), and pulsed field gel electrophoresis of *Sma*I DNA digests (69).

IV.   CONCLUSIONS

Numerous methods have been described in an attempt to diagnose catheter-related infections accurately. Comparison of these methods is difficult, as different criteria are used for catheter-related infections, different catheter types are used, and different patient populations are being studied. Diagnosis of catheter-associated infections with the catheter in situ should be based on careful clinical examination together with microbiological cultures. No single culture method diagnoses infected catheters with high sensitivity and specificity for all catheter types, and the selection of the method therefore often depends on the type of catheter.

1. Short peripheral catheters. If a short peripheral catheter is considered to be infected (after clinical examination), it should be removed. These catheters are intended to be used for only a few days, and the cultures to be taken are therefore intended to confirm the infection rather than to predict infection before removal. For that purpose the semiquantitative culture described by Maki and co-workers is suitable (7), but in addition the insertion site may also be cultured if it is considered infected.

2. Central venous catheters. When a central venous catheter is considered to be infected, the decision to remove the catheter depends on its importance for the patient. If it is not necessary for further treatment, it should be removed and cultures taken only to confirm infection. However, if the catheter is important for further treatment, especially if insertion of a new catheter is likely to be problematic, then attempts should be made to predict the likelihood of infection to avoid unnecessary removal. This is probably best done by quantitative blood cultures taken through the catheter and from a peripheral vein. If the exit site of the catheter appears infected, then cultures should be taken from the exit site. Cultures from the exit site or the surrounding skin are not likely to be useful on their own if the exit site is not infected, but may be used as an adjunct to other cultures. Likewise, cultures from the catheter hub may be performed, especially from catheters that have been in situ for a long time.

No single method will identify all infected catheters accurately, but the decision which method to choose will have to be taken locally in collaboration with the microbiology laboratory. Quantitative cultures of catheter tips after ultrasonication are regarded to be most sensitive and have an acceptable specificity, but the equipment needed is not available in many laboratories. Semiquantitative cultures of the external surface are totally acceptable, but ideally the number of colony-forming units needed to indicate infection should be evaluated by local studies. If the semiquantitative method is chosen, then additional cultures of the internal surface should be considered for tunneled catheters that have been in situ for long periods. This rough guideline is shown graphically in Figure 2.

It is important to realize the real value of catheter cultures for the patients. The clinical impact of the routine use of the semiquantitative culture technique has been studied (70). It was defined as a change in diagnosis or therapy on the basis of the culture result. For 96% of 157 catheter cultures there was no impact. Careful selection of culture methods together with a good cooperation between clinicians and the laboratory are likely to increase the impact. It may also be important to define which patient population is most likely to benefit from such

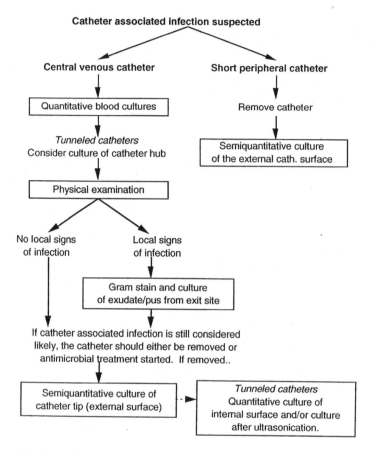

Figure 2 Flow diagram suggesting appropriate methods to diagnose catheter-related infections. It should be noted that this is not intended as a guide on how to manage catheter-associated infections.

cultures. Routine cultures of central venous catheters, using either a quantitative or a semiquantitative method, can be useful if the results are recorded as a part of an infection control program. The recorded infection rates can then be used as an important measure of the quality of catheter care.

REFERENCES

1. Raad II, Bodey GP. Infectious complications of indwelling vascular catheters. Clin Infect Dis 1992; 15:197–210.

2. Peters G, Locci R, Pulverer G. Adherence and growth of coagulase-negative staphylococci on surfaces of intravenous catheters. J Infect Dis 1982; 146:479–482.

3. Hoshal VL, Ause RG, Hoskins PA. Fibrin sleeve formation on indwelling subclavian central venous catheters. Arch Surg 1971; 102:353–358.

4. Goeäu-Brissonière O, Leport C, Guidoin R, et al. Experimental colonization of an expanded polytetrafluoroethylene vascular graft with *Staphylococcus aureus:* A quantitative and morphologic study. J Vasc Surg 1987; 5:743–748.

5. Raad I, Davis S, Khan A, Tarrand J, Elting L, Bodey GP. Impact of central venous catheter removal on the recurrence of catheter-related coagulase negative staphylococcal bacteremia. Infect Control Hosp Epidemiol 1992; 13:215–221.

6. Maki DG, Goldman DA, Rhame FS. Infection control in intravenous therapy. Ann Intern Med 1973; 79:867–887.

7. Maki DG, Weise CE, Sarafin HW. A semiquantitative culture method for identifying intravenous-catheter-related infection. N Engl J Med 1977; 296:1305–1309.

8. Armstrong CW, Mayhall CG, Miller KB, et al. Clinical predictors of infection of central venous catheters used for total parenteral nutrition. Infect Control Hosp Epidemiol 1990; 11:71–78.

9. Press OW, Ramsey PG, Larson EB, Fefer A, Hickman RO. Hickman catheter infections in patients with malignancies. Medicine 1984; 63:189–200.

10. Maki DG. Infections associated with intravascular lines. In: Remington JS, Swartz MN, eds. Current Clinical Topics in Infectious Diseases. Vol. 3. New York: McGraw-Hill, 1983:309–363.

10a. Pruitt BA, McManus WF, Kim SH, Treat RC. Diagnosis and treatment of cannula-related intravenous sepsis in burn patients. Ann Surg 1980; 191:546–554.

11. Collignon RJ, Munro R. Laboratory diagnosis of intravascular catheter associated sepsis. Eur J Clin Microbiol Infect Dis 1989; 8:807–814.

12. Henderson DK. Bacteremia due to percutaneous intravascular devices. In: Mandell GL, Bennett JE, Dolin R, eds. Principles and Practice of Infectious Diseases. Vol. 2. New York: Churchill Livingstone, 1995:2587–2599.

13. Maki DM. Epidemic nosocomial bacteremias. In: Wenzel RP, ed. CRC Handbook of Hospital Acquired Infections. Boca Raton: CRC Press, 1981:371–512.

14. Kloos WE, Bannerman TL. Update on clinical significance of coagulase-negative staphylococci. Clin Microbiol Rev 1994; 7:117–140.

15. Bjornson HS, Colley R, Bower RH, Duty VP, Schwartz-Fulton JT, Fischer JE. Association between microorganism growth at the catheter insertion site and colonization of the catheter in patients receiving total parenteral nutrition. Surgery 1982; 92:720–727.

16. Snydman DR, Murray SA, Kornfeld SJ, Majka JA, Ellis CA. Total parenteral nutrition-related infections. Prospective epidemiologic study using semiquantitative methods. Am J Med 1982; 73:695–699.

17. Linares J, Sitges-Serra A, Garau J, Perez JL, Martin R. Pathogenesis of catheter sepsis: a prospective study with quantitative and semiquantitative cultures of catheter hub and segments. J Clin Microbiol 1985; 21:357–360.

18. Adam RD, Edwards LD, Becker CC, Schrom HM. Semiquantitative cultures and routine tip cultures on umbilical catheters. J Pediatr 1982; 100:123–126.

19. Moyer MA, Edwards LD, Farley L. Comparative culture methods on 101 intravenous catheters. Routine, semiquantitative, and blood cultures. Arch Intern Med 1983; 143:66–69.
20. Wilkins EGL, Manning D, Roberts C, Davidson DC. Quantitative bacteriology of peripheral venous cannulae in neonates. J Hosp Infect 1985; 6:209–217.
21. Jones PG, Hopfer RL, Elting L, Jackson JA, Fainstein V, Bodey GP. Semiquantitative cultures of intravascular catheters from cancer patients. Diagn Microbiol Infect Dis 1986; 4:299–306.
22. Collignon PJ, Soni N, Pearson IY, Woods WP, Munro R, Sorrell TC. Is semiquantitative culture of central vein catheter tips useful in the diagnosis of catheter-associated bacteremia? J Clin Microbiol 1986; 24:532–535.
23. Kristinsson KG, Burnett IA, Spencer RC. Evaluation of three methods for culturing long intravascular catheters. J Hosp Infect 1989; 14:183–191.
24. Rello J, Coll P, Prats G. Evaluation of culture techniques for diagnosis of catheter-related sepsis in critically ill patients. Eur J Clin Microbiol Infect Dis 1992; 11:1192–1193.
25. Cleri DJ, Corrado ML, Seligman SJ. Quantitative culture of intravenous catheters and other intravascular inserts. J Infect Dis 1980; 141:781–786.
26. Brun-Buisson C, Abrouk F, Legrand P, Huet Y, Larabi S, Rapin M. Diagnosis of central venous catheter-related sepsis. Critical level of quantitative tip cultures. Arch Intern Med 1987; 147:873–877.
27. Raad I, Costerton W, Sabbarwal U, Sacilowski M, Anaissie E, Bodey GP. Ultrastructural analysis of indwelling vascular catheters: a quantitative relationship between luminal colonization and duration of placement. J Infect Dis 1993; 168:400–407.
28. Sherertz RJ, Raad II, Belani A, et al. Three-year experience with sonicated vascular catheter cultures in a clinical microbiology laboratory. J Clin Microbiol 1990; 28:76–82.
29. Cooper GL, Hopkins CC. Rapid diagnosis of intravascular catheter-associated infection by direct Gram staining of catheter segments. N Engl J Med 1985; 312:1142–1147.
30. Braunstein H. Rapid diagnosis of intravascular catheter-associated infection by direct Gram staining of catheter segments. N Engl J Med 1985; 313:754–755.
31. Kristinsson KG, Spencer RC. Failure to diagnose intravascular-associated infection by direct Gram staining of catheter segments. J Hosp Infect 1986; 7:305–306.
32. Collignon P, Chan R, Munro R. Rapid diagnosis of intravascular catheter-related sepsis. Arch Intern Med 1987; 147:1609–1612.
33. Zufferey J, Rime B, Francioli P, Bille J. Simple method for rapid diagnosis of catheter-associated infection by direct acridine orange staining of catheter tips. J Clin Microbiol 1988; 26:175–177.
34. Coutleé F, Lemieux C, Paradis J-F. Value of direct catheter staining in the diagnosis of intravascular-catheter-related infection. J Clin Microbiol 1988; 26:1088–1090.
35. Tonnesen A, Peuler M, Lockwood WR. Cultures of blood drawn by catheters vs venipuncture. JAMA 1976; 235:1877.
36. Tafuro P, Colbourn D, Gurevich I, et al. Comparison of blood cultures obtained

simultaneously by venepuncture and from vascular lines. J Hosp Infect 1986; 7:283–288.

37. Bryant JK, Strand CL. Reliability of blood cultures collected from intravascular catheter versus venipuncture. Am J Clin Pathol 1987; 88:113–116.

38. Wing EJ, Norden CW, Shadduck RK, Winkelstein A. Use of quantitative bacteriologic techniques to diagnose catheter-related sepsis. Arch Intern Med 1979; 139:482–483.

39. Raucher HS, Hyatt AC, Barzilia A, et al. Quantitative blood cultures in the evaluation of septicemia in children with Broviac catheters. J Pediatr 1984; 104:29–33.

40. Weightman NC, Simpson EM, Speller DCE, Mott MG, Oakhill A. Bacteremia related to indwelling central venous catheters: prevention, diagnosis and treatment. Eur J Clin Microbiol Infect Dis 1988; 7:125–129.

41. Flynn PM, Shenep JL, Barrett FF. Differential quantitation with a commercial blood culture tube for diagnosis of catheter-related infection. J Clin Microbiol 1988; 26:1045–1046.

42. Capdevila JA, Planes AM, Palomar M, et al. Value of differential quantitative blood cultures in the diagnosis of catheter-related sepsis. Eur J Clin Microbiol Infect Dis 1992; 11:403–407.

43. Benezra D, Kiehn TE, Gold JWM, Brown AE, Turnbull ADM, Armstrong D. Prospective study of infections in indwelling central venous catheters using quantitative blood cultures. Am J Med 1988; 85:495–498.

44. Andremont A, Paulet R, Nitenberg G, Hill C. Value of semiquantitative cultures of blood drawn through catheter hubs for estimating the risk of catheter tip colonization in cancer patients. J Clin Microbiol 1988; 26:2297–2299.

45. Paya CV, Guerra L, Marsh HM, Farnell MB, Washington J II, Thompson RL. Limited usefulness of quantitative culture of blood drawn through the device for diagnosis of intravascular-device-related bacteremia. J Clin Microbiol 1989; 27:1431–1433.

46. Dorn GL, Smith K. New centrifugation blood culture device. J Clin Microbiol 1978; 7:52–54.

47. Henry NK, McLimans CA, Wright AJ, Thompson RL, Wilson WR, Washington JA II. Microbiological and clinical evaluation of the isolator lysis-centrifugation blood culture tube. J Clin Microbiol 1983; 17:864–869.

48. Whimbey E, Wong B, Kiehn TE, Armstrong D. Clinical correlations of serial quantitative blood cultures determined by lysis-centrifugation in patients with persistent septicemia. J Clin Microbiol 1984; 19:766–771.

49. Fan ST, Teoh-Chan CH, Lau KF, Chu KW, Kwan AKB, Wong KK. Predictive value of surveillance skin and hub cultures in central venous catheters sepsis. J Hosp Infect 1988; 12:191–198.

50. Cercenado E, Ena J, Rodríguez-Créixems M, Romero I, Bouza E. A conservative procedure for the diagnosis of catheter-related infections. Arch Intern Med 1990; 150:1417–1420.

51. Jakobsen C-JB, Hansen V, Jensen JJ, Grabe N. Contamination of subclavian vein catheters: an intraluminal culture method. J Hosp Infect 1989; 13:253–260.

52. Guidet B, Nicola I, Barakett V, et al. Skin versus hub cultures to predict colonization

and infection of central venous catheter in intensive care patients. Infection 1994; 22:43–48.

53. Raad II, Baba M, Bodey GP. Diagnosis of catheter-related infections: the role of surveillance and targeted quantitative skin cultures. Clin Infect Dis 1995; 20:593–597.

54. Sitges-Serra A, Linares J, Garau J. Catheter sepsis: the clue is the hub. Surgery 1985; 97:355–357.

55. Rushforth JA, Hoy CM, Kite P, Puntis JWL. Rapid diagnosis of central venous catheter sepsis. Lancet 1993; 342:402–403.

56. Ishak MA, Gröschel DHM, Mandell GL, Wenzel RP. Association of slime with pathogenicity of coagulase-negative staphylococci causing nosocomial septicemia. J Clin Microbiol 1985; 22:1025–1029.

57. Christensen GD, Simpson WA, Bisno AL, Beachey EH. Adherence of slime-producing strains of *Staphylococcus epidermidis* to smooth surfaces. Infect Immun 1982; 37:318–326.

58. Davenport DS, Massanari RM, Pfaller MA, Bale MJ, Streed SA, Hierholzer WJ. Usefulness of a test for slime production as a marker for clinically significant infections with coagulase-negative staphylococci. J Infect Dis 1986; 153:332–339.

59. Younger JJ, Christensen GD, Bartley DL, Simmons JCH, Barrett FF. Coagulase-negative staphylococci isolated from cerebrospinal fluid shunts: importance of slime production, species identification, and shunt removal to clinical outcome. J Infect Dis 1987; 156:548–554.

60. Kotilainen P. Association of coagulase-negative staphylococcal slime production and adherence with the development and outcome of adult septicemias. J Clin Microbiol 1990; 28:2779–2785.

61. Kristinsson KG, Spencer RC, Brown CB. Clinical importance of production of slime by coagulase negative staphylococci in chronic ambulatory peritoneal dialysis. J Clin Pathol 1986; 39:117–118.

62. Ludlam HA, Noble WC, Marples RR, Bayston R, Phillips I. The epidemiology of peritonitis caused by coagulase-negative staphylococci in continuous ambulatory peritoneal dialysis. J Med Microbiol 1989; 30:164–174.

63. Parisi JT. Coagulase-negative staphylococci and the epidemiological typing of *Staphylococcus epidermidis*. Microbiol Rev 1985; 49:126–139.

64. Schumacher-Perdreau F, Jansen B, Peters G, Pulverer G. Typing of coagulase-negative staphylococci isolated from foreign body infections. Eur J Clin Microbiol Infect Dis 1989; 7:270–273.

65. Thomson-Carter FM, Pennington TH. Characterization of coagulase-negative staphylococci by sodium dodecyl sulfate-polyacrylamide gel electrophoresis and immunoblot analyses. J Clin Microbiol 1989; 27:2199–2203.

66. Burnie JP, Lee W. A comparison of DNA and immunoblot fingerprinting of the SII biotype of coagulase negative staphylococci. Epidemiol Infect 1989; 101:203–212.

67. Pennington TH, Harker C, Thomson-Carter F. Identification of coagulase-negative staphylococci by using sodium dodecyl sulfate-polyacrylamide gel electrophoresis and rRNA restriction patterns. J Clin Microbiol 1991; 29:390–392.

68. Walcher-Salesse S, Monzon-Moreno C, Aubert S, Névine ES. An epidemiological

assessment of coagulase-negative staphylococci from an intensive care unit. J Med Microbiol 1992; 36:321–331.

69. Proctor RA, van Langevelde P, Kristjansson M, Maslow JN, Arbeit RD. Persistent and relapsing infections associated with small-colony variants of *Staphylococcus aureus*. Clin Infect Dis 1995; 20:95–102.

70. Widmer AF, Nettleman N, Flint K, Wenzel RP. The clinical impact of culturing central venous catheters. Arch Intern Med 1992; 152:1299–1302.

3

Catheter-Related *Staphylococcus aureus* Infection

Barry M. Farr

University of Virginia, Charlottesville, Virginia

I. INTRODUCTION

Staphylococcus aureus is a virulent pathogen that continues to cause significant morbidity and mortality in the antimicrobial era (1). Infection of a vascular catheter due to this organism may cause dramatic illness with bloodstream infection and hematogenous spread to other sites resulting in serious secondary infections such as osteomyelitis, epidural abscess, and endocarditis. Patients with relatively minor predisposing illness occasionally succumb to such lethal infection.

II. PATHOGENESIS

Most vascular catheter-related infections of short-term catheters appear to derive from cutaneous flora entering the catheter tract and moving distally along the exterior of the catheter to reach the bloodstream (2–5). Experiments in a guinea pig model suggested that such migration can occur rapidly perhaps by capillary action once microbes are present at the catheter skin interface in sufficient numbers (6). For long-term catheters, intraluminal spread from a contaminated hub appears to be a more important mode of infection (5,7,8). Electron microscopy of an *S. aureus*-infected catheter shows 1 μm diameter cocci clumped in an extensive amorphous matrix on the surface of the catheter (9).

Catheter composition appears to be an important factor in the pathogenesis of infection since modern Teflon and polyurethane catheters are associated with extremely low rates of catheter infection, as compared with polyvinyl chloride catheters used previously (10–13). Studies of adherence of different microbial species to various catheter materials have shown significantly greater adherence to polyvinyl chloride catheters than to Teflon catheters (14). An animal model of *S. aureus* catheter infections found that silicone catheters could be infected with a lower inoculum than polyurethane, Teflon, or polyvinyl chloride catheters during the first 2 days after insertion (15).

The efficiency of phagocytes operating in the vicinity of different catheter materials may also be important, as one study has shown impairment of the respiratory burst of polymorphonuclear neutrophils in the presence of polyvinyl chloride, Teflon, and siliconized latex catheters or their eluates; such impairment was not demonstrated with polyurethane catheters (16). A chemotactic defect has been demonstrated in patients receiving interleukin-2 (IL-2), who appear to have a higher risk for *S. aureus* infection of catheters (17). Impaired bactercidal activity of polymorphonuclear neutrophils has also been documented in patients with AIDS (18), who also have a higher rate of *S. aureus* catheter infections.

Fibronectin appears to be more active than fibrin or fibrinogen in promoting adherence of *S. aureus* to catheter surfaces (19). Polyurethane catheters removed from patients showed significantly less adherence for *S. aureus* ($P < 0.01$) and contained significantly less fibronectin than polyvinyl chloride or Hickman catheters (19). Another study found that polyvinyl chloride catheters bound significantly more fibronectin than heparin-bonded polyurethane catheters, but also found that *S. aureus* bound significantly more to heparin-bonded polyurethane than to the polyvinyl chloride catheters if fibronectin was not present in vitro (20). Thrombospondin, a glycoprotein stored in platelets, also appears to promote adherence of *S. aureus* to catheter surfaces (21,22).

S. aureus and *Candida albicans* appear to be more likely to cause infection of a catheter once colonization has occurred, as compared with other colonizing microbes. For catheters growing at least 100 CFU on quantitative culture of the catheter tip, *S. aureus* resulted in bloodstream infection in 69% of cases as compared with 75% for *C. albicans*, 38% for *Staphylococcus epidermidis*, and 41% for *Enterobacter faecalis* (23). *S. aureus* was also more likely to result in purulence at the catheter site than other microbes (40% of cases of *S. aureus* colonization vs. 10% of cases of colonization with other microbes, $P = 0.007$) (23). *S. aureus* produces a variety of enzymes and toxins which may contribute to this enhanced virulence such as catalase, hyaluronidase, nuclease, β-lactamase, toxic shock syndrome toxin, enterotoxin, staphylococcal superantigens, α-toxin, β-toxin, γ-toxin, δ-toxin and leukocidin (24). When introduced into subcutaneous tissue in the presence of a foreign body such as a silk suture, the mean infectious dose is tremendously reduced (25).

III. INCIDENCE

The incidence of primary bloodstream infection in hospitals reporting data to the Centers for Disease Control and Prevention's National Nosocomial Infection Surveillance (NNIS) program from 1980 to 1989 was 0.28 per 100 discharges (26). The same rate was documented in a 1-year prospective study in a Danish university hospital (27). The incidence of primary bloodstream infection due to *S. aureus* in NNIS hospitals increased significantly during the 1980s (26). The rate also increased significantly in each of the four types of reporting hospitals: Large teaching hospitals reported a 176% increase (95% confidence interval, 72% to 343%), from 4/10,000 discharges in 1980 to 1.13/1000 discharges in 1989. Small teaching hospitals reported a 122% increase (95% CI, 58% to 211%) during the same period. Small nonteaching reported a 283% increase (95% CI, 139% to 514%), and large nonteaching hospitals reported a 272% increase (95% CI, 115% to 544%).

Fifteen percent to 20% of endemic nosocomial bloodstream infections are due to *S. aureus,* which accounts for 8% of epidemics of nosocomial bloodstream infection (28). Approximately one-third of endemic nosocomial bloodstream infections appeared to be related to indwelling catheters in one study, with vascular catheters accounting for a large majority of these infections (29). One-third to one-half of *S. aureus* nosocomial bacteremias have been due to vascular catheters in other studies (30,31).

IV. MORTALITY

The virulence of *S. aureus* has been recognized in many studies of catheter-related infections (4,32–40). A review of 25 studies of catheter-related *S. aureus* bacteremia found that 24% of patients suffered an infectious complication (95% CI, 19.9% to 28.1%) (41). Overall 59 of 177 patients in these 25 studies died (33.3%, 95% CI, 26.4% to 40.2%) (41). Almost half of the deaths in these studies were attributed to the catheter infection by the authors of the individual studies (14.8%, 95% CI, 10.8% to 18.8%) (41).

A meta-analysis of the case fatality rate associated with catheter related infections, which included 187 studies and 3569 catheter infections, found an overall case fatality rate of 14.0% (95% CI, 12.4% to 15.6%) (42). The authors of the individual studies attributed death to the catheter infection in 2.7% (95% CI, 2.0% to 3.4%) of cases, accounting for approximately 19% of all of the deaths in these studies. For cases of *S. aureus* catheter infection included in this meta-analysis, the overall case fatality rate was 18.2%; death was attributed to the catheter infection in 11.1% of cases, accounting for 61% of the deaths. The proportion of deaths attributed to catheter infection was significantly higher for *S. aureus* than for other etiologic agents (odds ratio = 3.81, 95% CI, 2.70 to 5.41). A prospective epidemiologic study in a Danish hospital demonstrated a case fatality rate of 38% for nosocomial bacteremia overall, but the case fatality rate for *S. aureus* was 65%, with 25% being attributed to the infection (27).

V. RISK FACTORS

The risk of bloodstream infection in patients with a vascular catheter is related to the type of catheter, with modern peripheral venous catheters being associated with extremely low rates of infection and central venous catheters accounting for up to 90% of such infections (43). An increased risk for *S. aureus* infection of central venous catheters has been described for several patient groups. Patients with end-stage renal disease requiring hemodialysis or peritoneal dialysis have long been recognized as being at higher risk of *S. aureus* catheter infections; almost all of the higher risk occurs in patients who are nasal carriers of *S. aureus* (44). In one study of patients undergoing chronic ambulatory peritoneal dialysis (CAPD), patients with diabetes mellitus were significantly more likely to be carriers of *S. aureus* (77% vs. 36%) (45); catheter exit site infections were four times more frequent among carriers than noncarriers (0.4 episodes per patient-year vs. 0.1 per patient-year, $P = 0.012$). A separate study of CAPD patients found only a modest increase in infections among diabetic patients (1.4 per patient-year vs. 1.2 per patient-year) and concluded that diabetes was not an important risk factor for catheter infection in these patients. A third study of patients undergoing CAPD followed 30 patients for 13 months, with periodic cultures for *S. aureus* carriage (44). *S. aureus* accounted for 8 of 25 episodes of peritonitis and 12 of 20 episodes of exit site infection during the study, and patients with nasal colonization were at higher risk of infection than noncarriers (44).

In a study of patients undergoing hemodialysis, nasal carriage of *S. aureus* was associated with a higher rate of bacteremia (0.095 per patient-year vs. 0.0417 per patient-year), but the presence of diabetes was an even more important risk factor (relative risk = 11.4, $P = 0.004$). The presence of a central venous catheter was a significant predictor of bacteremia (RR = 14.3, $P = 0.002$) (46).

Therapy with IL-2 has been shown to increase the risk of staphylococcal catheter-related bacteremia (47); a dose gradient was demonstrated for increasing exposure to IL-2, with no bacteremias being documented during 320 catheter days before therapy, 18% of patients becoming infected during 343 catheter days of low-dose therapy, and 38% of patients becoming infected during 96 catheter days of high-dose therapy ($P = 0.01$). Another study found that 19% of IL-2-treated patients developed sepsis as compared with 2.8% of patients receiving total parenteral nutrition, 4.1% of patients in the surgical intensive care unit, and 1.9% of patients with solid tumors. *S. aureus* was the etiologic agent in 13 of 20 episodes of sepsis. *S. aureus* colonization significantly increased the risk of *S. aureus* (RR = 6.3, 95% CI, 2.8% to 14.5%, *P* < 0.001). Skin desquamation at the catheter site also significantly increased the risk (RR = 2.0, 95% CI, 1.3% to 3.1%). The simultaneous occurrence of *S. aureus* colonization and desquamation at the catheter site was associated with a relative risk of 14.5 for *S. aureus* bacteremia (95% CI, 4.1% to 50.9%) (48). A third study found sepsis in 9% of patients receiving IL-2 without antibiotic prophylaxis; in that study *S. aureus* accounted for seven of eight episodes of sepsis (49).

Human immunodeficiency virus infection appears to be another risk factor for *S. aureus* infection. In one study excluding patients with a history of intravenous drug abuse or lymphedema, the incidence of *S. aureus* bacteremia in a population of patients with AIDS or AIDS-related complex was 5.4/1000 patient-years. Seventy-three percent of cases were catheter-related (50). In another study *S. aureus* accounted for 24% of catheter-related infections in AIDS patients as compared with 16% in other immunocompromised patients (51).

VI.   CLINICAL MANIFESTATIONS

Central venous catheter-related bloodstream infection is most often manifested by fever alone, with up to 70% of cases showing no local inflammation at the catheter site (52). A study of catheter-related *S. aureus* bloodstream infection found fever in all of 21 cases with a mean temperature of 39.6°C (range, 37.8° to 41.1°) (32). The clinical onset was described as "dramatic," with sudden high temperature and often rigors. Those with bacteremia due to a peripheral catheter usually had cellulitis at the catheter site, often with a purulent exudate. Eighty-one percent of patients had leukocytosis ranging as high as 31,000/mm^3. Two chronically leukopenic patients showed an increase above their baseline count associated with a left shift (i.e., an increasing percentage of immature polymorphonuclear neutrophils). The mean number of positive blood cultures per patient was 3.7 (range, 1 to 7). Although rare with modern peripheral venous catheters, a recent case report described a patient with *S. aureus* infection of a peripheral venous catheter which progressed to suppurative phlebitis complicated by lethal endocarditis (53). By contrast, most patients with inflammation at the site of a peripheral venous catheter appear to have only a bland physicochemical phlebitis that is unrelated to infection (54) and that does not occur more frequently in *S. aureus* carriers (55).

Infectious complications occur in approximately one-quarter of cases of catheter-related *S. aureus* bacteremia (41). Perhaps the most important complication to consider is endocarditis because of the frequent lack of specific signs

(56–58) and because short-course therapy for bacteremia with up to 2 weeks of antibiotics will often fail if endocarditis is present. A recent review of studies of short-course therapy of catheter-related *S. aureus* bacteremia found that 6.1% relapsed after therapy, usually with endocarditis or a metastatic infection such as epidural abscess (41). Most such relapses have occurred within 9 weeks (59). A more recent study reported that two of 21 patients receiving short-course therapy relapsed; both of the relapses were noted to occur among three patients receiving less than 10 days of therapy (60). Adding this experience to the pooled experience with short-course therapy from 11 previous studies would yield 10 relapses among 153 patients (6.5%) (41). If the three patients receiving less than 10 days of therapy are excluded, the pooled rate would be eight relapses among 150 patients (5.3%).

The classical manifestations of endocarditis such as new or changing murmur, splenomegaly, and embolic lesions are each present in only a minority of cases (61). Nolan and Beatty therefore attempted to develop criteria for differentiating patients with *S. aureus* bacteremia from those with endocarditis (59). Community acquisition, lack of an obvious primary site of infection, and presence of metastatic sequelae (e.g., intrabdominal, renal or cerebral abscess) were each associated with a high risk for endocarditis in their study. By contrast only two of the 26 cases of *S. aureus* endocarditis that they studied had an obvious primary site of infection, which was acquired in the hospital and had no metastatic sequelae (59). The lower risk of endocarditis among nosocomial cases has been confirmed in several more recent studies (33,62,63).

New criteria for diagnosing infective endocarditis using echocardiography were recently published (63a). According to this scheme a definite diagnosis can be made by either pathologic or clinical criteria. The pathologic diagnosis requires culture of an organism from a vegetation or histologic confirmation of a vegetation or intracardiac abscess. The clinical criteria include major and minor criteria, and a definite diagnosis would require the presence of two major criteria, one major and three minor criteria, or five minor criteria. The major criteria include blood culture results suggestive of endocarditis, either because of the species involved or the continuousness of the positive cultures, and evidence of endocardial involvement by echocardiography such as (1) intracardiac mass on valve or supporting structure, (2) abscess, or (3) new partial dehiscence of prosthetic valve or new valvular regurgitation. Minor criteria include a predisposing heart condition, fever (>38°C), valvular phenomena (e.g., emboli or mycotic aneurysms), immunologic phenomena (e.g., Osler's nodes or Roth spots), microbiologic evidence (e.g., blood cultures showing pathogen not meeting major criteria or serologic test consistent with endocarditis), and echocardiographic evidence suggestive of endocarditis but not meeting major criteria.

Other manifestations of catheter-related *S. aureus* infections have included such diverse presentations as sternoclavicular arthritis and clavicular osteomyelitis after *S. aureus* infection of a subclavian catheter (64); mycotic aneurysms and osteomyelitis after umbilical artery catheterization in a neonate (65); endarteritis with pseudoaneurysm, septic arthritis, osteomyelitis, and distal emboli after femoral artery catheterization (60,66); and an infected atrial thrombus following placement of a right atrial catheter (67). Most reported cases of infected pseudoaneurysm have involved *S. aureus* infection (68–72). A self-limited, sterile reactive arthritis has been reported as a rare complication following catheter-related *S. aureus* bacteremia in HLA-B27-negative patients (73).

Persistent high-grade bacteremia despite antibiotic therapy and removal of the catheter suggests the presence of septic phlebitis (74). Septic phlebitis related to a peripheral catheter may be associated with local inflammation and induration overlying the vein, but this is not present in all cases. With central venous catheters, septic phlebitis is usually not associated with local signs of inflammation or with clinical signs of venous obstruction, which are present in only a minority of radiographically documented cases. Deep venous thrombosis in such cases may be documented by venography, sonography, or CT scan.

VII. THERAPY

Catheter-related bloodstream infection has generally been treated with 1 to 2 weeks therapy for most etiologic agents. For *S. aureus,* however, there has been concern about the risk of complicating endocarditis, and until recently many have routinely treated for at least 4 weeks (75–77). During the past two decades several studies have suggested that the risk of complicating endocarditis is sufficiently low (<10% of cases) that short-course therapy (10 to 14 days) is safe for patients with apparently uncomplicated catheter-related bacteremia (33,35,59, 60,78–80). A meta-analysis of 11 studies of short-course therapy found a relapse rate of 6.1% (95% CI, 2.0% to 10.2%). Two studies have found that most relapses after short-course therapy occurred when therapy lasted less than 10 days (35,60).

Delayed removal of the catheter was associated with persistence of *S. aureus* bacteremia in a recent study (60). A retrospective study of *S. aureus* infections of Hickman catheters reported that failure to remove the catheter was associated with a worse outcome (34). Of 37 evaluable episodes of *S. aureus* bacteremia, 22 were cured with catheter removal plus antibiotics, while for the 15 patients whose catheters were not removed, eight were cured with antibiotics and seven failed antibiotic therapy (four relapses and three deaths due to progressive catheter-related sepsis (34).

Fever or bacteremia persisting more than 3 days after catheter removal were associated with an increased risk of endocarditis in one study, suggesting the need for a longer course of therapy in such patients (35). Placement of a central catheter tip into the right atrium or into the pulmonary artery has also been related to an increased risk for development of endocarditis, presumably due to trauma to endocardial surfaces by the catheter followed by seeding of these roughened surfaces during subsequent bacteremia (81).

AIDS and AIDS-related complex have also been found to be adverse prognostic factors in catheter-related *S. aureus* bacteremia, as six (35%) of 17 patients relapsed with late metastatic complications after a mean of 18 days of antibiotic therapy (50). Some authors have recommended that patients with HIV infection who develop catheter-related *S. aureus* bloodstream infection should routinely receive a longer course of therapy, such as 3 to 4 weeks (82).

The drug of choice for *S. aureus* bacteremia has been a beta lactam to which the isolate is susceptible. For the rare penicillin-susceptible isolates, high-dose penicillin would be the drug of choice (e.g., 20 million units IV per day for an adult with normal renal function). For the majority of isolates that are penicillin-resistant, a penicillinase-resistant penicillin would be the choice (e.g., nafcillin 1.5 g IV every 4 hours for an adult). In cases of penicillin allergy a first-generation cephalosporin has frequently been used with success (e.g., cefazolin 100 mg/kg/day intravenously in three divided doses). For those unable to tolerate a beta lactam and those with methicillin-resistant *S. aureus*, vancomycin is the drug of choice (30 mg/kg/day intravenously in two divided doses). Vancomycin should not be used as a drug of convenience because of its long half-life and consequent infrequent dosing for treating beta lactam-susceptible *S. aureus* infection in non-allergic patients. Such systematic overuse of vancomycin would add further pressure for selection of vancomycin resistance among organisms such as *Enterococcus faecium*, which has caused multiple nosocomial epidemics during the past decade (83). An additional concern with such overreliance on vancomycin for treatment of *S. aureus* bacteremia derives from several studies reporting higher failure rates and slower clearance of bacteremia in patients with *S. aureus* endocarditis treated with vancomycin (84–88).

Antibiotic lock therapy provides a new approach to treatment without removing the catheter, by infusing antibiotics through the catheter and then locking a high concentration into the catheter over a 12-hour period each night (89–97). Such therapy has been successful in curing the infection and salvaging the infected catheter in 97% of patients requiring long-term vascular access with infections due to a variety of pathogens (90,91), but the success rate was only 43% when this method was applied to infected subcutaneous ports (89). Vancomycin has been shown to be stable in both total parenteral nutrition solutions and heparin solutions at room temperature for a 24-hour period allowing for concurrent therapy during TPN infusion and/or for antibiotic lock with heparin overnight if indicated (98).

Therapy of superficial catheter-related septic phlebitis has generally consisted of ligation and venectomy coupled with antimicrobial therapy for 2 to 3 weeks.

Incision and drainage with antibiotics, but without venectomy, has been reported to work in some cases. For central venous septic phlebitis, catheter removal and prolonged antibiotic therapy are necessary, coupled with anticoagulation (99).

VIII. PREVENTION

Prevention of catheter-related *S. aureus* infection depends on the principles used for prevention of catheter infections in general (100). Placement of catheters with maximal barriers (cap, mask, sterile long-sleeved gown and gloves, and large drapes) was associated with a significantly lower rate of infection than when only a mask, sterile gloves, and a small drape were used in a randomized trial (101). A cohort study found similar protection using the same barriers except that a cap was not used (102). The importance of technique during insertion was additionally confirmed in a study by Armstrong et al., which found a significant association between catheter colonization and inexperience of the clinician inserting the catheter (103).

Site selection also may have an important effect as subclavian vein placement has been associated with lower infection rates than internal jugular vein placement in some cohort studies (102,104). Peripherally inserted central catheters have been associated with very low rates of infection but have been used primarily in outpatients (105,106). Only limited data are available for their use in hospitalized patients (107,108). Lower infection rates with this approach may relate to lower concentrations of resident bacteria on the arm than the neck or chest (109,110).

Tunneling of catheters has been done partly to reduce the risk of catheter infection, but three recent studies have raised questions as to the effectiveness of tunneling for preventing infection (111–113). By contrast, subcutaneous ports appear to be associated with significantly lower infection rates (114).

Dressing the catheter with povidone iodine ointment resulted in significant prevention of *S. aureus* bacteremia in a randomized trial involving subclavian dialysis catheters (115). An older study, however, found no benefit with povidone iodine ointment, and further studies are needed (116). By contrast, use of polymyxin-neomycin-bacitracin ointment should be avoided on central venous catheters because of a fivefold increase in *Candida* colonization with this product (117). Mupirocin ointment applied to central venous catheter sites resulted in a reduction in the frequency of significant colonization of catheter tips from 25% in controls receiving no antimicrobial ointment to 5% among those receiving mupirocin (118). Although no *Candida* were cultured from catheters in that study, it should be noted that mupirocin, like PNB ointment, lacks antifungal activity, and further studies are needed to confirm that a similar problem with *Candida* colonization will not occur (119).

Transparent dressings have been associated with a higher risk of infection in a randomized trial (120) and a higher risk of significant colonization in a meta-analysis (121), but a more recent trial found no difference (122). Further studies of transparent dressings are needed before they are routinely recommended, especially given their higher cost.

Antimicrobial catheters and catheter cuffs have been shown to exert significant protection against catheter-related bloodstream infection (117,123–126). While antibiotic coating has been shown to work (127–129), concern has been expressed regarding the use of clinically current antibiotics for this purpose because of the potential for selecting antibiotic-resistant flora (126). Use of an antiseptic-impregnated catheter may obviate this concern because of the common use of antiseptics in large numbers of patients without selection of resistance to clinically useful antibiotics.

Scheduled replacement of central venous catheters has proven ineffective in preventing catheter infection in multiple randomized trials and should no longer be recommended (49,130–133). Scheduled replacement appears to significantly increase the risk of major mechanical complications if new site puncture is used and, paradoxically, to increase the rate of bloodstream infection if guide wire exchange is employed (133).

Multiple studies have suggested a benefit for the use of a special IV team for caring for total parenteral nutrition catheters as compared with care by the regular ward team (134–137). Another study showed benefit from the use of an IV team for care of peripheral IVs (37). In that study the IV team cared for 90% of peripheral venous catheters that were followed during the study, but these catheters were associated with only 11% of the related bloodstream infections. The remaining catheters were the responsibility of resident physicians.

Specific prevention of *S. aureus* infection was demonstrated in a randomized trial of intravenous oxacillin prophylaxis in patients undergoing interleukin-2 therapy; by contrast, changing the catheter every 3 days was not effective in lowering the rate of infection in this trial (49). Prevention of *S. aureus* bacteremia has also been demonstrated among hemodialysis patients by weekly application of nasal creams containing mupirocin (138). Similar therapy using chlorhexidine and neomycin nasal cream has significantly reduced the risk of *S. aureus* peritonitis among CAPD patients colonized with *S. aureus* (139–141). In one study this strategy led to a reduction in the number of CAPD catheters that had to be removed during a year because of infection from 28% to 13% ($P < 0.001$) (139).

Recent in vitro studies have suggested novel mechanisms for preventing catheter infection. One study showed that copper- or silver-copper-coated catheters decrease adherence of *S. aureus* to Teflon, polyvinyl chloride, and silicon rubber catheters (142). Similarly, a negatively charged direct electric current of 10 µA reduced *S. aureus* adherence to catheters while a positively charged current had no effect (143). The use a 20-µA current flowing through a silver wire wrapped helically around the proximal segment of catheters has resulted in lower rates of adherence of *S. aureus, S. epidermidis,* and *C. albicans* in vitro and lower rates of colonization in an animal model, when compared with regular catheters and chlorhexidine-silver sulfadiazine-impregnated catheters (144). A minocycline-EDTA flush solution has been shown to have broad antimicrobial activity in vitro (145) and was successfully used to prevent catheter infection in three patients who required prolonged catheterization and had had repeated bouts of catheter sepsis before use of the flush solution (145).

REFERENCES

1. Sheagren JN. *Staphylococcus aureus:* the persistent pathogen. N Engl J Med 1984; 310:1368–1373.
2. Maki DG, Stolz S. The epidemiology of central-venous catheter-related bloodstream infection (BSI). In: Programs and Abstracts of the 34th Interscience Conference of Antimicrobial Agents and Chemotherapy. Orlando, 1994. Abstract 547.
3. Bjornson HS, Colley R, Bower RH, Duty VP, Schwartz-Fulton JT, Fisher JE. Association between microorganism growth at the catheter insertion site and colonization of the catheter in patients receiving total parenteral nutrition. Surgery 1982; 92:720–727.
4. Cheesbrough JS, Finch RG, Burden RP. A prospective study of the mechanisms of infection associated with hemodialysis catheters. J Infect Dis 1986; 154:579–589.
5. Linares J, Sitges-Serra A, Garau J, Perez JL, Martin R. Pathogenesis of catheter sepsis: a prospective study with quantitative and semiquantitative cultures of catheter hub and segments. J Clin Microbiol 1985; 21:357–360.
6. Cooper GL, Schiller AL, Hopkins CC. Possible role of capillary action in pathogenesis of experimental catheter-associated dermal tunnel infections. J Clin Microbiol 1988; 26:8–12.
7. Moro ML, Vigano EF, Lepri AC, et al. Risk factors for central venous catheter-related infections in surgical and intensive care units. Infect Control Hosp Epidemiol 1994; 15:253–264.
8. Raad I, Costerton W, Sabharwal U, Sacilowski M, Anaissie E, Bodey G. Ultrastructural analysis of indwelling vascular catheters: a quantitative relationship between luminal colonization and duration of placement. J Infect Dis 1993; 168:400–407.
9. Marrie TJ, Costerton JW. Scanning and transmission electron microscopy of in situ bacterial colonization of intravenous and intraarterial catheters. J Clin Microbiol 1984; 19:687–693.
10. Tully JL, Griedland GH, Baldini LM, Goldmann DA. Complications of intravenous therapy with steel needles and Teflon catheters a comparative study. Am J Med 1981; 70:702–706.
11. Tager IB, Ginsberg MB, Ellis SE, et al. An epidemiologic study of the risks associated with peripheral intravenous catheters. Am J Epidemiol 1983; 118:839–851.
12. Maki DG, Ringer M. Evaluation of dressing regimens for prevention of infection

with peripheral intravenous catheters gauze, a transparent polyurethane dressing, and an iodophor-transparent dressing. JAMA 1987; 258:2396–2403.

13. Garland JS, Nelson DB, Cheah T, Hennes HH, Johnson TM. Infectious complications during peripheral intravenous therapy with Teflon catheters: a prospective study. Pediatr Infect Dis J 1987; 6:918–921.

14. Sheth NK, Rose HD, Franson TR, Buckmire FL, Sohnle PG. In vitro quantitative adherence of bacteria to intravascular catheters. J Surg Res 1983; 34:213–218.

15. Sherertz RJ, Carruth WA, Marosok RD, Espeland MA, Johnson RA, Solomon DD. Contribution of vascular catheter material to the pathogenesis of infection: the enhanced risk of silicone in vivo. J Biomed Mater Res 1995; 29:635–645.

16. Lopez-Lopez G, Pascual A, Perea EJ. Effect of plastic catheters on the phagocytic activity of human polymorphonuclear leukocytes. Eur J Clin Microbiol Infect Dis 1990; 9:324–328.

17. Klempner MS, Noring R, Mier JW, Atkins MB. Acquired chemotactic defect in neutrophils from patients receiving interleukin-2 immunotherapy. N Engl J Med 1990; 322:959–965.

18. Murphy PM, Lane HC, Fauci AS, Gallin JI. Impairment of neutrophil bactericidal capacity in patients with AIDS. J Infect Dis 1988; 158:627–630.

19. Vaudaux P, Pittet D, Haeberli A, et al. Fibronectin is more active than fibrin or fibrinogen in promoting *Staphylococcus aureus* adherence to inserted intravascular catheters. J Infect Dis 1993; 167:633–641.

20. Russell PB, Kline J, Yoder MC, Polin RA. Staphylococcal adherence to polyvinyl chloride and heparin-bonded polyurethane catheters in species dependent on and enhanced by fibronectin. J Clin Microbiol 1987; 25:1083–1087.

21. Herrmann M, Lai QJ, Albrecht RM, Mosher DF, Proctor RA. Adhesion of *Staphylococcus aureus* to surface-bound platelets: role of fibrinogen/fibrin and platelet integrins. J Infect Dis 1993; 167:312–322.

22. Herrmann M, Suchard SJ, Boxer LA, Waldvogel FA, Lew PD. Thrombospondin binds to *Staphylococcus aureus* and promotes staphylococcal adherence to surfaces. Infect Immun 1991; 59:279–288.

23. Sherertz RJ, Raad II, Belani A, et al. Three year experience with sonicated vascular catheter cultures in a clinical microbiology laboratory. J Clin Microbiol 1990; 28:76–82.

24. Waldvogel FA: *Staphylococcus aureus* (including toxic shock syndrome). In: Mandell GL, Bennett JE, Dolin R, eds. Principles and Practice of Infectious Diseases. New York: Churchill Livingstone, 1995:1754–1777.

25. Elek SD, Conen PE. The virulence of *Staphylococcus pyogenes* for man: a study of the problems of wound infection. Br J Exp Pathol 1961; 42:266–277.

26. Bannerjee SN, Emori TG, Culver DH, et al. Secular trends in nosocomial primary bloodstream infections in the United States, 1980–1989. Am J Med 1991; 91(suppl 3B):87S–89S.

27. Eliasen K, Nielsen PB, Espersen F. A one-year survey of nosocomial bacteraemia at a Danish university hospital. J Hyg Camb 1986; 97:471–478.

28. Maki DG. Nosocomial bacteremia: a epidemiologic overview. Am J Med 1981; 70:719–732.

29. McGowan JE, Parrott PL, Duty VP. Nosocomial bacteremia. Potential for prevention of procedure-related cases. JAMA 1977; 237:2727–2729.

30. Libman H, Arbeit RD. Complications associated with *Staphylococcus aureus* bacteremia. Arch Intern Med 1984; 144:541–545.

31. Mylotte JM, McDermott C. *Staphylococcus aureus* bacteremia caused by infected intravenous catheters. Am J Infect Control 1987; 15:1–6.

32. Watanakunakorn C, Baird IM. *Staphylococcus aureus* bacteremia and endocarditis associated with a removable infected intravenous device. Am J Med 1977; 63:523–256.

33. Mylotte JM, McDermott C, Spooner JA. Prospective study of 114 consecutive episodes of *Staphylococcus aureus* bacteremia. Rev Infect Dis 1987; 9:891–907.

34. Dugdale DC, Ramsey PG. *Staphylococcus aureus* bacteremia in patients with Hickman catheters. Am J Med 1990; 89:137–141.

35. Raad I, Sabbagh MF. Optimal duration of therapy for catheter-related *Staphylococcus aureus* bacteremia: a study of 55 cases and review. Clin Infect Dis 1992; 14:75–82.

36. Rahal JJ, Chan YK, Johnson G. Relationship of staphylococcal tolerance, teichoic acid antibody, and serum bactericidal activity to therapeutic outcome in *Staphylococcus aureus* bacteremia. Am J Med 1986; 81:43–52.

37. Bentley DW, Lepper MH. Septicemia related to the indwelling venous catheter. JAMA 1968; 206:1749–1752.

38. Ryan JAJ, Abel RM, Abbott WM, et al. Catheter complications in total parenteral nutrition: a prospective study of 200 consecutive patients. N Engl J Med 1974; 290:757–761.

39. Bryan CS, Kirkhart B, Brenner ER. Staphylococcal bacteremia: current patterns in nonuniversity hospitals. South Med J 1984; 77:693–696.

40. Collignon PJ, Munro R, Sorrell TC. Systemic sepsis and intravenous devices. A prospective survey. Med J Aust 1984; 141:345–348.

41. Jernigan JA, Farr BM. Short-course therapy of catheter-related *Staphylococcus aureus* bacteremia: a meta-analysis. Ann Intern Med 1993; 119:304–311.

42. Byers KE, Adal KA, Anglim AM, Farr BM. Case fatality rate for catheter-related bloodstream infections (CRSBI): a meta-analysis. Infect Control Hosp Epidemiol 16:P23, 1995. Abstract 43.

43. Maki DG. Nosocomial bloodstream infections [abstract 3]. In: Third Decennial International Conference on Nosocomial Infections. Atlanta, GA, July 31–Aug 3, 1990.

44. Sewell CM, Clarridge J, Lacke C, Weinmna EJ, Young EJ. Staphylococcal nasal carriage and subsequent infection in peritoneal dialysis patients. JAMA 1982; 248:1493–1495.

45. Luzar MA, Coles GA, Faller B, et al. *Staphylococcus aureus* nasal carriage and infection in patients on continuous ambulatory peritoneal dialysis. N Engl J Med 1990; 322:505–509.

46. Roubicek C, Brunet P, Mallet MN, et al. Nasal carriage of *Staphylococcus aureus:* prevalence in a hemodialysis center and effect on bacteremia (French). Nephrologie 1995; 16:229–232.

47. Richards JM, Gilewski TA, Vogelzang NJ. Association of interleukin-2 therapy with staphylococcal bacteremia. Cancer 1991; 67:1570–1575.
48. Snydman DR, Sullivan B, Gill M, Gould JA, Parkinson DR, Atkins MB. Nosocomial sepsis associated with interleukin-2. Ann Intern Med 1990; 112:102–107.
49. Bock SN, Lee RE, Fisher B, et al. A prospective randomized trial evaluating prophylactic antibiotics to prevent triple-lumen catheter-related sepsis in patients treated with immunotherapy. J Clin Oncol 1990; 8:161–169.
50. Jacobson MA, Gellermann H, Chambers H. *Staphylococcus aureus* bacteremia and recurrent staphylococcal infection in patients with acquired immunodeficiency syndrome and AIDS-related complex. Am J Med 1988; 85:172–176.
51. Skoutelis AT, Murphy RL, MacDonell KB, VonRoenn JH, Sterkel CD, Phair JP. Indwelling central venous catheter infections in patients with acquired immune deficiency syndrome. J Acquired Immune Deficiency Syndromes 1990; 3:335–342.
52. Pittet D, Chuard C, Rae AC, et al. Clinical diagnosis of central venous catheter line infections: a difficult job. In: Programs and Abstracts of the 31st Interscience Conference of Antimicrobial Agents and Chemotherapy. Chicago, 1991. Abstract 453.
53. Widmer A, Zimmerli W. Fatal peripheral catheter phlebitis. (German). Schweizerische Medizinische Wochenschrift. Journal Suisse de Medecine 1988; 118:1053–1055.
54. Maki DG, Ringer M. Risk factors for infusion-related phlebitis with small peripheral venous catheters a randomized controlled trial. Ann Intern Med 1991; 114:845–854.
55. Lipsky BA, Peugeot RL, Boyko EJ, Kent DL. A prospective study of *Staphylococcus aureus* nasal colonization and intravenous therapy-related phlebitis. Arch Intern Med 1992; 152:2109–2112.
56. Hedstrom SA, Christensson B. *Staphylococcus aureus* septicaemia and endocarditis at the University Hospital in Lund 1976–1980. Scand J Infect Dis Suppl 1983; 41:38–48.
57. Watanakunakorn C, Tan JS. Diagnostic difficulties of staphylococcal endocarditis in geriatric patients. Geriatrics 1973; 28:168–173.
58. Watanakunakorn C, Tan JS, Phair JP. Some salient features of *Staphylococcus aureus* endocarditis. Am J Med 1973; 54:473–481.
59. Nolan CM, Beaty HN. *Staphylococcus aureus* bacteremia. Current clinical patterns. Am J Med 1976; 60:495–500.
60. Malanoski GJ, Samore MH, Pefanis A, et al. *Staphylococcus aureus* bacteremia: minimal effective therapy and unusual infectious complications associated with arterial sheath catheters. Arch Intern Med 1995; 155:1161–1166.
61. Scheld WM, Sande MA. Endocarditis and intravascular infections. In: Mandell GL, Bennett JE, Dolin R, eds. Principles and Practice of Infectious Diseases. 4th ed. New York: Churchill Livingstone, 1995:740–783.
62. Bayer AS, Lam K, Ginzton L, Norman DC, Chiu CY, Ward JI. *Staphylococcus aureus* bacteremia. Clinical serologic, and echocardiographic findings in patients with and without endocarditis. Arch Intern Med 1987; 147:457–462.
63. Cooper R, Platt R. *Staphylococcus aureus* bacteremia in diabetic patients. Am J Med 1982; 73:658–662.

63a. Durack DT, Lukes AS, Bright DK, Service DE. New criteria for diagnosis of infective endocarditis: Utilization of specific echocardiographic findings. Am J Med 1994; 96:200–209.

64. Moreno Guillen S, Eiros Bouza JM, Espinosa Parra EJ, Fernandez Guerrero ML, Rivera MT. Osteoarticular infections associated with catheterization of the subclavian vein (Spanish). Enfermedades Infecciosas y Microbiologia Clinica 1991; 9: 33–34.

65. Lim MO, Gresham EL, Franken EA, Leake RD. Osteomyelitis as a complication of umbilical artery catheterization. Am J Dis Child 1977; 131:142–144.

66. Frazee BW, Flaherty JP. Septic endarteritis of the femoral artery following angioplasty (Review). Rev Infect Dis 1991; 13:620–623.

67. Horner SM, Bell JA, Swanton RH. Infected right atrial thrombus—an important but rare complication of central venous lines. Eur Heart J 1993; 14:138–140.

68. Soderstrom CA, Wasserman DH, Ransom KJ, Caplan ES, Cowley RA. Infected false femoral artery aneurysms secondary to monitoring catheters. J Cardiovasc Surg 1983; 24:63–68.

69. Arnow PM, Costas CO. Delayed rupture of the radial artery caused by catheter-related sepsis. Rev Infect Dis 1988; 10:1035–1037.

70. Cohen A, Reyes R, Kirk M, Fulks RM. Osler's nodes, pseudoaneurysm formation and sepsis complicating percutaneous radial artery cannulation. Crit Care Med 1984; 12:1078–1079.

71. Falk PS, Scuderi PE, Sheretz RJ, Motsinger SM. Infected radial artery pseudoaneurysms occurring after percutaneous cannulation. Chest 1992; 101:490–495.

72. Fanning WL, Aronson M. Osler node, Janeway lesions and splinter hemmorrhages. Arch Dermatol 1977; 113:648–649.

73. Siam AR, Hammoudeh M. *Staphylococcus aureus* triggered reactive arthritis. Ann Rheumatic Dis 1995; 54:131–133.

74. Farr BM. Nonendocardial vascular infections. In: Hoeprich PD, Jordan MC, Ronald AR, eds. Infectious Diseases. 5th ed. Philadelphia: J.B. Lippincott, 1994:1248–1258.

75. Rabinovich S, Smith IM, January LE. The changing patterns of bacterial endocarditis. Med Clin North Am 1968; 52:1091–1101.

76. Lerner PI, Weinstein L. Infective endocarditis in the antibiotic era. N Engl J Med 1966; 274:388–393.

77. Hamburger M. Treatment of bacterial endocarditis. Mod Treat 1964; 1:1003–1015.

78. Iannini PB, Crossley K. Therapy of *Staphylococcus aureus* bacteremia associated with a removable focus of infection. Ann Intern Med 1976; 84:558–560.

79. Bayer AS, Tillman DB, Concepcion N, et al. Clinical value of teichoic acid antibody titers in the diagnosis and management of the staphylococcemias. West J Med 132:294–300, 1980.

80. Ehni WF, Reller LB. Short-course therapy for catheter-associated *Staphylococcus aureus* bacteremia. Arch Intern Med 149:533–536, 1989.

81. Sasaki TM, Panke TW, Dorethy JF, Lindberg RB, Pruitt BA. The relationship of central venous and pulmonary artery catheter position to acute right-sided endocarditis in severe thermal injury. J Trauma 19:740–743, 1979.

82. Mortara LA, Bayer AS. *Staphylococcus aureus* bacteremia and endocarditis. Infect Dis Clin North Am 7, 1993.
83. Anonymous. Recommendations for preventing the spread of vancomycin resistance. Hospital Infection Control Practices Advisory Committee (HICPAC) (Review). Infect Control Hosp Epidemiol 16:105–113, 1995.
84. Harstein AI, Mulligan ME, Morthland VH, et al. Recurrent *Staphylococcus aureus* bacteria. J Clin Microbiol 30:670, 1992.
85. Markowitz N, Quinn EL, Saravolatz LD. trimethoprim-sulfamethoxazole compared to vancomycin for the treatment of *Staphylococcus aureus* infection. Ann Intern Med 1992; 117:390.
86. Levine DP, Fromm BS, Reddy BR. Slow response to vancomycin or vancomycin plus rifampin therapy among patients with methicillin-resistant Staphylococcus aureus. Ann Intern Med 1991; 115:674.
87. Small PM, Chambers HF. Vancomycin for *Staphylococcus aureus* endocarditis in intravenous drug abusers. Antimicrob Agents Chemother 1990; 94:505.
88. Chambers HF, Miller T, Newman MD. Right-sided *Staphylococcus aureus* endocarditis in intravenous drug abusers—two week combination therapy. Ann Intern Med 1988; 109:619.
89. Longuet P, Douard MC, Maslo C, Benoit C, Arlet G, Leport C. Limited efficacy of antibiotic lock technique (ALT) in catheter related bacteremia of totally implanted ports (TIP) in HIV infected and oncologic patients. In: Programs and Abstracts of the 35th Interscience Conference of Antimicrobial Agents and Chemotherapy. San Francisco, 1995. Abstract J5.
90. Krzywda EA, Gotoff RA, Andris DA, Marciniak TF, Edmiston CE, Quebbeman EJ. Antibiotic lock treatment (ALT): impact on catheter salvage and cost savings. In: Programs and Abstracts of the 35th Interscience Conference of Antimicrobial Agents and Chemotherapy. San Francisco, 1995. Abstract J4.
91. Capdevila JA, Segarra A, Planes AM, Gasser I, Gavalda J, Pahissa A. Long term follow-up of patients with catheter related sepsis (CRS) treated without catheter removal. In: Programs and Abstracts of the 35th Interscience Conference of Antimicrobial Agents and Chemotherapy. San Francisco, 1995. Abstract J3.
92. Messing B, Peitra-Cohen S, Debure A, Beliah M, Bernier JJ. Antibiotic-lock technique: a new approach to optimal therapy for catheter-related sepsis in home-parenteral nutrition patients. JPEN 1988; 12:185–189.
93. Gaillard JL, Merlino R, Pajot N, et al. Conventional and nonconventional modes of vancomycin administration to decontaminate the internal surface of catheters colonized with coagulase-negative staphylococci. JPEN 1990; 14:593–597.
94. Arnow PM, Kushner R. *Malassezia furfur* catheter infection cured with antibiotic lock therapy (Letter). Am J Med 1982; 90:128–130.
95. Douard MC, Arlet G, Leverger G, et al. Quantitative blood cultures for diagnosis and management of catheter-related sepsis in pediatric hematology and oncology patients. Intens Care Med 1991; 17:30–35.
96. Elian JC, Frappaz D, Ros A, et al. Study of serum kinetics of vancomycin during the "antibiotic-lock" technique (French). Arch Fr Pediatr 1992; 49:357–360.
97. Cowan CE. Antibiotic lock technique. J Intravenous Nurs 1992; 15:283–287.

98. Yao JD, Arkin CF, Karchmer AW. Vancomycin stability in heparin and total parenteral nutrition solutions: novel approach to therapy of central venous catheter-related infections. JPEN 1992; 16:268–274.

99. Verghese A, Widrich WC, Arbeit RD. Central venous septic thrombophlebitis—the role of medical therapy. Medicine 1985; 64:394–400.

100. Farr BM. Understaffing: a risk factor for infection in the era of downsizing? Infect Control Hosp Epidemiol 1996; 17:147–149.

101. Raad II, Hohn DC, Gilbreath BJ, et al. Prevention of central venous catheter-related infections by using maximal sterile barrier precautions during insertion. Infect Control Hosp Epidemiol 1994; 15:231–238.

102. Mermel LA, McCormick RD, Springman SR, Maki DG. The pathogenesis and epidemiology of catheter-related infection with pulmonary artery Swan-Ganz catheters: a prospective study utilizing molecular subtyping. Am J Med 1991; 91(suppl 3B):3B-197S–3B-205S.

103. Armstrong CW, Mayhall CG, Miller KB, et al. Prospective study of catheter replacement and other risk factors of infection of hyperalimentation catheters. J Infect Dis 1986; 154:808–816.

104. Richet H, Hubert B, Nitemberg G, et al. Prospective multicenter study of vascular-catheter-related complications and risk factors for positive patients. J Clin Microbiol 1990; 28:2520–2525.

105. Raad I, Davis S, Becker M, et al. Low infection rate and long durability of nontunneled silastic catheters. Arch Intern Med 1993; 153:1791–1796.

106. Tice AD, Bonstell RP, Marsh PK, Craven PC, McEniry DW, Harding S. Peripherally inserted central venous catheters for outpatient intravenous antibiotic therapy. Infect Dis Clin Pract 1993; 2:186–190.

107. Linblad B, Wolff T. Infectious complications of percutaneously inserted central venous catheters. Acta Anaesthesiol Scand 1985; 29:587–589.

108. Bottino J, McCredie K, Groschel DHM, Lawson M. Long-term intravenous therapy with peripherally inserted silicone elastomer central venous catheters in patients with malignant diseases. Cancer 1979; 43:1937–1943.

109. Maki DG. Marked differences in skin colonization of insertion sites for central venous, arterial and peripheral IV catheters. The major reason for differing risks of catheter-related infection? In: Programs and Abstracts of the 30th Interscience Conference of Antimicrobial Agents and Chemotherapy. Atlanta, GA, 1990. Abstract 712.

110. Noble WC. Dispersal of skin microorganisms. Br J Dermatol 1975; 93:477–485.

111. Andrivet P, Bacquer A, Vu Ngoc C, et al. Lack of clinical benefit from subcutaneous tunnel insertion of central venous catheters in immunocompromised patients. Clin Infect Dis 1994; 18:199–206.

112. Guichard I, Nitemberg G, Abitbol JL, Andremont A, Leclercq B, Escudier B. Tunnelled versus non-tunnelled catheters for parenteral nutrition in an intensive care unit: a controlled prospective study of catheter-related sepsis. Clin Nutr 1986; 5(suppl I):169. Abstract 129.

113. Raad I, Gilbreath J, Suleiman N, et al. Maximal sterile barriers (MSB) during the insertion of central venous catheters (CVC) for the prevention of infections: a

prospective randomized study. In: Programs and Abstracts of the 32nd Interscience Conference of Antimicrobial Agents and Chemotherapy. 1992. Abstract 264.

114. Howell PB, Walters PE, Donowitz GR, Farr BM. Risk factors for infection of adult patients with cancer who have tunneled central venous catheters. Cancer 1995; 75:1367–1375.

115. Levin A, Mason AJ, Jindal KK, Fong IW, Goldstein MB. Prevention of hemodialysis subclavian vein catheter infections by topical povidone iodine. Kidney Int 1991; 40:934–938.

116. Prager RL, Silva J. Colonization of central venous catheters. South Med J 1984; 77:458–461.

117. Flowers RH, Schwenzer KJ, Kopel RF, Fisch MJ, Tucker SI, Farr BM. Efficacy of an attachable subcutaneous cuff for the prevention of intravascular catheter-related infection: a randomized, controlled trial. JAMA 1989; 216:878–883.

118. Hill RLR, Fisher AP, Ware RJ, Wilson S, Casewell MW. Mupirocin for the reduction of colonization of internal jugular cannulae—a randomized controlled trial. J Hosp Infect 1990; 15:311–321.

119. Tunkel AR: Topical antibacterials. In: Mandell GL, Bennett JE, Dolin R, eds. Principles and Practice of Infectious Diseases. 4th ed. New York: Churchill Livingstone, 1995:381–389.

120. Conly JM, Grieves K, Peters B. A prospective, randomized study comparing transparent and dry gauze dressings for central venous catheters. J Infect Dis 1989; 159:310–319.

121. Hoffman KK, Weber DJ, Samsa GP, Rutala WA. Transparent polyurethane film as an intravenous catheter dressing: a meta-analysis of the infection risks. JAMA 1992; 267:2072–2076.

122. Maki DG, Stolz SM, Wheeler SJ, Mermel LA. A prospective, randomized trial of gauze and two polyurethane dressings for site care of pulmonary artery catheters: implications for catheter management. Crit Care Med 1994; 22:1729–1737.

123. Romano G, Berti M, Goldstein BP, Borghi A. Efficacy of a central venous catheter (Hydrocath) loaded with teicoplanin in preventing subcutaneous staphylococcal infection in the mouse. Int J Med Microbiol Virol, Parasitol Infect Dis 1993; 279:426–433.

124. Maki DG, Cobb L, Garman JK, Shapiro JM, Ringer M, Helgerson RB. An attachable silver-impregnated cuff for prevention of infection with central venous catheters: a prospective randomized multicenter trial. Am J Med 1988; 85:307–314.

125. Clemence MA, Anglim AM, Jernigan JA, et al. A study of prevention of catheter related bloodstream infection with an antiseptic impregnated catheter. In: Programs and Abstracts of the 34th Interscience Conference of Antimicrobial Agents and Chemotherapy. Orlando, FL, 1994. Abstract J199.

126. Maki DG, Wheeler SJ, Stolz SM, Mermel LA. Clinical trial of a novel antiseptic central venous catheter In: Programs and Abstracts of the 31st Interscience Conference of Antimicrobial Agents and Chemotherapy. Chicago, IL, 1991. Abstract 461.

127. Kamal GD, Pfaller MA, Rempe LE, Jebson PJR. Reduced intravascular catheter infection by antibiotic bonding. JAMA 1991; 265:2364–2368.

128. Trooskin SZ, Donetz AP, Harvey RA, Greco RS. Prevention of catheter sepsis by antibiotic bonding. Surgery 1985; 97:547–551.

129. Sherertz RJ, Carruth WA, Hampton AA, Byron MP, Solomon DD. Efficacy of antibiotic-coated catheters in preventing subcutaneous *Staphylococcus aureus* infection in rabbits. J Infect Dis 1993; 167:98–106.

130. Uldall PR, Merchant N, Woods F, Yarworski U, Vas S. Changing subclavian haemodialysis cannulas to reduce infection. Lancet 1981; 1373.

131. Powell C, Kudsk KA, Kulich PA, Mandelbaum JA, Fabri PJ. Effect of frequent guidewire changes on triple-lumen catheter sepsis. JPEN 1988; 12:462–464.

132. Eyer S, Brummitt C, Crossley K, Siegel R, Cerra F. Catheter-related sepsis: prospective, randomized study of three methods of long-term catheter maintenance. Crit Care Med 1990; 18:1073–1079.

133. Cobb DK, High KP, Sawyer RG, et al. A controlled trial of scheduled replacement of central venous and pulmonary-artery catheters. N Engl J Med 1992; 327:1062–1068.

134. Faubion WC, Wesley JR, Khalidi N, Silva J. Total parenteral nutrition catheter sepsis: impact of the team approach. JPEN 1986; 10:642–645.

135. Freeman JB, Lemire A, Maclean LD. Intravenous alimentation and septicemia. Surg Gynecol Obstet 1972; 135:708–712.

136. Nehme AE. Nutritional support of the hospitalized patient. The team concept. JAMA 1980; 243:1906–1908.

137. Nelson DB, Kien CL, Mohr B, Frank S, Davis SD. Dressing changes by specialized personnel reduce infection rates in patients receiving central venous parenteral nutrition. JPEN 1986; 10:220–222.

138. Boelaert JR, Van Landuyt HW, De Baere YA, et al. Epidemiology and prevention of *Staphylococcus aureus* infections during hemodialysis (Review) (French). Nephrologie 1994; 15:157–161.

139. Wilson AP, Scott GM, Lewis C, Neild G, Rudge C. Audit of infection in continuous ambulatory peritoneal dialysis. J Hosp Infect 1994; 28:264–271.

140. Ludlam HA, Young AE, Berry AJ, Phillips I. The prevention of infection with *Staphylococcus aureus* in continuous ambulatory peritoneal dialysis. J Hosp Infect 1989; 14:293–301.

141. Ludlam H, McCann M. The prevention of infection with *Staphylococcus aureus* in continuous ambulatory peritoneal dialysis. J Hosp Infect 1991; 17:325–326.

142. McLean RJ, Hussain AA, Sayer M, Vincent PJ, Hughes DJ, Smith TJ. Antibacterial activity of multilayer silver-copper surface films on catheter material. Can J Microbiol 1993; 39:895–899.

143. Liu WK, Tebbs SE, Byrne PO, Elliott TS. The effects of electric current on bacteria colonizing intravenous catheters. J Infect 1993; 27:261–269.

144. Bodey GP, Zermeno A, Raad I. Novel approach for the prevention of catheter infections: iontophoretic catheter using silver wire. In: Programs and Abstracts of the 34th Interscience Conference on Antimicrobial Agents and Chemotherapy. Orlando, FL, 1994. Abstract J197.

145. Raad I, Darouiche R, Hachem R, Bodey GP. The broad-spectrum activity of catheters coated with minocycline and rifampin against bacteria and fungi. In: Pro-

grams and Abstracts of the 34th Interscience Conference on Antimicrobial Agents and Chemotherapy. Orlando, FL, 1994. Abstract J195.

146. Raad I, Hachem R, Sherertz R. Minocycline-EDTA (M-EDTA) flush solution for the prevention of vascular catheter infection. In: Programs and Abstracts of the 34th Interscience Conference of Antimicrobial Agents and Chemotherapy. Orlando, FL, 1994.

4

Catheter-Associated Infections Caused by Coagulase-Negative Staphylococci
Clinical and Biological Aspects

Mathias Herrmann and Georg Peters
University of Münster, Münster, Germany

I. INTRODUCTION

A variety of intravascular and other catheters are being used increasingly in diagnostic and therapeutic procedures of modern medicine. These devices are manufactured from various polymers, like polyvinylchloride (PVC), polyethylene (PE), silicon rubber (SR), and polyurethane (PUR). The use of such catheters has undoubtedly led to medical progress for the benefit of many patients. On the other hand, special complications associated with the use of foreign body materials have occurred, introducing new clinical syndromes. Besides thrombosis, one of the most frequent complications, which is now considered to be the major problem, is infection. These "polymer-associated" infections are nowadays clinical routine phenomena, yet they present possibly severe consequences for the individual patient—e.g., the development of sepsis with the possible necessity for removal of the catheter. A wide spectrum of bacteria such as *Pseudomonas* sp., nonfermenting gram-negative rods, Enterobacteriaceae, diphteroids, and streptococci, as well as fungi of the *Candida* group can be involved in this type of infection. However, by far the most frequently isolated group of bacteria are staphylococci, in particular coagulase-negative staphylococci.

The following chapter deals with recent knowledge concerning the underlying pathomechanisms as well as certain clinical, epidemiological, and general bacteriological aspects of catheter-associated infections caused by coagulase-negative staphylococci.

II. CLINICAL ASPECTS

Based on the data from an enormous amount of case reports and clinical studies extensively reviewed elsewhere (1–5), there is no doubt that staphylococci are the most frequently isolated organisms involved in most of the possible polymer-associated infections. Furthermore, it is obvious that coagulase-negative staphylococci (CoNS) generally predominate over *S. aureus*, especially also in infections associated with intravascular catheters (6). While the normal flora of the skin and mucous membranes of the patient and medical personnel serves as the main source for infection (7), hematogenous infections may also occur due to a short-term, clinically usually inapparent bacteremia which is often procedure-related but appears to be frequent even in healthy persons. The severity of the underlying disease and subsequently the frequence and invasiveness of disease-related interventions have been demonstrated to be independent risk factors (8), whereas others (such as the duration of catheterization or hospitalization) appear to be cofactors for catheter-related infections rather than independent risk factors (9).

From the clinical point of view one can examine staphylococcal catheter-associated infections according to their onset—i.e., the time of the first clinical manifestation of disease: early-onset infections occur within days or weeks after implantation (Hickman-Broviac) or insertion (Sheldon, pulmonary, central venous catheter) of an intravascular catheter. In these cases, the inoculation of the pathogen has taken place at the time of the respective procedure; late-onset infections occur after a much longer interval of several weeks or even months, according to some authors as long as 6 months later. Late-onset infections may be caused by true late hematogenous infection, but it may also be possible that the inoculation of the pathogen occurs at the time of surgical or nonsurgical insertion of the catheter followed by a long latent phase.

The clinical picture of catheter-related infections due to CoNS varies. However, in contrast to catheter-related infections caused by other, more virulent species, infections with CoNS often present a clinical picture characterized by a paucity of symptoms (10). Even in the case of bacteremia only moderate fever and only rarely chill episodes do occur. The long-lasting nature of the infection is a further characteristic, especially if the infected device is not removed. In these cases, other signs of chronic infection like anemia or splenomegaly may appear. It should be mentioned, that extensive CoNS colonization of an intravascular catheter can be found during routinely performed cultures, although clinical symptoms are absent in the patient. In fatal cases, multiple microabscesses are found in parenchymatous organs, especially in spleen, liver, and lung, at autopsy. While this severe course of a CoNS catheter infection is rather an exception, more frequently the diagnosis of catheter-related CoNS bacteremia may be difficult because CoNS isolates in the blood are frequent contaminants (11) and only approximately 50% of patients with CoNS catheter infections exhibit local signs of inflammation such as redness, warmth, tenderness, or purulence at the catheter exit site (10). Furthermore, while many CoNS catheter infections can be cured by antimicrobial therapy alone, in some cases a clinical response cannot be obtained despite the use of substances with proven high in vitro activity, and the host is often not able to overcome the infection despite a normal immune system and despite the low virulence of CoNS.

III. GENERAL BACTERIOLOGICAL ASPECTS

In the past, most of the numerous studies reporting on catheter infections have dealt with clinical aspects rather than with the differentiation of the staphylococci, especially the CoNS, involved. Usually, coagulase-negative staphylococcal species are referred to as *S. albus* or *S. epidermidis*, or simply as CoNS. Today the Kloos-Schleifer system is the accepted scheme for the differentiation of human *Staphylococcus* sp. According to the studies available, most CoNS involved in polymer associated infections belong to the *S. epidermidis* group (*S. epidermidis sensu stricto, S. hominis, S. haemolyticus, S. warneri, S. capitis*). Within the *S. epidermidis* group, *S. epidermidis* sensu stricto accounts for about two-thirds of all strains (1,12). This observation reflects the situation present in the normal human microflora and is also known from other coagulase-negative staphylococcal infections—for instance, in immunocompromised patients.

It is to date an open question whether all or at least the majority of CoNS strains causing catheter-related infections belong to the *S. epidermidis* group or just a special group of strains are able to cause catheter infections. A useful tool in answering this question can be isolate typing, since the recovery of identical isolates from various sites (i.e., catheter tip, blood, catheter exit site) be may reliably establish this isolate as the cause for infection. Several typing methods have been put forward: antibiotic resistance profiles, biotyping, and phage typing are often of limited help in differentiating isolates due to typical CoNS resistance pattern (13–15), similar biochemical reactions, or the necessity for phage susceptibility (13,16). Plasmid profile, SDS-PAGE patterns of extracellular proteins, and DNA restriction analysis have been successfully used for epidemiological studies or other purposes (13,16); however, some strains are not typable using these assays. Modern genomic methods with a high discriminatory power include arbitrarily primed PCR (17) and pulsed field gel electrophoresis (18). All these methods have been shown to be extremely useful for unrevealing epidemiologic or etiologic links associated with CoNS infections (19–21); however, they are of limited value in distinguishing catheter-associated from commensal CoNS strains.

The role of other properties such as slime production, surface hydrophobicity and hydrophilicity, and other specific properties like fibrinogen or fibronectin binding capacity are discussed in the pathogenesis chapter. However, to date no safe marker(s) are known defining strains with the potential to cause foreign body infections and thus to predict or confirm their clinical relevance. This counts also for tests measuring adherence to polymers or slime production (15,22–25). The application of these tests in various clinical studies has led to controversial results (26–33).

IV. PATHOGENESIS

The basic pathogenesis of CoNS polymer associated and thus also of catheter-related infections is generally characterized by a two-step process: adherence to the surface and accumulation with slime and biofilm production on the surface (see also Chapter 1). The following section will discuss first some morphological aspects regarding surface colonization, then the present knowledge of the mechanisms of adherence to and accumulation on polymer surfaces and of the physicochemical characteristics of the extracellular slime substance. Finally, the biological consequences concerning host response and antibiotic activity are presented, including animal data. Where applicable, these aspects are discussed in conjunction with their possible clinical relevance.

A. Morphological Aspects

Morphological investigations on various types of intravascular catheters using scanning electron microscopy (SEM) and transmission electron microscopy (TEM) have gained the first insight into the pathogenesis of these infections. Due to the nature of these techniques, these investigations have to be considered as descriptive rather than confirmative.

It is important to note that the inner and outer surfaces of catheters and other implant materials are not totally smooth but show various types of surface irregularities (34). These irregularities can be found on every polymer material so far investigated, but they vary in quantity, size, and appearance in different materials. Most of the irregularities are of a size that could trap one or more staphylococcal cells. If catheters were perfused in vitro with a buffer solution inoculated with CoNS, staphylococcal cells could be seen preferentially adhering to surface defects a few minutes after starting the perfusion experiment (Fig. 1). With increasing time, adherent and dividing cells forming microcolonies could be

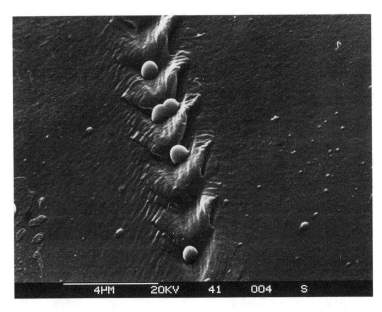

Figure 1   Scale-like scraping in the inner surface of a polyethylene catheter show-ing adherent staphylococci after perfusion with saline inoculated with *S. epider-midis.* (From Ref. 169, © Gustav Fischer Verlag.)

observed (35). Thus, staphylococci seem to be able to adhere irreversibly to the polymer surface despite the continuous flow in the in vitro perfusion system. Hereby the surface defects obviously serve as starting points for colonization.

In a stationary in vitro catheter colonization model a similar process occur-ring could be seen (36,37). The staphylococcal cells adhere to the polymer sur-face, now independently of the presence of surface irregularities. With increasing incubation time, microcolonies and finally multiple cell layers are formed on the polymer surface. Starting with an incubation time of about 12 hours, the adherent cells become covered by a thin film of material that steadily increases in thick-ness (Fig. 2). Most of the attached cells are then covered by this slime matrix pro-duced by the stapylococci. Similar observations have been made when investi-gating transvenous endocardial pacemaker leads (38).

SEM and TEM investigations have also been carried out on intravenous catheters isolated from patients with *S. epidermidis*-related sepsis, CAPD catheters obtained from patients with CAPD-related peritonitis, infected transve-nous endocardial pacemaker leads and aggregates, and infected CSF shunts (38–42). Deposits up to 160 mm thick could be shown on the surface of the respective polymers with a morphology identical to the slime matrix observed

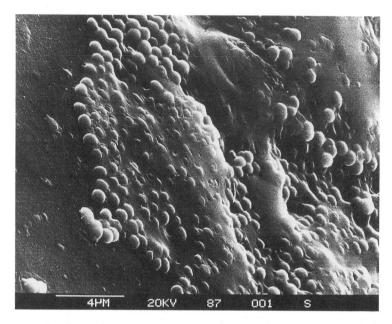

Figure 2 Slimy material produced by S. epidermidis of the inner surface of a poly-ethylene catheter after incubation for 48 hours. (From Ref. 37, © The University of Chicago.)

during in vitro experiments (Fig. 3). In artificial cracks in the matrix due to the preparation for EM, embedded coccal cells are visible. Although reasonable amounts of this matrix may be built out of staphylococcal extracellular slime, one has to consider that host products are also involved.

Some important aspects of the pathogenesis of staphylococcal foreign body infections can already be described from these morphological data: staphylococci are obviously able to adhere to and grow on polymer surfaces. In the course of surface colonization they produce an extracellular slime substance in which they become entirely embedded, and a biofilm is produced. The morphology of this surface colonization is identical both in vivo and in vitro, suggesting similar mechanisms. These observations lead to the hypothesis that the slime matrix or biofilm, respectively, may protect the embedded staphylococci against host response mechanisms as well as against antibiotics (43).

B. Adherence to Polymer Surfaces

The first step in the colonization or infection of a polymer device is the (probably irreversible) adherence of a bacterial cell to the polymer surface (44–47). This

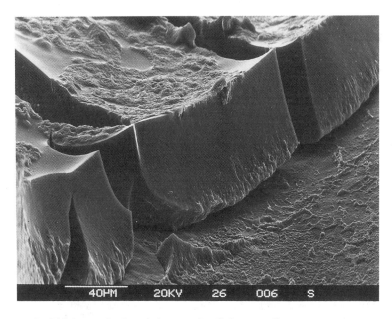

Figure 3 Thick matrix (staphylococcal cell layers, slime, serum components) deposited on the inner surface of a catheter infected by *S. epidermidis* obtained from a patient with *S. epidermidis* sepsis. (From Ref. 41, © Gustav Fischer Verlag.)

process occurs very quickly and is mediated by nonspecific and specific mechanisms. Regarding the nonspecific interaction, the adhesion of a bacterial cell to a polymer surface can be described as adhesion of a colloid particle to a solid surface in a liquid environment. Besides the hydrodynamic forces of the liquid medium that influence the transport of the particle to the surface, the process is governed by attractive or repulsive forces including electrostatic, van der Waals, and dipole-dipole interactions. The main nonspecific forces mediating attachment in saline, buffer, or other nutrient- and protein-free media are electrostatic and hydrophobic interactions (43,44,46–49). The DLVO theory of lyophobic colloid stabilization regards adhesion as a balance between van der Waals attraction and electrostatic repulsion, and has frequently been used to describe bacterial adherence to solid surfaces. The thermodynamic model for adhesion of cells to solid surfaces excludes electrostatic interactions and takes into account parameters such as surface tension of the polymer, bacterial cell, and liquid environment. The adherence is the net result of all forces active and is dependent on the surface properties of both the bacterial cell and the polymer in a given liquid environment. In general, the more hydrophobic strains adhere more strongly to hydrophobic polymers than hydrophilic strains. Regarding surface charge it can be stated that bacterial adhesion is highest on positively charged polymers and strongly reduced on negatively charged polymers, due to a repulsion effect between the two negatively charged surfaces.

If polymer surfaces are in contact with colloidal fluids such as serum or blood plasma, proteins such as albumin are immediately adsorbed to the surface, resulting in a major change of the physicochemical surface characteristics (50,51). In fact, many physical forces contributing to "nonspecific" adhesion such as hydrophobic interaction are greatly reduced after this surface modification, and when tested in vitro, adhesion of CoNS to hydrophobic polymer surfaces is generally largely diminished compared with adhesion to unadsorbed surfaces (35,44,47,52,53). It should be noted, however, that CoNS cells may adhere to a certain extent even to albumin-adsorbed polymers, and that physicochemical interactions may play a role also in "specific" adhesion mediated by a surface-adsorbed ligand and a bacterial adhesin.

As numerous in vitro studies have shown, upon surface adsorption certain "adhesive" proteins may greatly promote adhesion even in the presence of albumin in the milieu. Fibrinogen, fibronectin, laminin, collagen, thrombospondin, and vitronectin have been shown to interact with *S. aureus* and certain strains of CoNS species (54–61), and, while these proteins are able to adsorb to polymer surfaces, it has been shown that they greatly promote staphylococcal adhesion to polymer surfaces in albumin milieu (55,62,63). Fibronectin promotes adhesion of a large number of *S. epidermidis* strains to polymer surfaces in vitro (52), and fibronectin in vivo adsorbed on catheter material does also promote adhesion of *S. epidermidis* strain RP62A (64). In contrast to *S. aureus*, only limited information is available on the nature and genetic organization of adhesins on *S. epidermidis* recognizing extracellular matrix proteins. Also, in noncolloidal buffer systems, preadsorption of adhesive proteins may rather reduce adhesion of CoNS compared to adhesion to unadsorbed plastic, probably due to above-mentioned modification of physicochemical interaction (65). Taken together, while CoNS may adhere to polymeric surfaces due to physicochemical binding forces, specific "ligand-adhesin"-type mechanisms may involve certain extracellular matrix and plasma proteins. This interaction may even happen in a quite complex "cooperative" binding.

At least three different antigens have been described as being present in several strains of *S. epidermidis*, which are responsible for adherence to polymer surfaces: one is designated as a capsular polysaccharide adhesin (PS/A) (66,67), another one is characterized as a proteinaceous adhesin (68,69). For both antigens it could be shown that polyclonal or monoclonal antibodies, respectively, are able to block adherence of *S. epidermidis* to "native" (protein-free!) polymer surfaces. Just recently, a 60-KDa protein in a *S. epidermidis* strain was described which is also functioning as adhesin for binding to plastic (70). Tn*917* transposon insertion mutants of this strain were affected in primary adherence but not in biofilm formation. It is so far unclear, however, what role these antigens play in vivo and how they may act in the situation, in which the polymer surface is coated with host proteins.

C. Accumulation on Polymer Surfaces, Production of Extracellular Slime, and Biofilm Formation

The rapid process of primary adherence is followed by a more time-consuming step, namely, the accumulation on the polymer surface. The morphological studies described above have revealed that staphylococcal cells are able to grow on the polymer surface and to produce copious amounts of an extracellular slime substance during the course of polymer colonization. This leads to the buildup of an amorphous matrix of multiple staphylococcal cell layers embedded in extracellular slime. If plasma or serum is present during an experiment or in vivo, host serum proteins may also be involved in the buildup of this matrix. Obviously, in this accumulation phase the staphylococci seem to be able to grow in the free space by means of a strong intercellular adherence, and thus form a biofilm.

The importance of this second substantial step of surface accumulation could be shown by the discovery of a polysaccharide antigen associated with the ability for biofilm formation (71). This polysaccharide could be isolated from the slime-producing strain *S. epidermidis* RP62A. It seems to function in intercellular adherence. Thus, it was designated as "polysaccharide intercellular adhesin" (PIA). Very recently, its chemical structure could be discovered as a linear β-1, 6-linked glucosamino-glycan (72).

However, besides PIA other factors seem to be necessary for intercellular adherence and biofilm formation. This could be demonstrated by polymer surface colonization experiments using a pair of isogenic *S. epidermidis* strains. A slime-negative mutant *S. epidermidis* M7 was derived by chemical mutagenesis with mitomycin C from its slime positive parent *S. epidermidis* RP62A (73). Despite its inability to produce slime in the tube test, the mutant differed in two further properties (74). The mutant lacked the ability to accumulate on the surface whereas its growth in liquid culture was equal to that of the parent. Its ability for primary adherence was also not impaired, the rate of adherence being equal to the parent strain. The second differing property was the lack of a single protein band at approximately 115 kDa after separation of the extracellular proteins on SDS-PAGE. However, the ability to produce PIA was not impaired in the mutant (D. Mack, Hamburg, personal communication). Thus, it has to be considered that this 115-kDa protein is also necessary for accumulation and biofilm formation on a surface. Using antibodies directed against the 115-kDa protein (now shown to be a 140-kDa protein), most recently we could show that this protein is essential for accumulation of *S. epidermidis* strains on polymer surfaces (Hussain M, Herrmann M, von Eiff C, Perdreau-Remington F, Peters G. Infect Immun 1997, in press) and refer to it as accumulation-associated protein (AAP). Another antigen has been described as being associated with proliferative growth of *S. epidermidis* on the surface. It has been designated as slime-associated antigen (SAA), a polysaccharide with a molecular weight greater than 50 kDa (75). The functional role of this antigen has not been elucidated yet.

The extracellular slime substance (ESS) produced by *S. epidermidis* during its proliferation and accumulation on the polymer surface is still undefined (15,22,24,76–81). It is water-soluble—at least in vitro—and therefore removable from cells by washing with water or buffer. Thus, the extracellular slime is different from true capsules as defined for gram-positive cocci (24,82). The production or formation of slime is dependent on the environmental situation: it is enhanced in the presence of several sugars such as glucose, galactose, lactose, and mannose; amino acids are also required (15,22,24,79); it is inhibited if subinhibitory concentrations of tunicamycin are present during growth (15,24).

Several attempts have been made to chemically characterize ESS from *S. epidermidis*. It seems to be a complex mixture of various sugars and proteins. Thus, it appears to be quite unlikely that slime can be restricted to just one macromolecule. Regarding the carbohydrate composition, glucose, mannose, galactose, aminosugars, and glucuronic acid are found to be present (15,24,78,80). Of these, mannose, galactose, and glucuronic acid seem to be genuine constituents of the slime substance, since these monosaccharides are not present in the peptidoglycan or teichoic acid of the cell wall of *S. epidermidis*. However, other molecules excluded from the staphylococcal cell during normal growth turnover, such as cell wall components and extracellular proteins, may be present, even DNA or RNA (24,78,80). The main component, at least in a quantitative manner, is teichoic acid (80). Thus, the interpretation of experimental results has to be done very careful by considering these possibilities.

A further question is whether all *S. epidermidis* strains produce extracellular slime substance and to what extent if at all the slime produced may be different in chemical composition and in its immunogenicity. The same must be considered for other CoNS species. The situation is further complicated by the fact that slime production by *S. epidermidis* may be subject to phenotypic variation (83). Thus, it is still not possible to define clear markers for extracellular slime. A 30-kDa protein has been described as being present in the slime of most *S. epidermidis* strains but in no other *Staphylococcus* species so far investigated (84). Its biological role as well as its usefulness as a general marker for slime has yet to be defined.

D. Resistance of Surface-Grown Staphyloccoci Against Host Defense Mechanisms

The clinical experience with polymer-associated staphylococcal infections clearly shows that the host seems to be unable in many cases to handle the infection and, in particular, to eliminate the staphyloccoci from the infected polymer device (1,2,4,85). From various morphological investigations it has been postulated that this may be associated with the surface mode of growth and the production of extracellular slime and biofilms. Opsonization and subsequent phagocytosis by polymorphonuclear neutrophils (PMN) and macrophages are the major host response mechanisms of the human host against staphyloccoci. Therefore, several investigations have addressed the question as to whether surface-grown staphyloccoci resist opsonophagocytosis and whether extracellular slime and biofilm production, respectively, may contribute to this resistance.

Nearly all experimental data available have been derived using *S. epidermidis* and extracellular slime produced by *S. epidermidis*. Crude extracellular slime substance (ESS) of *S. epidermidis*—produced in chemically defined medium and free of contaminants, i.e., other microorganisms and endotoxin, and free of alpha-toxin and enterotoxins—has several effects on the function of PMN (86–92). ESS itself has been found to induce a significant chemotactic response in human PMN which was dose-dependent and not altered by heating (87,89). On the other hand, PMN preincubated with increasing amounts of ESS showed a decreased responsiveness to known chemotactic stimuli such as FMLP and zymosan-activated serum (ZAS) (87,89). This effect was especially pronounced and dose-dependent with ZAS, which leads to the speculation that ESS might interfere with a C5a receptor on the PMN membrane. A simple cytotoxic effect could be excluded since random migration was not decreased by any slime concentration used and since lactic dehydrogenase release and trypan blue dye exclusion were not affected (91). Preincubated PMN also showed enhanced adherence to plastic wells and a decrease in chemiluminescence response, again in a dose-response manner. On the other hand, preincubation of PMN with ESS stimulates PMN degranulation, especially after prior cytochalasin B treatment (87,89). This effect was pronounced and dose-dependent for lactoferrin. This may effectively lead to the waste of cellular products after contact with slime in addition to the decreased chemotactic responsiveness, all this resulting in a decreased ability for intracellular killing. The interference of *S. epidermidis* slime with PMN function may even be enhanced by negative effects of the polymer itself on PMN function (93).

Due to the water solubility of the extracellular slime substance, it is difficult to investigate resistance of slime covered staphylococcal cells in conventional uptake and killing assays. Consequently, no differences could be shown in respective studies (29,94). Isolated slime has been used to investigate a possible interference with opsonization or uptake of bacteria (91). In these experiments uptake and killing were markedly inhibited if slime was present during opsonization, suggesting a possible interference with bacterial opsonization. The new model of surface phagocytosis (95)—an assay more similar to the in vivo situation of a polymer-associated infection—first provided the possibility to investigate opsonization, uptake, and killing of *S. epidermidis* growing on a surface. If radiolabeled *S. epidermidis* was grown for 2 hours or 18 hours in plastic wells, then subjected to phagocytosis by PMN, a remarkable difference in uptake could be seen: with or without prior opsonization, the uptake of *S. epidermidis* grown for 18 hours was markedly diminished when compared to equal numbers of cells grown for only 2 hours (87,89). The non-slime-producing control strain—*S. aureus* COWAN I—showed no difference in uptake after 2 or 18 hours of growth under the same conditions. The reason for this difference in *S. epidermidis* uptake is supposedly due to the fact that after 18 hours of incubation the adhering cells are protected by the slime substance produced. This is further supported by the observation that phagocytosis of *S. epidermidis* was similarly decreased if the strain was incubated for 18 hours in a medium with supplementation to promote slime production but not without supplementation (87,89). This is also congruent with morphological studies showing that slime is not present in *S. epidermidis* incubated for 6 hours or less whereas the slime is visible after 12 hours' growth or longer on a polymer surface (37). Using a further modification of the surface phagocytosis model, an extended number of *S. epidermidis* and *S. haemolyticus* strains has been investigated (35,96). The results of this investigation confirmed that surface-grown and biofilm-producing staphyloccoci are markedly more resistant to phagocytosis by PMN than liquid-grown staphyloccoci.

It appears that interference with opsonization seems to be crucial, with the extracellular slime substance acting as a physical barrier for the deposition of complement or IgG on the cell surface (35,91). This is supported by the finding of another experimental study that the extracellular slime substance clearly interferes with the opsonization of surface-grown staphylococci measured by a decrease in superoxide production and in extracellular killing (86,88). In very recent investigations it could be finally shown using the above-mentioned isogenic *S. epidermidis* strains that the slime-negative mutant is significantly more effectively killed than its slime-positive parent. This effect was again especially pronounced if prior opsonization with pooled human serum was performed (Johnson GM, Schumacher-Perdreau F, Peters G. *Staphylococcus epidermidis* resistance to phagocytic bactericidal mechanisms: the role of accumulative growth and formation of a biofilm. Submitted). These in vitro studies appear to provide substantial evidence to support the view that the accumulative surface growth and the production of extracellular slime of CoNS interferes significantly with opsonophagocytosis of these bacteria by PMN.

The extracellular slime substance derived from *S. epidermidis* seems also to interfere with other host defense mechanisms as shown in in vitro experiments (90,97,98). Crude extracellular slime substance inhibited the proliferation of human peripheral mononuclear cells—which are mainly T-cells—after stimulation with polyclonal immunomodulators in a dose- and time-dependent manner (97). In these experiments, increasing levels of slime reduced both, the blastogenic response of peripheral mononuclear cells to phytohaemaglutinin as well as streptococcal blastogen A, indicated by the incorporation rate of ^{3}H-thymidine and the number of blastic cells in the cell cultures. This effect requires an extended incubation time and thus seems to be mediated by a gradual lysis of the mononuclear cells. Besides the inhibition of proliferation, obvious alterations in the cell surface antigen expression on remaining cells are found: the proportion of non-T, non-B-cells is greater with increasing culture time (98). In addition, fewer cells could be recognized as CD4 or CD8 cells. However, the decrease in CD4 cells was more pronounced than in CD8 cells. The CD4/CD8 ratio was markedly altered by 4 days of culture. The underlying mechanisms are still quite unclear, as is the relevance in the host response to foreign body infections by *S. epidermidis*. Nevertheless, the proportional decrease of T helper cells would suggest an alteration of the immune function dependent upon these cells by the action of slime. The results of another investigation could mainly confirm these results (99). However, it has been derived from these results that slime does not have a direct inhibitory effect on T-cells but that the slime can activate monocyte prostaglandine E2 production, which may contribute to the inhibition of T-cell proliferation (99,100).

The presence of slime in culture also inhibits the NK activity of mononuclear cells directed against a human leukemia cell line (98). Further, the slime substance interferes with B-cell blastogenesis: if mononuclear cell cultures were incubated with pokeweed mitogen and increasing amounts of slime, fewer B-cells and fewer B-cell blasts could be identified in these cultures (98). Parallel to this, decreasing amounts of immunoglubulin could be measured. These results are preliminary and still not yet confirmed by other investigations.

E. Resistance of Polymer Surface-Grown Staphylococci Against Antibiotics

Another fact based on clinical experience is that antibacterial chemotherapy is often not able to cure catheter-associated staphylococcal infections despite the use of antibiotics with proven in vitro activity. From the aforementioned morphological investigations it has been postulated that staphylococci growing on a polymer surface and embedded in a biofilm matrix may be protected against the action of antibiotics administered. Indeed, from a mechanical point of view, biofilms up to 160 mm thick, observed in infected prostheses and intravascular catheters by scanning electron microscopy, could serve as a diffusion or penetration barrier. This view is supported by investigations showing the reduction of antibiotic activity on surface-grown, slime- or biofilm-covered bacteria (101–104). CoNS adhering to PVC catheters could be shown to be phenotypically resistant to nafcillin but sensitive in the normal MIC test assay (104). The same findings could be obtained with vancomycin on staphylococci growing on a silicon catheter (102). Also, staphylococci growing on a polyethylene catheter survived 18 hours of oxacillin exposure

(15). Furthermore, it could be shown that the minimal inhibitory concentration (MIC) of various antibiotics was significantly higher for *S. epidermidis* adherent to a polymer surface than in a liquid growth medium. This could also be demonstrated for *S. epidermidis* grown in a medium promoting slime production compared to *S. epidermidis* grown in Mueller-Hinton medium, which does not stimulate slime production (15). Respective bacterial killing experiments revealed similar results: *S. epidermidis* grown in a medium promoting slime production was significantly less well killed than the same strain grown in Mueller-Hinton. This effect was especially pronounced for vancomycin, clindamycin, ciprofloxacin, gentamicin, and netilmicin. The medium used for promoting the production of extracellular slime did not have any negative effect on the activity of the antibiotics. From these results it can be hypothesized that extracellular slime may be responsible for the reduction of antibiotic activity.

For aminoglycosides this could be further supported by experimental data showing a significant reduction in the uptake of ^{3}H-labeled gentamicin (15,105). *S. epidermidis* cells grown in a medium promoting slime production and then exposed to the labeled gentamicin showed a reduced intracellular uptake of gentamicin: the cell wall/cell membrane-associated radioactivity and the cytoplasma associated radioactivity were significantly lower in cells growing in the medium promoting slime production than in cells grown in a standard Mueller-Hinton medium. Thus, the extracellular slime substance present on cell surface seems to interfere with the uptake of gentamicin into the cytoplasma of staphylococcal cells. The molecular mechanisms, however, are still unknown. One may speculate that membrane transport systems may be affected, since gentamicin uptake is an active process of the staphylococcal cell.

Further, it has been shown that slime extracted from *S. epidermidis* inhibits the antistaphylococcal action of the glycopeptide antibiotics vancomycin and teicoplanin during in vitro MIC experiments (106). Therefore, one may speculate not only that the uptake of antibiotics with intracellular targets is inhibited, but also that cell wall active antibiotics may not be able to reach their target if the slime substance is present on the staphylococcal cell surface.

These experimental findings could at least partially explain the clinical experience of antibiotic failure in cases of catheter-associated CoNS infections. Probably, surface-grown CoNS exhibit a special type of surface growth-associated phenotypic resistance which does not appear in liquid growth.

F. Animal Experimental Data

Only few animal data are available regarding the pathogenesis of staphylococcal polymer-associated infections. Furthermore, some of the results available are quite controversial. A tissue cage model using subcutaneously implanted perforated polytetrafluorethylene cylinders in guinea pigs has been introduced to study adherence mechanisms, host response mechanisms, and antibiotic treatment of experimental infections (107). With this model it could be shown that a polymer itself can depress bactericidal functions of polymorphonuclear leucocytes in vivo (93). Experiments performed with the protein A-deficient *S. aureus* strain WOOD 46 elucidated the in vivo role of fibrinogen and fibronectin as possible mediators of specific adherence of *S. aureus* and *S. epidermidis* to polymer surfaces (62).

Active immunization of rabbits with purified PS/A (67) and passive therapy with polyclonal and monoclonal antibodies to PS/A protect against bacteremia in a model of intravascular catheter infection (66) and against development of endocarditis in such rabbits when a second catheter is placed through the aortic valve producing local valve trauma (108). Using PS/A-deficient transposon insertion mutants, it could be shown that these strains did not produce endocarditis nor sustained bacteremia in the rabbit model (109). Supposedly, a capsule-like antiphagocytic effect of PS/A is mediated through an inhibition of complement deposition on the bacterial surface; thus, PS/A-positive strains appear to be more resistant to opsonic killing and therefore more virulent.

In a subcutaneous catheter infection model in mice it was shown that the incidence of infection is significantly greater when slime producing strains were used for infection than if non or weak slime producing strains were used (110). These experiments indicate that the foreign body is necessary to enable *S. epidermidis* to cause a subcutaneous infection and that extracellular slime seems to be an important factor. However, another study published obtained contradictory results in mice experiments using a similar model (111). Here no differences could be found between slime-producing and non- or weak slime-producing *S. epidermidis* strains in the ability to cause catheter tunnel tract infections despite the presence of the catheter. If the catheter was not present, even a higher abscess rate in mice infected with non- or weak slime-producing *S. epidermidis* strains was found. A further model has been described in which silastic catheters covered with preformed *S. epidermidis* biofilms are intraperitoneally implanted in mice (112). In this model, in about 18% of the mice a "chronic" *S. epidermidis* foreign body infection could be introduced within a period of 6 months.

Using an intraperitoneal infection model it could be clearly shown that slimy *S. epidermidis* strains have a higher mouse virulence than *S. epidermidis* without extracellular slime substance (15). Non-slime-producing *S. epidermidis* has practically no virulence in this intraperitoneal mouse model even when large inocula are used.

S. epidermidis 10^9 CFU grown in a medium promoting slime production and then vigorously washed were not capable of causing death in young female mice. In contrast, the same number of cells unwashed and thus with a slimy surface caused death in more than half the mice injected, whereas vigorously washed cells suspended in 1% slime killed more than 90% of the mice challenged. All mice died of sepsis within 48 hours without showing any abscess formation in the peritoneal cavity; the infecting strain could always be cultivated from this site. Slime obviously does not act like hog gastric mucin. The slime substance itself appeared to be not toxic for the mice; thus the slime substance seems to overwhelm the host defense mechanisms in the peritoneal cavity (opsonophagocytosis by peritoneal macrophages and invading PMN), leading to early sepsis and subsequently to death. This view is supported by the further observation that smaller inocula of the infecting strain together with the extracellular slime substance did not lead to death of the mice but to a significantly delayed clearance of the staphylococci from the peritoneal cavity and from heart blood. Although the exact underlying mechanisms are still unclear, these observations may correlate with the aforementioned in vitro findings regarding inhibition of PMN function and opsonophagocytosis.

Catheter-induced endocarditis in rabbits or rats is widely used, for example, to test the efficacy of antibiotic regimens in vivo. A few studies are available dealing with the role of extracellular slime in the development and curability of such endocarditis (113,114). In these studies, no correlation could be found between the ability of the strains used for slime production and the development of endocarditis. Preliminary studies using an isogenic pair of a slime-negative and a slime-positive S. epidermidis strain did not reveal differences in the establishment of experimental endocarditis in rabbits (74,115). The experimental data regarding polymer-associated staphylococcal infections have still to be considered as too insufficient and controversial to allow definite conclusions. Thus, there is an essential need for further animal experiments to support or confirm the numerous in vitro findings.

V. MANAGEMENT

Approximately 30% to 40% of central venous catheter-related infections are caused by coagulase-negative staphylococcal species (116). If such an infection is suspected either because of local signs of infection with or without positive superficial cultures or because of fever and/or positive blood cultures, several aspects have to be considered for optimal management: (1) the type and severity of infection (exit site infection, deep tunnel infection, or systemic catheter-related bacteremia); (2) the type of underlying disease; and (3) the necessity or at least the interest to maintain the catheter.

Local signs of superfical inflammation are unspecific (117) unless frank pus is present at the insertion site (which is highly indicative of a local infection; 118) or in the presence of positive targeted skin cultures (119,120). Deep-seated tunnel infections may be characterized by a spreading cellulitis around the subcutaneous tunnel tract of long-term catheters; however, tunnel infections due to CoNS may be locally asymptomatic or accompanied only by discrete inflammatory signs. Local infection of the intraluminal catheter segment (tip) is usually assert-ed by culture of the removed catheter portion. CoNS species can be isolated from 8% to 40% of removed catheters (10); however, only a small percentage of these catheters will become the source for catheter-related bacteremia. Thus, several quantitative catheter culture techniques have been developed to identify catheters being "contaminated" and only rarely associated with catheter-related, and to contrast these with catheter "colonization" or "local infection" more frequently associated with bacteremia (6,121–127) (see also Chapter 2 on the diagnosis of catheter-related infections). Quantitative culture techniques are now widely employed and have been validated in multiple clinical studies. In order to search for methods to identify or exclude catheter colonization without catheter removal, superficial culture techniques either of the skin surrounding the catheter wound, of the hub, or of both sites have been developed, some of them using quantitative techniques. Using these techniques, it has been shown that sterile skin exit site cultures and/or hub cultures allow to rule out catheter colonization (and systemic catheter infection) with a negative predictive value approaching 100% (120, 128–130); however, the presence of microorganisms at any superficial site is associated only with a modest positive predictive value for catheter colonization.

The clinical diagnosis of systemic catheter-related bacteremia of a central venous line is difficult in the absence of a purulent exit site and due to the impos-sibility to examine the perfused catheter without removal. Whereas the definitive diagnosis of catheter-related sepsis is based on the recovery of the same organism on the catheter segments and in the blood together with corresponding clinical symptoms, several studies have shown that between 70% and 90% of catheters removed for suspicion of catheter-related bacteremia were not infected and, in fact, could have been maintained (7,116,131–135). In addition, the placement of a new catheter carries significant risks (7,136) and elevated costs. Therefore, several non-invasive methods including rapid techniques (137), quantitative hemocultures drawn both peripherically and through the implicated catheter (118,138–144), and the aforementioned combined use of superficial hub and skin cultures (138,139) have been developed to allow a diagnosis of catheter infection with the catheter maintained. In most instances, however, catheter-related bacteremia caused by CoNS is suspected due to one or several positive conventional blood cultures in a patient with vascular access and fever. Upon isolation of skin commensals such as *S. epidermidis* from the blood, more than one blood culture for the same species is required to establish the diagnosis of true bacteremia (145). In addition, modern typing techniques may be useful for proof of identity of the isolates, particularly if a "precious" catheter such as a Broviac/Hickman or a Port catheter is suspected for infection (146). Another explanation for positive blood cultures is transient benign bacteremia due to translocation of CoNS from mucous membranes. Thus, CoNS isolated in conventional blood cultures may not necessarily be due to an infected intravascular catheter. Previously, in the presence of bacteremia, it was deemed necessary to remove the implicated catheter both as a therapeutic and diagnostic measure (147–149), yielding the intravascular catheter as the most reliable specimen segment. Recent data, however, suggest that patients with catheter-related bacteremia due to CoNS can be successfully (in >80% of the cases) treated without catheter removal (132,133,150–153). This now more generally accepted approach, however, carries a 20% chance that bacteremia will recur, whereas only a 3% risk of recurrence is present when the catheter is removed.

Taken together, the results from the various studies amount to the following approach to the patient with suspected or proven catheter-related infection due to CoNS. Local exit site inflammation usually does not require catheter ablation and can be treated with local care (152). Purulent tunnel infections are usually an indication for catheter removal (152), particularly if *Pseudomonas* sp., atypical mycobacteria (133) or a polymicrobial tunnel infection (152) is suspected. However, if *S. epidermidis* is suspected, e.g., using quantitative superficial cultures, it may be treated with antibiotherapy alone. In the case of CoNS sepsis suspected to be catheter-related, one of the following approaches may be possible according to the clinical circumstances:

1. In the case of shock or of underlying severe immunodeficiency (such as the pediatric neonatal or the neutropenic host), the suspect catheter should be removed, preferably after application of a first antibiotic dose through the device before insertion of a new catheter at a new site. The same approach may be opted for in patients with risk factors for endovascular CoNS infections such as patients with endovascular grafts. In addition, systemic antimicrobial therapy should be given—usually a glycopeptide, because most (50% to 80%) of the strains are resistant to antistaphylococcal penicillins. The optimal duration of therapy has not yet been defined; usually, however, a course of treatment of 5 to 7 days should be adequate (135). At any rate, upon presence of CoNS bacteremia the need for further vascular catheterization should be reevaluated and unnecessary vascular accesses should be removed and cultured.

2. If the catheter is "valuable," it may be maintained, and exit site and hub cultures as well as additional quantitative blood cultures may help to estimate the probability of establishing catheter-related bacteremia. In the case of isolation of CoNS from the blood and suspicion of its relatedness to an infected catheter, systemic therapy may be initiated even without these diagnostic procedures, since the cure rate of a CoNS-infected catheter by systemic antimicrobials is high. Alternatively, the catheter may be treated using the so-called antibiotic-lock technique. This technique, although not yet widely applied, consists of "locking" a highly concentrated solution of antibiotic (usually of vancomycin or an aminoglycoside—e.g., 3 to 5 mg of either or both compounds in 2 ml physio-

logical saline) within the catheter lumen for 12 hours a day, for 1 to 2 weeks (154–157). The technique proves to be efficient in 90% to 100% of the cases, particularly if CoNS are the cause, while cure rates of Port-a-cath® catheters appear to be inferior (158). Of course, the catheter must be dispensable at least for several hours. Multiple lumen catheters may be cured using a "rotative" lock technique. The use of thrombolytic agents, such as streptokinase or urokinase, for infected catheters (159,160) has still to be considered experimental. If the clinical situation does not improve, or if blood cultures remain positive, the removal of the catheter is imperative.

3. A compromise between a conclusive diagnostic and therapeutic approach and the need to maintain the vascular access may consist in catheter change over guide wire. This technique significantly reduces the risk of a new venous puncture (136) and has been employed for various catheter types (136,161–164). The principal drawbacks are the risks of embolization or of seeding of microorganisms to the new catheter (165–167). Until availability of catheter tip culture results, systemic antimicrobial therapy should be employed; the first dose should preferentially be given through the old catheter, which diminishes the risk of transfer of microorganisms without affecting the microbiological diagnosis (116). If the removed catheter is shown to be colonized by CoNS, a systemic therapy may be choosen as outlined above, or, if the quantitative culture remains negative, simple surveillance measure may be employed (other approaches may have to be used upon culture of pathogens other than CoNS). Using this approach, the "infection-free interval" of catheters with a significant infectious risk after definite insertion periods (e.g., Swan-Ganz catheters) may be increased by gaining a new infection-free interval upon catheter exchange (168).

Which of the above alternatives is opted for is highly influenced by the individual patient situation but also by the diagnostic possibilities provided by the microbiology laboratory. At any rate, over the past years, the previously uniform approach to the patient with CoNS vascular catheter infection has become considerably nuanced. This implies new diagnostic and therapeutic challenges for both the clinician and the clinical microbiology laboratory, yet it helps to optimize treatment of patients who rely on increasingly sophisticated vascular access devices for monitoring and therapy.

VI. CONCLUDING REMARKS

Catheter-associated infections are a rapidly growing problem in modern medicine. Especially if CoNS—ubiquitous inhabitants of human skin and mucous membranes and not pathogenic for the normal host—are concerned, these infections have to be regarded as a special type of "iatrogenic nosocomial" infections. Clinically, these infections are characterized by the obvious inability of the host to clear the infectious focus and by major problems to cure the infected device and the related infection by chemotherapy. The ability of staphylococci, at least of most strains of human origin, to adhere to and accumulate on polymer (i.e., catheter) surfaces and to produce an extracellular slime substance is the cornerstone in the pathogenesis of catheter-associated staphylococcal infections. The ability for surface growth and biofilm production may be a phylogenetically old property acquired during the evolution process. Here it enables the staphylococci to stick together in large cell clusters, allowing close contact and substance exchange. It may further enable them to stay in a dormant state thereby permitting survival in suboptimal environmental conditions.

It could be essential for staphylococci to live on their natural surface of skin and mucous membranes of humans or animals, without injuring the host. However, if a polymer foreign body, i.e., intravascular catheter is introduced into the host, a new surface is presented to the staphylococci. The natural mode of growth on this surface may subsequently result in infection of the tissue surrounding the device as well as in sepsis. Since the staphylococci are protected against host response mechanisms as well as against the action of antibiotics, this may lead to the maintenance of the infectious focus and thus to systemic infection.

Some important clinical consequences can be drawn from present knowledge on the pathogenesis of staphylococcal catheter-associated infections. The indication for insertion of an intravascular catheter of whatever type must be carefully considered. Since antibiotic therapy may fail, prevention of infection is crucial. Optimal performance of surgical or nonsurgical insertion and the most rigid aseptic procedures are required. A promising modern approach is to synthesize polymers with intrinsic antiadhesive and/or anti-infectious properties or to coat polymers with or incorporate into the polymer substances which inhibit bacterial adhesion or kill bacteria shortly after adherence. Finally, intravascular catheters with suspected or proven systemic catheter-related CoNS infection do not have to be automatically removed; on the contrary, an approach taking into account the type of microbiological data available, the risks of new catheter placement, the underlying disease, and the necessity for further vascular access all have to be considered in order to optimize an increasing choice of treatment modalities for these patients.

REFERENCES

1. Archer GL. *Staphylococcus epidermidis* and other coagulase-negative staphylococci. In: Mandell GL, Bennett JE, Dolin R, eds. Principles and Practice of Infectious Diseases. 4th ed. New York: Churchill Livingstone, 1995:1777–1783.

2. Bisno AL, Waldvogel FA. Infections Associated With Indwelling Medical Devices. 2nd ed. Washington, DC: American Society for Microbiology, 1994.

3. Pulverer G, Peters G, Schumacher-Perdreau F. Coagulase-negative staphylococci. Zbl Bakt Hyg I Abt Orig A 1987; 264:1–28.

4. Sugarman B, Young EJ. Infections Associated With Prosthetic Devices. Boca Raton: CRC Press, 1984.

5. Kloos WE, Bannerman TE. Update on clinical significance of coagulase-negative staphylococci. Clin Microbiol Rev 1994; 7:117–140.

6. Maki DG, Weise CE, Sarafin HW. A semiquantitative culture method for identifying intravenous-catheter infection. N Engl J Med 1977; 296:1305.

7. Maki DG. Infections due to infusion therapy. In: Bennett JV, Brachman PS, eds. Hospital Infections. 3rd ed. Boston: Little, Brown, 1992:849–898.

8. Henderson DK. Intravascular device-associated infection: current concepts and controversies. Infect Surg 1988; 7:365–371.

9. Stenzel JP, Green TP, Fuhrman BP, Carlson PE, Marchessault RP. Percutaneous central venous catheterization in a pediatric intensive care unit: a survival analysis of complications. Crit Care Med 1989; 17:984–988.

10. Rupp ME, Archer GL. Coagulase-negative staphylococci: pathogens associated with medical progress. Clin Infect Dis 1994; 19:231–245.

11. Kirchoff LV, Sheagren JN. Epidemiology and clinical significance of blood cultures positive for coagulase-negative *Staphylococcus*. Infect Control 1985; 6:479–486.

12. Peters G, Schumacher-Perdreau F, Pulverer G. Adherence of coagulase-negative staphylococci to polymers. In: Medical Microbiology. 5th ed. London: Academic Press, 1986:209–226.

13. Christensen GD, Parisi JT, Bisno AL, Simpson WA, Beachey EH. Characterization of clinically significant strains of coagulase-negative staphylococci. J Clin Microbiol 1983; 18:258–269.

14. Kotilainen P, Nikoskelainen J, Houvinen P. Antibiotic susceptibility of coagulase-negative staphylococcal blood isolates with special reference to adherent, slime-producing *Staphylococcus epidermidis* strains. Scand J Infect Dis 1991; 23:325–332.

15. Peters G, Schumacher-Perdreau F, Jansen B, Bey M, Pulverer G. Biology of *Staphylococcus epidermidis* extracellular slime. In: Pulverer G, Quie PG, Peters G, eds. Pathogenicity and Clinical Significance of Coagulase-Negative Staphylococci. New York: Gustav Fischer Verlag, 1987:15–32.

16. Schumacher-Perdreau F, Jansen B, Peters G, Pulverer G. Typing of coagulase-negative staphylococci isolated from foreign body infections. Eur J Clin Microbiol Infect Dis 1988; 7:270–273.

17. Van Belkum A, Kluytmans J, van Leeuwen W, et al. Multicenter evaluation of arbitrarily primed PCR for typing of *Staphylococcus aureus* strains. J Clin Microbiol 1995; 33:1537–1547.

18. Goering RV. The application of pulsed field gel electrophoresis to analysis of the global dissemination of methicillin-resistant *Staphylococcus areus*. In: Brun-Buisson C, Casewell MW, El Solh N, Régnier B, eds. Methicillin Resistant Staphylococci. Paris: Flammarion Médecine-Sciences, 1995:76–81.

19. Jansen B, Hartmann C, Schumacher-Perdreau F, Peters G. Late onset endophthalmi-

tis associated with intraocular lens:a case of molecularly proved *Staphylococcus epidermidis* aetiology. Br J Ophthalmol 1991; 75:440–441.

20. Perdreau-Remington F, Stefanik D, Peters G, et al. Microbial ecology of explanted prosthetic hips: a four year prospective study of 52 patients with "aseptic" prosthetic joint loosening. Eur J Clin Microbiol Infect Dis 1996; 15:160–165.

21. Schumacher-Perdreau F, Peters G, Digon-Guzman F, Jansen B, Pulverer G. Incidence of coagulase-negative staphylococci (CNS) in fibrous capsular contracture (FCC) after augmentation mammoplasty with silicone. Interscience Conference on Antimicrobial Agents and Chemotherapy 1988. Abstract 996.

22. Christensen GD, Simpson WA, Bisno AL, Beachey EH. Adherence of slime-producing strains of *Staphylococcus epidermidis* to smooth surfaces. Infect Immun 1982; 37:318–326.

23. Christensen GD, Simpson WA, Younger JJ, et al. Adherence of coagulase-negative staphylococci to plastic tissue culture plates: a quantitative model for the adherence of staphylococci to medical devices. J Clin Microbiol 1985; 22:996–1006.

24. Ludwicka A, Ulenbruck G, Peters G, et al. Investigation on extracellular slime substance produced by *Staphylococcus epidermidis*. Zbl Bakt Hyg I Abt Orig A 1984; 258:256–267.

25. Pfaller M, Davenport D, Bale M, Barrett M, Koontz F, Massanari RM. Development of the quantitative micro-test for slime production by coagulase-negative staphylococci. Eur J Clin Microbiol Infect Dis 1988; 7:30–33.

26. Davenport DS, Masanari RM, Pfaller MA, Bale MJ, Streed SA, Hierholzer WJ Jr. Usefulness of a test for slime production as a marker for clinically significant infections with coagulase-negative staphylococci. J Infect Dis 1986; 153:332–339.

27. Deighton MA, Balkau B. Adherence measured by microtiter assay as a virulence marker for *Staphylococcus epidermidis* infections. J Clin Microbiol 1990; 28:2442–2447.

28. Diaz-Mitoma F, Harding GKM, Hoban DJ, Roberts RS, Low DE. Clinical significance for slime production in ventriculoperitoneal shunt infections caused by coagulase-negative staphylococci. J Infect Dis 1987; 156:555–560.

29. Ishak MA, Gröschel DGM, Mandell GL, Wenzel RP. Association of slime with pathogenicity of coagulase-negative staphylococci causing nosocomial septicemia. J Clin Microbiol 1985; 22:1025–1029.

30. Kotilainen P. Association of coagulase-negative staphylococcal slime production and adherence with the development and outcome of adult septicemias. J Clin Microbiol 1990; 28:2779–2785.

31. Kristinsson KG, Spencer RC, Brown CB. Clinical importance of production of slime by coagulase-negative staphylococci in chronic ambulatory peritoneal dialysis. J Clin Pathol 1986; 39:117–118.

32. Kristinsson KG, Spencer RC, Hastings JG, Brown CB. Slime production by coagulase-negative staphylococci—a major virulence factor? Contrib Nephrol 1987; 57:79–84.

33. Younger JJ, Christensen GD, Bartley DL, Simmons JCH, Barrett FF. Coagulase-negative staphylococci isolated from cerebrospinal fluid shunts: importance of slime production, species identification, and shunt removal to clinical outcome. J Infect Dis 1987; 156:548–554.

34. Locci R, Peters G, Pulverer G. Microbial colonization of prosthetic devices. I. Microtopographical characteristics of intravenous catheters as detected by scanning electron microscopy. Zbl Bakt Hyg I Abt Orig B 1981; 173:285–292.

35. Jansen B, Schumacher-Perdreau F, Peters G, Pulverer G. New aspects in the pathogenesis and prevention of polymer-associated foreign body infections caused by coagulase-negative staphylococci. J Invest Surg 1989; 2:361–380.

36. Franson TR, Sheth NK, Rose HD, Sohnle PG. Scanning electron microscopy of bacteria adherent to intravascular catheters. J Clin Microbiol 1984; 20:500–505.

37. Peters G, Locci R, Pulverer G. Adherence and growth of coagulase-negative staphylococci on surfaces of intravenous catheters. J Infect Dis 1982; 146:479–482.

38. Peters G, Saborowski F, Locci R, Pulverer G. Investigations on staphylococci infection of transvenous endocardial pacemakerelectrodes. Am Heart J 1984; 108:359–365.

39. Marrie TJ, Costerton JW. Scanning and transmission electron microscopy of in situ bacterial colonization of intravenous and intraarterial catheters. J Clin Microbiol 1984; 19:687–693.

40. Marrie TJ, Nelligan J, Costerton JW. A scanning and transmission electron microscope study of an infected pacemaker lead. Circulation 1982; 66:1339–1341.

41. Peters G, Locci R, Pulverer G. Microbial colonization of prosthetic devices. II. Scanning electron microscopy of naturally infected intravenous catheters. Zbl Bakt Hyg I Abt Orig B 1981; 173:293–299.

42. Peters G, Pulverer G. Microbiology of staphylococcal pacemaker lead infection. Clin Prog Electrophysiol Pacing 1986; 4:205–215.

43. Peters G. Adherence and proliferation of bacteria on artificial surfaces. In: Jackson GG, Schlumberger HD, Zeiler HJ, eds. Perspectives in Antiinfective Therapy. Wiesbaden: Friedrich Vieweg & Sohn, 1988:209–215.

44. Dankert J, Hogt AH, Feijen J. Biomedical polymers: bacterial adhesion, colonization and infection. In: Williams DF, ed. Critical Reviews in Biocompatibility. 2nd ed. Boca Raton: CRC Press, 1986:219–301.

45. Espersen F, Wilkinson BJ, Gahrn-Hansen B, Thamdrup Rosdahl V, Clemensen I. Attachment of staphylococci to silicone catheters in vitro. APMIS 1990; 98:471–478.

46. Hogt AH, Dankert J, Hulstaert CE, Feijen J. Cell surface characteristics of coagulase-negative staphylococci and their adherence to fluorinated poly(etylenepropylene). Infect Immun 1986; 51:294–301.

47. Jansen B, Peters G, Pulverer G. Mechanisms and clinical relevance of bacterial adhesion to polymers. J Biomater Appl 1988; 2:520–543.

48. Ludwicka A, Jansen B, Wadström T, Pulverer G. Attachment of staphylococci to various synthetic polymers. Zbl Bakt Hyg I Abt Orig A 1984; 256:479–489.

49. Ludwicka A, Jansen B, Wadström T, Switalski LM, Peters G, Pulverer G. Attachment of staphylococci to various synthetic polymers. In: Shalaby SW, Hoffmann AS, Ratner BD, Horbett TA, eds. Polymers as Biomaterials. New York; Plenum, 1984:241–255.

50. Cottonaro CN, Roohk HV, Shimizu G, Sperling DR. Quantitation and characterization of competitive protein binding to polymers. Transact Am Soc Artif Organs 1981; 27:391–395.

51. Kochwa S, Litwak RS, Rosenfield RE, Leonard EF. Blood elements at foreign surfaces: a biochemical approach to the study of the adsorption of plasma proteins. Ann NY Acad Sci 1977; 283:37–49.

52. Herrmann M, Vaudaux PE, Pittet D, et al. Fibronectin, fibrinogen, and laminin act as mediators of adherence of clinical staphylococcal isolates to foreign material. J Infect Dis 1988; 158:693–701.

53. Pascual A, Fleer A, Westerdaal NAC, Verhoef J. Modulation of adherence of coagulase-negative staphylococci to teflon catheters in vitro. Eur J Clin Microbiol Infect Dis 1986; 5:518–522.

54. Hawiger J, Hammond DK, Timmons S. Human fibrinogen possesses binding site for staphylococci on Aa and Bb polypeptide chains. Nature 1975; 258:643–645.

55. Herrmann M, Suchard SJ, Boxer LA, Waldvogel FA, Lew PD. Thrombospondin binds to *Staphylococcus aureus* and promotes staphylococcal adherence to surfaces. Infect Immun 1991; 59:279–288.

56. Kuusela P. Fibronectin binding to *Staphylococcus aureus*. Nature 1978; 276:718–720.

57. Lopes JD, dos Reis M, Brentani RR. Presence of laminin receptors in *Staphylococcus aureus*. Science 1985; 229:275–277.

58. Mosher DF, Proctor RA. Binding and factor XIIIa-mediated cross-linking of a 27 kilodalton fragment of fibronectin to *Staphylococcus aureus*. Science 1980; 209: 927–929.

59. Paulsson M, Wadström T. Vitronectin and type-I collagen binding by *Staphylococcus aureus* and coagulase-negative staphylococci. FEMS Microbiol Immunol 1990; 65:55–62.

60. Switalski LM, Rydén C, Rubin K, Ljungh A, Hook M, Wadstrom T. Binding of fibronectin to *Staphylococcus* strains. Infect Immun 1983; 42:628–633.

61. Watts JL, Naidu AS, Wadström T. Collagen binding, elastase production, and slime production associated with coagulase-negative staphylococci isolated from bovine intramammary infections. J Clin Microbiol 1990; 28:580–583.

62. Vaudaux PE, Suzuki R, Waldvogel FA, Nydegger UE. Foreign body infection: role of fibronectin as a ligand for the adherence of *Staphylococcus aureus*. J Infect Dis 1984; 150:546–553.

63. Vaudaux PE, Waldvogel FA, Morgenthaler JJ, Nydegger UE. Adsorption of fibronectin onto polymethylmethacrylate and promotion of *Staphylococcus aureus* adherence. Infect Immun 1984; 45:768–774.

64. Vaudaux PE, Pittet D, Haeberli A, et al. Host factors selectively increase staphylococcal adherence on inserted catheters: a role for fibronectin and fibrinogen/fibrin. J Infect Dis 1989; 160:865–875.

65. Muller E, Takeda S, Goldman DA, Pier GB. Blood proteins do not promote adherence of coagulase-negative staphylococci to biomaterials. Infect Immun 1991; 59:3323–3326.

66. Kojima Y, Tojo M, Goldmann DA, Tosteson TD, Pier GB. Antibody to the capsular polysaccharide/adhesin protects rabbits against catheter-related bacteremia due to coagulase-negative staphylococci. J Infect Dis 1990; 162:435–441.

67. Tojo M, Yamashita DA, Goldman DA, Pier GD. Isolation and characterization of a

capsular polysaccharide adhesin from *Staphylococcus epidermidis*. J Infect Dis 1988; 157:713–722.

68. Timmermann CP, Besnier JM, de Graaf L, et al. Characterisation and functional aspects of monoclonal antibodies specific for surface proteins of coagulase-negative staphylococci. J Med Microbiol 1991; 35:65–71.

69. Timmermann CP, Fleer A, Besnier JM, de Graaf L, Cremers F, Verhoef J. Characterization of a proteinaceous adhesion of *Staphylococcus epidermidis* which mediates attachment to polystyrene. Infect Immun 1991; 59:4187–4192.

70. Heilmann C, Gerke C, Perdreau-Remington F, Götz F. Characterization of Tn917 insertion mutants of *Staphylococcus epidermidis* affected in biofilm formation. Infect Immun 1996; 64:277–282.

71. Mack D, Siemssen N, Laufs R. Parallel induction by glucose of adherence and a polysaccharide antigen specific for plastic-adherent *Staphylococcus epidermidis*. Infect Immun 1992; 60:2048–2057.

72. Mack D, Fischer W, Krokotsch A, et al. The intercellular adhesin involved in biofilm accumulation of *Staphylococcus epidermidis* is a linear b-1,6-linked glucosaminoglykan: purification and structural analysis. J Bacteriol 1996; 178:175–183.

73. Schumacher-Perdreau F, Stefanik D, Hasbach H, Jansen B, Peters G. Description of a slime negative mutant of *Staphylococcus epidermidis*. Annual Meeting, American Society for Microbiology 1990. Abstract D-111.

74. Schumacher-Perdreau F, Heilmann C, Peters G, Götz F, Pulverer G. Comparative analysis of a biofilm forming *Staphylococcus epidermidis* strain and its adhesion-positive, accumulation-negative isogenic mutant. FEMS Microbiol Lett 1994; 117: 71–78.

75. Christensen GD, Barker LP, Mawhinney TP, Baddour LM, Simpson WA. Identification of an antigenic marker of slime production for *Staphylococcus epidermidis*. Infect Immun 1990; 58:2906–2911.

76. Bayston R, Penny SR. Excessive production of mucoid substance in *Staphylococcus* SII A, a possible factor in colonization of Holter shunts. Dev Med Child Neurol 1972; 14(suppl):25–28.

77. Bayston R, Rodgers J. Production of extra-cellular slime by *Staphylococcus epidermidis* during stationary phase of growth: its association with adherence to implantable devices. J Clin Pathol 1990; 43:866–870.

78. Drewry DT, Galbraith L, Wilkinson BJ, Wilkinson SG. Staphylococcal slime: a cautionary tale. J Clin Microbiol 1990; 28:1292–1296.

79. Hussain M, Hastings JGM, White PJ. A chemically defined medium for slime production by coagulase-negative staphylococci. J Med Microbiol 1991; 34:143–147.

80. Hussain M, Hastings JGM, White PJ. Isolation and composition of the extracellular slime made by coagulase-negative staphylococci in a chemically defined medium. J Infect Dis 1991; 163:534–541.

81. Schmidt DD, Bandyk DF, Pequet AJ, Malangoni MA, Towne JB. Mucin production by *Staphylococcus epidermidis:* a virulence factor promoting adherence to vascular grafts. Arch Surg 1986; 121:89–95.

82. Ohshima Y, Schumacher-Perdreau F, Peters G, Quie PG, Pulverer G. Antiphagocyt-

ic effect of the capsule of *Staphylococcus simulans*. Infect Immun 1990; 58:1350–1354.

83. Christensen GD, Baddour LM, Simpson WA. Phenotypic variation of *Staphylococcus epidermidis* slime production in vitro and in vivo. Infect Immun 1987; 55:2870–2877.

84. Kotilainen P, Maki J, Oksman P, Viljanen MK, Nikoskelainen J, Huovinen P. Immunochemical analysis of the extracellular slime substance of *Staphylococcus epidermidis*. Eur J Clin Microbiol Infect Dis 1990; 9:262–270.

85. Quie PG, Belani KK. Coagulase-negative staphylococcal adherence and persistence. J Infect Dis 1987; 156:543–547.

86. Johnson GM, Carparas LS, Peters G. Slime production enhances resistance of *Staphylococcus epidermidis* to phagocytic killing: interference with opsonization and oxidative burst. Pediatr Res 1989; 25:181A.

87. Johnson GM, Lee PE, Regelmann WE, Gray ED, Peters G, Quie PG. Interference with granulocyte function by *Staphylococcus epidermidis* slime. Infect Immun 1986; 54:13–20.

88. Johnson GM, Regelmann WE, Gray ED, Peters G, Quie PG. *S. epidermidis* slime effects on neutrophil oxidative burst and adherence. Evidence of membrane and receptor interactions. Spring Meeting of the American Pediatric Society/Society for Pediatric Research, San Francisco, 1987. Abstract.

89. Johnson CM, Regelmann WE, Gray ED, Peters G, Quie PG. Staphylococcal slime and host-defenses—effects on polymorphonuclear granulocytes. In: Pulverer G, Quie PG, Peters G, eds. Pathogenicity and Clinical Significance of Coagulase-Negative Staphylococci. New York: Gustav Fischer Verlag, 1987:33–44.

90. Peters G, Gray ED, Johnson GM. Immunomodulating properties of extracellular slime substance. In: Bisno AL, Waldvogel FA, eds. Infections Associated With Indwelling Medical Devices. Washington, DC: American Society for Microbiology, 1989:61–74.

91. Regelmann WE, Gray ED, Thomas P, Peters G. *Staphylococcus epidermidis* slime effects on bacterial opsonization and PMN leucocyte function. Pediatr Res 1984; 18 (part 2):1131.

92. Schumacher-Perdreau F, Peters G, Pulverer G, Quie PG. Effect of cell wall components and extracellular slime substance of *S. epidermidis* on the chemiluminescence of human polymorphonuclear granulocytes. 3rd European Congress of Clinical Microbiology, 1987. Abstract 61.

93. Zimmerli W, Lew PD, Waldvogel FA. Pathogenesis of foreign body infection. Evidence for a local granulocyte defec. J Clin Invest 1984; 73:1191–1200.

94. Kristinsson KG, Hastings JG, Spencer RC. The role of extracellular slime in opsonophagocytosis of *Staphylococcus epidermidis*. J Med Microbiol 1988; 27:207–213.

95. Lee DA, Hoidal JR, Clawson CC, Quie PG, Peterson PK. Phagocytosis by polymorphonuclear leukocytes of *Staphylococcus aureus* and *Pseudomonas aeruginosa* adherent to plastic, agar, or glass. J Immunol Methods 1983; 63:103–114.

96. Schumacher-Perdreau F, Peters G, Jansen B, Pulverer G. A new model for evaluation of phagocytosis of catheter surface grown coagulase-negative staphylococci (CNS)

by human granulocytes (PMN). 4th European Congress of Clinical Microbiology, 1989. Abstract 380.

97. Gray ED, Peters G, Verstegen M, Regelmann WE. Effect of extracellular slime substance from *Staphylococcus epidermidis* on the human cellular immune response. Lancet 1984; 1:365–367.

98. Gray ED, Regelmann WE, Peters G. Staphylococcal slime and host defenses—effects on lymophocytes and immune function. In: Pulverer G, Quie PG, Peters G, eds. Pathogenicity and Clinical Significance of Coagulase-Negative Staphylococci. New York: Gustav Fischer Verlag, 1987:45–54.

99. Stout RD, Ferguson KP, Yi-Ning L, Lambe DW. Staphylococcal eopolysaccharides inhibit lymphocyte proliferative responses by activation of monocyte proliferative responses by activation of monocyte prostaglandin production. Infect Immun 1992; 60:922–927.

100. Stout RD, Miller AR, Lambe DW. Staphylococcal glycocalix activates macrophage prostaglandin E2 and interleukin 1 production and modulates tumor necrosis factor a and nitric oxide production. Infect Immun 1994; 62:4160–4166.

101. Elliott TS, D'Abrera VC, Dutton S. The effect of antibiotics on bacterial colonisation of vascular cannulae in a novel in-vitro model. J Med Microbiol 1988; 26:229–235.

102. Evans RC, Holmes CJ. Effect of vancomycin hydrochloride on *Staphylococcus epidermidis* biofilm associated with silicone elastomer. Antimicrob Agents Chemother 1987; 31:889–894.

103. Christina AG, Hobgood CD, Webb LX, Myrvik QN. Adhesive colonization of biomaterials and antibiotic resistance. Biomaterials 1987; 8:423–426.

104. Sheth NK, Franson TR, Sohnle PG. Influence of bacterial adherence to intravascular catheters on in vitro antibiotic susceptibility. Lancet 1985; II:1266–1268.

105. Schumacher-Perdreau F, Bey M, Peters G, Jansen B, Pulverer G. Extracellular slime substance (ESS) of *S. epidermidis* inhibits gentamicin uptake into the staphylococcal cells. Annual Meeting, American Society for Microbiology, 1988. Abstract B 223.

106. Farber BF, Kaplan MH, Clogston AG. *Staphylococcus epidermidis* extracted slime inhibits the antimicrobial action of glycopeptide antibiotics. J Infect Dis 1990; 161:37–40.

107. Zimmerli W, Waldvogel FA, Vaudaux PE, Nydegger UE. Pathogenesis of foreign body infection: description and characteristics of an animal model. J Infect Dis 1982; 146:487–497.

108. Takeda J, Pier GB, Kojima Y, et al. Protection against endocarditis due to *Staphylococcus epidermidis* by immunization with capsular polysaccharide/adhesin. Circulation 1991; 84:2539–2546.

109. Shiro H, Muller E, Guttierez N, et al. Transposon mutants of *Staphylococcus epidermidis* deficient in elaboration of capsular polysaccharide/adhesin and slime are avirulent in a rabbit model of endocarditis. J Infect Dis 1994; 169:1042–1049.

110. Christensen GD, Simpson WA, Bisno AL, Beachey EH. Experimental foreign-body infections in mice challenged with slime-producing *Staphylococcus epidermidis*. Infect Immun 1983; 40:407–410.

111. Patrick CC, Plaunt R, Hetherington SV, May SM. Role of the *Staphylococcus epidermidis* slime layer in experimental tunnel tract infections. Infect Immun 1992; 60:1363–1367.
112. Gallimore B, Gagnon RF, Subang R, Richards GK. Natural history of chronic *Staphylococcus epidermidis* foreign body infection in a mouse model. J Infect Dis 1991; 164:1220–1223.
113. Baddour LM, Christensen GD, Schadow KH. The effect of slime production on vancomycin efficacy in the treatment of experimental endocarditis due to *Staphylococcus epidermidis*. J Antimicrob Chemother 1989; 24:365–373.
114. Steckelberg JM, Keating MR, Rouse MS, Wilson WR. Lack of extracellular slime effect on treatment outcome of *Staphylococcus epidermidis* experimental endocarditis. J Antimicrob Chemother 1989; 23:117–121.
115. Chambers HF, Schumacher-Perdreau F, Wilcox MH, Peters G, Sande MA, Pulverer G. *Staphylococcus epidermidis* wild type and its slime-negative mutant equally induce endocarditis in rabbits. Interscience Conference on Antimicrobial Agents and Chemotherapy, 1993. Abstract 148.
116. Widmer AF. IV-related infections. In: Wenzel RPB, ed. Prevention and Control of Nosocomial Infections. Baltimore: Williams and Wilkins, 1993:556–579.
117. Moyer MA, Edwards LD, Farley L. Comparative culture methods on 101 intravenous catheters. Routine, semiquantitative, and blood cultures. Arch Intern Med 1983; 143:66–69.
118. Armstrong CW, Mayhall G, Miller KB, et al. Clinical predictors of infection of central venous catheters used for total parenteral nutrition. Infect Control Hosp Epidemiol 1990; 11:71–78.
119. Raad II, Baba M, Bodey GP. Diagnosis of catheter-related infections: the role of surveillance and targeted quantitative skin cultures. Clin Infect Dis 1995; 20:593–597.
120. Guidet B, Nicola I, Barakett V, et al. Skin versus hub cultures to predict colonization and infection of central venous catheter in intensive care patients. Infection 1994; 22:43–48.
121. Colligon PG, Soni N, Pearson IY, Woods WP, Munro R, Sorrell TC. Is semiquantitative culture of central vein catheter tips useful in the diagnosis of catheter-associated bacteremia? J Clin Microbiol 1986; 24:532–535.
122. Moyer MA, Edwards LD, Farley L. Comparative culture methods on 101 intravenous catheters. Arch Intern Med 1983; 143:66–69.
123. Snydman DR, Murray SA, Kornfeld SJ, Majka JA, Ellis CA. Total parenteral nutrition-related infections: prospective epidemiologic study using semiquantitative methods. Am J Med 1982; 73:695–699.
124. Cleri DJ, Corrado ML, Seligman SJ. Quantitative culture of intravenous catheters and other intravascular inserts. J Infect Dis 1980; 141:781–786.
125. Bjornson HS, Colley R, Bower RH, Duty VP, Schwartz-Pulton JT, Fisher JE. Association between microorganism growth at the catheter insertion site and colonization of the catheter in patients receiving total parenteral nutrition. Surgery 1982; 92:720–726.
126. Brun-Buisson C, Abrouk F, Legrand P, Huet Y, Larabi S, Rapin M. Diagnosis of cen-

tral venous catheter-related sepsis: critical level of quantitative tip cultures. Arch Intern Med 1987; 147:873–877.

127. Sherertz RJ, Raad II, Balani A, et al. Three-year experience with sonicated vascular catheter cultures in a clinical microbiology laboratory. J Clin Microbiol 1990; 28: 76–82.

128. Snydman DR, Pober BR, Murray SA, Gorbea HF, Majka JA, Perry LK. Predictive value of surveillance skin cultures in total parenteral nutrition-related infections. Lancet 1982; 2:1385–1388.

129. Fan ST, Teoh-Tchan CH, Lau KF. Predictive value of surveillance skin and hub cultures in central venous catheter sepsis. J Hosp Infect 1988; 12:191–198.

130. Cercenado EJ, Rodriguez-Creixems M. A conservative procedure for the diagnosis of catheter-related infections. Arch Intern Med 1990; 150:1417–1420.

131. Corona ML, Peters SG, Narr BJ, Thompson RL. Infections related to central venous catheters. Mayo Clin Proc 1990; 65:979–986.

132. Nitenberg G, Antoun S, Escudier B, Leclercq B. Complications infectieuses liées aux abords veineux centraux. In: Nitenberg G, Cordonnier C, eds. Infections Graves en Onco-Hématologie. Paris: Masson, 1991:55–73.

133. Raad II, Bodey GP. Infectious complications of indwelling vascular catheters. Clin Infect Dis 1992; 15:197–208.

134. Clarke DE, Raffin TA. Infectious complications of indwelling long-term central venous catheters. Chest 1990; 97:966–972.

135. Hampton AA, Sherertz RJ. Vascular-access infections in hospitalized patients. Surg Clin North Am 1988; 68:57–71.

136. Cobb DK, High KP, Sawyer RG, et al. A controlled trial of scheduled replacement of central venous and pulmonary-artery catheters. N Engl J Med 1992; 327:1062–1068.

137. Rushforth JA, Hoy CM, Kite P, Puntis JW. Rapid diagnosis of central venous catheter sepsis. Lancet 1993; 342:402–403.

138. Fan ST, Teoh-Tchan CH, Lau KF. Evaluation of central venous catheter sepsis by differential quantitative blood cultures. Eur J Clin Microbiol Infect Dis 1989; 8:142–144.

139. Paya CV, Guerra L, Marsh HM, Farnell MB, Washington J II, Thompson RL. Limited usefulness of quantitative culture of blood drawn through the device for diagnosis of intravascular-device-related bacteremia. J Clin Microbiol 1989; 27:1431–1433.

140. Douard MC, Clementi E, Arlet G, et al. Negative catheter-tip culture and diagnosis of catheter-related bacteremia. Nutrition 1994; 10:397–404.

141. Flynn PM, Shenep JL, Barret FF. Differential quantitation with a commercial blood culture tube for diagnosis of catheter-related infection. J Clin Microbiol 1988; 26:1045–1046.

142. Raucher HS, Hyatt AC, Barzilai A, et al. Quantitative blood cultures in the evaluation of septicemia in children with Broviac catheters. J Pediatr 1984; 104: 29–33.

143. Flynn PM, Shenep JL, Stokes DC, Barrett FF. In situ management of confirmed central venous catheter-related bacteremia. Pediatr Infect Dis J 1987; 6:729–734.

144. Mosca R, Curtas S, Forbes B, Meguid MM. The benefits of isolator cultures in the management of suspected catheter sepsis. Surgery 1987; 102:718–723.
145. Garner JS, Jarvis WR, Emori TG, Horan TC, Hughes JM. CDC definition for nosocomial infections. Am J Infect Control 1988; 16:128–140.
146. Maslow JN, Slutsky AM, Arbeit R. Application of pulsed-field gel electrophoresis to molecular epidemiology. In: Persing DH, Smith TF, Tenover FC, White TJ, eds. Diagnostic Molecular Microbiology: Principles and Applications. Washington, DC: American Society for Microbiology, 1993:563–572.
147. Pollack PF, Kadder M, Byrne WJ, et al. One hundred patient years' experience with the Broviac silastic catheter for central venous nutrition. J Parenter Enteral Nutr 1981; 5:32–36.
148. Ladefoged K, Efsen F, Christoffersen JK, et al. Long-term parenteral nutrition in catheter-related complications. Scand J Gastroenterol 1981; 16:913–919.
149. Riella MC, Scribner BH. Five years' experience with a right atrial catheter for prolonged parenteral nutrition at home. Surg Gynecol Obstet 1976; 143:205–208.
150. Wang EEL, Prober CG, Ford-Jones L, Gold R. The management of central intravenous catheter infections. Pediatr Infect Dis J 1984; 3:110–113.
151. Hiemenz J, Skelton J, Pizzo PA. Perspective on the management of catheter-related infections in cancer patients. Pediatr Infect Dis J 1986; 5:6–11.
152. Benezra D, Kiehn TE, Gold JW, Brown AE, Turnbull AD, Armstrong D. Prospective study of infections in indwelling central venous catheters using quantitative blood cultures. Am J Med 1988; 85(4):495–498.
153. Karmochkine M, Brunet F, Lanore JJ, et al. Recovery from staphylococcal septicaemia in neutropenic patients without removal of the previously inserted central venous catheter. Eur J Med 1993; 2(3):143–147.
154. Messing B, Thuillier F, Alain S, et al. Traitement par verrou local d'antibiotique des infections bactériennes liées aux cathéters centraux en nutrition parentérale. Nutr Clin Metabol 1991; 5:105–112.
155. Messing B, Peitra-Cohen S, Debure A, Beliah M, Bernier J-J. Antibiotic-lock technique: a new approach to optimal therapy for catheter-related sepsis in home-parenteral nutrition patients. J Parenter Enteral Nutr 1988; 12:185–189.
156. Douard MC, Leverger G, Paulien R, et al. Quantitative blood cultures for diagnosis and management of catheter-related sepsis in pediatric hematology and oncology patients. Intens Care Med 1991; 17:30–35.
157. Krzywda EA, Gotoff RA, Andris DA, Marciniak TF, Edmiston CE, Quebbeman EJ. Antibiotic lock treatment: impact on catheter salvage and cost savings. 35th Interscience Conference on Antimicrobial Agents and Chemotherapy, San Francisco, 1995. Abstract J4.
158. Longuet P, Douard MC, Maslo C, Benoit C, Arlet G, Leport C. Limited efficacy of antibiotic lock technique in catheter related bacteremia of totally implanted ports in HIV infected and oncologic patients. 35th Interscience Conference on Antimicrobial Agents and Chemotherapy, San Francisco, 1995. Abstract J5.
159. Jones GR, Konsler GK, Dunaway RP, Lacey SR, Azizkhan RG. Prospective analysis of urokinase in the treatment of catheter sepsis in pediatric hematology-oncology patients. J Pediatr Surg 1993; 28:350–357.

160. Schuman ES, Winters V, Gross GF, Hayes JF. Management of Hickman catheter sepsis. Am J Surg 1985; 149:627–628.
161. Norwood S, Jenkins G. An evaluation of triple-lumen catheter infections using a guidewire exchange technique. J Trauma 1990; 30:706–712.
162. Senagore A, Waller JD, Bonell BW, Bursch LR, Scholten DJ. Pulmonary artery catheterization: a prospective study of internal jugular and subclavian approaches. Crit Care Med 1987; 15:35–37.
163. Blake PG, Huraib S, Wu G, Uldall PR. The use of dual lumen jugular venous catheters as definitive long term access for hemodialysis. Int J Artif Organs 1990; 13:26–31.
164. Carlisle EJ, Blake PG, McCarthy F, Vas S, Uldall R. Septicemia in long-term jugular hemodialysis catheters: eradicating infection by changing the catheter over a guidewire. Int J Artif Organs 1991; 14:150–153.
165. Isenberg HD, Cleri DJ. Comparaison de l'utilisation des cathéters mono et multi-lumiepres. Limite de la technique d'échange du cathéter sur guide métallique. Nutr Clin Metabol 1991; 5:73–80.
166. Pettigrew RA, Lang SD, Haydock DA, Parry BR, Bremner DA, Hill GL. Catheter-related sepsis in patients on intravenous nutrition: a prospective study of quantitative catheter cultures and guidewire changes for suspected sepsis. Br J Surg 1985; 72: 52–55.
167. Johnson CW, Miller DL, Ognibene FP. Acute pulmonary emboli associated with guidewire change of a central venous catheter. Intens Care Med 1991; 17:115–117.
168. Mermel LA, Maki DG. Infectious complications of Swan-Ganz pulmonary artery catheters. Am J Respir Crit Care Med 1994; 149:1020–1036.
169. Locci R, Peters G, Pulverer G. Microbial colonization of prosthetic devices. III. Adhesion of staphylococci to lumina of intravenous catheters perfused with bacterial suspensions. Zbl Bakt Hyg I Abt Orig B 1981; 173:300–307.

5

Catheter-Related Infections Due to Gram-Negative Bacilli

Harald Seifert

Institute of Medical Microbiology and Hygiene, University of Cologne,
Cologne, Germany

I. INTRODUCTION

The past two decades have witnessed a marked change of the distribution of pathogens reported to cause nosocomial bloodstream infections (BSI) (1–3). There was a constant increase in the proportion of gram-positive versus gram-negative organisms implicated in nosocomial BSI, and this shift was mainly due to significant increases of infections with coagulase-negative staphylococci (CoNS), *Staphylococcus aureus*, and enterococci (4,5). These organisms currently account for over 40% of the recovered bloodstream pathogens (3). A considerable part of these infections is associated with the increasing use of intravascular catheters.

The problem of bacteremia caused by aerobic gram-negative bacilli has received less attention in the recent literature. Little is known, in particular, about the impact of gram-negative bacilli associated with device-related infections. This holds true with regard to the factors involved in the pathogenesis of catheter-related infections (CRI) since the vast majority of studies investigating the pathogenesis of foreign body infections have focused on gram-positive organisms (6).

There is an ever increasing number of gram-negative species causing infections due to indwelling devices (7). This chapter attempts to summarize the current knowledge of gram-negative microorganisms as a cause of CRI, their contribution to infections due to specific devices, and specific considerations regarding the pathogenesis and management of CRI due to gram-negative bacilli. It will focus on CRI due to three major groups of gram-negative organisms: members of the family Enterobacteriaceae, *Pseudomonas aeruginosa*, and *Acinetobacter* spp. CRI due to other gram-negative organisms such as nonaeruginosa pseudomonads and other nonfermenting gram-negative bacilli is covered in Chapter 7, "Miscellaneous Organisms."

II. EPIDEMIOLOGY

A. General Aspects—Source of Data

Since only very few studies have specifically addressed the issues related to CRI caused by gram-negative bacilli, it is difficult to obtain the necessary data from the literature. Various studies have analyzed the epidemiology of BSI in different settings and in different types of hospitals (1,8–10). Other investigators have focused on nosocomial bacteremia (11,12); polymicrobial bacteremia (13); bacteremia in specific patient populations such as cancer patients (7,14), critically ill patients (12), and burn patients (15,16); bacteremia of unknown origin (17); BSI due to gram-negative organisms in general (18,19) or due to specific gram-negative pathogens such as *Acinetobacter* spp. (20), Enterobacteriaceae (21–24), and *P. aeruginosa* (25–27). Information regarding CRI due to gram-negative bacilli may also be derived from retrospective or prospective studies that specifically address device-related infections (14,28–30). Both approaches, however, have major limitations. The various reports on bacteremia and BSI in different epidemiological settings provide information of the epidemiology of the microorganisms involved, patient characteristics, and mortality, and often include also the presumed sources or portals of entry of the bacteremia. However, the vast majority of these retrospective case series have not employed stringent definitions and microbiological methods to accurately identify a device as the cause of bacteremia. If a pathogen is recovered from the bloodstream but not concomitantly from a distant site including an indwelling vascular catheter, bacteremia is usually considered of unknown origin. This may lead to an underestimate of catheter-related BSI since catheters are often removed but not always cultured if signs and symptoms of sepsis evolve.

Prospective clinical studies of CRI that have addressed different issues such as different types of catheters and catheter design (30,31), antibiotic bonding (32), different types of dressings (33), and the consequences (34) and the prevention of these infections (35,36) also suffer from the different definitions and microbiological methods used by different investigators. In addition, device-related infections due to gram-negative bacilli have only rarely been analyzed separately with regard to their specific contribution to morbidity and mortality as well as to their specific management problems, and the reported numbers of these infections are usually too small to allow for statistical evaluation.

Consequently, the data presented in this review that are obtained from different types of studies published over a period as long as two decades may aid to cope with the special problem posed by CRI due to gram-negative bacilli. However, prospective clinical studies are needed that address the specific issues related to these infections in more detail.

B. Catheter-Related Bacteremia Due to Gram-Negative Organisms

Kreger et al. evaluated 612 episodes of gram-negative bacteremia over the 10-year period 1965 to 1974 (18). The urinary tract was the most frequent source of bacteremia, and *Escherichia coli* was the most frequent etiologic agent. The source of bacteremia remained unknown in 30% of cases, but intravascular catheters were not implicated. Bryan and co-workers studied 1186 episodes of gram-negative bacteremia over a 5-year period 1977 to 1981 (19). Again, intravascular devices as a source of bacteremia were not evaluated. In a study of 500 episodes of clinically significant bacteremia and fungemia conducted by Weinstein and collegues (9), gram-negative bacteremia arose mainly from genitourinary, respiratory, and gastrointestinal sources; in only five episodes (2%) was an intravascular catheter the definite source of bacteremia. However, a portal of entry could not be identified in nearly one-third of episodes.

In more recent series, 30% to 40% of all bacteremias were due to members of the family Enterobacteriaceae or to *P. aeruginosa* and related genera (8,10). In a 3-year study of positive blood cultures Roberts et al. found that of 1504 isolates from 1244 episodes of clinically significant bacteremia, 727 (47%) were gram-negative bacilli (10). The urinary tract was the most frequent portal of entry, accounting for 16% of episodes; an intravascular catheter was considered the source of bacteremia in 8%; and the source remained unknown for another 9%. The proportion of gram-negative bacilli causing CRI is not reported. Mortality for cases of bacteremia from intravascular sources was 20%. Similar results were reported from Geerdes et al. (8). Among 980 episodes of both community- and hospital-acquired clinically significant bacteremia, 159 (16%) were related to intravascular devices; 10% of these were due to gram-negative organisms.

However, the incidence and causative agents of intravascular-device-related infections may vary considerably with the patient population studied and the methods and definitions employed. Using strict criteria, Kiehn and Armstrong investigated the spectrum of organisms causing 933 episodes of bacteremia and fungemia associated with surgically implanted intravascular devices in immunocompromised patients (7). Fifty percent of bacteremic episodes in these patients were vascular access-related; 46% of these were caused by gram-negative organisms. Among the major organism groups, the percentages of septic episodes that were device-related were 44% for Enterobacteriaceae and 69% for *P. aeruginosa*. In a recent study of the incidence of bacteremia in organ transplant patients, gram-negative bacilli constituted 47% of the pathogens found in 125 cases of clinically significant bacteremia. The most common portals of entry were the abdominal site (18%) and the urinary tract (15%). Only 6% of bacteremias were attributed to intravascular catheters; the source was unidentified in 38% (37).

Bacteremia is reported to be polymicrobial in 6% to 14% of cases and is most often associated with increased mortality (38,39). In a recent review extending over 17 years, polymicrobial bacteremia due to gram-negative bacilli most commonly occurred in intra-abdominal, urinary tract, and wound infections, whereas catheters were the presumed source of infection in only 3% to 5% (38,39). Conversely, in a prospective study of polymicrobial bacteremia in ICU patients that employed adequate microbiologic methods to detect catheter-related bacteremia, intravascular devices (43%) were the most common source of polymicrobial bacteremia (13). Catheter replacement in patients who develop polymicrobial bacteremia was therefore suggested by the authors.

C. Infections Due to Gram-Negative Bacilli Related to Specific Devices

The incidence and etiologic organisms of intravascular-device related infections may be strongly influenced by the type and intended use of the device. The rate of infections related to different intravascular devices may range from < 0.2% for small peripheral catheters to > 50% for central venous catheters (CVCs) used in burn patients (15,40). Infections related to specific devices are dealt with in the respective chapters in this book. Herein, the incidence of gram-negative bacilli as causative agents of CRI is summarized for different types of intravascular catheters.

1. Devices Used for Short-Term Vascular Access

a. Peripheral Intravenous Catheters

The lowest rates of infection are now with small peripheral intravenous catheters. The risk for bacteremia due to these devices is very low (< 0.2%). Gram-negative bacteria are rarely implicated and usually range in frequency between 0% and 4% (41–43). In a prospective study by Richet and co-workers, however, 28% of the pathogens isolated from peripheral catheters were gram-negative bacilli (28).

b. Nontunneled Central Venous Catheters

Nontunneled, percutaneously inserted CVCs are the most commonly used central catheters and account for the majority of catheter-related bloodstream infections. Prospective studies investigating the epidemiology, associated risk factors, and means for prevention of infections related to these devices have found rates of catheter-related BSI in the range of 3% to 5% (36,44,45).

In a prospective study, Gil and collegues found gram-negative organisms in 22 of 41 (54%) colonized catheters and in 6 of 11 (55%) associated bacteremias (30). Other investigators reported gram-negative bacilli implicated in CRI to

Table 1   Frequency of Gram-Negative Organisms Associated With Central
Venous Catheters Compiled From Recent Studies

	Haslett et al. (46)	Yeung et al. (45)	Gil et al. (30)	Eyer et al. (44)	Richet et al. (28)	Sheretz et al. (29)
No. of isolates recovered	76	42	41	43	123	1032
Gram-negative bacilli (%)	17 (22)	5 (12)	22 (54)	18 (42)	32 (26)	287 (28)
E. coli[a]	0	0	1 (5)	1 (6)	0	40 (14)
Enterobacter spp.	5 (29)	0	2 (10)	6 (33)	2 (6)	45 (16)
Klebsiella spp.	2 (12)	2 (40)	3 (14)	3 (17)	5 (16)	18 (6)
Serratia spp.	1 (6)	1 (20)	4 (19)	0	2 (6)	19 (7)
P. aeruginosa	5 (29)	0	6 (29)	4 (22)	13 (41)	143 (50)
Acinetobacter spp.	4 (24)	1 (20)	4 (19)	1 (5)	4 (13)	12 (4)

[a]Percent of gram-negative isolates.

range between 12% and 42% (28,29,44–46). *P. aeruginosa, Enterobacter* spp., *S. marcescens, K. pneumoniae,* and *Acinetobacter* spp. were the organisms most frequently encountered among gram-negative isolates. The results of several studies are summarized in Table 1.

c.   Pulmonary Artery (PA) Catheters

Flow-directed Swan-Ganz pulmonary artery (PA) catheters are widely used for hemodynamic monitoring of critically ill patients. The infectious complications of PA catheters have been reviewed by Mermel and Maki (47). The incidence of PA catheter-related BSI has been estimated to be in the range of one case of bacteremia per 100 catheters. CoNS were recovered from more than half of colonized catheters but only from one-third of catheter-related BSI. Gram-negative enteric bacilli were recovered from 20% of colonized catheters and from 11% of associated BSI, whereas *P. aeruginosa* accounted for 5% of colonized catheters and 5% of catheter-related BSI.

d.   Arterial Catheters

Arterial pressure monitoring has become indispensible in modern hospital care predominantly for ICU patients. In a prospective study of 130 arterial catheters used for hemodynamic monitoring, 23 (18%) produced local infection and five (3.8%) produced associated BSI (48). *Candida* spp. (31%), gram-negative bacilli (17%), and enterococci (17%) predominated in these infections; three of five bacteremias (60%) were due to Enterobacteriaceae. With more frequent replacement of the monitoring system, the risk of endemic BSI associated with arterial catheters used for hemodynamic monitoring has more recently been estimated to be in the range of 1% (40). One specific feature of these devices is that they have been frequently associated with epidemic BSI. Donowitz et al. investigated an outbreak of *S. marcescens* bacteremia and demonstrated the presence of the epidemic organism on all in-use transducer heads (49). The authors postulated transmission of bacteria from the hands of hospital personnel into the fluid column of the device during manipulation of the system. Beck-Sague and Jarvis reviewed 24 outbreaks of nosocomial BSI investigated by the Centers for Disease Control (50). Intravascular pressure monitoring devices were implicated as the source of infection in eight (33%) outbreaks, seven of which were due to gram-negative bacilli. In all outbreaks, improperly disinfected reusable transducers served as reservoirs.

2. Devices Used for Long-Term Vascular Access

a. Tunneled Central Venous Catheters

Surgically implanted silicone elastomer catheters, including Hickmans, Broviacs, Groshongs, and Quintons, have revolutionized the management of patients requiring prolonged central venous access, particularly for chemotherapy, total parenteral nutrition (TPN), and hemodialysis. The risk of infection due to these catheters is significantly lower than that reported with use of nontunneled catheters and has been estimated to be in the range of 0.2% bacteremias per 100 catheter-days (51,52).

Decker and Edwards reviewed 13 studies of BSIs associated with Broviac catheters in pediatric patients and found gram-negative bacilli as the etiologic agents in 28%, with *Klebsiella* spp., *E. coli*, and *Enterobacter* spp. the predominating organisms (53). Local infections such as exit site and tunnel infections in these patients were even more frequently due to gram-negative rods (41% of all organisms recovered). In adult patients with surgically implanted CVCs of the Hickman/Broviac type, the frequency of gram-negative bacteria involved in catheter-related BSI ranged from 26% to 55% (14,54–56). The results of several studies are summarized in Table 2. Gram-negative bacilli were also responsible for 12 of 23 (52%) exit site infections and for 12 of 20 (60%) tunnel infections reported by Benerza et al. (54). *P. aeruginosa* was the most common isolate (44%) from exit site infections reported by Johnson et al. (56). It was suggested that one reason for the predominance of waterborne organisms such as *P. aeruginosa* may have been related to the fact that patients were not restricted from bathing or swimming.

b. Totally Implantable Intravascular Devices (TIDs)

Surgically implanted subcutaneous ports have the lowest reported rates of catheter-related BSI among long-term catheters (14,57). In one of the largest prospective studies of the infectious complications associated with long-term vascular access devices involving 1431 cancer patients, Groeger et al. (14) demonstrated a risk of 0.21 infections per 1000 device-days for TIDs vs. 2.8 for central venous catheters.

Table 2 Frequency of Gram-Negative Organisms Associated With Long-Term Catheters Compiled From Recent Studies

	Johnson et al. (56)		Benerza et al. (54)		Decker et al. (53)[b]		Groeger et al. (14)		Rotstein et al. (55)	
	I[a]	II[a]	I	II	I	II	I	II	I	II
Total number of isolates recovered	47	27	37	43	326	100	346	60	148	99
Gram-negative bacilli[c]	19 (40)	15 (56)	18 (49)	25 (58)	91 (28)	41 (41)	191 (55)	12 (20)	38 (26)	16 (16)
E. coli[d]	4 (21)	0	0	0	16 (18)	5 (12)			11 (29)	3 (19)
Enterobacter spp.	4 (21)	1 (7)	7 (39)	0	12 (13)	5 (12)			5 (13)	2 (13)
Klebsiella spp.	2 (11)	0	0	0	16 (18)	9 (22)			4 (11)	1 (6)
Serratia spp.	0	0	0	0	1 (1)	0			2 (5)	1 (6)
P. aeruginosa	3 (16)	12 (80)	8 (44)	23 (92)	10 (11)	16 (39)	23 (12)		9 (24)	7 (44)
Acinetobacter spp.	3 (16)	1 (7)	3 (17)	0	9 (10)	5 (12)			3 (8)	0

[a]Number (%) of isolates recovered from (I) bacteremia or (II) local (exit site or tunnel) infection.
[b]Compiles 13 studies.
[c]Number (%) of isolates.
[d]Number (%) of gram-negative isolates.

The predominant organisms isolated in catheter-related bacteremia were gram-negative bacilli (55%); in port-related bacteremia gram-positive cocci (65%) were recovered more frequently than gram-negative organisms (21%).

D. Bloodstream Infections Due to Contamination of Infusate or Blood Products

1. Bacterial Contamination of Infusate

Although less frequently than from infection of the percutaneous catheter tract or from a contaminated catheter hub, device-related BSI may also arise from contamination of infusate—parenteral fluid, blood products, or intravenous medications. In fact, cases of infusion-related bacteremia may be falsely attributed to the intravascular cannula due to failure to culture the infusate (41).

Infusion-related sepsis has been reviewed extensively by Maki (11,40). Bacteria may be introduced both during manufacture of the infusate (extrinsic contamination) and during its preparation and administration in the hospital (intrinsic contamination). The pathogens implicated in the vast majority of nosocomial bacteremias related to contaminated infusate have been gram-negative bacilli. This may, at least in part, be due to the different growth properties of specific microorganisms in parenteral fluids (see below). Whereas contaminated infusate is a rare cause of endemic infusion-related infection with most intravascular devices, it is well documented as a common cause of epidemic nosocomial bacteremia (11,40). In fact, nosocomial BSI caused by specific gram-negative organisms such as *Enterobacter* spp. (particularly *E. cloacae* and *E. agglomerans*), *S. marcescens*, and *Burkholderia* (*Pseudomonas*) *cepacia* that are able to multiply at room temperature in the solution involved points toward contaminated fluid as a possible source and, if observed repeatedly, should prompt an in-depth epidemiological evaluation.

The problem and reported causes of epidemic infusion related bacteremia due to intrinsic contamination of infusate has been reviewed in detail by Maki (41). All of the outbreaks reported from U.S. and European hospitals, some of which have reached a nationwide scope, have involved gram-negative bacilli (41,58). The largest outbreak of this kind occurred in 1970–1971 and involved 378 patients in 25 U.S. hospitals. It was ultimately traced to the contamination of closures of unopened infusion bottles with *E. cloacae* and *E. agglomerans* during the manufacturing process (59). More recently, outbreaks of *Pseudomonas* bacteremia and pseudobacteremia due to intrinsic contamination of 10% povidone iodine, a widely used skin antiseptic, have been reported (60). However, the frequency of these outbreaks has declined considerably during the past decade due to improved control measures of the manufacturers.

Most epidemics of infusion-related bacteremia, however, have originated from a common source of extrinsic contamination in the hospital such as use of contaminated disinfectants, repeated use of contaminated multidose medication vials (61), or improper sterilization of medical equipment—in particular of transducers used for arterial pressure monitoring (49,62,63). There have been more than 30 epidemics of nosocomial BSI traced to contaminated fluid within the administration set of arterial pressure monitoring devices. Again, the majority of these outbreaks (90%) were caused by gram-negative bacteria, most frequently *S. marcescens*, *Enterobacter* spp., and *B. cepacia* (62). The authors discussed the various mechanisms of contamination of the arterial pressure monitoring system and speculated that the major reason for the predominance of gram-negative bacilli in these epidemics may be the specific growth properties of these organisms in heparinized saline and glucose-containing solutions. In many outbreaks, the hospital reservoir and the mode of transmission of the epidemic organism could not be determined, but the pathogen was found on the hands of healthcare workers involved in the care of patients receiving infusion therapy.

2. Bacterial Contamination of Blood Products

Bacterial infections transmitted by contaminated blood or blood products have been rare but may be associated with severe morbidity often culminating in septic shock and death. Various sources of contamination have been suggested such as infection of the donor or bacterial invasion of the blood product during collection, preparation, and storage (64). A wide spectrum of bacteria have been implicated but aerobic gram-negative rods were the organisms most commonly involved (61%), with *Pseudomonas* spp. accounting for 28% of episodes. Transfusion-related sepsis due to *Yersinia enterocolitica* was associated with diarrheal illness of the donor (65), whereas an outbreak of *Salmonella* sepsis from platelet transfusions was traced to a hematogenous carrier of *Salmonella cholera-suis* (66). Cold-growing (psychrophilic) bacteria such as *Yersinia* spp., *P. fluorescens*, and *Flavobacterium* spp. may play an important role in the contamination of blood products since, once introduced, even in small numbers, they may grow to massive numbers during storage of whole blood at 4°C (67). In contrast, platelets are stored at room temperature and may become contaminated with bacteria such as *Enterobacter* spp. that grow well at 25°C to 37°C (68).

III. CATHETER-RELATED INFECTIONS DUE TO SPECIFIC GRAM-NEGATIVE ORGANISMS

A. Enterobacteriaceae

The various members of the family Enterobacteriaceae taken together constitute the largest group of gram-negative organisms involved in all types of nosocomial infections including BSI and catheter-associated infections (14,47) and clearly predominate over *P. aeruginosa* and other nonfermenting gram-negative rods (69). If the different species are considered separately, *E. coli*, *Enterobacter* spp., *Klebsiella* spp., and *Serratia* spp. are the leading causes of nosocomial BSI, whereas *Citrobacter* spp., *Proteus* spp., *Morganella morganii*, and *Salmonella* spp. are only rarely encountered (8,9,19,69). Rare enterobacterial species that have been implicated in CRI include *Enterobacter amnigenus* (70), *Kluyvera cryocrescens* (71), and *Serratia odorifera* (72).

1. Escherichia coli

E. coli is the most common cause of enterobacterial bacteremia, ranging in frequency from 31% to 47% of all gram-negative bacteremias, and is predominantly associated with urinary tract infections (10,18,21,69). In light of the frequency with which *E. coli* is isolated from the bloodstream, it may be surprising that *E. coli* is an exceptionally rare cause of intravascular device-associated BSI. Grandsen and co-workers reviewed 861 cases of *E. coli* bacteremia observed during an 18-year survey (21). In more than half of all cases (57%), bacteremia originated in the urinary tract, but *E. coli* was never encountered infecting an intravenous line. Bodey and collegues, in a similar series of *E. coli* bacteremia in cancer patients, identified a catheter as the source of infection in only 1% (73).

In prospective studies of catheter-related infections *E. coli* is less often recovered than other Enterobacteriaceae. The frequency of *E. coli* among gram-negative infections associated with tunneled CVCs ranges from 15 to 26% (7,53–56), whereas nontunneled CVCs are rarely infected (0–14%) (28–30, 44,46).

2. Enterobacter spp.

Enterobacter bacteremia is usually nosocomial and accounts for 5% to 8% of reported gram-negative BSIs (9,10,18,19,74,75). In their large series of *Enterobacter* bacteremia in a cancer hospital including 281 patients, Bodey and colleages could identify a portal of entry in only 28%, and only two infections (<1%) were considered catheter-related (76). In contrast, in his review of 33 pediatric patients, Gallagher concluded that the biliary tract (18%) and central venous catheters (15%) were the most common sources of *Enterobacter* bacteremia (22). Chow and co-workers prospectively studied 129 patients with *Enterobacter* bacteremia. An abdominal source was the most common portal of entry (39%), followed by the urinary tract (13%) and intravascular catheters (11%) (75). Of special importance is the rapid development of resistance to cephalosporin antibiotics by *Enterobacter* (75).

Enterobacter spp. and *E. cloacae* in particular are among the most common gram-negative organisms involved in CRI, only rivaled by *Klebsiella* spp. and *P. aeruginosa*. *Enterobacter* spp. constituted 13% to 39% of gram-negative bacteria isolated from infections associated with long-term CVCs of the Hickman/Broviac type (7,53–56). *Enterobacter* spp. were also frequently found causing infections associated with short-term CVCs, ranging from 6% to 33% among gram-negative organisms (28–30,44,46). *Enterobacter* is rarely if ever recovered from infections related to small peripheral venous catheters (16,28), pulmonary artery catheters (47), and arterial catheters (48,62).

Another characteristic feature of *Enterobacter* is its association with epidemics of bacteremia caused by contaminated intravenous products (68). *Enterobacter* spp. are among the leading causes of epidemic nosocomial bacteremia, accounting for 9 of 97 epidemics reviewed by Maki (11). *Enterobacter* spp. were also involved in 5 of 23 nosocomial epidemics (22%) of bloodstream infection traced to arterial pressure monitoring that were reviewed by Mermel and Maki (62).

3.   Klebsiella *spp.*

Microorganisms of the genus *Klebsiella* are among the leading causes (11% to 16%) of gram-negative rod bacteremia, ranking second only to *E. coli* (9,10,18,19). *Klebsiella* bacteremia is most often a nosocomial disease with a strong association with septic shock (23). In an analysis of 100 episodes of *Klebsiella* bacteremia, Garcia de la Torre et al. demonstrated that the most frequent portals of entry were urinary, respiratory, and biliary tracts, whereas only four cases (4%) were considered catheter-related (23).

Klebsiella spp. have been implicated in intravascular device-associated infections with similar frequency as *Enterobacter* spp. *K. pneumonia* usually predominates over *K. oxytoca*. *Klebsiella* spp. constituted 6% to 17% of gram-negative bacteria isolated from infections associated with nontunneled CVCs (28–30, 44,46) and were also recovered from 11% to 18% of infections related to tunneled long-term CVCs that were due to gram-negative organisms (7,53,55,56). A *Klebsiella* species was the only gram-negative organism found to be responsible for catheter-related sepsis associated with short peripheral catheters (77), although these organisms are exceptionally rare in these infections (28).

Klebsiella spp. were also implicated—although less frequently than *Enterobacter* spp. and *Serratia* spp.—in nosocomial outbreaks associated with pressure transducers used for arterial pressure monitoring (50,62), as well as in epidemic nosocomial bacteremia related to contaminated infusate (11).

4.   Serratia *spp.*

Serratia bacteremia is hospital-acquired in nearly all instances and tends to be associated with especially long durations of hospitalization. *Serratia* spp. constitute between 2% and 6% of bacteremia cases in large surveys of gram-negative bacteremia (9,10,18,19). In recent reviews of *Serratia* bacteremia the respiratory tract, urinary tract, and surgical wounds served as the most important portals of entry. Catheters were implicated as the origin of infection in only 2% to 9% (24,77). Like *Enterobacter* spp., these organisms are often multidrug resistant.

Serratia spp. are considerably less often involved in CRI and catheter-related BSI than *Enterobacter* spp. and *Klebsiella* spp., ranging in frequency between 1% and 19% of all gram-negative organisms recovered from infections associated with nontunneled CVCs (28–30,44,46) as well as long-term tunneled CVCs

(7,53,55,56). However, *Serratia* spp. are among the organisms that should suggest the possibility of a contaminated infusion product if identified as a clear cause of device-associated bacteremia. *S. marcescens* accounted for 6 of 23 (26%) reported outbreaks of infection related to arterial pressure monitoring (62) and was the causative agent of nosocomial epidemic BSIs associated with a contaminated infusate reviewed by Maki (11).

B. *Pseudomonas aeruginosa*

P. aeruginosa is a ubiquitous organism that has been isolated from water, soil, and plants. It is also a frequent colonizer of human skin and mucous membranes, especially in hospitalized patients. The capability of *P. aeruginosa* to withstand adverse environmental conditions may have contributed to its role as a successful nosocomial pathogen. Hospital reservoirs of *P. aeruginosa* infection have included respiratory equipment, humidifiers, fluids for intravascular administration, ophthalmic solutions, soap, sinks, and disinfectants (78). Baltch recently gave a comprehensive historical review of the published literature on *P. aeruginosa* bacteremia (79). This bacteremia is nearly always nosocomial and typically occurs among patients with severe underlying disease. *P. aeruginosa* accounts for 8% to 17% of gram-negative bacteremia cases in large series (8–10,19,20) and has recently been ranked sixth among the pathogens causing nosocomial BSI in critical care unit patients reported to the CDC (69).

The urinary tract, respiratory tract, and skin appear to be the most common portals of entry for *P. aeruginosa* into the bloodstream. In their review of 108 cases of *P. aeruginosa* bacteremia, Flick and Cluff found the respiratory tract (20%) and the urinary tract (19%) to be the major sources followed by intravascular catheters (15%) and the skin (11%) (80). In the largest series of *P. aeruginosa* bacteremia reported to date, Bodey et al. could not identify the portal of entry in the majority of cases. *P. aeruginosa* was cultured concomitantly from an intravascular catheter in only five cases (1%) (25). In more recent reports the rate of catheter-related BSI among cases of *P. aeruginosa* bacteremia ranged between 7% and 14% (26,27,81,82).

P. aeruginosa is among the predominant gram-negative organisms causing CRI associated with various types of intravascular catheters such as tunneled CVCs (7,14,54–56), nontunneled CVCs (28–30,44,46), small peripheral venous catheters (16,28), and pulmonary artery catheters (47), ranging in frequency from 12% to 50% of all gram-negative isolates. Not surprisingly, these organisms appear to play a predominant role as etiologic agents of CRIs in burn patients (15,83).

Whereas *P. aeruginosa* bacteremia appeared to decrease in cancer patients in recent years (7), this infection is on the increase in patients with AIDS (84–86). Roilides and co-workers reviewed 13 bacteremias and 25 nonbacteremic infections caused by *Pseudomonas* spp. in children infected with HIV (85). Central venous catheter-related infections were most frequent and accounted for 10 of 13 bacteremias and 10 of 25 nonbacteremic infections. *P. aeruginosa* was the most common pathogen. Nelson et al. found 19 episodes of *Pseudomonas* bacteremia among 584 adult patients with AIDS (86). Association with central venous catheters in 11 of 19 cases (58%) and high mortality of CVC-unrelated bacteremias and in those patients whose central line was not removed, was noted.

Many investigators have noted the extremely high rate of mortality associated with hospital-acquired *P. aeruginosa* infections that may range between 50% and 80% (18,19,27,80) but appeared to decrease in the more recent past probably due to the introduction of antipseudomonal beta-lactam antibiotics (25,82). Mortality is most pronounced in bacteremia secondary to respiratory tract infection and skin/soft tissue infections (27,79,81) but appears to be considerably lower in catheter-related infections (27,87) and as low as 9% in patients with AIDS (85).

C. *Acinetobacter* spp.

Until recently, the genus *Acinetobacter* comprised a single species, *A. calcoaceticus*, and two subspecies, or biovars—*A. calcoaceticus* var. *lwoffii*, and *A. calcoaceticus* var. *anitratus*. Following extensive taxonomic reorganization of the genus (88), currently at least 18 DNA hybridization groups or genospecies are recognized including the named species *A. baumannii, A. calcoaceticus, A. haemolyticus, A. johnsonii, A. junii, A. lwoffii*, and *A. radioresistens* as well as 11 unnamed genomic species.

In recent years, *Acinetobacter* species have emerged as clinically important pathogens. Though the organisms are widely prevalent in nature, most human infections are hospital acquired, *A. baumannii* being the predominant species.

1. Acinetobacter baumannii

Nosocomial *A. baumannii* infections, such as respiratory tract infections, urinary tract infections, meningitis, and bacteremia mainly affect patients with severe underlying illnesses in the ICU (20,63,89). *Acinetobacter* spp. account for 1% to 4% of gram-negative bloodstream isolates in large surveys of bacteremia (8–10), with considerable regional differences. In 1991, at the Institute of Medical Microbiology and Hygiene, University of Cologne, Germany, *Acinetobacter* spp. were among the top five organisms isolated from blood cultures and among gram-negative pathogens were only second to *E. coli*.

A substantial part of *A. baumannii* bacteremia cases represent catheter-related infections that usually carry a more favorable prognosis. The association of *Acinetobacter* bacteremia with indwelling vascular access devices has been reported in early reviews dating back to the early 1960s (90). As reviewed by Seifert and colleagues (20), the number of catheter-related infections among bacteremia cases caused by *Acinetobacter* spp. varied considerably (8% to 90%) in more recent reports (20,63,91,92). Rolston et al. (91) noted an increase in the number of *A. calcoaceticus* septicemia cases in cancer patients that paralleled the increasing use of intravascular catheters over a 10-year period. Beck-Sagué and co-workers (63) recently described an outbreak of *A. baumannii* infections that was traced to contaminated pressure transducers and involved 75 patients. In the largest survey of *A. baumannii* bacteremia reported to date (20), intravascular catheters were the major portal of entry, accounting for 39 of 87 (45%) bacteremia cases, followed by respiratory tract infections (31%), and skin and soft-tissue infections (4%). The overall mortality was 44%, ranging from 21% in patients with catheter-related BSI to 100% in patients with pneumonia.

In large prospective studies *Acinetobacter* spp. were among the major organisms causing CRI, accounting for 7% to 12% of gram-negative bacteria isolated from infections associated with long-term CVCs of the Hickman/Broviac type (7,53,55,56). They were associated with similar frequency ranging from 4% to 24% with infections of short-term CVCs due to gram-negative organisms (28–30,46). Siegman-Igra et al. (89) reported 25 cases of nosocomial *Acinetobacter* meningitis secondary to invasive neurosurgical procedures. The majority of infections were associated with indwelling ventriculostomy tubes (52%) or CSF fistulae (28%). Galvao et al. (93) reported 23 cases of *Acinetobacter* peritonitis in chronic peritoneal dialysis. *Acinetobacter* represented the second most common gram-negative pathogen in CAPD peritonitis and was nearly as frequent as *Pseudomonas*. Catheter removal for cure of the infection was only rarely indicated.

Most of these studies, with the exception of the report by Seifert and co-workers (20), were not based on the current taxonomy of the genus *Acinetobacter*, and therefore bacteremia cases and CRI due to *A. baumannii* and due to other *Acinetobacter* species have never been clearly separated. In fact, the clinical significance and the propensity to cause device-related bacteremia of *A. baumannii* is clearly different from that of other *Acinetobacter* spp., as will be pointed out below.

2. Acinetobacter *spp. Other Than* Acinetobacter baumannnii

The clinical importance and hospital epidemiology of *Acinetobacter* spp. other than *A. baumannii* (formerly *A. calcoaceticus* var. *lwoffii*) is less well understood. These organisms are considered part of the normal flora of the human skin and mucous membranes and have only rarely been implicated in human disease. However, rare cases of meningitis, endocarditis, and bacteremia have been described (91,94–96).

Nosocomial bacteremia due to these organisms is mostly sporadic and almost exclusively related to intravascular devices (97). Seifert and colleges recently reviewed 55 episodes of true bacteremia due to *Acinetobacter* spp. other than *A. baumannii* occurring in 53 patients during a study period of 18 months (95). *Acinetobacter* spp. were not recovered from any other specimen obtained for culture in these patients except from catheter tips. The most frequently isolated species were *A. johnsonii* (n = 14), *Acinetobacter* species 3 (n = 12), and *A. lwoffii* (n = 10). These species are also the most common *Acinetobacter* spp. isolated from the skin of healthy volunteers and hospitalized patients (author's unpublished observation). Other *Acinetobacter* spp. (*A. junii*, *A. haemolyticus*, *Acinetobacter* spp. 6, 10, and 12) were only rarely recovered from blood specimens.

The clinical presentation was usually benign, and all but four patients (93%) were cured. Using strict criteria, 50 episodes (90.9%) of *Acinetobacter* bacteremia were considered definitely or probably catheter-related. Only six patients showed clinical signs of exit site infection. One episode was meningitis following neurosurgery and was felt to be related to an indwelling ventricular catheter.

The main differences regarding predisposing factors, epidemiologic features, and clinical characteristics of CRI due to *A. baumannii* and *Acinetobacter* spp. other than *A. baumannii* have recently been reviewed in detail by Seifert and coworkers (98).

IV. PATHOGENESIS

The complex pathogenesis of CRI is reviewed by Sherertz in Chapter 1. However, nearly all in vitro and animal studies investigating the pathogenesis of infections related to intravascular devices have focused on gram-positive organisms, in particular coagulase-negative staphylococci and *S. aureus* as well as *Candida* spp. (6). Little is known about the specific factors involved in the pathogenesis of CRI due to gram-negative organisms.

It is widely accepted that the largest proportion of catheter-related BSI derive from the cutaneous flora at the insertion site or from contamination of the catheter hub (40). As demonstrated earlier, if compared with gram-positive bacteria, enteric gram-negative rods rarely cause catheter-related infections, especially those associated with peripheral and nontunneled CVCs. This may be partly explained by the fact that gram-negative bacteria, with the exception of *Acinetobacter* spp., are not part of the resident human skin flora. However, with prolonged hospitalization patients are increasingly colonized with nosocomial pathogens, namely *P. aeruginosa*, *Enterobacter*, and *Klebsiella* spp., especially in areas with high endemic transmission such as ICUs. We recently showed in a prospective surveillance study that during a nosocomial outbreak due to *A. baumannii* in a surgical ICU 74% of patients hospitalized for more than 72 hours were colonized with the epidemic strain after a mean ICU stay of 4 days (99). Respiratory tract colonization was usually demonstrated initially and was followed by colonization of various body surface sites. The skin of the subclavian region, the area most commonly used for the insertion of CVCs, showed the highest colonization rates, followed by the axilla, groin, and antecubital fossa. Thus, in the epidemiological setting described here, nosocomial gram-negative pathogens may colonize intravascular catheters in the same way as common gram-positive bacteria usually present on human skin.

The adherence properties of staphylococci to intravascular catheters play a predominant role in the pathogenesis of device-related infections due to CoNS. Usually, gram-negative bacteria adhere less readily to polymer surfaces than CoNS, with the exception of *P. aeruginosa* and *Acinetobacter* spp. (100). SEM studies revealed that colonization of polyurethane catheters with different *Acinetobacter* spp. occurred in a similar time fashion and to a comparable extent as with CoNS (author's unpublished observation).

Like most environmental bacteria, *P. aeruginosa* lives predominantly in slime-enclosed biofilms adherent to available surfaces from which it periodically releases planctonic (free-swimming) cells. *P. aeruginosa* possesses a tremendous array of virulence factors that have been excellently reviewed by Woods and Vasil (101). As observed with CoNS, growth in biofilms protects *P. aeruginosa* cells from antibacterial factors produced by the host as well as from antibiotics and may account for its survival and extended persistence on foreign devices. *P. aeruginosa* embedded in thick biofilm has been seen on a variety of transcutaneous medical devices such as vascular catheters (102), peritoneal catheters (103), and urinary catheters (104). It has been suggested that polymer catheters made of PVC or silicone may favor survival and growth of *P. aeruginosa* (105).

Other mechanisms such as invasion of bacteria from a contaminated parenteral fluid are only rarely involved in CRI and catheter-related BSI due to staphylococci (42) but, as demonstrated above (II D), may play an important role in the pathogenesis of CRI due to gram-negative bacteria.

The contribution of hematogenous seeding of the catheter tip from remote unrelated sites of infection to catheter colonization and sepsis has only rarely been demonstrated (40). In patients with hematological disorders, however, especially in those with altered mucosal barriers following cytotoxic chemotherapy, there may be translocation of endogenous gut bacteria to the catheter (106). Groeger and co-workers suggested that this mechanism may explain the fact that device-related bacteremia in cancer patients was caused predominantly by gram-negative enteric bacilli (14).

The different growth properties of microbial pathogens in parenteral fluids may also play an important role. Though microbial growth in most solutions used for parenteral administration is rather poor, different infusion fluids may support the growth of specific organisms. Parenteral nutrition solutions are excellent substrates for the growth of certain microorganisms. Goldmann and co-workers demonstrated that *K. pneumonia and S. marcescens* grew exuberantly in peptone containing casein hydrolystate-dextrose solution whereas other bacteria tested such as *S. aureus, E. coli*, and *P. mirabilis* grew more slowly while *P. aeruginosa* slowly died (107). Distilled water may allow the proliferation of *B. cepacia* (108), *Acinetobacter* spp., and *Serratia* spp. (40). Glucose-containing solutions (5% dextrose in water) support the growth of *Klebsiella* spp., *Enterobacter* spp., *Serratia* spp., and *B. cepacia*, whereas *E. coli, Proteus* spp., and *P. aeruginosa* slowly loose viability (109). Sodium chloride solutions may support the growth of many gram-negative bacteria. These solutions, however, usually do not allow growth of gram-positive bacteria. Lipid emulsions, in contrast, allow rapid multiplication of nearly all microorganisms (110).

V. COMPLICATIONS

Arnow and co-workers recently assessed the consequences of intravascular catheter sepsis in 94 patients with 102 episodes of catheter-related BSI due to percutaneously inserted catheters (34). Major complications occurred in 33 (32%) of the episodes and included septic shock (12 episodes), sustained sepsis (12), suppurative thrombophlebitis (7), metastatic infection (2), endocarditis (2), and arteritis (2). The risk of major complications was highest in catheter-related BSI caused by *Candida* spp. (64%), *P. aeruginosa* (50%), and *S. aureus* (38%), followed by gram-negative enteric bacilli (20%).

Suppurative thrombophlebitis, defined as the presence of intraluminal pus, is an inflammation of the vein wall due to the presence of microorganisms and is frequently associated with thrombosis and sustained bacteremia. Suppurative thrombophlebitis is the most serious form of catheter-related infection and is a particular problem in burn and trauma patients. In recent years, most cases of septic thrombophlebitis have been due to gram-negative bacteria. Garrison and co-workers reviewed 29 cases of septic thrombophlebitis over a 7-year period (111). Gram-negative enteric bacilli, especially *Enterobacter* and *Klebsiella* spp. were the causative agents in 21 cases (72%) followed by *S. aureus* (24%). Similar results were reported by Johnson and co-workers who noted a correlation between the isolation of enteric organisms (gram-negative rods and enterococci) from the inflamed veins and recent abdominal surgery (112). Surgical intervention with excision of the inflamed vein is considered the treatment of choice for suppurative thrombophlebitis. For catheter-related central vein suppurative thrombophlebitis the recommended approach is catheter removal, anticoagulation with heparin, and prolonged antibiotic therapy (113).

Infective endocarditis is another serious complication of CRI. Terpenning et al. recently reviewed 22 patients with nosocomial endocarditis (114). Intravascular devices were the source of bacteremia resulting in endocarditis in 10 (45%) of these cases. Nosocomial endocarditis was due predominantly to *S. aureus* and CoNS, whereas only one episode was due a gram-negative pathogen, *P. aeruginosa*.

VI. MANAGEMENT

The management of device-related infection depends on the type of catheter, the underlying illness of the patient, the infecting microorganism, and the type of infection, and is covered in the respective chapters elsewhere in this book. This section attempts to summarize the currently recommended approaches to the management of intravascular device-related infection caused specifically by gram-negative organisms.

Although the infection of CVCs may be successfully treated without catheter removal, it is common practice to remove and culture a short-term, percutaneous, noncuffed intravascular catheter that is suspected of being infected irrespective of the pathogen cultured (115). This also holds true for peripheral catheters, pulmonary artery, and arterial catheters used for hemodynamic monitoring.

Uncomplicated BSI associated with surgically implanted Hickman or Broviac catheters usually responds well to intravenous antibiotic therapy with the catheter left in place. Most investigators did not observe that the type of pathogen was an important factor for cure of patients with catheter-related bacteremia without removal of the catheter (52,56,116). In contrast, Rotstein and associates recently demonstrated that a fungal or a gram-negative pathogen were most predictive for catheter removal (55). Twenty-five (24%) of 103 Hickman catheter-related infections due to gram-positive organisms resulted in catheter removal, in contrast to 13 (52%) of 25 infections caused by gram-negative bacilli. Certain organisms such as *S. aureus*, *Bacillus* spp., *Corynebacterium jeikeium*, yeasts, and atypical mycobacteria have been traditionally considered to be difficult to eradicate and may require catheter removal.

Various reports have demonstrated that catheter-related BSI including those caused by enteric gram-negative bacilli can be cured with intravenous antibiotics administered over the infected catheter (52,53,87,116). More recently, a new technique to treat central venous catheter infection called "antibiotic lock technique" has been proposed that involves instillation of a highly concentrated antimicrobial agent into the catheter lumen, where it remains in place for 12 hours. Successful management of CRI with this technique has been documented including infections caused by gram-negative organisms (117–119). In a similar protocol, Rao et al. successfully treated Broviac catheter infection caused by gram-negative bacilli with 8-hourly instillation of 1 ml of heparinized amikacin solution (120). However, these reports have not included infections with *P. aeruginosa*. Antibiotic therapy should be based on in vitro susceptibility of the infecting pathogen; however, superiority of a specific class of antibiotics in the treatment of gram-negative device-related BSI has not been demonstrated.

Catheter removal was significantly associated with survival in patients with bacteremia due to *A. baumannii* whereas appropriate antimicrobial therapy was not (20). The occurrence of multiresistant strains often limits therapeutic options (121). *Acinetobacter* spp. other than *A. baumannii*, in contrast, are usually susceptible to most antimicrobial agents and successful management of bacteremia due to these organisms in one series included catheter removal in 45 cases (82%) and appropriate antimicrobial therapy in 34 cases (62%). Seven patients were successfully treated with the catheter left in place (95).

The management of catheter-related infections due to *Pseudomonas* is less clear. Whereas some researchers have found *P. aeruginosa* among the organisms that more frequently have required catheter removal (55), others have not documented a correlation between specific gram-negative organisms and failure to eradicate these organisms from an infected catheter left in place (87,122). Elting and Bodey reviewed their experience with catheter-related bacteremia caused by *S. maltophilia* and non-aeruginosa *Pseudomonas* spp. (123). They noted a high rate of treatment failure and recurrence if the catheter was not removed, whereas all patients whose catheters were removed were cured. Similar observations were made by Nelson et al. in patients with catheter-related *P. aeruginosa* bacteremia associated with HIV (86). Conversely, 13 of 20 catheter-related *P. aeruginosa* infections (65%) reported by Roilides et al. (85) were successfully treated with appropriate antibiotics without removal of the involved catheter. Prompt initiation of appropriate therapy usually administered as a combination of an antipseudomonal beta-lactam and an aminoglycoside is considered crucial to improve survival.

Whereas exit site infections can usually be treated with antibiotics and local care without removal of the catheter (53,56), management with the catheter left in place is probably less successful in tunnel infections that require catheter removal if not responding promptly to intravenous antibiotics (54,124). This may be especially true if these infections are caused by *P. aeruginosa*. Of the 20 tunnel infections reported by Benerza and associates (54), only five were successfully treated with antibiotics; the other 15 required catheter removal for cure. Eleven of the cases requiring catheter removal were caused by *P. aeruginosa*.

VII. CONCLUSION

Though less often implicated than gram-positive organisms, gram-negative bacilli, in particular members of the family Enterobacteriaceae, *P. aeruginosa*, and *Acinetobacter* spp., account for up to one-third of infections associated with most intravascular devices. Rates as high as 50% have been observed in catheter-related BSI as well as in exit site and tunnel infections due to these organisms if surgically implanted catheters are involved. Of particular importance is the propensity of certain gram-negative organisms to cause infections associated with bacterial contamination of infusate and contamination of blood products, probably due to the specific growth properties of gram-negative bacilli in various infusion fluids. These organisms have also been implicated in the majority of hospital outbreaks of infusion-related bacteremia.

Factors involved in the pathogenesis of CRI associated with gram-negative bacilli have only rarely been investigated. As with CoNS, the adherence properties and the formation of biofilm of certain gram-negative organisms such as *P. aeruginosa* and *Acinetobacter* spp. may play an important role in the pathogenesis of these infections.

The treatment of CRI due to gram-negative organisms is usually not different from the general recommendations regarding the management of infections associated with intravascular devices, although this question has not been specifically addressed in prospective clinical trials. Treatment of gram-negative infections associated with surgically implanted catheters has been equally successful as with gram-positive organisms. Possible consequences such as sustained bacteremia and suppurative thrombophlebitis which is most often caused by gram-negative organisms have to be considered. There is evidence, however, that CRI due to *P. aeruginosa* usually requires catheter removal for cure.

REFERENCES

1. Banerjee SN, Emori TG, Culver DH, et al. Secular trends in nosocomial primary bloodstream infections in the United States, 1980–1989. Am J Med 1991; 91(suppl 3B):86S–89S.
2. Jarvis WR, Edwards JR, Culver DH, et al. Nosocomial infection rates in adult and pediatric intensive care units in the United States. Am J Med 1991; 91(suppl 3B):185S–191S.
3. Schaberg DR, Culver DH, Gaynes RP. Major trends in the microbial etiology of nosocomial infection. Am J Med 1991; 91(suppl 3B):72S–75S.
4. Dougherty SH. Pathobiology of infection in prosthetic devices. Rev Infect Dis 1988; 10:1102–1117.
5. Patterson JE, Sweeney AH, Simms M, et al. An analysis of 110 serious enterococcal infections. Epidemiology, antibiotic susceptibility, and outcome. Medicine (Baltimore) 1995; 74:191–200.
6. Goldmann DA, Pier GB. Pathogenesis of infections related to intravascular catheterization. Clin Microbiol Rev 1993; 6:176–192.
7. Kiehn TE, Armstrong D. Changes in the spectrum of organisms causing bacteremia and fungemia in immunocompromised patients due to venous access devices. Eur J Clin Microbiol Infect Dis 1990; 9:869–872.
8. Geerdes HF, Ziegler D, Lode H, et al. Septicemia in 980 patients at a university hospital in Berlin: prospective studies during 3 selected years between 1979 and 1989. Clin Infect Dis 1992; 15:991–1002.
9. Weinstein MP, Reller LB, Murphy JR, Lichtenstein KA. The clinical significance of positive blood cultures: a comprehensive analysis of 500 episodes of bacteremia and fungemia in adults. 1. Laboratory and epidemiologic observations. Rev Infect Dis 1983; 5:35–53.
10. Roberts FJ, Geere IW, Coldman A. A three-year study of positive blood cultures, with emphasis on prognosis. Rev Infect Dis 1991; 13:34–46.
11. Maki DG. Nosocomial bacteremia. An epidemiologic overview. Am J Med 1981; 70:719–732.
12. Smith RL, Meixler SM, Simberkoff MS. Excess mortality in critically ill patients with nosocomial bloodstream infections. Chest 1991; 100:164–167.
13. Rello J, Quintana E, Mirelis B, Gurgui M, Net A, Prats G. Polymicrobial bacteremia in critically ill patients. Inten Care Med 1993; 19:22–25.

14. Groeger JS, Lucas AB, Thaler HT, et al. Infectious morbidity associated with long-term use of venous access devices in patients with cancer. Ann Intern Med 1993; 119:1168–1174.

15. Franceschi D, Gerding RL, Philips G, Fratianne RB. Risk factors associated with intravascular catheter infections in burned patients: a prospective, randomized study. J Trauma 1989; 29:811–816.

16. Maki DG, Jarrett F, Sarafin HW. A semiquantitative culture method for identification of catheter-related infection in the burn patient. J Surg Res 1977; 22:513–520.

17. Leibovici L, Konisberger H, Pitlik SD, Samra Z, Drucker M. Bacteremia and fungemia of unknown origin in adults. Clin Infect Dis 1992; 14:436–443.

18. Kreger BE, Craven DE, Carling PC, McCabe WR. Gram-negative bacteremia. III. Reassessment of etiology, epidemiology and ecology in 612 patients. Am J Med 1980; 68:332–343.

19. Bryan CS, Reynolds KL, Brenner ER. Analysis of 1,186 episodes of gram-negative bacteremia in non-university hospitals: the effects of antimicrobial therapy. Rev Infect Dis 1983; 5:629–638.

20. Seifert H, Strate A, Pulverer G. Nosocomial bacteremia due to *Acinetobacter baumannii:* clinical features, epidemiology, and predictors of mortality. Medicine (Baltimore) 1995; 74:340–349.

21. Gransden WR, Eykyn SJ, Phillips I, Rowe B. Bacteremia due to *Escherichia coli:* a study of 861 episodes. Rev Infect Dis 1990; 12:1008–1018.

22. Gallagher PG. *Enterobacter* bacteremia in pediatric patients. Rev Infect Dis 1990; 12:808–812.

23. García de la Torre M, Romero-Vivas J, Martínez-Beltrán J, Guerrero A, Meseguer M, Bouza E. *Klebsiella* bacteremia: an analysis of 100 episodes. Rev Infect Dis 1985; 7:143–150.

24. Bouza E, García de la Torre M, Erice A, Cercenado E, Loza E, Rodriguez-Créixems M. *Serratia* bacteremia. Diagn Microbiol Infect Dis 1987; 7:237–247.

25. Bodey GP, Jadeja L, Elting L. *Pseudomonas* bacteremia: retrospective analysis of 410 episodes. Arch Intern Med 1985; 145:1621–1629.

26. Vázquez F, Mendoza MC, Villar MH, Vindel A, Méndez FJ. Characteristics of *Pseudomonas aeruginosa* strains causing septicemia in a spanish hospital 1981–1990. Eur J Clin Microbiol Infect Dis 1992; 11:698–703.

27. Bisbe J, Gatell JM, Puig J, et al. *Pseudomonas aeruginosa* bacteremia: univariate and multivariate analyses of factors influencing the prognosis in 133 episodes. Rev Infect Dis 1988; 10:629–635.

28. Richet H, Hubert B, Nitemberg G, et al. Prospective multicenter study of vascular-catheter-related complications and risk factors for positive central-catheter cultures in intensive care unit patients. J Clin Microbiol 1990; 28:2520–2525.

29. Sherertz RJ, Raad II, Belani A, et al. Three-year experience with sonicated vascular catheter cultures in a clinical microbiology laboratory. J Clin Microbiol 1990; 28:76–82.

30. Gil RT, Kruse JA, Thill-Baharozian MC, Carlson RW. Triple- vs single-lumen central venous catheters. A prospective study in a critically ill population. Arch Intern Med 1989; 149:1139–1143.

31. Pemberton LB, Lyman B, Lander V, Covinsky J. Sepsis from triple- vs single-lumen

catheters during total parenteral nutrition in surgical or critically ill patients. Arch Surg 1986; 121:591–594.

32. Kamal GD, Pfaller MA, Rempe LE, Jebson PJ. Reduced intravascular catheter infections by antibiotic bonding. A prospective, randomized, controlled trial. JAMA 1991; 265:2364–2368.

33. Hoffmann KK, Western SA, Kaiser DL, Wenzel RP, Groschel DH. Bacterial colonization and phlebitis-associated risk with transparent polyurethane film for peripheral intravenous site dressings. Am J Infect Control 1988; 16:101–106.

34. Arnow PM, Quimosing EM, Beach M. Consequences of intravascular catheter sepsis. Clin Infect Dis 1993; 16:778–784.

35. Maki DG, Ringer M, Alvarado CJ. Prospective randomised trial of povidon-iodine, alcohol, and chlorhexidine for prevention of infection associated with central venous and arterial catheters. Lancet 1991; 338:339–343.

36. Flowers RH, Schwenzer KJ, Kopel RF, Fisch MJ, Tucker SI, Farr BM. Efficacy of an attachable subcutaneous cuff for the prevention of intravascular catheter-related infection. JAMA 1989; 261:878–883.

37. Wagener MM, Yu VL. Bacteremia in transplant recipients: a prospective study of demographics, etiologic agents, risk factors, and outcomes. Am J Infect Control 1992; 20:239–247.

38. Weinstein MP, Reller LB, Murphy JR. Clinical importance of polymicrobial bacteremia. Diagn Microbiol Infect Dis 1986; 5:185–196.

39. Reuben AG, Musher DM, Hamill RJ, Broucke I. Polymicrobial bacteremia: clinical and microbiologic patterns. Rev Infect Dis 1989; 11:161–183.

40. Maki DG. Infections caused by intravascular devices. In: Bisno AL, Waldvogel FA, eds. Infections Associated With Indwelling Medical Devices. 2nd ed. Washington: ASM Press, 1994:155–212.

41. Maki DG. Infections due to infusion therapy. In: Bennet JV, Brachman PS, eds. Hospital Infections. 3rd ed. Boston; Little, Brown and Company, 1992:849–898.

42. Maki DG, Weise CE, Sarafin HW. A semiquantitative culture method for identifying intravenous-catheter-related infection. N Engl J Med 1977; 296:1305–1309.

43. Maki DG, Ringer M. Risk factors for infusion-related phlebitis with small peripheral venous catheters. A randomized controlled trial. Ann Intern Med 1991; 114:845–854.

44. Eyer S, Brummitt C, Crossley K, Siegel R, Cerra F. Catheter-related sepsis: prospective randomized study of three methods of long-term catheter maintenance. Crit Care Med 1990; 18:1073–1079.

45. Yeung C, May J, Hughes R. Infection rate for single lumen vs. triple lumen subclavian catheters. Infect Control Hosp Epidemiol 1988; 9:154–158.

46. Haslett TM, Isenberg HD, Hilton E, Tucci V, Kay BG, Vellozzi EM. Microbiology of indwelling central intravascular catheters. J Clin Microbiol 1988; 26:696–701.

47. Mermel LA, Maki DG. Infectious complications of Swan-Ganz pulmonary artery catheters. Pathogenesis, epidemiology, prevention, and management. Am J Respir Crit Care Med 1994; 149:1020–1036.

48. Band JD, Maki DG. Infections caused by arterial catheters used for hemodynamic monitoring. Am J Med 1979; 67:735–741.

49. Donowitz LG, Marsik FJ, Hoyt JW, Wenzel RP. *Serratia marcescens* bacteremia from contaminated pressure transducers. JAMA 1979; 242:1749–1751.

50. Beck-Sagué CM, Jarvis WR. Epidemic bloodstream infections associated with pressure transducers: a persistent problem. Infect Control Hosp Epidemiol 1989; 10: 54–59.

51. Press OW, Ramsey PG, Larson EB, Fefer A, Hickman RO. Hickman catheter infections in patients with malignancies. Medicine (Baltimore) 1984; 63:189–200.

52. Weightman NC, Simpson EM, Speller DC, Mott MG, Oakhill A. Bacteraemia related to indwelling central venous catheters: prevention, diagnosis and treatment. Eur J Clin Microbiol Infect Dis 1988; 7:125–129.

53. Decker MD, Edwards KM. Central venous catheter infections. Pediatr Clin North Am 1988; 35:579–612.

54. Benezra D, Kiehn TE, Gold JW, Brown AE, Turnbull AD, Armstrong D. Prospective study of infections in indwelling central venous catheters using quantitative blood cultures. Am J Med 1988; 85:495–498.

55. Rotstein C, Brock L, Roberts RS. The incidence of first Hickman catheter-related infection and predictors of catheter removal in cancer patients. Infect Control Hosp Epidemiol 1995; 16:451–458.

56. Johnson PR, Decker MD, Edwards KM, Schaffner W, Wright PF. Frequency of broviac catheter infections in pediatric oncology patients. J Infect Dis 1986; 154: 570–578.

57. Mueller BU, Skelton J, Callender DP, et al. A prospective randomized trial comparing the infectious and noninfectious complications of an externalized catheter versus a subcutaneously implanted device in cancer patients. J Clin Oncol 1992; 10:1943–1948.

58. Matsaniotis NS, Syriopoulou VP, Theodoridou MC, Tzanetou KG, Mostrou GI. *Enterobacter* sepsis in infants and children due to contaminated intravenous fluids. Infect Control 1984; 5:471–477.

59. Maki DG, Rhame FS, Mackel DC, Bennett JV. Nationwide epidemic of septicemia caused by contaminated intravenous products. 1. Epidemiologic and clinical features. Am J Med 1976; 60:471–485.

60. Jarvis WR. Nosocomial outbreaks: the Centers for Disease Control's Hospital Infections Program experience, 1980–1990. Epidemiology Branch, Hospital Infections Program. Am J Med 1991; 91(suppl 3B):101S–106S.

61. Jarvis WR, Highsmith AK, Allen JR, Haley RW. Polymicrobial bacteremia associated with lipid emulsion in a neonatal intensive care unit. Pediatr Infect Dis 1983; 2: 203–208.

62. Mermel LA, Maki DG. Epidemic bloodstream infections from hemodynamic pressure monitoring: signs of the times. Infect Control Hosp Epidemiol 1989; 10:47–53.

63. Beck-Sagué CM, Jarvis WR, Brook JH, et al. Epidemic bacteremia due to *Acinetobacter baumannii* in five intensive care units. Am J Epidemiol 1990; 132:723–733.

64. Morduchowicz G, Pitlik SD, Huminer D, et al. Transfusion reactions due to bacterial contamination of blood and blood products. Rev Infect Dis 1991; 13:307–314.

65. Bufill JA, Ritch PS. *Yersinia enterocolitica* serotype 0:3 sepsis after blood transfusion. N Engl J Med 1989; 320:810.

66. Rhame FS, Root RK, MacLowry JD, Dadisman TA, Bennett JV. *Salmonella* septicemia from platelet transfusions. Study of an outbreak traced to a hematogenous carrier of *Salmonella cholerae-suis*. Ann Intern Med 1973; 78:633–641.

67. Murray AE, Bartzokas CA, Shepherd AJN, Roberts FM. Blood transfusion-associat-

ed *Pseudomonas fluorescens* septicaemia: is this an increasing problem? J Hosp Infect 1987; 9:243–248.

68. Buchholz DH, Young VM, Friedman NR, Reilly JA, Mardiney MR Jr. Bacterial proliferation in platelet products stored at room temperature. Transfusion-induced *Enterobacter* sepsis. N Engl J Med 1971; 285:429–433.

69. Jarvis WR, Martone WJ. Predominant pathogens in hospital infections. J Antimicrob Chemother 1992; 29(suppl A):19–24.

70. Bollet C, Elkouby A, Pietri P, de Micco P. Isolation of *Enterobacter amnigenus* from a heart transplant recipient. Eur J Clin Microbiol Infect Dis 1991; 10:1071–1073.

71. Wong VK. Broviac catheter infection with *Kluyvera cryocrescens:* a case report. J Clin Microbiol 1987; 25:1115–1116.

72. Mermel LA, Spiegel CA. Nosocomial sepsis due to *Serratia odorifera* Biovar 1. Clin Infect Dis 1992; 14:208–210.

73. Bodey GP, Elting L, Kassamali H, Lim BP. *Escherichia coli* bacteremia in cancer patients. Am J Med 1986; 81(suppl 1A):85–95.

74. Bouza E, Garcia de la Torre G, Erice A, Loza E, Diaz-Borrego JM, Buzón L. *Enterobacter* bacteremia. An analysis of 50 episodes. Arch Intern Med 1985; 145:1024–1027.

75. Chow JW, Fine MJ, Shlaes DM, et al. *Enterobacter* bacteremia: clinical features and emergence of antibiotic resistance during therapy. Ann Intern Med 1991; 115:585–590.

76. Bodey GP, Elting LS, Rodriguez S. Bacteremia caused by *Enterobacter:* 15 years of experience in a cancer hospital. Rev Infect Dis 1991; 13:550–558.

77. Saito H, Elting L, Bodey GP, Berkey P. *Serratia* bacteremia: review of 118 cases. Rev Infect Dis 1989; 11:912–920.

78. Pollack M. *Pseudomonas aeruginosa.* In: Mandell GL, Douglas RG, Bennett J, eds. Principles and Practice of Infectious Diseases. 4th ed. New York: Churchill Livingstone, 1995:1980–2003.

79. Baltch AL. *Pseudomonas aeruginosa* bacteremia. In: Baltch AL, Smith RP, eds. *Pseudomonas aeruginosa* Infections and Treatment. New York: Marcel Decker, 1994:73–128.

80. Flick MR, Cluff LE. *Pseudomonas* bacteremia. Review of 108 cases. Am J Med 1976; 60:501–508.

81. Mallolas J, Gatell JM, Miró JM, et al. Analysis of prognostic factors in 274 consecutive episodes of *Pseudomonas aeruginosa* bacteremia. Antibiot Chemother 1991; 44:106–114.

82. Hilf M, Yu VL, Sharp J, Zuravleff JJ, Korvick JA, Muder RR. Antibiotic therapy for *Pseudomonas aeruginosa* bacteremia: outcome correlations in a prospective study of 200 patients. Am J Med 1989; 87:540–546.

83. McManus AT, Mason AD, McManus WF, Pruitt BA. Twenty-five year review of *Pseudomonas aeruginosa* bacteremia in a burn center. Eur J Clin Microbiol 1985; 4:219–223.

84. Fichtenbaum CJ, Woeltje KF, Powderly WG. Serious *Pseudomonas aeruginosa* infections in patients infected with human immunodeficiency virus: a case-control study. Clin Infect Dis 1994; 19:417–422.

85. Roilides E, Butler KM, Husson RN, Mueller BU, Lewis LL, Pizzo PA. *Pseudomonas*

infections in children with human immunodeficiency virus infection. Pediatr Infect Dis J 1992; 11:547–553.

86. Nelson MR, Shanson DC, Barter GJ, Hawkins DA, Garrard BG. *Pseudomonas* septicaemia associated with HIV. AIDS 1991; 5:761–763.

87. Rizzari C, Palamone G, Corbetta A, Uderzo C, Vigano EF, Codecasa G. Central venous catheter-related infections in pediatric hematology-oncology patients: role of home and hospital management. Pediatr Hematol Oncol 1992; 9:115–123.

88. Bouvet PJ, Grimont PA. Taxonomy of the genus *Acinetobacter* with the recognition of *Acinetobacter baumannii* sp. nov., *Acinetobacter haemolyticus* sp. nov., *Acinetobacter johnsonii* sp. nov., and *Acinetobacter junii* sp. nov. and emended descriptions of *Acinetobacter calcoaceticus* and *Acinetobacter lwoffii.* Int J Syst Bacteriol 1986; 36:228–240.

89. Siegman-Igra Y, Bar-Yosef S, Gorea A, Avram J. Nosocomial *Acinetobacter* miningitis secondary to invasive procedures: report of 25 cases and review. Clin Infect Dis 1993; 17:843–849.

90. Daly AK, Postic B, Kass EH. Infections due to organisms of the genus *Herella.* Arch Int Med 1962; 110:86–91.

91. Rolston K, Guan Z, Bodey GP, Elting L. *Acinetobacter calcoaceticus* septicemia in patients with cancer. South Med J 1985; 78:647–651.

92. Tilley PAG, Roberts FJ. Bacteremia with *Acinetobacter* species: risk factors and prognosis in different clinical settings. Clin Infect Dis 1994; 18:896–900.

93. Galvao C, Swartz R, Rocher L, Reynolds J, Starmann B, Wilson D. *Acinetobacter* peritonitis during chronic peritoneal dialysis. Am J Kidney Dis 1989; 14:101–104.

94. Reindersma P, Nohlmans L, Korten JJ. *Acinetobacter,* an infrequent cause of community acquired bacterial meningitis. Clin Neurol Neurosurg 1993; 95:71–73.

95. Seifert H, Strate A, Pulverer G. Bacteremia due to *Acinetobacter* species other than *Acinetobacter baumannii.* Infection 1994; 22:379–385.

96. Weinberger I, Davidson E, Rotenberg Z, Fuchs J, Agmon J. Prosthetic valve endocarditis caused by *Acinetobacter calcoaceticus* subsp. *lwoffii.* J Clin Microbiol 1987; 25:955–957.

97. Seifert H, Strate A, Schulze A, Pulverer G. Vascular catheter-related bloodstream infections due to *Acinetobacter johnsonii* (formerly *A. calcoaceticus* var. *lwoffii*): report of 13 cases. Clin Infect Dis 1993; 17:632–636.

98. Seifert H. *Acinetobacter* species as a cause of catheter-related infections. Zbl Bakt 1995; 283:161–168.

99. Seifert H, Schulze A, Hofmann R, Pulverer G. Skin and mucous membrane colonization is an important source of nosocomial *Acinetobacter baumannii* infection: a prospective surveillance study. 7th International Congress for Infectious Diseases, Hong Kong, June 10–13, 1996. Abstract 10656.

100. Peters G, Locci R, Pulverer G. Microbial colonization of prosthetic devices. II. Scanning electron microscopy of naturally infected intravenous catheters. Zbl Bakt 1981; 173:293–299.

101. Woods DE, Vasil ML. Pathogenesis of *Pseudomonas aeruginosa* infections. In: Baltch AL, Smith RP, eds. *Pseudomonas aeruginosa* Infections and Treatment. New York: Marcel Dekker, 1994:21–50.

102. Kowalewska-Grochowska K, Richards R, Moysa GL, Lam K, Costerton JW, King

EG. Guidewire catheter change in central venous catheter biofilm formation in a burn population. Chest 1991; 100:1090–1095.

103. Dasgupta MK, Costerton JW. Significance of biofilm adherent bacterial microcolonies on Tenckhoff catheters in CAPD patients. Blood Purif 1989; 7:144–155.

104. Nickel JC, Downey JA, Costerton JW. Ultrastructural study of microbiologic colonization of urinary catheters. Urology 1989; 34:284–291.

105. Martínez-Martínez, L, Pascual A, Perea EJ. Effect of three plastic catheters on survival and growth of *Pseudomonas aeruginosa.* J Hosp Infect 1990; 16:311–318.

106. Tancrede CH, Andremont AO. Bacterial translocation and gram-negative bacteremia in patients having hematological malignancies. J Infect Dis 1985; 15:99–103.

107. Goldmann DA, Martin WT, Worthington JW. Growth of bacteria and fungi in total parenteral nutrition solutions. Am J Surg 1973; 126:314–318.

108. Carson L, Favero M, Bond W, et al. Morphological biochemical and growth characteristics of *Pseudomonas cepacia* from distilled water. Appl Microbiol 1973; 25: 476–483.

109. Maki DG, Martin WT. Nationwide epidemic of septicemia caused by contaminated infusion products. IV. Growth of microbial pathogens in fluids for intravenous infusion. J Infect Dis 1975; 131:267–272.

110. Crocker KS, Noga R, Filibeck DJ, Krey SH, Markovic M, Steffee WP. Microbial growth comparisons of five commercial parenteral lipid emulsions. J Parenter Enteral Nutr 1984; 8:391–395.

111. Garrison RN, Richardson JD, Fry DE. Catheter-associated septic thrombophlebitis. South Med J 1982; 75:917–919.

112. Johnson RA, Zajac RA, Evans ME. Suppurative thrombophlebitis: correlation between pathogen and underlying disease. Infect Control 1986; 7:582–585.

113. Topiel MS, Bryan RT, Kessler CM, Simon GL. Case report: treatment of silastic catheter-induced central vein septic thrombophlebitis. Am J Med Sci 1986; 291: 425–428.

114. Terpenning MS, Buggy BP, Kauffmann CA. Hospital-acquired infective endocarditis. Arch Intern Med 1988; 148:1601–1603.

115. Raad II, Bodey GP. Infectious complications of indwelling vascular catheters. Clin Infect Dis 1992; 15:197–210.

116. Wang EEL, Prober CG, Ford-Jones L, Gold R. The management of central intravenous catheter infections. Pediatr Infect Dis 1984; 3:110–113.

117. Johnson DC, Johnson FL, Goldman S. Preliminary results treating persistent central venous catheter infections with the antibiotic lock technique in pediatric patients. Pediatr Infect Dis J 1994; 13:930–931.

118. Benoit JL, Carandang G, Sitrin M, Arnow PM. Intraluminal antibiotic treatment of central venous catheter infections in patients receiving parenteral nutrition at home. Clin Infect Dis 1995; 21:1286–1288.

119. Krzywda EA, Andris DA, Edmiston CE, Quebbeman EJ. Treatment of Hickman catheter sepsis using antibiotic lock technique. Infect Control Hosp Epidemiol 1995; 16:596–598.

120. Rao, JS, O'Meara A, Harvey T, Breatnach F. A new approach to the management of Broviac catheter infection. J Hosp Infect 1992; 22:109–116.

121. Seifert H, Baginski R, Schulze A, Pulverer G. Antimicrobial susceptibility of *Acinetobacter* species. Antimicrob Agents Chemother 1993; 37:750–753.

122. Flynn PM, Shenep JL, Stokes DC, Barrett FF. In situ management of confirmed central venous catheter-related bacteremia. Pediatr Infect Dis J 1987; 6:729–734.

123. Elting LS, Bodey GP. Septicemia due to *Xanthomonas* species and non-*aeruginosa Pseudomonas* species: increasing incidence of catheter-related infections. Medicine (Baltimore) 1990; 69:296–306.

124. Hiemenz J, Skelton J, Pizzo PA. Perspective on the management of catheter-related infections in cancer patients. Pediatr Infect Dis 1986; 5:6–11.

6

Fungal Infections of Catheters

Sergio B. Wey and Arnaldo Colombo
São Paulo Federal Medical School, São Paulo, Brazil

I. INTRODUCTION

The past three decades have witnessed major changes in hospital populations and in the technology used in healthcare. As a result, there has been an improvement in patient survival, but some of these patients are highly susceptible to infection. These patients often have diseases and complications that require the use of invasive techniques for both monitoring and treatment. Fungi are pathogens that can take advantage of these procedures, especially in the compromised host.

Multiple studies from various hospitals have reported an increasing rate of nosocomial fungal infections. Bloodstream infections are one of the most serious hospital-acquired infections and many are caused by the use of vascular catheters, which are widely used in hospitals for monitoring and intravenous therapy, especially in intensive care units.

Several factors interfere with an analysis of fungal infections caused by indwelling intravascular catheters. One is the widely differing criteria used to define fungal infection or colonization of vascular catheters. Another is that the vast majority of published articles do not differentiate between the ethiologic agents involved in such infections. Many studies do not specify catheter type or whether the catheter had been in use on a short-term or long-term basis. To complicate matters further, different populations of patients with a variety of different intravascular catheters have been analyzed together.

The incidence of nosocomial bloodstream infection has ranged from 1.2 to 13.9 per 1000 hospital admissions, and from 0.3 to 2.02 per 1000 days of care (1). Primary nosocomial candidemia rates ranged from 2.8 per 10,000 discharges in nonteaching hospitals to 6.1 per 10,000 discharges in large teaching hospitals in 1989 according to data collected by the National Nosocomial Infections Surveillance (NNIS) program (2). This represented a fivefold increase over the period 1980–1989. Beck-Sagué and co-workers (3) analyzed data collected by the NNIS program from 115 hospitals from January 1980 to December 1990. During this time, 30,477 nosocomial fungal infections were reported. The nosocomial fungal infection rate at the facilities increased from 2.0 infections per 1000 patients discharged in 1980 to 3.8 in 1990, while cases of nosocomial fungemia rose from 1.0 to 4.9 per 10,000 patients discharged. The proportion of nosocomial infections reported by all hospitals due to fungal pathogens at all major sites of infection, rose from 6% in 1980 to 10.4% in 1990, and the proportion of nosocomial bloodstream infections that were fungal increased from 5.4% to 9.9%. The proportion of bloodstream infections due to fungal pathogens varied depending on patient care characteristics. Patients who had a central intravascular catheter were more than three times as likely to have a fungus isolated as were patients with bloodstream infection who did not have such a catheter ($P < 0.001$).

Central line–associated bloodstream infection rates have varied among different types of intensive care units (ICUs). Device-associated bloodstream infections have accounted for more than 90% of the bloodstream infections reported to the NNIS (4). In a prospective study of five hospitals in Germany and Switzerland, Dashner and colleagues (5) reported that nosocomial bloodstream infections accounted for 14.2% to 28.8% of all nosocomial infections occurring in the ICUs.

Most of the species of microorganisms causing primary nosocomial bloodstream infections at NNIS hospitals did not change significantly from 1975 to 1983 (4). In 1975, *Candida* spp. did not appear on the list of the 10 leading pathogens, but in 1983 it was the seventh most common pathogen, representing 5.6% of cases. *Candida* accounted for 7.8% of cases for the period 1986–1989 and was the fourth most common etiologic agent in primary bloodstream infections. Morrison and colleagues (6), using a statewide surveillance network in Virginia, found that coagulase-negative staphylococci and *Candida* spp. were the only pathogens that demonstrated statistically significant increases in bloodstream infection rates over the period 1978–1984. Fungi accounted for 6% of bloodstream infections in a neonatal intensive care unit between 1976 and 1978, and 13% of bloodstream infections in the same unit between 1979 and 1981 (7).

Mortality due to fungal nosocomial bloodstream infection is significant. Miller and Wenzel (8), studying 385 episodes of nosocomial bloodstream infections, found that the presence of *Candida* spp. and *Pseudomonas* spp. were independent predictors of death. An NNIS analysis (3) showed that patients with fungemia were more likely to die during hospitalization [954 (29%) of 3256] than were patients with bloodstream infection due to nonfungal pathogens [5594 (17%) of 3882; relative risk, 1.8; 95% confidence interval, 1.7–1.9; $P < 0.001$].

A relationship between candidemia and indwelling vascular catheters has been recognized for decades. In 1962, Louria et al. (9) reported that 23 of the 29 patients who developed systemic candidiasis had indwelling vascular catheters. In four of these patients cultures from the skin around apparently uninfected cut-down sites, taken at the onset of fungemia, grew species of *Candida* that were identical to those found in the blood.

Fungi can cause important infections in long-term intravascular catheters such as Hickman and Broviac tunneled catheter and subcutaneous ports. Between January 1982 and December 1983, King and co-workers (10) studied 335 Broviac catheters placed in 270 infants and children. Blood culture-proven sepsis occurred on 77 occasions (23%), an average of one septic episode for every 434 days of catheter use. Eighty-three bacterial (94%) and five fungal isolates were recovered from blood culture. The fungemias included two *Candida* spp. and three patients with *Malassezia furfur.*

Uderzo et al. (11) studied infectious and mechanical complications occurring with long-term central venous catheters in children with hematological malignancies who underwent bone marrow transplantation. *Pseudomonas* and *Candida* species were more commonly isolated in hospital-managed patients whereas coagulase-negative staphylococci were more frequently isolated in domiciliary infections.

In summary, it is possible to conclude from the medical literature that during the past decade the overall incidence of nosocomial fungemia has steadily increased, with most cases involving *Candida* species, and that many such infections are related to the use of intravascular catheters.

II. PATHOGENESIS

The pathogenesis of fungal infections due to intravascular devices may be infusion-related or cannula-related. Infusion-related sepsis is very rare, but the lack of awareness of the problem can contribute to under reporting by healthcare workers (12–14).

The infusate can be contaminated during its manufacture (intrinsic contamination) or during its preparation and administration in the hospital (extrinsic contamination) (12). There are several reports of fungemias secondary to the contamination of parental nutrition formulations (15–17).

There is a strong relationship between *Candida parapsilosis* fungemia or systemic infection and hyperalimentation using intravascular devices (18). The adherence of *C. parapsilosis* to plastic materials exceeds that of *C. albicans.* The capability of *C. parapsilosis* isolates to proliferate and produce large amounts of slime in glucose-containing solutions may facilitate their ability to cause catheter-related fungemia (18–21).

Another example of systemic yeast infection specifically related to catheter use is *Malassezia furfur*. Fungemia due to *M. furfur*, which does not invade the gastrointestinal tract, almost invariably has an intravascular line as a portal of entry. This organism proliferates in fat emulsions and has been particularly associated with catheter-related fungemias in pediatric patients undergoing hyperalimentation (13,22). Occlusion of the catheter and adhesion of the central venous catheter to the wall of the vein has been reported in association with *M. furfur* infection (23,24).

Central venous catheters, particularly long-term catheters, are the intravascular devices most likely to cause infection (12). The source of catheter-related bacteremia has been investigated by several authors and is still a controversial subject. The skin surrounding the insertion site can be a source of the fungus and, as a consequence, catheter-related infections. Other investigators have highlighted the hub as an important source of catheter-related septicemia (12,25–27). Raad et al. (28) found that luminal colonization increased progressively with duration of catheterization and that in short-term central venous catheters the skin was the main source of catheter colonization; in long-term vascular catheters (>30 days), colonization was predominantly luminal.

Despite the paucity of published studies on the pathogenesis of catheter-related fungemia, it seems reasonable to discuss mechanisms of fungal infection according to the models that have been proposed to explain catheter-related bacteremia. Thus far, the site care during the catheter insertion and thereafter by healthcare workers, and the skin colonization appear to be potential sources for fungal infections.

Fungus can be found colonizing the site of catheter insertion and the subcutaneous tract created by the catheter in patients with infected intravascular devices (29,30). This is an indication that catheter-related fungemia can be the result of invasion of yeast at the site of catheter insertion and along the subcutaneous tract created by the catheter. It is likely that the administration of broad-spectrum antibiotics plays a role in eradicating endogenous competing flora and promoting overgrowth of yeast in the skin area surrounding the catheter entry site. Polymyxin-neomycin-bacitracin ointment placed at the catheter exit site results in a 50% decrease in the frequency of bacterial colonization but a fivefold increase in fungal colonization of the catheter (74), and has been associated with an increased risk of catheter-related candidiasis in some studies (30a). In addition, underlying diseases can contribute to local yeast catheter wound colonization and infection (30).

Another possibility is yeast colonization of the hub through contact of the device with the patient's skin flora or with the hands of healthcare personnel, with subsequent entry of fungi into the catheter lumen and migration along the luminal surface to the intravascular portion of the device. In support of this hypothesis, is the observation of an adherent biofilm, including hyphal elements, on the luminal surface of long-term intravascular catheters removed from patients who had developed *Candida* spp. fungemia (32,33).

Finally, hematogenous seeding of vascular catheters following secondary fungemia could cause catheter colonization and persistence of infection. According to Anaissie et al. (34), this phenomenon is uncommon, but it may be more common for *Candida* spp. than for other microorganisms causing catheter-related bloodstream infection (12).

Primary cutaneous aspergillosis has been reported as a cause of infection at the cutaneous catheter exit site. In this clinical situation, the source of infection appears to be the adhesive tape or arm boards (35–38). Other molds have been associated with infections related to intravascular devices, such as *Paecilomyces* spp. and *Fusarium* spp. (39,40).

Candida species can be a cause of suppurative peripheral thrombophlebitis. According to Walsh et al., the pathogenesis of this infection appears to be the result of preceding candidal colonization of the skin and inadequate intravenous site care in susceptible patients, permiting candidal infection of the catheter wound and progression to the venous wall. Additionally, candidemia from other sites could cause colonization of the catheter with subsequent candidal thrombophlebitis (41).

After colonization of the catheter, microbial factors and host immunity play a role in the progression to fungemia and clinical sepsis (31).

III. DIAGNOSIS

Gram staining and cultures must be performed from pus obtained from any superficial or subcutaneously infected site that is related to the use of peripheral or central intravenous lines. In cases of suppurative peripheral thrombophlebitis, histopathology and culture of the removed segment of thrombosed vein is usually helpful in diagnosing the causative agent (42,43).

Several methods have been described for the diagnosis of vascular catheter-related septicemia (44–46). Unfortunately, the accuracy of these methods for correctly identifying catheter-related fungal infections has not been demonstrated. A semiquantitative roll plate culture method and several quantitative methods that permit culturing of the internal surface of catheters have been applied to the diagnosis of catheter-related septicemia (44–48). However, the original data obtained in these studies were related to bacterial and not fungal infections. As a consequence, there is not a validated "gold standard" for diagnosing catheter related fungemia.

Recently, Khatib et al. (49) published data from a retrospective study in which 3544 intravavascular catheters had been cultured by a semiquantitative culture technique (SQC). *Candida* species were present in 80 catheters. Although the authors found a high rate of SQC-positive specimens among patients with invasive candidiasis, they also found positive results among catheters obtained from patients without corresponding clinical illness.

Tellenti et al. (50), studying the relationship between quantitative data from peripheral blood cultures and source of infection, found a good correlation between high-grade candidemia (>25 CFU/10 ml of blood) and an intravascular sources of fungemia. Of 48 episodes of high-grade fungemia, 43 (90%) were associated with an infected intravascular device. However, it is important to note that the authors used Maki's criteria as the "gold standard" to classify episodes of candidemia that were associated with an intravascular device (44).

Available culture methods are associated with low sensitivity for early recognition of systemic candidiasis. New diagnostic approaches have been attempted for identifying and monitoring the course of patients with disseminated candidiasis. These methods include the detection of cell wall mannan, cytoplasmic antigens such as *Candida* enolase antigens, and specific metabolites such as D-arabinitol. Another possibility is the detection of *Candida* spp. specific genomes by polymerase chain reaction. All these methods are currently under development and investigation, and are not routinely available in clinical microbiology laboratories (51).

IV. EPIDEMIOLOGY AND RISK FACTORS

Previous studies have identified several risk factors for the development of nosocomial fungemia. Among the clinical characteristics that most consistently increase this risk are neutropenia, use of wide-spectrum antibiotics, hyperalimentation, antecedent surgery (especially abdominal surgery), and indwelling catheters (13). In 1967, Ellis and Spivack (52) described a series of 12 patients with disseminated candidemia; all had intravenous catheters in place, and *Candida* was recovered from three of the catheters. In the same year, Louria et al. (53) presented a series of seven patients with fungemia due to yeasts other than C. albicans. All patients had intravascular catheters. Vic-Dupont et al. (54) found that intravascular catheters were the source for 16 out of 30 cases of candidemia. Between 1969 and 1970, Williams et al. (55) published a review of 27 cases of *Candida* septicemia; 25 of the patients had indwelling central venous catheters. More significantly, the authors found that 89% of these 25 patients had developed positive cultures after the central venous catheter had been in place for 2 weeks.

Long-term, indwelling, central venous catheters have facilitated the care of patients with cancer, but local and systemic infections remain a major cause of morbidity and catheter failure. Fungal infections have complicated the management of patients with these catheters for many years. Hickman et al. published an article in 1979 showing *Candida* spp. and *Nocardia* spp. colonization of Broviac catheters in bone marrow transplant recipients (56).

Lecciones and colleagues (13) reviewed a total of 155 episodes of fungemia associated with an indwelling central catheter that had developed in 149 inpatients with cancer during a 10-year period (January 1979 to December 1988). The majority of the patients had lymphoma or solid tumors, and most episodes of fungemia were associated with neutropenia, the use of wide-spectrum antibiotics, and/or hyperalimentation. Many patients had received chemotherapy or undergone surgery (usually abdominal) within the month preceding the diagnosis of fungemia. Ninety-eight percent of fungemic episodes were caused by *Candida* spp., with *C. albicans* accounting for approximately three-fourths of cases and *Candida tropicalis* accounting for 13%. One episode of *Malassezia furfur* and one of *Saccharomyces cerevisiae* fungemia were also found. Eighty percent of infected catheters were short-term catheters.

Moro and co-workers (17) observed 623 episodes of central venous catheterization among 607 patients admitted to intensive care units. Overall, 58 catheter-related infections were recorded (9.3/100 catheters); 47 were local infections (7.5/100 catheters) and 11 were septicemias (1.8/100 catheters). *Candida albicans* represented 3 (5.9%) of the local infections and *Candida* spp. were responsible for five of the 11 episodes of catheter-related sepsis. The authors found that colonization with *Candida* species was frequently associated with systemic infections.

Franceschi et al. (57) studied the risk factors associated with intravascular catheter colonization in burn patients. They analyzed 101 intravascular catheter sites from 89 patients. The overall incidence of colonized catheters was 25.7% (>15 CFU). The most frequent organisms recovered from the colonized tips were *Pseudomonas* spp. (30.7%), coagulase-negative staphylococci (27%), and *Candida albicans* (27%). The incidence of catheter colonization was inversely correlated with the distance of the catheter insertion from the site of the burn. A stepwise, logistic, multivariate analysis showed cutaneous colonization at the insertion site at the time of catheter removal to be a significant risk factor for catheter colonization.

Wey and colleagues (58) studied risk factors for nosocomial candidemia in 88 patients who had at least one blood culture positive for *Candida* spp. These patients were pair-matched using six criteria: age, period at risk, primary diagnosis, surgery, date of admission, and sex. Using a step-wise, logistic regression analysis, four independent variables were selected that predicted the acquisition of nosocomial candidemia. These were the number of antibiotics received before infection, prior use of a Hickman catheter, isolation of *Candida* spp. from other body sites, and prior hemodialysis. Bross et al. (59) studied adult patients without leukemia who acquired nosocomial candidemia. Each patient was matched to a control based on medical speciality and duration of hospitalization up to the first *Candida* spp.-positive blood culture. Seven risk factors were identified through a logistic regression including prior antibiotic use, candiduria, central catheter use, and azotemia. Karanabis et al. (60) compared 30 cancer patients with candidemia with 58 controls. The multivariate logistic model showed the following independent risk factors for candidemia: positive peripheral cultures for *Candida* spp. ($P = 0.002$), central venous catheterization ($P = 0.03$), and neutropenia ($P = 0.05$). These last three studies reached similar conclusions about the use of central lines and antibiotics as risk factors for candidemia.

Groeger and colleagues (61) followed 1430 cancer patients who had been submitted to long-term venous access devices for at least 500 days. Fungi were responsible for 11 (3.3%) of the bloodstream infections that were related to tunneled catheters and one (3.5%) of those related to subcutaneous ports. The fungi cultured were *C. parapsilosis* (5), *C. albicans* (2), *Rhodotorula rubra* (1), *Malassezia furfur* (1), *Torulopsis glabrata* (1), *Alternaria* spp. (1), and *Aspergillus niger* (1).

An important risk factor for infection/colonization of an indwelling intravascular catheter by a fungus is the utilization of total parenteral nutrition (TPN). This therapeutic measure has been associated with an appreciable risk of sepsis, with fungal sepsis being an especially serious complication (62). The incidence of catheter-associated bloodstream infection in patients receiving TPN ranges from 0% to 14% with an average of 3–5%. *Candida* spp. are the usual fungal isolates. *Malassezia furfur* is a rare but serious infection, associated with TPN in young children (63).

NNIS data from 1980 to 1990 (2) show that patients with bloodstream infections receiving total parenteral nutrition or those in intensive care units were more likely to develop fungemia (15.6% and 11.0%, respectively) than those not receiving total parenteral nutrition (6.4%) or not in intensive care units (8.1%). When parenteral nutrition was controlled for, central intravascular catheterization was significantly associated with fungemia. Among patients with central intravascular catheters receiving total parenteral nutrition who developed bloodstream infections, those in intensive care units were still somewhat more likely to have fungemia (relative risk, 1.2; 95% confidence interval, 1.1–1.4).

Outbreaks of *Candida parapsilosis* fungemia have been traced to contaminated vacuum pumps used to prepare parenteral nutrition solutions, central intravascular pressure monitoring, and use of parenteral nutrition in immunocompromised hosts (2). Solomon et al. described an outbreak of *Candida parapsilosis* bloodstream infection in patients receiving parenteral nutrition (16). Epidemiologic investigation showed an association with the use of an electrically powered vacuum pump to assist parenteral nutrition. Cultures from the vacuum pump showed heavy growth of *C. parapsilosis* from multiple sites. Laboratory investigation demonstrated that sterile solutions could be contaminated by the vacuum pump. Use of the vacuum pump was stopped, and no further cases occurred. *Candida parapsilosis* was also responsible for nosocomial fungemia in eight infants in a neonatal intensive care unit. A case control study compared the cases with 29 weight-matched controls. Logistic regression analysis indicated that the risk factors for candidemia were duration of umbilical artery catheterization, duration of parenteral nutrition, and estimated gestational age. Parenteral nutrition therapy was often administered through the umbilical artery catheter, which was also used for monitoring arterial pressure. The transducer domes thus contained parenteral nutrition fluid. Transducers were usually disinfected with alcohol. Laboratory investigation showed that the heads of six of 11 blood pressure transducers in use and one of four transducers in storage after disinfection were culture-positive for *C. parapsilosis.* After control measures were instituted, no further cases occurred (64).

V. CLINICAL SYNDROMES AND AGENTS

Unfortunately, there are no characteristic clinical signs and symptoms to indicate a diagnosis of disseminated fungal disease. There is the possibility that infected or colonized catheters may seed organisms to various body sites, resulting in a great variety of clinical presentation depending on the affected organs. For example, when *Candida* is disseminated, multiple organs are usually affected, especially the kidney, brain, myocardium, and eye.

Candida species are the most common fungi isolated from intravascular catheters. Horn and Conway (65) documented four cases of candidemia related to fully implantable venous access systems in patients with cystic fibrosis. These cases were successfully treated, but removal of the venous access device was necessary in each case. Tchekmedyian et al. (33) described a case of a patient with acute nonlymphocytic leukemia who developed *Staphylococcus epidermidis* bacteremia and candidemia after maintenance chemotherapy. The patient also developed an infected abdominal aortic aneurysm. The same organisms were cultured from the aneurysm as from the Hickman catheter. This suggests that the Hickman catheter was the source of the candidemia and may well have caused the infection in the aneurysm.

Fungal thrombophlebitis is a major concern for those with indwelling intravascular catheters. Both peripheral and deep vascular structures can be involved as well as the venous and arterial sides of the circulation (66). *Candida* species are not usually considered a cause of suppurative peripheral thrombophlebitis. Walsh et al. (41) described seven cases of suppurative peripheral thrombophlebitis during a 15-month period. They defined candidal peripheral thrombophlebitis by the following criteria: (1) clinical evidence of venous catheter-associated thrombophlebitis manifested by warmth, tenderness, erythema, palpable cord, and/or suppuration at the percutaneous catheter puncture site, and (2) microbiologic evidence of *Candida* spp. demonstrated by culture in resected vein specimens or pus expressed from the intravenous catheter exit site. The median duration of hospitalization until development of candidal peripheral thrombophlebitis was 27 days; subjects had a median age of 64 years. All patients were admitted to the surgical service and had underlying diseases, including cancer in three, diabetes mellitus in three, and ethanol abuse in two. All but one patient underwent surgery. None of the patients was receiving corticosteroids, cytotoxic therapy, or parenteral hyperalimentation when the thrombophlebitis developed. All patients had concomitant infections and all had received antibiotics for at least 2 weeks before candidal thrombophebitis was diagnosed. Five of the seven patients had had candidal colonization of urine, sputum, or wounds preceding their phlebitis. Gram stain and culture of expressed pus in three patients showed only *Candida* species. Five patients had veins resected surgically that were grossly purulent; all five grew *Candida* species. *C. albicans* was present in five patients, *C. tropicalis* in one, and *C. lipolytica* in another. Four had candidemia, but none had ocular or cutaneous manifestations of systemic candidiasis.

Fry et al. found 32 episodes of septic thrombophlebitis in 143 patients that had had an intravascular device (67). *Candida* spp. was isolated in two of them. In no case was it necessary to excise veins in the absence of local signs of infection and inflammation at the venous access site. None of the cases were related to central venous catheters.

Fungal infections of long-term catheters are difficult to differentiate clinically from bacterial infections. When nonpurulent erythematous lesions progress to radial necrotic lesions at the exit site of the catheter, *Aspergillus* infection should be suspected (37). If there is purulent discharge at the exit site, the pus should be examined microscopically and cultured. Fungal infection can also affect the pocket of fully implantable devices. Such infections may present with local inflammation, including erythema and necrosis over the reservoir. *Aspergillus* spp. are not often found in vascular catheters, but Allo et al. described nine cases of primary cutaneous aspergillosis at the entry site of Hickman catheters in immunocompromised patients (37). All patients had underlying hematologic cancer and the Hickman catheter had been placed to provide venous access for chemotherapy, hyperalimentation, or both. Clinical signs of infection included erythema, induration, and cutaneous or subcutaneous necrosis at the point of entry into the subclavian vein, in the subcutaneous tunnel, or at the exit site from the skin. Diagnosis was confirmed by positive wound culture for *Aspergillus flavus* in all but one patient.

Tan and colleagues (39) reported a case of an 18-month-old white male baby with obstructive uropathy secondary to embryonal rhabdomyosarcoma group III involving the bladder and prostate. A tunneled central venous catheter (Hickman) was in place at the time of tumor biopsy, but removed 3 months later after the patient developed a catheter-associated chest wall abscess and sepsis due to *K. pneumoniae*. A fully implantable central venous catheter (Portacath) was therefore inserted 1 month later to allow chemotherapy to continue. The blood cultures obtained from the Portcath and peripheral vein were positive for the same mold, subsequently identified as *Paecilomyces lilacinus*. The catheter was removed and amphotericin B was initiated. The patient was discharged without further clinical evidence of infection.

Right atrial thrombosis is a potentially lethal complication associated with central venous catheters, which are now used in nearly 70% of all patients in pediatric intensive care units (68). Paut et al. (69) reported a case of right atrial septic thrombosis due to catheter-related fungal sepsis in a young trauma victim. A 9-year-old boy with multiple trauma was submitted to surgery and received cefamandol for 5 days; a CVC was inserted on the second day posttrauma to allow total parenteral nutrition. The patient improved, but on day 12 sepsis developed and was treated empirically with antibiotics. On day 14 blood specimens, as well as the catheter tip, proved positive for *Candida albicans* and amphotericin B and 5 flucytosine were initiated. On day 17, candidal endophthalmitis was diagnosed and a large right atrial mass was confirmed by two-dimensional echocardiography. The patient was submitted to surgery, and a mass containing fungi was removed. The patient improved and was discharged from intensive care unit on day 36. Important sequelae of fungemia include endophthalmitis, endocarditis, and hepatosplenic candidiasis (13).

The compromised host is especially susceptible to infection due to uncommon microorganisms. Sycova-Milá et al. (70) reported a case of *Trichosporon capitatum* catheter-associated fungemia which followed a severe clinical course in a compromised host and was successfully treated with amphotericin B plus flucytosine. The yeast was found in both blood and catheter cultures. Kiehn and co-workers (71) reported 23 patients between 1985 and 1989 who had catheter-related *Rhodotorula* sepsis. All 23 had indwelling central venous catheters that had been in place from 1 to 22 months (average, 9.3 months). Blood was drawn from both the catheter and a peripheral source, but only one patient had a peripheral blood culture positive for *Rhodotorula* spp. Colony counts of yeast from the catheter cultures often exceeded 100 (15 patients) and even 1000 (seven patients) CFU/mL of blood.

The incidence of *Fusarium* spp. infection is increasing, especially among compromised patients. Disseminated fusariosis is an uncommon disease, and the reasons for the increasing incidence are multiple. Important factors include the use of intensive chemotherapeutic regimens for the treatment of malignancies and bone marrow transplant recipients, the empirical use of broad-spectrum antibiotics, the early use of amphotericin B in febrile neutropenic patients, and the increasing number of patients with impaired mucosal or skin barriers due underlying malignancy or chomotherapy. Ammari et al. (72) described a case of a 13-year-old boy with acute promyelocytic leukemia, in remission, who had a catheter-related *Fusarium solani* fungemia and pulmonary infection. The patient had many factors that predisposed him to opportunistic infection, including underlying malignancy, immunosuppressive chemotherapy, and an indwelling central venous line. The blood culture obtained by venipuncture and Broviac catheter were positive for *Fusarium solani*.

Malassezia furfur is the etiologic agent of tinea versicolor and is considered a relatively benign agent. However, some reports from the literature suggest a strong correlation between *M. furfur* sepsis and the use of intravascular catheters. It was cultured from the lumen of 32% of catheters removed from infants over 1 week of age in a neonatal intensive care unit (73). Two of these patients also had clinical evidence of systemic infection.

VI.   CONTROL MEASURES

Nosocomial infections have become increasingly more difficult to prevent and manage. The most important infection control measures for the prevention of fungal colonization of indwelling intravascular catheters are quite similar to those recommended for bacterial infections, which have been outlined elsewhere in this text. However, some peculiarities of fungal complications should be addressed.

Flowers et al. (74) performed a randomized controlled trial in order to evaluate the efficacy of an attachable subcutaneous cuff to prevent central vascular catheter-related infection among patients receiving intensive care. All catheters were dressed with polyantibiotic ointment containing polymyxin, neomycin, and bacitracin. They found that catheters with cuffs were associated with less frequent bloodstream infection than controls (0% vs. 13%). However, an unexpectedly large proportion (75%) of catheter infections were due to *Candida albicans*. This may have been due in part to the use of polyantibiotic ointment, as suggested by a pooled analysis of previous trials that demonstrated increased *Candida* colonization in catheters in which the ointment had been used.

Candidal peripheral thrombophlebitis can be prevented by vigorous skin preparation, site care, and routine rotation of intravenous catheter sites every 48 to 72 hours (41). Other infection control measures to prevent candidal peripheral thrombophlebitis include limiting the spectrum and duration of antimicrobial therapy to specific culture-defined organisms, short time intervals, and meticulous care of intravenous sites. New scientific approaches are needed to help establish better techniques for catheter management.

VII.   THERAPY

The aim of this chapter is not so much to address the use of specific antifungal agents as to outline some general therapeutic measures. Whether the infected catheter should always be removed is polemic. The major problem with candidemia or fungemia is determining which patients have tissue invasion and thus require antifungal therapy, and which can be treated by simply removing the catheter. Rose reported 55 cases of candidemia associated with venous catheters (75). Of the 35 patients who survived, 26 became afebrile within 72 hours after removal of the catheter. While most bacterial infections of long-term CVC can be cured without removal of the catheter, the same is not true of fungal catheter infections. There have been occasional reports of fungal infection associated with long-term CVCs that were cured with antifungal therapy alone. But the overwhelming experience of fungal infection (usually with *Candida* spp.) associated with the use of the long-term CVC, is that the catheter must be removed for resolution of the infection to occur (76).

The decision to remove the catheter must be formed on an individual basis because case-specific and patient-specific factors prevent general recommendations. Removal of the catheter system is indicated for the following situations: documented *Candida* or fungal catheter-associated infection, purulent tunnel infection, or persistent bloodstream infection after the third day of appropriate intravenous antimicrobial therapy (77).

Some authors state that is prudent to remove the long-term catheter and treat the patient with intravenous amphotericin B when catheter infection is due to *Candida* spp. or *Aspergillus* spp. Patients with fungal infections of their catheters should be monitored for dissemination. *Aspergillus* mainly disseminates to the lung, while *Candida* has a predeliction for the eye, necessitating frequent funduscopic examinations (78).

Kiehn et al. (71) studied 23 patients who had had catheter-related *Rhodotorula* sepsis. Thirteen were treated with antifungal therapy and removal of the catheter while five patients received antifungal therapy alone and another five had the catheter removed without antifungal therapy. All patients survived the fungemic episode and experienced no recurrence.

Allo et al. (37) treated nine cases of primary cutaneous aspergillosis at Hickman catheter sites. The treatment consisted of intravenous amphotericin B, oral fluocytosine, and local wound care. Three patients recovered completely without operative debridement, and a further three recovered after operative debridement and delayed grafting. Two patients died of disseminated aspergillosis, and one died of unrelated causes while still recovering from primary cutaneous aspergillosis. Successful treatment required resolution of aplasia or leukopenia, catheter removal, systemic treatment with amphotericin B, and local wound care.

The treatment of peripheral candidal thrombophlebitis also includes removal of the infected peripheral venous catheter. Walsh et al. (41) documented a cluster of seven cases of peripheral candidal thrombophlebitis, all of which resolved. Three received systemic therapy (amphotericin B), two topical care, and five venous resection.

Catheter-related candidiasis has in the past been managed in some cases by simply removing the catheter. Many patients were cured by this approach, but the attributable mortality of candidemia has been estimated at 38% (58). Fourteen percent of nonneutropenic patients developed endophthalmitis in a recent study (30a). Most authorities recommend amphotericin B for therapy of neutropenic patients with candidiasis. For nonneutropenic patients, fluconazole 400 mg qd and amphotericin B 0.6 mg/kg/day were equivalent in a recent randomized trial (30a).

Catheter infection was believed responsible for 72% of cases of candidiasis. Most authorities recommend removal of catheters infected with *Candida* (78).

REFERENCES

1. Hamory BH. Nosocomial bloodstream and intravascular device-related infections: In: Wenzel RP, ed. Prevention and Control of Nosocomial Infections. Baltimore: Williams & Wilkins, 1987:283–319.
2. Banerjee SN, Emori TG, Culver DH, et al. Secular trends in nosocomial primary bloodstream infections in the United States, 1980–1989. National Nosocomial Infections Surveillance System. Am J Med 1991; 91:86S–89S.
3. Beck-Sagué CM, Jarvis R, National Nosocomial Infections Surveillance System. Secular trends in the epidemiology of nosocomial fungal infections in the United States, 1980–1990. J Infect Dis 1993; 167:1247–1251.
4. Pittet D. Nosocomial bloodstream infections. In; Wenzel RP, ed. Prevention and Control of Nosocomial Infections. Baltimore: Williams & Wilkins, 1993:512–555.
5. Daschner FD, Frey P, Wolff G, Baumann PC, Suter P. Nosocomial infections in intensive care wards: a multicenter prospective study. Intens Care Med 1982; 8:5–9.
6. Morrison AJ Jr, Freer CV, Searcy MA, Landry SM, Wenzel RP. Nosocomial bloodstream infections: secular trends in a statewide surveillance program in Virginia. Infect Control 1986; 7:550–553.
7. Donowitz LG, Haley CE, Gregory WW, Wenzel RP. Neonatal intensive care unit bacteremia: emergence of gram-positive bacteria as major pathogens. Am J Infect Control 1987; 15:141–147.
8. Miller PJ, Wenzel RP. Etiologic organisms as independent predictors of death and morbidity associated with bloodstream infections. J Infect Dis 1987; 156:471–477.
9. Louria DB, Stiff DP, Bennett B. Disseminated moniliasis in the adult. Medicine 1962; 41:317–333.
10. King DR, Komer M, Hoffman J, et al. Broviac catheter sepsis: the natural history of an iatrogenic infection. J Pediatr Surg 1985; 20:728–733.
11. Uderzo C, D'Angelo P, Rizzari C, et al. Central venous catheter-related complications after bone marrow transplantation in children with hematological malignancies. Bone Marrow Transplant 1992; 9:113–117.
12. Maki DG. Pathogenesis, prevention and management of infections due to intravascular devices used for infusion therapy. In: Bisno AL, Waldvogel FA, eds. Infections Associated With Indwelling Medical Devices. Washington, DC: American Society for Microbiology, 1989:161–177.
13. Lecciones JA, Lee JW, Navarro EE, et al. Vascular catheter-associated fungemia in patients with cancer: analysis of 155 episodes. Clin Infect Dis 1992; 14:875–883.
14. Curry CR, Quie PG. Fungal septicemia in patients receiving parenteral hyperalimentation. N Engl J Med 1971; 285:1221–1225.
15. Plouffe JF, Brown DG, Silva J, Eck T, Stricof RL, Fekety R. Nosocomial outbreak of *Candida parapsilosis* fungemia related to intravenous infusions. Arch Intern Med 1977; 137:1686–1689.

16. Solomon SL, Khabbaz RF, Parker RH, et al. An outbreak of *Candida parapsilosis* bloodstream infections in patients receiving parenteral nutrition. J Infect Dis 1984; 149(1):98–102.

17. Moro ML, Maffei C, Manso E, Morace G, Polonelli L, Biavasco F. Nosocomial outbreak of systemic candidosis associated with parenteral nutrition. Infect Control Hosp Epidemiol 1990; 11(1):27–35.

18. Weems JJ. *Candida parapsilosis:* epidemiology, pathogenicity, clinical manifestations, and antimicrobial susceptibility. Clin Infect Dis 1992; 14:756–766.

19. Branchini ML, Pfaller MA, Rhine-Chalberg J, Frempong T, Isenberg HD. Genotypic variation and slime production among blood and catheter isolates of *Candida parapsilosis*. J Clin Microbiol 1994; 32(2):452–456.

20. Pfaller MA, Messer SA, Hollis RJ. Variations in DNA subtype, antifungal susceptibility, and slime production among clinical isolates of *Candida parapsilosis*. Diagn Microbiol Infect Dis. 1995; 21:9–14.

21. Critchley IA, Douglas LJ. Differential adhesion of pathogenic *Candida* species to epithelial and inert surfaces. FEMS Microbiol Lett 1985; 28:199–203.

22. Marcon MJ, Powell DA. Human infections due to *Malassezia* spp. Clin Microb Rev 1992; 5(2):101–119.

23. Kim EH, Cohen RS, Ramachandram P, Glasscock GF. Adhesion of percutaneously inserted silastic central venous lines to the vein wall associated with *Malassezia furfur* infection. J Parenter Enter Nutr 1993; 17(5):458–460.

24. Azimi PH, Levernier K, Lefrak LM, et al. *Malassezia furfur:* a cause of occlusion of percutaneous central venous catheters in infants in the intensive care nursery. Pediatr Infect Dis J 1988; 7:100–103.

25. Sitges-Serra A, Puig P, Linares J, et al. Hub colonization as the initial step in an outbreak of catheter-related sepsis due to coagulase-negative staphylococci during parenteral nutrition. J. Parenter. Ent. Nutr. 1984; 8:668–672.

26. Linares J, Sitges-Serra A, Garau J, Perez JL, Martin R. Pathogenesis of catheter sepsis: a prospective study with quantitative and semiquantitative cultures of catheter hub and segments. J. Clin. Microb. 1985; 21:357–360.

27. Cooper GL, Hopkins CC. Rapid diagnosis of intravascular catheter-associated infection by direct gram staining of catheter segments. N. Engl. J. Med. 1985; 312:1142–1147.

28. Raad II, Costeron W, Sabharwal U, Sacilowski M, Anaissie E, Bodey GP. Ultrastructural analysis of indwelling vascular catheters: a quantitative relationship between luminal colonization and duration of placement. J. Infect. Dis. 1993; 168: 400–407.

29. Bjornson HS, Colley R, Bower RH, et al. Association between microorganism growth at the catheter insertion site and colonization of the catheter in patients receiving total parenteral nutrition. Surgery 1982; 92(4):720–727.

30. McGeer A, Righer J. Improving our ability to diagnose infections associated with central venous catheters: value of Gram's staining and culture of entry site swabs. CMAJ 1987; 137:1009–1021.

30a. Rex JH, Bennett JE, Sugar AM, et al. A randomized trial comparing fluconazole with amphotericin B for the treatment of candidemia in patients without neutropenia. N Engl J Med 1994; 331:1125–1130.

31. Wade JC. Epidemiology of *Candida* infections. In: Bodey, GP, ed. Candidiasis: Pathogenesis, Diagnosis, and Treatment. New York: Raven Press, 1993:85–107.

32. Tenney JH, Moody MR, Newman KA, et al. Adherent microorganisms on luminal surfaces of long-term intravenous catheters. Arch Intern Med 1986; 146:1949–1954.

33. Tchekmedyian NS, Newman K, Moody MR, et al. Case report: special studies of the Hickman catheter of a patient with recurrent bacteremia and candidemia. Am J Med Sci 1986; 291(6):419–424.

34. Anaisse E, Samonis G, Kortoyianni D, et al. Role of catheter colonization and unfrequent hematogenous seeding catheter-related infections. Eur J Clin Microbiol Infect Dis 1995; 14:134–137.

35. Young RC, Bennett JE, Vogel CL, Carboni PR, DeVita VT. Aspergillosis: the spectrum of the disease in 98 patients. Medicine 1970; 49:147–173.

36. Khardori N, Hayat S, Rolston K, Bodey GP. Cutaneous *Rhizopus* and *Aspergillus* infections in five patients with cancer. Arch Dermatol 1989; 125:952–956.

37. Allo MD, Miller J, Townsend T, Tan C. Primary cutaneous aspergillosis associated with Hickman intravenous catheters. N Engl J Med 1987; 317:1105–1108.

38. Hunt SJ, Nagi C, Gross KG, Wong DS, Mathews WC. Primary cutaneous aspergillosis near central venous catheters in patients with the acquired immunodeficiency syndrome. Arch Dermatol 1992; 128:1229–1232.

39. Tan TQ, Ogden AK, Tillman J, Demmler GJ, Rinaldi MG. *Paecilomyces lilacinus* catheter-related fungemia in an immunocompromised pediatric patient. J Clin Microbiol 1992; 30(9):2479–2483.

40. Rabodonirina M, Piens MA, Monier MF, Guého E, Fière D, Mojon M. Fusarium infections in immunocompromised patients: case reports and literature review. Eur J Clin Microbiol Infect Dis 1994; 13:152–161.

41. Walsh TJ, Bustamente CI, Vlahov, Standiford HC. Candidal suppurative peripheral thrombophlebitis: recognition, prevention, and management. Infect Control 1986; 7(1):16–22.

42. Torres-Rojas JR, Stratton CW, Sanders CV, et al. Candidal suppurative peripheral thrombophlebitis. Ann Intern Med 1982; 96:431–435.

43. Johnson A, Oppenhein R. Vascular catheter-related sepsis: diagnosis and prevention. J Hosp Infect 1992; 20:67–78.

44. Maki DG, Weise CE, Sarafin HW. A semiquantitative culture method for identifying intravenous-catheter-related infection. N Engl J Med 1977; 296(23):1305–1309.

45. Cleri DJ, Corrado ML, Seligman SJ. Quantitative culture of intravenous catheters and other intravascular inserts. J Infect Dis 1980; 141:781–786.

46. Sherertz RJ, Raad II, Balani A, et al. Three year experience with sonicated vascular catheter cultures in a clinical microbiology laboratory. J Clin Microb 1990; 28:76–82.

47. Brun-Buisson C, Abrouk F, Legrand P, Houet Y, Larabi S, Rapin M. Diagnosis of central venous catheter-related sepsis. Critical levels of quantitative tip cultures. Arch Intern Med 1987; 147:873–877.

48. Raad II, Sabbagh MF, Rand KH, Sherertz RJ. Quantitative tip culture methods and the diagnosis of central venous catheter-related infections. Diagn Microbiol Infect Dis 1992; 15:13–20.

49. Khatib Riad, Clark JF, Briski LE, Wilson FM. Relevance of culturing *Candida* species from intravascular catheters. J Clin Microb 1995; 33(6):1635–1637.

50. Telenti A, Steckelberg JM, Stockman L, Edson RS, Roberts GD. Quantitative blood cultures in candidemia. Mayo Clin Proc 1991; 66:1120–1123.

51. Walsh TJ, Pizzo PA. Laboratory diagnosis of candidiasis. In: Bodey GP, ed. Candidiasis: Pathogenesis, Diagnosis, and Treatment. New York: Raven Press, 1993:109–135.

52. Ellis CA, Spivack ML. The significant of candidemia. Ann Intern Med 1967; 67(3): 511–522.

53. Louria DV, Blevins A, Armastrong D, Burdick R, Lieberman P. Fungemia caused by "nonpathogenic" yeasts. Arch Intern Med 1967; 119:247–252.

54. Vic-Dupont V, Coulaud JP, Delrieu F. Les septièmies a *Candida*. Presse Med 1968; 76:747–750.

55. Williams RJ, Chandler JG, Orloff MJ. *Candida* septicemia. Arch Surg 1971; 103: 8–11.

56. Hickman RO, Buckner CD, Clift RA, Sanders JE, Stewart P, Thomas ED. A modified right atrial catheter for access to the venous system in marrow transplant recipients. Surg Gynecol Obstet 1979; 148:871–875.

57. Franceschi D, Gerding RL, Phillips G, Fratianne RB. Risk factors associated with intravascular catheter infections in burned patients: a prospective, randomized study. J Trauma 1989; 29:811–816.

58. Wey SB, Mori M, Pfaller MA, Woolson RF, Wenzel RP. Risk factors for hospital-acquired candidemia. A matched case-control study. Arch Intern Med 1989; 149: 2349–2353.

59. Bross J, Talbot FH, Maislin G, Hurwitz S, Strom BL. Risk factors for nosocomial candidemia: a case-control study in adults without leukemia. Am J Med 1989; 87:614–620.

60. Karanabis A, Hill C, Leclercq B, Tancrede C, Baume D, Andremont A. Risk factors for candidemia in cancer patients: a case-control study. J Clin Microbiol 1988; 26: 429–432.

61. Groeger JS, Lucas AB, Thaler HT, et al. Infectious morbidity associated with long-term use of venous devices in patients with cancer. Ann Intern Med 1993; 119:1168–1174.

62. Armstrong CW, Mayhall CG, Miller KB, et al. Clinical predictors of infections of central venous catheters used for total parenteral nutrition. Infect Control Hosp Epidemiol 1990; 11:71–78.

63. Dankner WM, Spector SA, Ferier J, Davis CE. *Malassezia* fungemia in neonates and adults: complication of hyperalimentation. Rev Infect Dis 1987; 9:743–753.

64. Solomon SL, Alexander H, Eley JW, et al. Nosocomial fungemia in neonates associated with intravascular pressure-monitoring devices. Pediatr Infect Dis 1986; 5: 680–685.

65. Horn CK, Conway SP. Candidemia: risk factors in patients with cystic fibrosis who have totally implantable venous access systems. J Infect 1993; 26:127–132.

66. Widmer AF. IV-related infections. In: Wenzel RP, ed. Prevention and Control of Nosocomial Infections. Baltimore: Williams & Wilkins, 1993:556–579.

67. Fry DE, Fry RV, Borzotta AP. Nosocomial blood-borne infection secondary to intravascular devices. Am J Surg 1994; 167:268–272.
68. Bagwell CE, Marchildon MB. Mural thrombi in children: potentially lethal complication of central venous hyperalimentation. Crit Care Med 1989; 17:295–296.
69. Paut O, Kreitmann B, Silicani MA, et al. Successful treatment of fungal right atrial thrombosis complicating central venous catheterization in a critically ill child. Intens Care Med 1992; 18:375–376.
70. Sycova-Milá Z, Sufliarshy J, Trupl J, Jasendská Z, Blahvá M, Krcmery V Jr. Catheter-associated septicemia due to *Trichosporon capitatum.* J Hosp Infect 1992; 22:257–261.
71. Kiehn TE, Gorey E, Brown AE, Edwards FF, Armstrong D. Sepsis due to *Rhodotorula* related to use of indwelling central venous catheters. Clin Infect Dis 1992; 14: 841–846.
72. Ammari LK, Puck JM, McGown KL. Catheter-related *Fusarium solani* fungemia and pulmonary infection in a patient with leukemia in remission. Clin Infect Dis 1993; 16:148–150.
73. Aschner JL, Punsalang A, Maniscalco WM, Menegus MA. Percutaneous central venous catheter colonization with *Malassezia furfur:* incidence and clinical significance. Pediatrics 1987; 80:535–539.
74. Flowers III RH, Schwenzer KJ, Kopel RF, Fisch MJ, Tucker SI, Farr BM. Efficacy of an attachable subcutaneous cuff of th prevention of intravascular catheter-related infection. JAMA 1989; 261:878–883.
75. Rose HD. Venous catheter-associated candidemia. Am J Med Sci 1978; 275:265–269.
76. Clarke DE, Raffin TA. Infectious complications of indwelling long-term central venous catheters. Chest 1990; 97:966–972.
77. Press OW, Ramsey PG, Larson EB, Fefer A, Kickman RO. Hickman catheter infections in patients with malignancies. Medicine 1984; 63:189–200.
78. Mayhall G. Diagnosis and management of infections of implantable devices used for prolonged venous access. Curr Clin Top Infect Dis 1992; 12:83–110.

7

Miscellaneous Organisms

Andreas Voss
University Hospital St. Radboud, Nijmegen, The Netherlands

I. INTRODUCTION

Coagulase-negative staphylococci are still the most frequently isolated pathogens from patients with catheter-related infections. The increasing use of indwelling devices in an expanding population of immunocompromised patients may be the most important explanation for why the list of microorganisms involved in catheter-related infections continues to expand, since "nonpathogenic" microorganisms from the patient's skin, formerly regarded as contaminants, may cause infections. The improved microbiological diagnostic, especially the development of easy-to-use identification systems, may have also led to the recognition of "new" pathogens. Novel approaches in catheter design and materials may help to reduce colonization with *Staphylococcus epidermidis* and other gram-positive cocci (1), but may not always help to prevent infections due to other, frequently saprophytic microorganisms.

This chapter reviews case reports and small series of catheter-related infections (CRI) due to "miscellaneous" bacterial pathogens, i.e., microorganisms that rarely cause infection, as well as common pathogens which do not usually cause catheter-related infections. Rare fungal catheter-related infections such as those due to *Malassezia furfur* (2) or *Acremonium* (3) are discussed elsewhere in this book.

At the moment, case reports of catheter-related infections due to "miscellaneous" organisms are still rare enough to be reported in the medical literature, but in the above-mentioned situation we might encounter these organisms on a regular basis.

At Memorial Sloan-Kettering Cancer Center in New York, the extensive use of vascular access devices and associated device-related sepsis has resulted in changes in the type (and colony counts) of organisms causing bloodstream infections (4). The proportion of bacteremia caused by "miscellaneous" organisms increased from 12% to 19% in 1984 and 1988, respectively (Table 1).

II.   MISCELLANEOUS GRAM-NEGATIVE BACTERIA

In contrast to the "classical" bacteria causing CRI, among the miscellaneous pathogens, gram-negative organisms dominate over gram-positive organisms. For the purpose of this chapter, the organisms are classified as (1) "nonfermenters," (2) *Pseudomonas* spp. and related genera, and (3) other gram-negative bacilli (Table 2). The more common gram-negative organisms involved in CRI, such as Enterobacteriaceae, including rare species such as *Enterobacter amnigenus* (5) and *Klyvera cryocrescens* (6); *Pseudomonas aeruginosa*; and *Acinetobacter* species are covered elsewhere in this book.

A.   *Pseudomonas* Species and Related Genera

The taxonomy of *Pseudomonas* species and related genera was recently changed. Some of the microorganisms now belong to the genus *Stenotrophomonas* and *Burkholderia*. Bacteremia due to *Stenotrophomonas (Xanthomonas) maltophilia* and non-*aeruginosa Pseudomonas* species occurs rarely but may be increasing. At the M.D. Anderson Cancer Center the rate of bacteremia due to these bacteria significantly increased from three cases per 10,000 admissions in 1974 to 14 cases per 10,000 admissions in 1986 (7). About 50% of these infections were caused by *S. maltophilia*, whereas *P. stutzeri* and *P. putida* each accounted for about 10%. Other species, such as *P. fluorescens*, *P. paucimobilis*, *P. testosteroni*, *P. vesicularis*, *P. picketti*, or *Burkholderia (Pseudomonas) cepacia*, were seen occasionally. The most important predisposing factor in the immunocompromised patients was the presence of an indwelling central venous or arterial line, present in 83% of the patients for an average of 3 months before the onset of bacteremia. Catheters were proven to be the source of the infection in 57 of 83 patients (69%) in whom the portal of entry was identified. Ninety-five percent of these patients responded to therapy.

It was shown that the removal of the central venous catheter resulted in a 100% cure rate, irrespective of the appropriateness of the antibiotic therapy. Recurrent catheter-related infections were seen in 29% of patients who had

Table 1 Microorganisms Causing Bacteremia at Memorial Sloan-Kettering Cancer Center

	No. (%) of episodes	
Organisms	1984 (n = 64)	1988 (n = 190)
Anaerobes	42 (8)	35 (4)
Bacteroides spp.	21 (4)	18 (2)
Clostridium spp.	14 (3)	16 (2)
Others	7 (1)	1
Non-*aeruginosa Pseudomonas* spp.	3 (1)	59 (5)
P. fluorescens		3 (0.5)
P. (Stenotrophomonas) maltophilia		32 (3)
P. putida		14 (1.5)
Others	19 (3)	96 (10)
Aeromonas spp.	2	2
Alcaligenes spp.	0	3
Bacillus spp.	3 (1)	26 (3)
Corynebacterium spp.	8 (2)	45 (5)
Flavobacterium spp.	0	4
H. influenzae	0	4
Listeria spp.	5 (1)	5 (1)
Micrococcus spp.	0	7 (1)
Vibrio spp.	1	0

Source: Adapted from Ref. 4.

received appropriate antibiotics but in whom the catheter, or the site of catheter insertion (during guide wire exchange), had not been changed. Thus, removal of the catheter and, if still necessary, insertion at a new site, seems to be of utmost importance in successfully managing CRI due to these microorganisms. In contrast to these findings, Decker et al. (8) reported two cases of *P. paucimobilis* CRI which were successfully treated without removal of the Groshong catheters. Of interest, one of the patients was treated with TMP/SMZ, since the strain was resistant to ceftazidime.

B. cepacia is widely distributed throughout the environment, especially water and soil. Outbreaks of infection have been reported as a result of exposure to contaminated povidone-iodine solutions, parenteral fluids, and invasive pressure-monitoring devices (9,10). After contact with a contaminated heparin flush

Table 2 Miscellaneous Gram-Negative Bacteria Causing Catheter-Related Infection

Gram-negative bacteria	Species	Reference
Pseudomonas species and related genera	Stenothrophomonas maltophilia	Elting and Bodey (7)
	Pseudomonas stutzeri	Elting and Bodey (7)
	Pseudomonas paucimobilis	Decker et al. (8)
	Pseudomonas putida	Anaissie et al. (11)
	Pseudomonas pickettii	Raveh et al. (12)
	Pseudomonas fluorescens	Elting and Bodey (7)
	Burkholderia cepacia	Pegues et al. (10)
	Comamonas acidovorans	Castagnola et al. (14)
	Methylobacterium extorquens	Poirier et al. (16); Kaye et al. (17)
	Chryseomonas luteola (CDC group Ve-1)	Kostman et al. (19)
	Flavimonas oryzihabitans (CDC group Ve-2)	Kostman et al. (19); Conlu et al. (22)
	CDC group IV c-2	Arduino et al. (18)
Other "nonfermenters" (nonfermentative gram-negative bacteria)	Alcaligenes xylosoxidans (=Achromobacter xylosoxidans)	Legrand and Anaissie (30); Cieslak and Raszak (25)
	Ochrobactrum anthropi (= Achromobacter, CDC group Vd)	Cieslak et al. (24); Gransden and Eykyn (26); Kern et al. (23); Alnor et al. (28)
	Agrobacterium spp.	Edmond et al. (31); Alnor et al. (28)
	Flavobacterium spp.	Stamm et al. (34)
Other gram-negative bacilli	Aeromonas hydrophila	Siddiqui et al. (36); Rello et al. (35)
	Bordetella bronchiseptica	Qureshi et al. (38)
	Kingella kingae	Goutzmanis et al. (40)
	Moraxella osloensis	Buchman et al. (39)

solution, 15 patients with catheter-associated *B. cepacia* bacteremia were identified in a U.S. oncology center (10). The findings emphasize the importance of avoiding multiple use of solutions intended for single use.

P. putida is a ubiquitous environmental saprophyte found in soil, in water, and on plants. The organism may also be a part of the normal human oropharyngeal flora. In 1987, *P. putida* was described as a newly recognized pathogen causing bacteremia in cancer patients at the M.D. Anderson Hospital, Texas (11). Between 1980 and 1985 the organism was isolated from blood culture specimens of 15 patients, including five cases considered to have polymicrobial bacteremia. The bloodstream infection appeared to be catheter-related in three patients who had phlebitis, cellulitis, or both at the catheter insertion site. The increase in *P. putida* infections during the study period was paralleled by a similar increase in the number of intravascular devices. In cases of catheter-related bacteremia, removal of the catheter in addition to antimicrobial treatment—e.g., ceftazidime, ciprofloxacin, imipenem, or piperacillin—was necessary to control the infection.

CRI due to *P. pickettii* were reported for the first time by Raveh et al. (12), who described four cases, all of which were associated with long-term indwelling intravascular devices, such as Infuse-a-port, Broviac, and Hickman catheters.

So far, *P. putrefaciens* has not been reported to cause catheter-related bacteremia, but three patients were described with CAPD-peritonitis, which was probably associated with the Tenckhoff catheter (13).

Comamonas acidovorans is ubiquitous in the environment, including soil and foodstuffs. Recently, a boy with non-Hodgkin's lymphoma was reported with *C. acidovorans* CRI (14). The child was admitted for treatment of a herpes simplex virus ocular infection and experienced symptoms of sepsis during infusion therapy. Treatment with ceftazidime and vancomycin was started; amikacin was added the next day when *C. acidovorans* was recovered from blood cultures. Despite a clinical response, bacteremia persisted until the Broviac catheter was removed.

Methylobacterium extorquens was originally isolated from the surface of a leaf (15). Various synonyms have been used for *Methylobacterium*, such as *Pseudomonas mesophilica*, *Protaminobacter rubra*, *Pseudomonas methanolica*, *Vibrio extorquens*, and *Mycoplana rubra*. *M. extorquens* is an opportunistic pathogen of low virulence, causing CRI, fever, pulmonary infiltrates, ulcers and uveitis, among the 16 cases reported so far in the literature (16,17). Blood isolates were shown to be susceptible to TMP/SMZ, tetracycline, imipenem, ciprofloxacin, and aminoglycosides. The indolent nature of the infection might justify antibiotic treatment without removal of the catheter, even though this recommendation is based on the results of only three cases (16).

Other genera related to *Pseudomonas* that are known to cause bacteremia include CDC Group IV c-2, *Chryseomonas luteola* (CDC Group VE-1), and *Flavimonas oryzihabitans*, formerly know as CDC Group Ve-2, *Pseudomonas oryzihabitans*, or *Chromobacterium typhiflavum* (18–22). Reported cases are generally associated with the presence of prosthetic material or catheters in immunocompromised patients.

F. oryzihabitans is a relatively avirulent, nonfermenting, gram-negative bacillus that has been isolated from skin, wounds, sputum, urine, and blood, but was not classified as clinically significant until the first report of infection in 1977

(21). Since then, *F. oryzihabitans* has been reported to cause CAPD-related peritonitis, indwelling venous catheter-related infections, and occasionally bacteremia (19–22). Of 36 cases reported until 1993, 22 episodes of *F. oryzihabitans* sepsis came from one center (20). Most of the patients had significant underlying medical problems, especially malignancies, and the source of infection was unclear since no environmental cultures or cultures from other body sites of infected patients yielded the organism. The CRIs were treatable with TMP/SMZ and antipseudomonal antibiotics. With some exceptions the majority of reviewed cases (81%) did not require the removal of the catheter to control bacteremia.

B. "Nonfermenters" (Nonfermentative Gram-Negative Bacteria)

In general the group of nonfermentative gram-negative bacteria includes a variety of heterogeneous organisms. An overview on colonization or infections due to these organisms is further complicated by the fact that they have undergone frequent taxonomic changes in recent years.

Nonfermentative, nonfastidious, gram-negative bacilli, formerly classified as *Achromobacter* spp. or *Achromobacter*-like organisms, have been assigned to *Ochrobactrum anthropi*, *Alcaligenes* spp., and *Agrobacterium* spp. The organisms have been isolated from clinical specimens, the environment, and hospital water supplies. As far as the confusing taxonomy allows interpretation, it is only recently that these microorganisms have been recognized as pathogens in humans associated with intravascular catheter infections (23–26).

The first case of bacteremia caused by *Ochrobactrum anthrophi* (formerly *Achromobacter*, CDC group Vd) was reported by Kish et al in 1984 (27). Since then, 15 other, mainly catheter-related bacteremia cases have been published (23,24,26,28). Cieslak et al. described the first case of CRI due to *O. anthropi* in a neutropenic, pediatric patient (24). The extensive resistance of these microorganisms to a wide range of antimicrobial agents, including penicillins, cephalosporins, and aminoglycosides, was discussed. Hospital water supplies and translocation from the gut were discussed as possible sources. This publication led to another of seven cases of CRI with *O. anthropi* (26). All the isolates were susceptible to aminoglycosides, ciprofloxacin, imipenem, and trimethoprim-sulfamethoxazole (TMP/SMZ). According to the authors, the infections were managed solely by removing the infected catheters. Interestingly, only two of the seven patients were immunosuppressed. Kern et al. (23) observed four cancer patients with multiple blood cultures yielding *O. anthropi*. The patients presented clinical symptoms consistent with catheter-related bacteremia. In three of the patients, the infection appeared to be unrelated to chemotherapy-associated neutropenia and occurred shortly after hospital admission, or was the reason for it. The antimicrobial susceptibility of the isolates varied, with some of the isolates being resistant to aminoglycosides, newer fluoroquinolones, and TMP/SMZ.

Despite the initial isolates being susceptible to imipenem, treatment with this agent failed to eradicate the organism in two cases, one of which relapsed with bacteremia shortly after treatment was discontinued; the other remained persistently febrile and bacteremic. In general, the choice of antibiotic treatment seems to depend on the individual antibiogram. Removal of the catheter is probably necessary.

Infections, including catheter-associated bacteremia, due to *Alcaligenes xylosoxidans* subsp. *xylosoxidans* (formerly *Achromobacter xylosoxidans* and *Alcaligenes denitrificans* subsp. *xylosoxidans*) were observed in cancer patients (29,30) and in a child with AIDS (25). Despite resistance to aminoglycosides, the patients were successfully treated with a combination of ceftazidime and amikacin, without removing the catheter. The antimicrobial resistance of *Alcaligenes* spp. appears to be unpredictable, and the optimal therapeutic management is unknown. After reviewing the literature, Legrand and Anaissie (30) came to the conclusion that infections usually respond to therapy with TMP/SMZ or an appropriate β-lactam antibiotic. The use of multiple antibiotics (including combinations with aminoglycosides) has also been recommended, but whether the infected device has to be removed or not remains unclear.

Agrobacterium species are nonfermentative saprophytic bacilli, found in aqueous environments and appear to be nonindigenous to human beings. Until 1993, 19 cases of systemic infections had been reported. Infections were strongly related to the presence of plastic foreign material (31). *Agrobacterium radiobacter* may produce copious amounts of slime, and forms biofilms, characteristics that may enhance its pathogenic ability to cause infections in patients requiring intravenous access and peritoneal dialysis (28). Community-acquired CRI may arise through handling plants; most patients reported by Alnor et al. (28) and Hulse et al. (32) acquired their infection at home. Restriction enzyme analysis of *Agrobacterium* isolates from eight patients of one hospital revealed unique patterns in each case, thus excluding a common nosocomial source (32). In patients with mucositis and breakdown of the intestinal barrier, translocation of the organism from the patient's gut might be another possible source. Antimicrobial susceptibility is variable and treatment must be based on individual antibiograms. Most cases responded to treatment only after removal of the indwelling device.

Flavobacterium spp. are found in water and in the hospital environment. Bacteremia was shown to be related to the infusion of contaminated blood (33). In 1973, *Flavobacterium* bloodstream infections occurred in 14 ICU patients in a 5-month-period (34). The infection occurred only in patients with an arterial monitoring system, and *Flavobacterium* spp. were isolated from in-use arterial catheters and stopcocks. Syringes cooled on ice before being used to obtain arterial blood specimens for blood gas determination were suggested as a possible cause of this outbreak. Subsequent cultures from ice in the ice machine grew

Flavobacterium spp., supporting the hypothesis. Fever and positive blood cultures persisted in 8 of 14 patients, despite antibiotic treatment. The symptoms resolved in 5 of 6 patients after the arterial catheter has been removed. No deaths were directly related to *Flavobacterium* bacteremia.

C. Other Gram-Negative Bacilli

Aeromonas hydrophila is a facultative anaerobe, oxidase-positive, gram-negative rod, belonging to the family Vibrionaceae. *Aeromonas* spp. can be found in water, soil, and foodstuffs. *Aeromonas* spp. may cause wound infections, septicemia, diarrheal disease, and extraintestinal infections such as meningitis, osteomyelitis, peritonitis, and urinary tract infections. So far most cases of bacteremia have occurred in patients with hepatic or pancreatic diseases and leukemia. One case of *A. hydrophila* bacteremia was reported among a group of 15 patients with pulmonary artery catheter infections, described by Rello et al. (35). The strain probably originated from the IV system, since the hubs were contaminated with the organism. Siddiqui et al. (36) published a case report of a 50-year-old patient who died of a myonecrosis. The gas gangrene-like presentation due to *A. hydrophila* followed the insertion of an IV catheter into the long saphenous vein.

   Bordetella spp. cause infections in humans and animals. Whereas *B. pertussis* and *B. parapertussis* are restricted to humans, *B. bronchiseptica* mainly causes respiratory infections in animals (37). *B. bronchiseptica* bacteremia is extremely rare. So far only one case of catheter-related bacteremia has been reported (38). At the time of infection, a 33-year-old patient with AIDS received ganciclovir maintenance treatment via an indwelling Broviac catheter. Several weeks after experiencing a CRI due to *Bacillus subtilis* which was cured without removing the catheter, the patient presented with high fever and chills. *Achromobacter* spp. were isolated from blood cultures, and the patient received imipenem. After 2 weeks of treatment the patient was discharged with the Broviac catheter still in place. However, another episode of CRI occurred 3 weeks later. This time, *B. bronchiseptica* was isolated from blood cultures, and despite treatment with imipenem, bacteremia only cleared after the catheter was removed. The authors presumed that the initial identification as *Achromobacter* spp., done in a commercial laboratory, may have been incorrect, since *B. bronchiseptica* and *Achromobacter* spp. differ only by a few biochemical reactions, and the susceptibility tests of the two isolates were very similar (susceptible to aminoglycosides, ciprofloxacin, and imipenem; resistant to all tested penicillins and cephalosporins). The second episode of CRI may therefore represent a relapse. As a possible source of the infection, close contact to an animal vector (cat) was suggested.

   Moraxella osloensis is a gram-negative, oxidase positive, aerobic coccobacillus that is considered to be a part of the normal resident respiratory tract flora and has only rarely been implicated as a human pathogen. The first report of central venous catheter infection was published in 1993 (39). A 71-year-old woman receiving long-term total parenteral nutrition for her short-bowel syndrome and suffering of chronic sinusitis, experienced a sudden-onset fever and rigors after flushing of her Hickman line. No signs of exit site infection were present, but multiple blood cultures drawn through the line grew *M. osloensis*. The authors supposed that the organism had been introduced into the bloodstream either directly from the sinuses or through contamination of catheter hubs with sinus secretions. Treatment with vancomycin and gentamicin was started for presumptive CRI. Clinical signs resolved within a day, and the patient was discharged after 4 weeks of IV treatment. *Moraxella* spp. are usually susceptible in vitro to penicillin, cephalosporins, aminoglycosides, chloramphenicol, and erythromycin, and, as shown in the above report, treatment of CRI may be possible without removing the infected catheter.

Kingella kingae is another uncommon resident of the upper respiratory tract that has been reported to cause CRI (40). This fastidious coccobacillus is part of the so-called HACEK group of microorganisms (*Haemophilus* spp., *Actinobacillus actinomycetemcomitans*, *Cardiobacterium hominis*, *Eikenella corrodens*, *Kingella* spp.) which may cause endocarditis. *K. kingae* mainly causes bacteremia and osteomyelitis, and since the organism does not colonize the skin, CRI is probably secondary to systemic infections. Treatment with penicillins, cephalosporins, aminoglycosides, or TMP/SMZ is recommended (40).

Haemophilus influenzae has not yet been reported to cause CRI, but by 1993, 27 CSF shunt infections have been published including the case described by Wong et al. (41). The reported cases were treated with antibiotics alone, and removal of the shunt was not necessary. The exact pathogenesis of this infection remains unclear, but seeding of bacteria to the meninges and the shunt in the presence of bacteremia seems to be the most probable cause.

III.   MISCELLANEOUS GRAM-POSITIVE BACTERIA

Gram-positive pathogens causing CRI may be divided into (1) *Corynebacterium* spp. and related organisms. (2) gram-positive cocci other than staphylococci, (3) *Bacillus* spp. and other gram-positive rods, (4) mycobacteria, and (5) actinomycetes (Table 3).

A.   *Corynebacterium* spp. and Related Genera

Corynebacterium afermentans var. *afermentans* is a gram-positive rod, formerly referred to as *Corynebacterium* CDC group ANF-1. Like other coryneform bacteria, the microorganism is part of the normal resident skin flora. Two case reports of intravenous line infections with this organism have been published in the literature (42,43). Both authors concluded that the bacteremia in their patients was due to the *Corynebacterium*, even though the organism was only isolated from

Table 3 Misellaneous Gram-Positive Bacteria Causing Catheter-Related Infection

Gram-positive bacteria	Species	Reference
Coryneforms and related organisms	*Corynebacterium afermentans*	Dealler et al. (42); Kerr et al. (43)
	Corynebacterium minutissimum	Cavendish et al. (44)
	Corynebacterium jeikeium	Riebel et al. (45); Fish and Danziger (46)
	Corynebacterium urealyticum	Wood and Pepe (47)
	Corynebacterium striatum	Tumbarello et al. (48)
	Coryneform CDC group A-5	Campbell et al. (49)
	Brevibacterium epidermidis	McCaughey and Damani (50)
Gram-positive cocci	*Enterococcus casseliflavus*	van Goethem et al. (53)
	Enterococcus faecalis	Patterson et al. (51)
	Enterococcus faecium	Patterson et al. (51)
	Enterococcus gallinarum	Patterson et al. (51)
	Pediococcus pentosaceus	Atkins et al. (55)
	Stomatococcus mucilaginosus	Ascher et al. (54)
Bacillus spp. and other gram-positive rods	*Bacillus* spp.	Tuazon et al. (56); Richard et al. (58); Sliman et al. (57); Cotton et al. (59)
	Rothia dentocariosa	Nivar-Aristy et al. (64)
	Listeria monocytogenes	Katner and Joiner (65); Fish and Danziger (46)
Mycobacteria	*Mycobacterium neoaurum*	Davison et al. (67); Holland et al. (68)
	Mycobacterium fortuitum complex	Raad et al. (69)
	Mycobacterium avium complex	Schelonka et al. (70)
Actinomycetes	*Nocardia nova*	Miron et al. (72)
	Nocardia asteroides	Rubin et al. (71)
	Nocardia otitidis-caviarum	Lee et al. (73)
	Tsukamurella paurometabolum	Shapiro et al. (74); Lai (75)
	Gordona rubropertincta	Buchman et al. (76)
	Gordona terrae	Buchman et al. (76)

blood cultures or the line tip, not from both sites. In a patient with cancer reported by Kerr et al. (43) the "failure" to isolate *C. afermentans* from the line was probably attributed to the use of vancomycin at the time the catheter was removed, since the organism was susceptible to glycopeptides, gentamicin, and rifampin. Despite adequate antibiotic treatment, fever resolved only after the Hickman line was removed. Intravenous lines are a likely source of this organism since in vitro experiments show *C. afermentans* to grow in large numbers on the surface of intravenous lines (Dealler, unpublished; in reply to 43).

Cavendish et al. (44) reported a polymicrobial catheter-related bacteremia involving a multiresistant strain of *C. minutissimum*, isolated from blood cultures and the tip of a femoral central venous catheter, together with *C. jeikeium* and *Staphylococcus aureus*. All three microorganisms including *C. minutissimum*, which is usually susceptible to penicillin, cephalosporins, doxycycline, and clindamycin, were only susceptible to vancomycin. It was suggested that the placement of the catheter through a skin lesion (erythrasma?) was responsible for the catheter colonization and subsequent infection (44).

Infections due to *C. jeikeium* (group JK) are reported most frequently in neutropenic or otherwise immunocompromised patients, including AIDS patients, with central venous catheters in place (45,46).

C. urealyticum (formerly group D2) is a skin commensal known to cause urinary tract infections but rarely bacteremia. A CRI due to *C. urealyticum* was reported in a neutropenic patient who did not respond to empiric treatment with imipenem and vancomycin (47). The patient recovered only after removal of the Hickman catheter, which was shown to be heavily contaminated with *C. urealyticum*. Isolates from the catheter and the blood culture were resistant to aminoglycosides and β-lactam antibiotics (including imipenem) but susceptible to vancomycin. This report underlines the importance of removing any device that might be the source of infection due to a skin commensal when bacteremia persists despite apparently appropriate antibiotics.

Until now, a total of five patients with systemic *C. striatum* infections have been described, including one patient with bacteremia. Tumbarello et al. (48) provided the first report of *C. striatum* bacteremia in a patient with AIDS, and believed that the presence of a central venous catheter was the cause of the infection.

Of special interest is a case report of a 11-year-old patient with acute myeloblastic leukemia, who developed catheter-related sepsis caused by a vancomycin-resistant *Corynebacterium* CDC group A-5 (49). The natural habitat and clinical significance of this organism are unknown, but resistance to vancomycin, which is commonly used to treat CRI in neutropenic patients, may cause clinical failure. The boy was successfully treated with cefotaxime, without removal of the catheter.

Brevibacterium epidermidis is part of the normal resident skin flora. Until 1991, no cases of *B. epidermidis* causing illness in man have been reported. However, in 1992 a 40-year-old man receiving total parenteral nutrition developed a subclavian catheter-related infection, with erythema at the insertion site. Peripheral blood cultures and a culture of the catheter tip yielded coryneform bacteria, later identified as *B. epidermidis* (50). As most of the other CRI caused by *Corynebacterium* species, the case reflects the tendency of so-called nonpathogenic skin organisms to cause central venous catheter infections.

B.   Gram-Positive Cocci

During the past decade the prevalence and importance of *Enterococcus* species causing infections has increased significantly. In a prospective, observational study of 110 patients with serious enterococcal infections, such as endocarditis, bacteremia, cholangitis, pancreatitis, osteomyelitis, pneumonia, and empyema, catheter-related bacteremia was the single most common infection, accounting for 28% of all infections (51). In infants, all infections were catheter-related bacteremias. Overall, 78% of the enterococcal isolates were identified as *E. faecalis*, 20% as *E. faecium*, and 1% as *E. gallinarum* and *E. casseliflavus*. *E. faecium* was the most common species accounting for relapse. In one of these patients with CRI due to high-level vancomycin-resistant *E. faecium*, bacteremia reoccurred after the development of ciprofloxacin resistance, which was the only antibiotic initially still susceptible.

Enterococcus casseliflavus is a motile, yellow-pigmented enterococcus, accounting for less than 1% of all human enterococcal isolates (52). Recently, the organism was isolated from multiple blood cultures drawn through both lumina of a Hickman catheter inserted into a 19-year-old patient with leukemia (53). The girl developed fever of unknown origin during aplasia following remission induction therapy and was treated empirically with penicillin, ceftazidime, and vancomycin. Once the organism's identity and susceptibility were known, treatment was switched to ampicillin and teicoplanin since *Enterococcus casseliflavus* is intrinsically resistant to low levels of vancomycin, and after 48 hours of treatment the patient became afebrile. Unfortunately, it was not reported whether or not the colonized Hickman line was removed.

Ascher et al. (54) described 10 cases of bacteremia due to *Stomatococcus mucilaginosus* (formerly *Staphylococcus salivarius*, or *Micrococcus mucilaginosus*) and reviewed eight other case reports of bacteremia due to this organism. Mucositis and catheter-related infections were among the most common clinical presentations, and bacteremia was frequently associated with risk factors such as intravenous drug abuse, cardiac valve disease, presence of foreign bodies (especially indwelling vascular catheters), and an immunocompromised state. *S. mucilaginosus* bacteremia is readily treatable with antibiotics, such as erythromycin, cefazolin, or vancomycin. This organism is of low virulence. Treatment of CRI or foreign-body-related infections might be successful without removal of the device.

Pediococcus spp. are ubiquitous, facultative, anaerobic gram-positive cocci, which were formerly considered to be clinically irrelevant. *Pediococcus* spp. are widely used in the food-processing industry and are normal inhabitants of the gastrointestinal tract. So far, only two of the eight *Pediococcus* spp. known have been reported to cause infections in humans, but with the ongoing attempts to improve the diagnosis of vancomycin-resistant gram-positive cocci, these organisms are being increasingly recovered from clinical specimens. Atkins et al. (55) presented an infant who required a central venous catheter for total parenteral nutrition secondary to gastroschisis. The infant developed a polymicrobial catheter-related bacteremia due to *Klebsiella pneumoniae*, coagulase-negative staphylococci, and a nonhemolytic streptococcus, later identified as *P. pentosaceus*. Since the catheter became obstructed it was removed, and cure was achieved following treatment with vancomycin and amikacin. The recent recognition of *P. pentosaceus* as a pathogen is probably due to an improved diagnosis rather than an increase in frequency or virulence. Its intrinsic resistance to vancomycin may lead to complications, especially during the treatment of nosocomial infections for which glycopeptides are often empirically used.

C. *Bacillus* spp. and Other Gram-Positive Rods

Bacillus spp. are aerobic, gram-positive or gram-variable, spore-forming rods which are found in decaying organic matter, dust, soil, and water. They are frequent culture contaminants and, with the exception of *Bacillus anthracis*, often not considered to be clinically significant when recovered from clinical specimens. *Bacillus* spp. have been occasionally reported to cause meningitis, pneumonia, and bacteremia (56). Bacteremia has been detected among IV drug abusers with endocarditis (56,57) and after administration of an oral preparation (Bactisubtil) containing *Bacillus subtilis* spores to immunocompromised patients (58). However, *Bacillus* bacteremia seems to be mainly related to the use of IV devices (57). If *Bacillus* spp. are isolated from blood cultures of a patient with sepsis, IV devices should be considered as the most probable source. Indwelling vascular catheters should be promptly removed, especially among immunocompromised patients, and empiric antibiotic treatment should be started (59). Among nonimmunocompromised patients the clinical course is indolent, and bacteremia may even be self-limiting. In this setting antibiotic treatment should be delayed until the antibiotic susceptibility is known. Whereas most *Bacillus* spp. are susceptible to β-lactam antibiotics, *B. cereus* is frequently resistant. Imipenem, ciprofloxacin, and gentamicin are highly active, as is vancomycin, which is also bactericidal at the MIC (60). In a patient with AIDS, *B. subtilis* bacteremia resolved with vancomycin therapy without removing the indwelling Broviac catheter (58).

Rothia dentocariosa is a coccal to rod-shaped, anaerobic bacterium, morphologically resembling *Actinomyces, Corynebacterium,* and *Nocardia* spp. It is part of the normal oral and upper respiratory tract flora and in general is susceptible to penicillins, cephalosporins, erythromycin, vancomycin, aminoglycosides, chloramphenicol, and TMP/SMZ. However, susceptibility results are limited to a few isolates and were determined using different methods (61,62). Infections are rare but may range from peridontal inflammation (62) and other infections of the oral cavity to endocarditis with brain abscess (63). An infection due to *R. dentocariosa* associated with an intravascular device was reported in a 46-year-old diabetic suffering multiple postsurgery complications, including renal failure that required hemodialysis. During hospitalization when the patient was treated with vancomycin and gentamicin for CRI During the first months after discharge, the arteriovenous shunt, despite being implicated as the source of the infection, was still used for vascular access without evidence of local or systemic infection (64).

Fish et al. (46) reported 4.8% of all pathogens causing bacteremia in HIV-infected patients to be *Listeria monocytogenes.* The authors did not describe whether these infections were catheter-related or not, but Katner et al. (65) reported an AIDS patient whose bacteremia was traced to an indwelling IV catheter. Among U.S. cancer patients, 1% of bacteremia cases were due to this organism (4). *L. monocytogens* was furthermore shown to cause a ventriculoperitoneal shunt infection in a patient with brain tumor, who was successfully treated with TMP/SMZ after removal of the device (66).

D. Mycobacteria

Mycobacteria are acid-fast, aerobic, nonmotile bacteria. At least 25 species are associated with the development of granulomatous infections in humans. *Mycobacterium neoaurum* is a rapidly growing mycobacterium, primarily found in soil but also being recovered from dust and water, that had not been described to cause infections in humans until Davison et al. (67) reported the isolation of *M. neoaurum* from the Hickman catheter of an immunocompromised patient. Six years later, Holland et al. (68) reported a bone marrow transplant recipient who suffered from bacteremia and insertion site infection due to *M. neoaurum* during aplasia. Despite rapid clinical response during treatment with ticaracillin/clavulanate and tobramycin, bacteremia persisted until the catheter was removed. Microbiological cultures of the tip indeed revealed *M. neoaurum.*

M. fortuitum and *M. chelonae* (the *M. fortuitum* complex) are rapidly growing ubiquitous mycobacteria found in soil and water. Both mycobacteria have been identified as the cause of skin/soft-tissue abscesses, wound infections, pulmonary infections, keratitis, peritonitis, endocarditis, and bacteremia. Bacteremia occurred in association with prosthetic valves, sternal wounds, and reused hemodialyzers. Until 1991, 29 cases of CRI have been reported in the literature (69). The incidence was reported to follow the increasing use of central venous catheters but in general was low (1.2 cases per year). None of the patients with *M. fortuitum* complex CRI showed signs of a disseminated cutaneous form of the infection, except at the catheter insertion site. Another indication that the infections in the described patients were strictly catheter-related rather than due to disseminated disease, is that none of the patients died and even those who initially failed treatment recovered after catheter removal. In addition to appropriate antibiotics (TMP/SMZ or amikacin, depending on in vitro susceptibility) removal of the catheter is essential. Furthermore, in cases with tunnel infections, surgical excision of the infected tissue (skin and tunnel track) is recommended.

In contrast to the localized *M. fortuitum* complex infection, Schelonka et al. (70), described two cases of secondary catheter-related *M. avium* complex (MAC) infections in patients with disseminated disease. The CRI was probably due to seeding of the catheter by hematogenous spread of MAC. Sterilization of the blood was only possible after removal of the catheter (Port-a-cath). The treatment included rifampin, ethambutol, amikacin, clarithromycin, clofazimine, and ciprofloxacin. The last three drugs were continued for 14 and 20 months, respectively.

E. Actinomycetes

Actinomycetes are aerobic, catalase-producing branched filamentous bacteria. The organisms are ubiquitous, having been found on human and animal body surfaces and in soil and plants.

Catheter-related bacteremia has been reported with three different *Nocardia* species (71–73). A Tenckhoff catheter-associated infection due to *N. asteroides* (71) in a CAPD-patient and an implantable central venous catheter infection with *N. nova* (72) were successfully treated with antibiotics and removal of the catheter. In one case report, Hickman catheter-related bacteremia caused by *N. otitidis-caviarum* in a bone marrow transplant patient was successfully treated without removing the catheter, after switching from vancomycin to imipenem treatment (73).

Tsukamurella paurometabolum (formerly *Corynebacterium paurometabolum*, *Gordona aurantiaca*, *Rhodococcus aurantiacus*) is a pleomorphic, gram-positive bacillus that is weakly acid-fast. Until the case reports of Shapiro et al. (74), only a handful of human infections had been published, and none included bacteremia. The authors described three cases of *T. paurometabolum* bacteremia related to long-term use of central venous catheters in cancer patients. In all cases, the persistence of positive blood cultures during antibiotic therapy necessitated the removal of the catheter. (A detailed case report of one of the patients was published by Lai, 75, a year later.)

Table 4 Alphabetical List, Natural Source, and Clinical Data of Miscellaneous Organisms Causing Catheter-Related Infections

Microorganism	Reference	Natural source	Clinical infections	Recommended antibiotics[a]	Catheter removal
Aeromonas hydrophila	36,76	Water sources, environment, food	CRI, cellulitis, bacteremia, UTI, endocarditis, osteomyelitis, peritonitis, meningitis, diarrhea	TMP/SMZ, ciprofloxacin, tetracycline, aminoglycosides, piperacillin, 2nd + 3rd gen. cephalosporins	+ / –
Agrobacterium spp.	28,31,32	Environment, water sources, plants	CRI, endocarditis, UTI, peritonitis, bacteremia	Ciprofloxacin, TMP/SMZ, imipenem, aminoglycosides	+
Alcaligenes xylosoxidans	25,29,30	Water sources, hospital environment, human GI tract	CRI, bacteremia, peritonitis, meningitis	TMP/SMZ, antipseudomonal penicillins, ceftazidime, imipenem, aminoglycosides	?/–
Bacillus spp.	56–59	Environment, water sources	CRI, meningitis, wound infection, pneumonia, bacteremia, osteomyelitis	Imipenem, vancomycin, ciprofloxacin, aminoglycosides, β-lactam antibiotics depending on species	+ / –
Bordetella bronchiseptica	38	Animal (rarely human) respiratory tract	CRI, CAPD peritonitis, meningitis, pneumonia, endocarditis	Ciprofloxacin, imipenem, aminoglycosides	+
Brevibacterium epidermidis	50	Human skin	CRI (insertion site)	Penicillins, erythromycin, tetracycline, cephalosporins, aminoglycosides, vancomycin	?
Burkholderia cepacia	7,9,10,11	Water sources, environment, food (onions), animal sources, hospital equipment including disinfectants	CRI, pneumonia, UTI, meningitis, endocarditis, wound infection, arthritis	Ceftazidime, piperacillin, imipenem, TMP/SMZ	+
CDC group IV 2-c	18	Water sources	CRI	Ciprofloxacin, imipenem, ceftazidime	+ / –

Organism	Ref.	Source	Infections	Treatment	
Chryseomonas luteola	19	Primarily human saprophyte, water sources	CRI, endocarditis, bacteremia	Ureidopenicillins, 3 gen. cephalosporins, aminoglycosides	+
Comamonas acidovorans	14	Water sources, environment, food	CRI, bacteremia	(Not mentioned)	+
Corynebacterium afermentans	42,43	Human skin and mucous membranes	CRI, endocarditis, bacteremia	Glycopeptide, rifampin, aminoglycosides	+
Corynebacterium jeikeium	45,46	Human skin and mucous membranes	CRI, endocarditis, bacteremia, UTI, pneumonia, meningitis	Glycopeptide, doxycycline, rifampin	+ / −
Corynebacterium minutissimum	44	Human skin and mucous membranes	CRI, erythrasma, endocarditis	Glycopeptide, cephalosporins, penicillin, erythromycin, clindamycin, doxycycline	?
Corynebacterium urealyticum	47	Human skin and mucous membranes	CRI, UTI, endocarditis, bacteremia	Glycopeptides, rifampin, aminoglycosides	+
Corynebacterium striatum	48	Human skin and mucous membranes, cattle	CRI, pneumonia, endocarditis, arthritis, wound infection, bacteremia	Glycopeptides, rifampin, aminoglycosides	+/?
Coryneform CDC group A-5	49	Human skin (?)	CRI	3rd gen. cephalosporins, (vancomycin-resistant!)	−
Enterococcus casseliflavus	52	Human GI tract	CRI, bacteremia	Ampicillin, teicoplanin (vancomycin-resistant!)	?
Enterococcus faecalis/faecium	51	Human GI tract	CRI, bacteremia, endocarditis, cholangitis, pancreatitis, pneumonia	Glycopeptides, ampicillin (+ aminoglycoside)	?
Flavimonas oryzihabitans	19,20,21,22	Natural and hospital environment, water sources, human	CRI, wound infection, CAPD peritonitis, abscess, bacteremia	TMP/SMX, ureidopenicillins, 3 gen. cephalosporins, aminoglycosides, imipenem, ciprofloxacin	− / +

Table 4 Continued

Microorganism	Reference	Natural source	Clinical infections	Recommended antibiotics[a]	Catheter removal
Flavobacterium spp.	34	Water sources, hospital environment	CRI, bacteremia	?, commonly multiresistant incl. aminoglycosides	+
Gordona spp.	76	Environment	CRI, meningitis, (sternal) wound infections, pulmonary infections	TMP/SMZ, imipenem, 3rd gen. cephalosporins, amikacin, ciprofloxacin	– / +
Kingella kingae	40	Human respiratory tract	CRI, endocarditis, bacteremia, osteomyelitis, endophthalmitis	Penicillins, cephalosporins, TMO/SMZ, aminoglycosides, erythromycin	?
Listeria monocytogenes	65,66	Environment, water sources, food, human and animal GI tract	CRI, endocarditis, CNS-infections including CSF-shunt infection	Penicillin + aminoglycosides, TMP/SMZ, erythromycin, tetracycline, rifampin	?
Methylobacterium extorquens	16,17	Plants, environment, water sources, air	CRI, RTI, peritonitis, skin ulcers, uveitis	TMP/SMX, imipenem, ciprofloxacin, aminoglycosides, tetracycline	–
Moraxella osloensis	39	Human respiratory tract	CRI, septic arthritis, meningitis, endocarditis	Penicillins, cephalosporins, aminoglycosides, erythromycin	–
Mycobacterium neoaurum	67,68	Environment, water sources	CRI	(?)	+
Mycobacterium furtuitum complex	69	Environment, water sources	CRI, bacteremia, endocarditis, RTI, abscesses, wound inf., peritonitis	Rifampin, ethambutol, amikacin, clarithromycin, clofazimine, ciprofloxacin	+

Mycobacterium avium complex	70	Environment, water sources	CRI, bacteremia, endocarditis, RTI, abscesses, wound inf., peritonitis	Rifampin, ethambutol, amikacin, clarithromycin, clofazimine, ciprofloxacin	+
Nocardia asteroides	71	Environment, animals, humans, plants	CRI, pulmonary abscess, CNS infection, mycetoma	Sulfonamides + tetracycline or aminoglycoside, minocycline, β-lactams	+ / –
Nocardia nova	72	Environment, water sources	CRI, mycetoma	Sulfonamides + tetracycline or aminoglycosides, minocycline, β-lactams	+ / –
Nocardia otitidis-caviarum	73	Environment, water sources	CRI, mycetoma	Imipenem, sulfonamides + tetracycline or aminoglycosides, minocycline, β-lactams	–
Ochrobactrum anthropi	23,24,26,28	Environment, water sources, human GI tract	CRI, endocarditis, peritonitis, bacteremia	TMP/SMZ, ciprofloxacin, imipenem, aminoglycosides	+ / –
Pediococcus pentosaceus	54	GI tract (used in food-processing industry)	CRI, bacteremia	Penicillin + β-lactam-inhibitors, aminoglycosides (vanocmycin-resistant)	?
Pseudomonas paucimobilis	7,8,11	Water sources, plants, air, hospital equipment	CRI, peritonitis, UTI, meningitis, empyema, wound infection, splenic abscess, bacteremia	Ceftazidime, piperacilline, imipenem, TMP/SMZ	+
Pseudomonas putida	7,11	Water sources, plants, animal sources, general and hospital environments, oral flora	CRI, UTI, wound infection, septic arthritis	Imipenem, ceftazidime, piperacillin, ciprofloxacin, polymyxin	+

Table 4 Continued

Microorganism	Reference	Natural source	Clinical infections	Recommended antibiotics[a]	Catheter removal
Pseudomonas pickettii	12	Water sources, (wet) hospital equipment and solutions	CRI, bacteremia, meningitis, UTI, RTI	Imipenem, ceftazidime, piperacillin, tobramycin	+
Pseudomonas stutzeri	7	Water sources, plants, animal sources, general and hospital environments	CRI, pneumonia, bacteremia, otitis media, corneal ulcers, endocarditis, osteomyelitis	Polymyxin, imipenem, ceftazidime, piperacillin, aminoglycosides	+
Rothia dentocariosa	64	Oral flora/upper respiratory tract, dental caries and plaque	CRI, oral cavity infection, endocarditis	Penicillin, erythromycin, aminoglycosides, TMP/SMZ, vancomycin	– / +
Stenotrophomonas maltophilia	7	Water sources, plants, animal sources, natural and hospital environments	CRI, pneumonia, UTI, endocarditis, wound infection, corneal ulcers	Ceftazidime, TMP/SMZ, (imipenem-resistant)	+
Stomatococcus mucilaginosus	53	Human respiratory tract	CRI, pneumonia, bacteremia, endocarditis, mucositis	Cephalosporins, erythromycin, vancomycin, aminoglycosides, ciprofloxacin, tetracycline	– / +
Tsukamurella paurometabolum	74,75	Environment	CRI, pneumonia, meningitis	TMP/SMZ, imipenem, 3rd gen. cephalosporins, amikacin, ciprofloxacin	+

[a]Antibiotics successfully employed or in vitro susceptible.

Abbreviations: GI = gastrointestinal tract, CRI = catheter-related infection, UTI = urinary tract infection, TMP/SMZ = trimethoprim-sulfamethoxazole, CNS = central nervous system, CSF = cerebrospinal fluid, RTI = respiratory tract infection.

Catheter removal (based on case reports): + necessary, + / – probably necessary, – / + possible necessary, – probably not necessary, ? unclear.

Gordona (Rhodococcus) species are rarely reported organisms causing skin and pulmonary infections. Buchman et al. (76) described two immunocompetent patients with long-term parenteral nutrition with catheter-related infections due to *G. rubropertincta* and *G. terrae*, respectively. It was assumed that the microorganisms gained access to the bloodstream through manipulation and contamination of home TPN catheters. Both cases were successfully treated with antimicrobial therapy, and removal of catheters does not seem necessary, even though this was done in one case.

IV. POLYMICROBIAL INFECTIONS

Clusters of nosocomial infections focusing on a single organism, either because it is an unusual pathogen or because it appears in a large cluster, are easily identified and frequently reported. Ponce de Leon et al. (77) were the first to report a cluster of epidemiologically related polymicrobial bloodstream infections, related to indwelling catheters, involving two or more common organisms such as *S. epidermidis, S. aureus, Pseudomonas* spp., *Enterobacter* spp., and *Candida albicans*. Bacteremia due to several different organisms (in place of a single causative pathogen) may be a first hint to consider CRI. In another study, polymicrobial bacteremia was shown to be especially frequent in neutropenic patients; 34% (29/86) of all bacteremic episodes versus 3% (1/30) in nonneutropenic patients (78). Intravascular catheters were the most common source of bacteremia in these cases, but the higher incidence of polymicrobial bacteremia was also assumed to be due to the repeated occurrence of cutaneous and mucosal lesions in these patients. Among ICU patients, the incidence of true polymicrobial bacteremia was 8.4%, with Enterobacteriaceae being the most common pathogens (79). The prognosis of patients with polymicrobial bacteremia was not any worse than for those with monomicrobial bloodstream infections. Mortality was even significantly lower than in a cohort of patients with bacteremia due to a single organism. Since intravascular devices were the most common source (42.8%), the authors recommended removing these devices, even though they did not compare the outcome in patients with or without catheters left in place.

V. CONCLUSIONS

The review of the different case reports and case series illustrates that saprophytic and environmental organisms can realize their potential for causing catheter-related infections. So-called avirulent or saprophytic organisms from the patient's own skin flora or from the environment that are present on the hands of healthcare workers inserting or handling the catheter may cause CRI, especially in the immunocompromised host. Therefore, the catalog of miscellaneous pathogens summarized in Table 4 may only represent the tip of the iceberg. Bacteremia due to uncommon pathogens is frequently reported, but information is seldom given as to whether the infection might have been catheter-related or not, even though intravascular devices seem to be the main source of bacteremia due to these organisms. The rapid development of medical technology leading to the use of new indwelling medical devices in patients increasingly at high risk for any noso-comial infection will furthermore increase the incidence of this newcomers among pathogens causing CRI. Under such circumstances *Peptostreptococcus anaerobius* (78), *Propionibacterium* spp. (78), and probably others, including other anaerobe bacteria (80), might already now be added to the list of pathogens causing CRI. Mortality and the rate of complication such as endocarditis or sep-tic thrombophlebitis seems to be low in cases with CRI due to these organisms. Still, a therapeutic dilemma could occur, since some of these pathogens express intrinsic resistance against standard antibiotics used in the empiric treatment of CRI, such as vancomycin. At present, no general advice whether the device should be removed or not, or if and which antibiotic is needed, can be given.

Despite their rising importance, infections due to miscellaneous pathogens are likely to stay underreported, since the organisms can be easily misidentified in the laboratory. The lack of prolonged incubation times, specific atmospheric conditions, special media, and complete databases of automated microbiologic identification systems are factors contributing to this diagnostic problem. Efforts should be made to differentiate unusual organisms isolated from blood cultures or catheter tips of patients with assumed CRI to species level, in order to identify pathogens that might often be considered contaminants.

REFERENCES

1. Tebbs SE, Elliott TSJ. Modification of central venous catheter polymers to prevent invitro microbial colonization. Eur J Clin Microbiol Infect Dis 1994; 13:111–117.
2. Dankner WM, Spector SA, Fierer J, Davis CE. *Malassezia fungemia* in neonates and adults: complication of hyperalimentation. Rev Infect Dis 1987; 9:743–753.
3. Brown NM, Blundell E, Chown SR, Warnock DW, Hill JA, Slade RR. Acremonium infection in a neutropenic patient. Case report J Infect 1992; 25:7376.
4. Kiehn TE, Armstrong D. Changes in the spectrum of organisms causing bacteremia and fungemia in immunocompromised patients due to venous access devices. Eur J Clin Microbiol Infect Dis 1990; 12:869–872.
5. Bollet C, Elkouby A, Pietri P, Micco de P. Isolation of *Enterobacter amnigenus* from a heart transplant recipient. Eur J Clin Microbiol Infect Dis 1991; 10:1071–1073.
6. Wong VK. Broviac catheter infection with *Kluyvera cryocrescens:* a case report. J Clin Microbiol 1987; 25:1115–1116.

7. Elting SE, Bodey GP. Septicemia due to *Xanthomonas* species and non-*aeruginosa* *Pseudomonas* species: increasing incidence of catheter-related infections. Medicine 1990; 5:296–306.

8. Decker CF, Hawkins RE, Simon GL. Infections with *Pseudomonas paucimobilis*. Clin Infect Dis 1992; 14:783–784.

9. Panlilio AL, Beck-Sague CM, Siegel JD, et al. Infections and pseudoinfections due to povidone-iodine solution contaminated with *Pseudomonas cepacia*. Clin Infect Dis 1992; 14:1078–1083.

10. Pegues DA, Carson LA, Anderson RL, et al. Outbreak of *Pseudomonas cepacia* bacteremia in oncology patients. Clin Infect Dis 1993; 16:407–411.

11. Anaissie E, Fainstein V, Miller P, et al. *Pseudomonas putida*. Newly recognized pathogen in patients with cancer. Am J Med 1987; 82:1191–1194.

12. Raveh D, Simhon A, Gimmon Z, Sacks T, Shapiro M. Infections caused by *Pseudomonas pickettii* in association with permanent indwelling intravenous devices: four cases and a review. Clin Infect Dis 1993; 17:877–880.

13. Dan M, Gutman R, Biro A. Peritonitis caused by *Pseudomonas putrefaciens* in patients undergoing continuous ambulatory peritoneal dialysis. Clin Infect Dis 1992; 14:359–360.

14. Castagnola E, Tasso L, Conte M, Nantron M, Barretta A, Giacchino R. Central venous catheter-related infection due to *Comamonas acidovorans* in a child with non-Hodgkin's lymphoma. Clin Infect Dis 1994; 19:559–560.

15. Austin B, Goodfellow M. *Pseudomonas mesophilica*, a new species of pink bacteria isolated from leaf surfaces. Int J Syst Bacteriol 1979; 29:373–378.

16. Poirier A, Lapointe R, Claveau S, Joly JR. Bacteremia caused by *Pseudomonas mesophilica*. Can Med Assoc J 1988; 139:411–412.

17. Kaye KM, Macone A, Kazanjian PH. Catheter infection caused by *Methylobacterium* in immunocompromised hosts: report of three cases and review of the literature. Clin Infect Dis 1992; 14:1010–1014.

18. Arduino S, Villar H, Veron MT, Koziner B, Dictar M. CDC Group IV c-2 as a cause of catheter-related sepsis in an immunocompromised patient. Clin Infect Dis 1993; 17:512–513.

19. Kostman JR, Solomon F, Fekete T. Infections with *Chryseomonas luteola* (CDC Groep Ve-1) and *Flavimonas oryzihabitans* (CDC Groep Ve-2) in neurosurgical patients. Rev Infect Dis 1991; 13:233–236.

20. Lucas KG, Kiehn TE, Sobeck KA, Armstrong D, Brown AE. Sepsis caused by *Flavimonas oryzihabitans*. Medicine 1994; 73:209–303.

21. Pien FD. Group Ve-2 (*Chromobacterium typhiflavum*) bacteremia. J Clin Microbiol. 1977; 6:435–436.

22. Conlu A, Rothman J, Staszewski H, et al. *Flavimonas oryzihabitans* (CDC group Ve-2) bacteraemia associated with Hickman catheters. J Hosp Infect 1992; 20:293–299.

23. Kern WV, Oethinger M, Kaufhold A, Rozdzinski E, Marre R. Ochrobactrum anthropi bacteremia: report of four cases and short review. Infection 1993; 21:306–310.

24. Cieslak TJ, Robb ML, Drabick CJ, Fischer GW. Catheter-associated sepsis caused

by *Ochrobactrum anthropi:* report of cases and review of related nonfermentative bacteria. Clin Infect Dis 1992; 14:902–907.

25. Cieslak TJ, Raszak WV. Catheter-associated sepsis due to *Alcaligemes xylosoxidans* in a child with AIDS (letter). Clin Infect Dis 1993; 16:592–593.

26. Grandsen WR, Eykyn SJ. Seven cases of bacteremia due to *Ochrobactrum anthropi* (Letter). Clin Infect Dis 1992; 15:1068–1069.

27. Kish MA, Buggy BP, Forbes BA. Bacteremia caused by *Achromobacter* species in an immunocompromised host. J Clin Microbiol 1984; 19:947–948.

28. Alnor D, Frimodt-Moller N, Espersen F, Frederiksen W. Infections with unusual human pathogens: *Agrobacterium* species and *Ochrobactrum anthropi.* Clin Infect Dis 1994; 18:914–920.

29. Gröschel D, Cody LD, Tieman C. Nosocomial infections with *Achromobacter xylosoxidans* in cancer patients. In: Program and Abstracts of the 19th ICAAC. Washington, DC: American Society of Microbiology, 1979:1458–1459.

30. Legrand C, Anaissie E. Bacteremia due to *Achromobacter xylosoxidans* in patients with cancer. Clin Infect Dis 1992; 14:479–484.

31. Edmond MB, Riddler SA, Baxter CM, Wicklund BM, Pasculle AW. *Agrobacterium radiobacter:* a recently recognized opportunistic pathogen. Clin Infect Dis 1993; 16: 388–391.

32. Hulse M, Johnson S, Ferrieri P. *Agrobacterium* infections in humans: experience at one hospital and review. Clin Infect Dis 1993; 16:112–117.

33. Maki DG. Nosocomial bacteremia. An epidemiologic overview. Am J Med 1981; 70:719–732.

34. Stamm WE, Colella JJ, Anderson RL, Dixon RE. Indwelling arterial catheters as a source of nosocomial bacteremia. An outbreak caused by *Flavobacterium* species. N Engl J Med 1975; 292:1099–1102.

35. Rello J, Coll P, Net A, Prats G. Infection of pulmonary artery catheters. Epidemiologic characteristics and multivariate analysis of risk factors. Chest 1993; 103:133–136.

36. Siddiqui MN, Ahmed I, Farooqi BJ, Ahmed M. Myonecrosis due to *Aeromonas hydrophila* following insertion of an intravenous cannula: case report and review. Clin Infect Dis 1992; 14:619–620.

37. Papasian CJ, Downs NJ, Talley RL, Romberger DJ, Hodges GR. *Bordetella bronchiseptica* bronchitis. J Clin Microbiol 1981; 25:575–577.

38. Qureshi MN, Lederman J, Neibart E, Bottone EJ. *Bordetella bronchiseptica* recurrent bacteremia in the setting of a patient with AIDS and indwelling Broviac catheter. Intern J STD AIDS 1992; 3:291–293.

39. Buchman AI, Pickett MJ, Mann L, Ament ME. Central venous catheter infection caused by *Moraxella osloensis* in a patient receiving home parenteral nutrition. Diagn Microbiol Infect Dis 1993; 17:163–166.

40. Goutzmanis JJ, Gonis G, Gilbert GL. *Kingella kingae* infection in children: ten cases and a review of the literature. Pediatr Infect Dis 1991; 10:677–683.

41. Wong GWK, Oppenheimer SJ, Vaudry W. CSF shunt infection by uncapsulated *Haemophilus influenzae.* Clin Infect Dis 1993; 17:519–520.

42. Dealler S, Malnick H, Cammish D. Intravenous line infection caused by *Corynebacterium afermentans* CDC group ANF-1. J Hosp Infect 1993; 23:319–320.

43. Kerr KG, Anson JJ, Patmore R, Smith G. Intravenous line infections (letter). J Hosp Infect 1993; 24:73–75.
44. Cavendish J, Cole JB, Ohl CA. Polymicrobial central venous catheter sepsis involving a multiantibiotic-resistant strain of *Corneybacterium minutissimum.* Clin Infect Dis 1994; 19:204–205.
45. Riebel W, Frantz N, Adelstein D, Spagnuolo PJ. *Corynebacterium* JK: a cause of nosocomial device-related infection. Rev Infect Dis 1986; 8:42–49.
46. Fish DN, Danziger LH. Neglected pathogens: bacterial infections in persons with human immunodeficiency virus infection. A review of the literature. (First of two parts.) Pharm 1993; 13:415–439.
47. Wood CA, Pepe R. Bacteremia in a patient with non-urinary tract infection due to *Corynebacterium urealyticum.* Clin Infect Dis 1994; 19:367–368.
48. Tumbarello M, Tacconelli E, Del Forno A, Caonera S, Cauda R. *Corynebacterium striatum* bacteremia in patient with AIDS. Clin Infect Dis 1994; 18:107–1008.
49. Campbell PB, Palladino S, Flexman JP. Catheter-related septicemia caused by a vancomycin-resistant coryneform CDC group A-5. Pathology 1994; 26:56–58.
50. McCaughey C, Damani NN. Central line infection caused by *Brevibacterium epidermidis.* J Hosp Infect 1991; 23:211–212.
51. Patterson JE, Sweeney AH, Simms M, et al. An analysis of 110 serious enterococcal infections. Epidemiology, antibiotic susceptibility and outcome. Medicine 1995; 74: 191–200.
52. Ruoff KL, de la Maza L, Murtagh MJ, Sparago JD, Ferraro MJ. Species identities of enterococci from clinical specimens. J Clin Microbiol 1990; 28:435–437.
53. van Goethem GF, Louwagie BM, Simoens MJ, Vandeven JM, Verhaegen JL, Boogaerts MA. *Enterococcus casseliflavus* septicaemia in a patient with acute myeloid leukaemia. Eur J Clin Microbiol Infect Dis 1994; 13:519–520.
54. Ascher DP, Zbick C, White C, Fischer GW. Infections due to *Stomatococcus mucilaginosus:* 10 cases and review. Rev Infect Dis 1991; 13:1048–1052.
55. Atkins JT, Tillman J, Tan TQ, Demmler GJ. *Pediococcus pentosaceus* catheter-associated infection in an infant with gastroschisis. Ped Infect Dis J 1994; 13:75–76.
56. Tuazon CU, Murray HW, Levey C, Solny MN, Curtin JA, Sheagren JN. Serious infections from *Bacillus* spp. JAMA 1979; 241:1137–1140.
57. Sliman R, Rehm S, Shlaes DM. Serious infections by *Bacillus* species. Medicine 1987; 66:218–223.
58. Richard V, Van der Auwera P, Snoeck R, Daneau D, Meunier F. Nosocomial bacteremia caused by *Bacillus* species. Eur J Clin Microbiol Infect Dis 1988; 7:783–785.
59. Cotton DJ, Gill VJ, Marshall DJ, Gress J, Thaler M, Pizzo P. Clinical features and therapeutic interventions in 17 cases of *Bacillus* bacteremia in an immunosuppressed patient population. J Clin Microbiol 1987; 25:672–674.
60. Weber DJ, Saviteer SM, Rutala W, Thomann C. In vitro susceptibility of *Bacillus* spp. to selected antimicrobial agents. Antimicrob Agents Chemother 1988; 32:642–645.
61. Schafer FJ, Wing EJ, Norden CW. Infectious endocarditis caused by *Rothia dentocariosa.* Ann Intern Med 1979; 91:747–749.
62. Dzierzanowska D, Miksza-Zytkiewicz R, Czerniawska M, Borowski LH, Borowski J. Sensitivity of *Rothia dentocariosa.* J Antimicrob Chemother 1979; 4:469–473.

63. Isaacson H, Genko R. *Rothia dentocariosa* endocarditis complicated by brain abscess. Am J Med 1988; 84:352–355.
64. Nivar-Aristy RA, Krajewski LP, Washington JA. Infection of an arteriovenous fistula with *Rothia dentocariosa*. Diagn Microbiol Infect Dis 1991; 14:167–169.
65. Katner HP, Joiner TA. *Listeria monocytogenes* sepsis from an indwelling IV catheter in a patient with AIDS (letter). South Med J 1989; 82:94–95.
66. Dominguez EA, Patil AA, Johnson WM. Ventriculoperitoneal shunt due to *Listeria monocytogenes*. Clin Infect Dis 1994; 19:223–224.
67. Davison MB, McCormack JG, Blacklock ZM, Dawson DJ, Tilse MH, Crimmins FB. Bacteremia caused by *Mycobacterium neoaurum*. J Clin Microbiol 1988; 26:762–764.
68. Holland DJ, Chen SC, Chew WW, Gilbert GL. *Mycobacterium neoaurum* infection of a Hickman catheter in an immunosuppressed patient. Clin Infect Dis 1994; 18:1002–1003.
69. Raad II, Vartivarian S, Khan A, Bodey GP. Catheter-related infections caused by the *Mycobacterium fortuitum* complex: 15 cases and review. Rev Infect Dis 1991; 13:1120–1125.
70. Schelonka RL, Ascher DP, McMahon DP, Drehner DM, Kuskie MR. Catheter-related sepsis caused by *Mycobacterium avium* complex. Pediatr Infect Dis J 1994; 13:236–238.
71. Rubin J, Kirchner K, Wash D, Greeen M, Bower J. Fungal peritonitis during continuous peritoneal dialysis: a report of 17 cases. Am J Kidney Dis 1987; 10:361–368.
72. Miron D, Dennehy PH, Josephson SL, Forman EN. Catheter-associated bacteremia with *Nocardia nova* with secondary pulmonary involvement. Pediatr Infect Dis J 1994; 13:416–417.
73. Lee ACW, Yuen KY, Lau YL. Catheter-associated nocardiosis. Pediatr Infect Dis J 1994; 13:1023–1024.
74. Shapiro CL, Haft RF, Gantz NM, et al. *Tsukamurella paurometabolum:* a novel pathogen causing catheter-related infections. Clin Infect Dis 1992; 14:200–203.
75. Lai KK. A cancer patient with central venous catheter-related sepsis caused by *Tsukamurella paurometabolum* (*Gordona aurantiaca*) (letter). Clin Infect Dis 1993; 17:285–287.
76. Buchman AI, McNeil MM, Brown JM, Lasker BA, Ament ME. Central venous catheter sepsis caused by unusual *Gordona* (*Rhodococcus*) species: identification with a digoxigenin-labeled rDNA probe. Clin Infect Dis 1992; 15:694–697.
77. Ponce de Leon S, Critchley S, Wenzel RP. Polymicrobial bloodstream infections related to prolonged vascular catheterization. Crit Care Med 1984; 12:856–859.
78. D'Antonio D, Pizzigallo E, Jacone A, et al. Occurrence of bacteremia in hematolgic patients. Eur J Epidemiol 1992; 8:687–692.
79. Rello J, Quintana E, Mirelis B, Gurgui M, Net A, Prats G. Polymicrobial bacteremia in critically ill patients. Intens Care Med 1993; 19:22–25.
80. Haug JB, Harthug S, Kalager T, Digranes A, Solberg CO. Bloodstream infections at a Norwegian university hospital, 1974–1979 and 1988–1989: Changing etiology, clinical features and outcome. Clin Infect Dis 1994; 19:246–256.

8

Central Venous Catheters

Andreas F. Widmer
University Hospital Basel, Basel, Switzerland

I. INTRODUCTION

Intravascular devices are indispensable for the administration of fluids and electrolytes, blood products, drugs, and nutritional support. Central venous access is necessary for chemotherapy for malignant diseases or serious infectious diseases and for total parenteral nutrition. In addition, intensive care units use these devices for continuous hemodynamic monitoring of their critically ill patients (e.g., pulmonary artery catheters). Most catheters are made of polyurethane, silicon, or Teflon. A more recent development is the coating of catheters that may prevent microbial colonization and subsequent infection. More than 20 million patients admitted to U.S. hospitals (over 50%) receive infusion therapy each year (1), and a figure of 63% was noted in a European multicenter study (2). Unfortunately, complications arising from intravascular access catheters are frequently observed and generally underestimated. The occurrence of infectious complications was first published only 2 years after the introduction of plastic catheters in 1945 (3). This chapter focuses on epidemiology, microbiologic treatment, and prevention of infectious complications associated with central venous catheters.

II. EPIDEMIOLOGY

Central venous catheters (CVCs) have gained widespread use in hospitals, especially in intensive care units (ICUs) (Fig. 1). Approximately 3 million CVCs are inserted annually in the United States, and 200,000 in the U.K. (4). Catheter-related infection (CRI) belongs to the most frequently observed complication of intravascular catheterization (see below for definitions). Of all intravascular catheters, CVCs are responsible for 80% to 90% of catheter-related bloodstream infections (CR-BSIs) (5). In the United States approximately 850,000 CRIs, and more than 50,000 CR-BSIs occur annually (1,6). The attributable mortality of CR-BSIs ranges from 14% to 28% (1,7–9). Thus, an estimated 7000 to 14,000 deaths annually may be attributable to CR-BSIs. A recent European prevalence study on nosocomial infections underlined the importance of devices as risk factors for nosocomial infections (10). ICU patients with CVCs have a fivefold risk to develop a BSI compared to ICU patients without a CVC (11).

Nosocomial bloodstream infections account for an estimated $6000 increase in hospital costs per infection (12) or $40,000 per survivor in an ICU (7), an extra week of hospital stay (7,13), and a case fatality of more than 20% (7,14). The attributable mortality for bloodstream infections in surgical ICUs has recently been estimated to be 35% (7,15). For the subgroup of CR-BSIs, the attributable mortality was 25%, an excess length of ICU stay of 6.5 days, and attributable costs of almost $30,000 (16). These infections are largely preventable.

At the University of Iowa Hospitals and Clinics, bloodstream infections increased linearly from 6.7 to 18.4 per 1000 discharges (0.83 to 1.72 episodes per 1000 patient-days) from 1980 to 1992 ($r = .87$). Increases in infection rates were due to gram-positive cocci ($r = .96$) and yeasts ($r = .95$) and essentially explained by infections caused by coagulase-negative staphylococci (CoNS), *Staphylococcus aureus*, enterococci, and *Candida* species, respectively (15). Not surprisingly, large teaching institutions (>500 beds) report higher rates of BSIs than do smaller, nonteaching hospitals (<200 beds). In large teaching institutions, every fifth nosocomial infection is a BSI (17). The most recent report from 1993 to 1995 by the CDC shows that between 10% and 20% of all reported nosocomial infections are primary BSIs (17). Primary bloodstream infection is defined as laboratory-confirmed bloodstream infection and clinical sepsis not related to infection at another site (18). By definition, intravascular CR-BSIs are classified as primary BSIs (18).

The risk of acquiring CR-BSI ranges from 0.9% to 8% (19–23). A rate of 15% has recently been reported in a study from Spain that primarily enrolled patients on total parenteral nutrition (24). These differences partly result from including different subjects in the study population (e.g., patients from burn units, intensive care, patients on long-term total parenteral nutrition), catheter care, and duration of catheterization. In addition, the type of ICU (e.g., coronary care unit

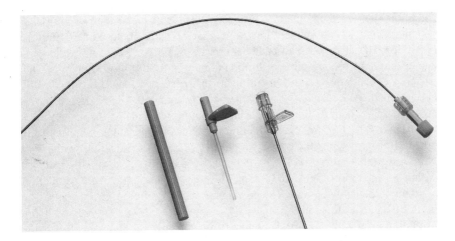

Figure 1   Polyurethane central venous catheter.

or burn unit) may contribute to the variation in the observed incidence of CR-BSIs. Therefore, the CDC stratifies the data collected by the national nosocomial infections surveillance (NNIS) into the different types of ICUs (17). In the European study on nosocomial infections in intensive care units (EPIC) involving 10,038 patients, the presence of a central venous line was a statistically significant risk factor (OR 4.6, Cl_{95} 3.1–6.8) for bloodstream infections (25). The risk of CR-BSIs increases over time if measured as infections per catheter (26–28), but remains remarkably stable if measured as incidence density (infections per catheter-days) (29,30). To adjust for this potential confounder, the CDC recommends to report nosocomial device-associated infections as number of infections per 100 or 1000 device-days. This issue is clinically important because it has been recommended that CVCs in an ICU should be replaced at least every 3 to 7 days (1,31). Recent prospective, randomized clinical trials did not show a difference in the rate of CR-BSI if CVCs were routinely changed or left in place as long as clinically indicated (30,32).

CR-BSIs are largely preventable and are part of most surveillance systems for infection control. The current guidelines for prevention of CR-BSIs were issued in 1981 by the Centers for Disease Control (CDC) (33). It took more than a decade for an update: The CDC have issued a draft proposal in September 1995; a final publication is expected in fall 1996 (34).

III. MICROBIOLOGY

The spectrum of microorganisms causing CRIs largely depends on the type of hospital care (e.g., intensive care), infusate (e.g., glucose 40%, lipids), patient condition such as a immunocompromised host (e.g., bone marrow transplant patients), or patients undergoing hemodialysis and many other variables (1,35–38). The distribution of pathogens varies by hospital size and affiliation— e.g., teaching vs. nonteaching institution (Table 1). A shift toward gram-positive bacteria and fungi was observed over the past two decades in CR-BSIs (17,39,40). CoNS, *Candida* spp., enterococci, and, less frequently, *S. aureus* emerged as frequent pathogens associated with intravascular catheters in the last decade (41–43). For CoNS, methicillin-resistance is present in approximately 50% of European, and 80% of U.S. strains (43). The rate of infections with methicillin-resistant *S. aureus* (MRSA) depends on the prevalence of this pathogen within an institution. Between 0% and 40% of *S. aureus* strains are methicillin-resistant in the United States. The prevalence of MRSA in Europe increases from north (0% to 5%) to south (30% to 60%) (25,44) and differs from institution to institution even within a city. Therefore, it is imperative to know the distribution of microorganisms within an institution.

Information about the patient and his or her underlying disease, the endemic hospital flora, the county and the country must be taken into account before starting empirical therapy or to comply a set of recommendations for diagnosis and therapy of CR-BSI at an individual institution. Detailed information about the importance of individual pathogens is provided in the previous chapters.

IV. DIAGNOSIS OF CVC-RELATED INFECTIONS

A. Definitions and Terminology

The definitions are based on the 1996 guideline of the CDC for the prevention of intravascular device-related infections (34). They take into account that the definition may vary depending on the type of catheter (e.g., peripheral catheter, short-term catheter, long-term catheter). For more detailed information, see Chapter 2, by K.G. Kristinsson.

For short-term CVCs, the following definitions were suggested.

1. Colonized Catheter

Growth of >15 colony forming units (CFU) by the roll-plate technique (45) or $\geq 10^3$ (quantitative culture) from a proximal or distal catheter segment in the absence of accompanying clinical symptoms.

2. Catheter-Related Infection

Growth of ≥ 15 CFU from a catheter by semiquantitative culture with accompanying signs of inflammation (e.g., erythema, warmth, swelling, or tenderness) at the device site is indicative of local catheter-related infection.

Table 1   Microbiology of Short-Term Central Venous Catheters

Where short-term CVCs used	Most frequently isolated pathogen		Other typical pathogens	
Intensive care unit	Gram-negative bacteria	30–40%	Staphylococci	≈30%
Immunocompromised host	Coagulase-negative staphylococci	> 50%	*S. aureus* Gram-negative bacilli	≈10% < 10%
Total parenteral nutrition	*S. aureus*	> 30%	CoNS *Candida* spp.	≈20% ≈10%

The relative frequency is an overall estimation, and the range is very broad. The spectrum of microorganisms causing CRIs largely depends on the type of hospital care (e.g., intensive care), infusate (e.g., glucose 40% and lipids), immunosuppression, and many other variables. (See details in Chapters 3–6.)
Source: From Refs. 79, 170, 177, 181–189.

3.   Catheter-Related Bloodstream Infection

CR-BSI is defined as isolation of the same organism (i.e., identical species, antibiogram) from a semiquantitative or quantitative culture of a catheter segment and from the blood (preferably drawn from a peripheral vein) of a patient with accompanying clinical symptoms of bloodstream infection and no other apparent source of infection. In the absence of laboratory confirmation, defervescence after removal of an implicated catheter from a patient with bloodstream infection may be considered *indirect* evidence of CR-BSI.

The term "sepsis" was recently redefined as systemic inflammatory response syndrome (SIRS) due to an infection, and "severe sepsis" as SIRS plus signs of organ failure (46). The term catheter-related infection (CRI) would belong to the term sepsis according to this definition suggested by R. Bone (46,47). Importantly, the definition does not necessarily require microbiologic documentation of infection because mortality and the progression of sepsis are very similar, dependent on microbiologic documentation of infection (48). Therefore, the draft guidelines of the CDC include defervescence after removal of an implicated catheter as indirect evidence for CR-BSI. The term catheter-related bacteremia is frequently used to describe episodes of CR-BSI. However, short-term bacteremia such as after a dental procedure is not always accompanied by a response of the host and, most importantly, do not require treatment (49). Therefore, only CRI and CR-BSI are used exclusively in this chapter to describe episodes of local and systemic infection associated with intravascular catheters.

B.   Signs and Symptoms of Central Venous CR-BSI

In contrast to peripheral catheters, central venous CR-BSI rarely presents with the classical signs of infection: redness, induration, and pain (29). Clinical sepsis without obvious source of infection is the most frequent symptom observed in cases with CR-BSI. However, it is important to look for evidence of CR-BSI if a patient has fever of unknown source and a central venous line. Therefore, a workup in a febrile patient with a central venous line must always include a check of the insertion site and the duration of catheterization. A rare but very serious complication is septic thrombophlebitis (Fig. 2). Typically, a large area around the insertion site is inflamed, and distension of superficial veins and prominent venous collaterals are observed. Pathogens such as *S. aureus* frequently cause

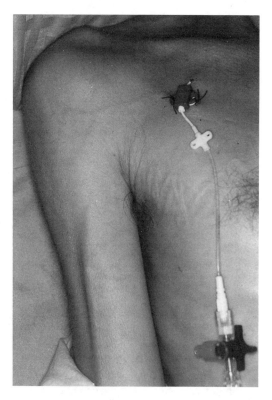

Figure 2   *S. aureus* catheter-associated bloodstream infection. Erythema, distension of superficial veins, and appearance of prominent venous collaterals as clinical evidence of septic thrombophlebitis. Photograph taken by T. Bregenzer, M.D.

such serious infections, but CoNS can also induce septic shock within hours even in immunocompetent hosts.

C. Microbiologic Methods for Diagnosis of CRI

Sensitivity and specificity of microbiological methods for diagnosis of CRI and CR-BSI depend on the method used in the routine microbiology laboratory. Sieg-man-Igra and Farr calculated a pooled estimate of the sensitivity, specificity, and cost of the methods (50). If the catheter has been removed, sensitivity and specificity were best for quantitative catheter segment cultures (94% and 92%, respectively). However, since there is no gold standard for the diagnosis of CRI, the results of this meta-analysis must be interpreted with caution. The author's personal opinion is that quantitative cultures with vortex ± sonication are the most appropriate methods for the time being, if the catheter has been removed. The different methods are described in a previous chapter. For long-term catheters, quantitative blood cultures with an automated dilution and reading system may be the optimal diagnostic technique. Microbiological methods requiring removal of the catheter and in situ methods are recommended for short-term CVCs. Removal of the catheter is still the safe strategy to eliminate this potential source of infection if a febrile episode of unknown source is observed. Diagnostic methods using the catheter tip are most accurate for such cases. However, removal or even guidewire replacement might set the patient at risk (e.g., in cases with severe thrombocytopenia). A method with the catheter left in place is more suitable for such patients (51–53). Examples are quantitative blood cultures taken through the catheter and a peripheral vein, or targeted skin cultures if the patient is on TPN (52,54). Most quantitative cultures have a higher sensitivity to detect microorganisms on the catheter than the semiquantitative method. Catheters are either flushed with broth or saline, or placed in broth and vortexed and/or sonicated (55,56), a method that detects microorganisms on the external and internal surface of the catheter. Sonication releases microorganisms adherent to the catheter and may therefore have greater sensitivity than flushing the catheter only from the surface. However, these methods are not routinely available in many microbiology laboratories and are much more time-consuming. Therefore, the microbiologist should be consulted in such cases to discuss the most appropriate culture technique given the patient's condition and the resources of the microbiology laboratory.

V. CATHETER MATERIALS

A. Catheter Composition

Most catheters used in the U.S. are made of polyurethane, polyvinyl chloride (PVC), polyethylene, or silicone. As for peripheral catheters, silicone catheters are associated with a lower risk of infection than PVC catheters (57). Therefore, PVC catheters are rarely used today. Surface modification of polymer intravascular catheters attenuates tissue response against the foreign material (58). A hydrophilic surface was achieved by introducing hydroxyethylmethacrylate into polyurethane catheters. These hydrophilic surfaces reduced in vitro adhesion of *S. epidermidis* compared to hydrophobic polyurethane catheters (59). Host protein and other substances may coat the surface of the catheter and limit the influence of the catheter composition (60). However, lacking randomized controlled clinical trials, definite conclusions about the contribution of catheter material to CVC-related infection can not be drawn.

B.   Outer Surface–Modified Catheters and Cuffs

Microorganisms can adhere to any implanted device. Once adhered and embedded in a glycocalix (called slime), they become resistant to most antimicrobial agents even if standard susceptibility testing reveals high sensitivity (61). The mode of growth, the influence of bacterial products such as slime for CoNS, and the different susceptibility of planctonic versus adherent microorganisms partly explain why microorganisms become resistant in the presence of a foreign body (61–63). In animal models, several investigators succeeded to reduce bacterial adherence by coating the catheters with antimicrobials or antiseptics (64,65). Colonization of the skin at the insertion site is a well-recognized risk factor for the development of CRI and CR-BSI (52). In addition, bacteria on exit sites of percutaneous catheters can migrate rapidly from the entry site into the dermal tunnel along the external catheter surface, perhaps suspended in a fluid phase and propelled by capillary action (66). Therefore, research was started on cuffs hindering bacteria from moving along the catheter from the surface to the intradermal part of the catheter. In addition, polymers with antiadherence properties were developed, followed by impregnated catheters.

1.   Cuffs

A cuff acts as a tissue-interface barrier. A commercially available example is a biodegradable collagen cuff impregnated with silver ions (VitaCuff) attached to a catheter just prior to insertion. Multiple prospective, randomized clinical trials have shown that cuffed catheters lower the risk of CRI and CR-BSI more than threefold compared to noncuffed catheters (26,27,67). However, their efficacy wanes after 2 weeks of catheterization (67). The cuff does not prevent intraluminal transmission of pathogens from contaminated hubs or infusates because the cuff is on the outside of the catheter. If guidewire exchange is attempted with a cuffed catheter, early colonization will occur carrying a high risk of subsequent infection. The importance of the hub as source of infection augments as time of catheterization increases. Therefore, protection of the VitaCuff wanes over time due to loss of silver ions and increasing importance of the intraluminal pathway.

2. Coated Catheters

In animal studies, catheters coated with an antiseptic, antimicrobial agent (65,68) or even with nonsteroidal anti-inflammatory agents (69) reduced bacterial colonization of the catheter. Chlorhexidine-coated catheters decreased biofilm formation and bacterial adherence on catheters (68). Benzalkonium chloride also lowers the degree of bacterial colonization in vitro (59). In elegant animal studies performed by Sherertz, coating with dicloxacillin, clindamycin, and fusidic acid decreased the risk of infection compared with uncoated control catheters ($P < 0.05$) (64).

Most Swan-Ganz pulmonary artery catheters used in the U.S. are heparin bonded to maintain patency and coated with benzalkonium chloride, which also provides short-term but broad-spectrum antimicrobial activity (70). In a study by Kamal et al, central venous catheters pretreated with a cationic surfactant and the antibiotic cefazolin lowered the rate of CRI from 14% to 8% in a surgical ICU ($P < 0.004$) (71); however, the catheter must be coated immediately before use, which is time-consuming and needs special training. A commercially available CVC impregnated with sulfadiazine and chlorhexidine (Arrowgard, Arrow International, Reading, PA) reduced the rate of CR-BSI from 5% (uncoated catheters) to 1% (coated catheters) in a randomized study that included 405 catheters (72). However, only the outer surface is coated. As mentioned above, the internal lumen becomes more important with time of catheterization as risk factor for CRI or CR-BSI (73), a factor which this type of catheter and attachable cuffs will not influence. Most recently, catheter precoated with rifampin and minocycline demonstrated excellent efficacy against CRI in vitro (74) and in vivo (75). A clinical study with 234 patients, randomized to receive a triple-lumen catheter precoated with rifampin-minocycline or without, showed that none of the patients with a precoated catheter had CR-BSI compared to seven in the control group ($P = 0.01$) (75). In addition, this protective effect exceeds 14 days (76). Coated catheters will likely become catheters of choice for high-risk patients. The microbiology laboratory should be informed about the type of coating because inactivation of the impregnation (e.g., for chlorhexidine) is necessary to avoid false-negative culture results.

3. Electrically Powered Catheters

Adherent bacteria become resistant against antimicrobial agents by the mode of growth, biofilm formation, and other, ill-known factors (61). If exposed to an electric field, these adherent bacteria respond similarly to antibiotics as planctonic pathogens (77). Consecutively, electrically charged catheters were developed to prevent binding and colonization of bacteria. However, this has been tested in a rabbit model and clinical data are scarce. One major advantage is the long-term effect because batteries can be replaced without removing the catheter (78). Given the complexity of such a device, they probably will not replace catheters precoated with antiseptics or antibiotics.

VI.   OPTIMAL SITE OF INSERTION

CVCs can be inserted from a peripheral vein [e.g., midline catheters, peripherally inserted central catheters (PICCs)] or directly into a large vein (subclavian, jugular, axilla, femoral access). The jugular access is associated with a statistically significant increased risk of infection compared with subclavian vein insertion (28,79–84). These studies report an average colonization of CVCs inserted into the jugular vein of 27% compared to 4% in CVCs inserted into the subclavian vein ($P < 0.05$). The differences may be due to increased colonization by respiratory pathogens at the internal jugular insertion site (85), the difficulty of fixation, the mechanical burdening by head movements, and insufficient adherence of catheter dressings. This long-term complication must be weighed against the noninfectious risks at the time of insertion such as pneumothorax and severe bleeding by inadvertent puncture of the A. subclavia. The subclavian catheter is easier to keep dry and clean—factors associated with a lower risk of infection. For patients undergoing surgery such as coronary bypass surgery, the jugular access is probably the better choice because short-time catheterization is anticipated (< 3 to 7 days), and acute complication rates during insertion are of concern. For prolonged catheterization, infectious complications probably outweigh those associated with insertion. Therefore, the subclavian access may be preferable for medical ICU patients, who frequently require prolonged catheterization.

Many authors observed a higher risk of CRI with femoral central venous lines. Recent studies, however, demonstrated a similar risk of femoral central venous catheterization as known for the jugular or subclavian access, providing a reasonable alternative if the jugular or subclavian site cannot be used (86,87). This discrepancy may be explained by selection bias in observational studies: The femoral access is frequently chosen in ICU patients with protracted shock or after unsuccessful attempts to access the jugular or subclavian vein. Such patients have an inherent high risk for nosocomial infections (88). Therefore, higher rates of CRI with femoral catheters must be interpreted with caution. It is crucial to try to control for these variables or, even better, to balance these factors by a randomized clinical trial. Noninfectious risks should also be considered if choosing the femoral access: In a randomized clinical trial, deep-vein thrombosis occurred in 25% of subjects after femoral catheterization, compared to 0% in the jugular/subclavian group (89).

VII. THERAPY OF INFECTIONS

A. Suspected CRI or CR-BSI

Clinicians are most frequently faced with an acute febrile episode with unknown source of infection rather than an infectious complication known to be catheter-related. Removal of the catheter is recommended if few risks are anticipated for the patient. Advantages and disadvantages of early catheter removal are summarized in Table 2. In >70% of such episodes, fever can be traced down to a different source, and the catheter is unnecessarily replaced (29,90,91). In addition, CRIs due to CoNS can be successfully treated with antibiotics without removal of the device (92). Therefore, the British guidelines for good practice in central venous catheterization recommend to obtain entry site swabs and blood cultures via the CVC and a separate peripheral venipuncture (93) before catheter removal is considered.

Table 2 Suspected Catheter-Related Bloodstream Infection: Pros and Cons for Catheter Removal

	Removal	No or delayed removal
Microbiological diagnostic for CRI or CR-BSI	Easy; several established methods	Difficult; limited data for in situ methods
Complications	Can prevent septic complications	Risk of septic complications
Advantage	Recommended procedure if little risks are anticipated with exchange	Many unnecessary changes prevented
	Guide wire exchange with culture of the removed catheter possible if catheter was in place < 1 week, and insertion site normal	Avoids any risk due to catheter exchange
Disadvantage	Risk for noninfectious complications such as pneumothorax, short-term interruption of fluid administration, bleeding	Increased risk for septic complications such as septic thrombophlebitis, endocarditis, and perpetuation of ongoing CR-BSI, relapse of bacteremia

However, this procedure requires quantitative blood cultures, a regimen rarely available around the clock in the clinical microbiology laboratory. In addition, failure to remove the catheter puts the patient at high risk for sustained bacteremia, septic thrombosis, and endocarditis (94–96). Serious complications after an episode of CR-BSI with *S. aureus* or fungi are frequent: 25% of patients with *S. aureus* CR-BSI develop complications and 68% of patients with fungal CR-BSI have persistent fungemia (95,97,98). The crude mortality is reported to be 16% for *S. aureus* and 52% for fungal CR-BSIs (95,98). Given the possibility of severe complications, it is wise to replace a short-term CVC if clinically possible. Hemato-oncology units may follow a less strict policy because CoNS are the most common pathogens that allow antimicrobial treatment with the catheter in situ with very little risk for the patient. However, recurrent bacteremia occurs in 20% even with CoNS if the catheter is not removed (92). In summary, removal of the catheter should always be attempted for short-term CVCs unless a high risk is associated with the exchange or CRI, or CR-BSI is less likely (Table 2). Guide wire exchange is not recommended if there is purulence at the insertion site, or CRI or CR-BSI are very probable.

The empiric antimicrobial regimen for CR-BSI depends on the resistance rates of the predominant nosocomial pathogens observed at the institution. The guidelines of the University of Basel Hospitals/Switzerland recommend a second-generation cephalosporin because cases with methicillin-resistant *S. aureus* (MRSA) CR-BSI were not observed during the previous 5 years. In institutions with a high prevalence of MRSA, a combination of a glycopeptide such as vancomycin with an aminoglycoside or a quinolone is appropriate against the bacterial pathogens likely to be encountered with an infected catheter.

B.   Treatment of Established Infections

Antimicrobial treatment depends on the microorganism(s) isolated from the catheter tip or with other culture techniques. In most instances, removal of the devices and an antimicrobial treatment for 7 to 10 days is appropriate for short-term central venous lines. Persistent bacteremia may indicate septic thrombosis and should prompt immediate diagnostic procedures. It is the author's personal opinion that immediate removal of a catheter is necessary for *S. aureus* and fungal episodes of CR-BSI, recommended for gram-negative pathogens, and rarely indicated for CoNS (Table 2). A proposal for the clinical approach to patients presenting with suspected CR-BSI is given in Figure 3.

1.   Coagulase-Negative Staphylococci

CoNS are the most frequently involved pathogens in CR-BSI. Most infections with long-term catheters can be treated without removal of the device (54,99). This also appears to be true for short-term CVCs. Raad et al. investigated 70 cases

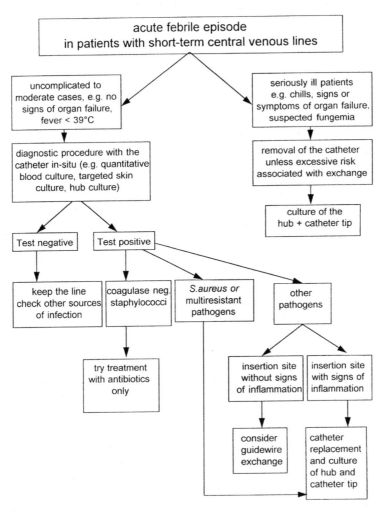

Figure 3 Proposal for the management of febrile episodes of patients with suspected catheter-related infection or catheter-related bloodstream infection.

with CR-BSI due to CoNS (92). Recurrent bacteremia was observed in 20% of patients when the catheter was not removed. However, 80% were successfully treated with the catheter left in place. In addition, mortality was not influenced by treatment with or without catheter removal ($P > 0.1$). Therefore, the only risk with this kind of management is recurrent bacteremia without serious complications, which makes catheter removal necessary.

A glycopeptide such as vancomycin or teicoplanin is the treatment of choice because most CoNS are methicillin-resistant (43). However, an antistaphylococcal penicillin should be used if the the organism turns out to be methicillin-susceptible. CoNS adhere to plastic surfaces and produce a glycocalix, called slime. They become embedded in a biofilm layer that provides a measure of protection from antibacterial agents (100). Failure of glycopeptide antibiotics to cure device-related infection is not due to poor penetration of drugs into biofilm but likely due to diminished antimicrobial effect on bacteria in the biofilm environment (101).

Rifampin is highly efficacious against adherent CoNS. Antibiotic combinations with rifampin are much more effective against device-related infections than those without rifampin (61,63). Outcome may be improved by addition of rifampin, but few data are available for intravascular catheters. However, minocycline and rifampin have been suggested for coating the plastic surface of the catheter, resulting in a significant reduction of CR-BSI episodes (102). Alternatively, the antibiotic lock technique for long-term catheters probably kills even adherent CoNS by its high intraluminal concentration, well above peak levels in blood. The optimal treatment is still controversial.

Treatment should last 5 to 7 days if the catheter is removed. If the catheter is not removed, treatment should be extended to ≥14 days. However, the optimal duration of treatment is not well established.

2. S. aureus

S. aureus CR-BSI frequently leads to septic complications; 25% of patients experiencing an episode of *S. aureus* CR-BSI develop complications. One in seven will die (98). These data have been collected from patients with the catheter removed. Therefore, CR-BSI with *S. aureus* is a very serious disease, and the catheter should be removed whenever possible. Raad et al. recommended 10 days of antibiotic therapy for uncomplicated cases (96), but this has been questioned by other authors (103). Uncomplicated cases were defined as those who became afebrile within ≤3 days of therapy *and* negative blood cultures. Fourteen days of antimicrobial therapy appears to suffice for noncomplicated cases (1). Complicated cases (e.g., those with septic metastasis or suppurative thrombophlebitis) require an antimicrobial treatment of 4 to 6 weeks (104).

3. Gram-Negative Rods

Gram-negative rods can be treated with a short course of appropriate antibiotics, unless there is evidence for *Pseudomonas* spp. CR-BSI. Bacteremia with *Pseudomonas aeruginosa* have a higher mortality than those with other bacteria (105), and treatment should include an anti-*Pseudomonas* β-lactam and an aminoglycoside, preferably tobramycin. A promising alternative against *P. aeruginosa* CR-BSI is the combination of high-dose ciprofloxacin and piperacillin-tazobactam (106). However, only limited clinical data are available as for meropenem, which may be another option.

There are no randomized clinical trials to determine the optimal duration of therapy. Uncomplicated cases respond to a 7- to 10-days course of appropriate antibiotics if the catheter is removed.

4. Candida spp.

Candida spp. are isolated from episodes of CR-BSI in up to 20% (107). In cancer patients, overall mortality after an episode of fungal CR-BSI exceeds 50%. Treatment with fluconazole appears to be as effective as amphotericin B (108). However, fluconazole-resistant *Candida* spp. emerged in recent years, mainly after previous treatment in HIV-positive patients. However, these pathogens were recently observed also without previous exposure to fluconazole (109). Therefore, the microbiology laboratory should always identify genus and species to guide appropriate treatment. If a patient did receive fluconazole prophylaxis, susceptibility testing may be considered before fluconazole treatment. Isolation of *Candida* spp. or other fungi always requires a change of catheter, because a higher mortality and a prolonged period of fungemia has been observed if the catheter remains in place (95,108). However, some authors dare to treat candidal BSI with the catheter in place (110). Fluconazole is appropriate if *C. albicans* is isolated. For most other fungal pathogens, amphotericin B is probably still treatment of choice unless fluconzole susceptibility has been tested. However, susceptibility testing for fungi is not well established, and limited data are available for the correlation between the in vitro results and clinical outcome. New compounds such as voriconazole may improve antifungal treatment options, specifically for rare molds.

VIII. TOTAL PARENTERAL NUTRITION

Total parenteral nutrition (TPN) differs in many ways from other modes of intravascular therapy: (1) Catheters used for TPN are needed much longer than other catheters; (2) TPN solutions support the growth of microorganisms, especially gram-negative bacteria, and *Candida* spp. (111–113); and (3) the underlying disease of the patient increases the risk of acquiring nosocomial infections, and remote infections are frequently present that expose the catheter to hematogenous seeding. A second episode of a nosocomial infection is observed 11 times more frequently if a patient has already been diagnosed with a nosocomial infection (88).

The incidence of CR-BSI in patients receiving TPN ranges from 0% to 14%, on the average 3% to 5% (114–119). Common organisms isolated are CoNS, *S. aureus*, *Candida* spp., *Serratia* spp., and *Enterobacter* spp. (23,120,121). *Malassezia furfur* is a rare but serious infection strongly associated with TPN in young children (122). In such cases of suspected CR-BSI, the clinician should advise the microbiology laboratory about the patient being on TPN. *Malassezia furfur* requires specific supplements to grow in standard media (122–124). CRI or CR-BSI caused by *Candida* spp. has been a particular problem in patients on TPN. These patients often receive multiple antibiotics for other infections, a factor that is independently associated with an increased risk for *Candida* infection (125).

Catheter care is a crucial factor in TPN. Ryan and colleagues (91) related CRIs to violation of the infusion delivery system. Snydman estimated the risk of developing CRI six times higher for catheters that were exposed to violations of the catheter care guidelines compared with those that were not (120).

As mentioned above, a risk factor for all catheters is skin colonization (114,119,126). Fan et al. performed routine surveillance cultures of skin and hubs to predict cases of CRI (127). When either a positive skin or hub culture was considered as an indicator for CRI, the sensitivity of the test was almost 80%. However, the positive predictive value was only 44%, an unreliable and expensive parameter in clinical practice (126,128,129). In a recently published study, the so-called targeted quantitative skin cultures—cultures that are done only when CRI or CR-BSI is clinically suspected—had specificities and negative predictive values well above 90% and sensitivities and positive predictive values of 75% and 100%, respectively (52). However, routine cultures even in this study were of little clinical value (sensitivity 18%).

The optimal catheter type for short-term (<1 month) TPN is probably the single-lumen catheter without stopcocks (120,130,131). If a triple-lumen catheter is used, the distal port should be avoided for TPN solutions, to minimize the risk of contamination if guide wire exchange should be necessary. Howard and colleagues reported that patients prefer a totally implantable, subcutaneous infusion port for long-term TPN (>3 months) rather than regular central venous lines (132) (see chapter on long-term catheters).

Needleless and protected-needle intravascular access system have been recommended for use with intravenous lines to reduce the risk of needlestick injuries in healthcare workers. However, these devices have higher rates of CR-BSI than regular devices (risk ratio 14.9; $P < 0.05$), specifically for patients with TPN. These devices bear critical reevaluation for its use (133). They may protect the healthcare worker, but at the same time put the patient at higher risk for CR-BSI (134).

Mermel et al. reported severe adverse reaction associated with midline catheters (135): Acute hypersensitivity reactions have been reported in four patients still lacking an appropriate explanation. Therefore, this type of catheter should be reevaluated before it can be recommended for TPN.

A difficult clinical task is to decide when to remove a TPN catheter for suspected sepsis. Quantitative cultures are appropriate if a long-term catheter is in place. For short-term central venous lines, exchange to a new site or by guide wire is frequently recommended (90); however, in one study, over 90% of the catheters removed for suspected sepsis were not the source of that sepsis (90,131). Bonadimani and colleagues reported successful treatment of CRI in 91% with guide wire exchange (121). Semiquantitative cultures of the blood taken through the catheter may help in deciding when to keep the line or to change it (negative predictive value 100%, positive predictive value 60%) (136). As mentioned above, targeted skin cultures may help in making the correct diagnosis (134). There is no consensus on this issue, but guide wire exchange seems to be a reasonable step in the early management of episodes of patients on TPN. Antimicrobial agents should be given sequentially through the different ports to expose all inner lumens to high concentrations of the antimicrobial agent (99).

IX. PREVENTION STRATEGIES

As mentioned above, most CRIs and CR-BSIs are preventable: The different strategies have been covered in Chapter 16, by B. Jansen. Specific prevention strategies for short-term CVCs are summarized below.

A. Barrier Precautions

Full barrier precautions including the use of mask, cap, sterile gloves, gown, and large sterile drape have been shown to significantly reduce the risk of CRI and CR-BSI (38,83). Strict asepsis at the time of insertion is a crucial step for effective infection control. It is unknown if mask and cap are mandatory, but they might provide an additional level of safety. The environment where the catheter is inserted does not play a major role: two randomized studies could not demonstrate a difference in the infection rate between the study group (insertion in the operating theater) and the control group (insertion in wards) (38,83).

B. Disinfection of the Skin

Cutaneous antisepsis of the insertion site is regarded as one of the most important measures for preventing CRI and CR-BSI (34). However, the disinfectant to be preferred to use for catheter insertion sites is still debated. The use of highly concentrated acetone for defatting the catheter insertion site is unwarranted (114). In 1981, Maki and Band demonstrated that an ointment containing polymyxin, neomycin, and bacitracin reduced the rate of CRI from 6.5% to 2.2% (137); however, three *Candida* infections including one case of fungemia occurred in this treatment arm. In addition, topical ointments do not have to be sterile under the pharmacopeia's requirement, and a large outbreak of fungal infections was caused by a contaminated topical ointment (138). Maki et al. prospectively tested three different disinfectants—alcohol, povidone-iodine, and chlorhexidine—to evaluate their efficacy in reducing CRI and CR-BSI (19). Alcohol and povidone-iodine had clearly higher rates of CRI and CR-BSI than chlorhexidine—7.1% and 9.3% vs. 2.3%, respectively ($P < 0.02$); however, the differences were seen in CR-BSIs due to CoNS, and only by pooling of the data.

Daily application of povidone-iodine did not reduce colonization of central-venous lines in another large study (84). A hand-washing system using chlorhexidine at the University of Iowa reduced the rate of nosocomial infections significantly compared to one using alcohol (139), supporting the preference for chlorhexidine. However, in a randomized clinical trial addressing the effectiveness of alcohol versus chlorhexidine for surgical scrub, alcohol was significantly more efficacious than chlorhexidine (140). Alcoholic preparations are most suitable because of their rapid action (within $\approx$30 sec), broad spectrum, and minimal side effects. However, there is no residual effect after evaporation of the alcohol. Therefore, chlorhexidine or povidone-iodine might be added to extend the antimicrobial effect (remanent effect). Unfortunately, there are no commercially available preparations of alcoholic chlorhexidine approved for use at intravenous catheter insertion sites in the U.S. Disinfectants without alcohol need 3 to 5 min for microbial killing, a waiting time frequently not observed in a busy hospital. Therefore, the chlorhexidine gluconate patch that significantly reduces the incidence of epidural catheter colonization may not be suitable for intravascular catheters (141).

C.   Catheter Dressings

In the early 1980s, transparent dressings were frequently used to allow visual inspection of the insertion site at all times. Furthermore, only weekly changes were considered to be necessary, saving nursing time and dressing supply. A well-designed, randomized prospective study showed a higher risk for CRI with the transparent dressing than with gauze (RR 2.6) (142). Other studies that included mainly patients on total parenteral nutrition did not confirm these results (143–146). However, moisture under the dressing increased the risk for CRI (RR > 3), a factor more frequently seen in the transparent dressing group (143). A metaanalysis found that transparent dressings led to a threefold increased risk for CR-BSI compared with gauze dressings (147). In addition, four independent studies demonstrated higher bacterial counts under transparent dressings than under gauze (28,142,147,148). Today, the new, highly permeable transparent dressings are not associated with higher rates of CRI or CR-BSI (36), even if they still are associated with higher levels of microbial colonization. Dressing changes every 2 days are recommended in the hospital (149). This interval can be extended for highly permeable transparent dressings up to 5 days (36); however, daily inspection of the insertion site is crucial to detect early signs of CRI. Gauze still has some advantages, but the highly permeable transparent dressing may be preferred by patients and nurses.

D. Routine Exchange of CVCs

The recent literature supports the idea of *not* routinely changing CVCs (Fig. 3) (32,150,151), as do the latest recommendations by the CDC (34). The hazard for CRI or CR-BSI linearly increases with the duration the catheter remains in place (152). Noninfectious complications are more frequent with routine change than with a policy to keep the line as long as clinically indicated (32). However, a policy including routine changes always lets physicians reconsider the indication for continuous central venous access. This regular check will not work with a policy of keeping the line as long as clinically indicated. It is important to train the staff to strictly limit time of catheterization because each day of catheterization puts the patient at risk for CRI and CR-BSI (153).

E. Guide Wire vs. New Puncture

Guide wire exchange is the preferred method to change a pulmonary artery catheter to a CVC or to replace a malfunctioning catheter (34). The risk of infection after guide wire exchange is not yet established; one large randomized clinical trial showed an increased risk (Fig. 4) (32). Other studies do not support this finding (20,30,154,155). For patients on total parenteral nutrition, Bonadimani and colleagues reported successful treatment in 91% of CRI episodes by guide-wire exchange (121). The draft guideline for prevention of intravascular device-related infections from the CDC allows for guide wire exchange for suspected CRI if clinical signs of local inflammation are absent (34). Another exchange to a new site becomes necessary if the culture result of the removed catheter indicates local infection. Other authors do not support guide wire exchange for febrile patients with suspected CRI or CR-BSI (1,90). Therefore, the clinician must weigh the risks for complication for the procedure against the risks of recurrent infection. A purulent discharge at the insertion site precludes guide wire exchange.

F. IV Teams

Prospective studies demonstrated a significantly higher incidence rate of phlebitis among catheters inserted and maintained by floor staff than among those devices inserted or maintained by an IV therapy team (156–158). In addition, these catheter teams have also been found to be highly cost-effective (118,156,158). Randomized controlled trials have been performed with peripheral catheters only

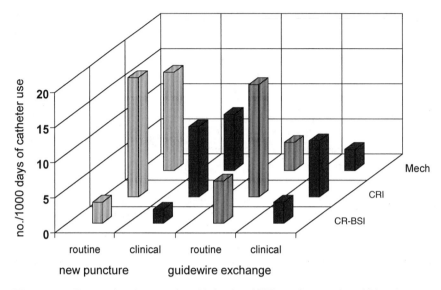

Figure 4   Rates of catheter-related infection (CRI), catheter-related bloodstream infection (CR-BSI), and mechanical complications (Mech) according to the method of catheter replacement. Routine: scheduled exchange of catheter every 3 days by the respective method (new puncture or guide wire exchange). Clinical: replacement of catheter only as clinically indicated. Adapted from Ref. 32.

(156). The rate of phlebitis was 1% in the staff-inserted groups and 0.2% in the team-inserted group (relative risk 5); however, as mentioned above, catheter material and catheter care have changed over time, and these older study findings do not necessarily apply for today's conditions. As pointed out by Puntis and colleagues, staff training is a key factor in reducing catheter-related infections (153). It is conceivable that professional teams are less likely to inadvertently contaminate the catheter than nurses on the ward without specific training. However, most CVCs are inserted in ICUs where all healthcare workers should have appropriate training in catheter care.

G.   Antimicrobial Prophylaxis

Several studies have indicated that systemic antimicrobial prophylaxis at the time of insertion of long-term catheters reduced the risk for CR-BSI (159–162). However, two randomized trials failed to show a benefit of such prophylaxis (163,164). This issue remains controversial for long-term catheters, but prophylaxis is not recommended for short-term CVCs. Some data indicate that prophylaxis may be warranted for neonates weighing <1000 g or for patients undergoing bone marrow transplantation (165). However, glycopeptides are generally used for prophylaxis, and their use has been associated with the emergence of vancomycin-resistant enterococci (166,167).

X. HOST-SPECIFIC ISSUES

A. Burns

After a serious burn, the skin area is initially almost sterile. Therefore, a catheter can be introduced immediately after the trauma through a burned skin area and left in place for 2 or 3 days if intravascular access sites are limited. Because burned skin becomes always colonized by multiple, frequently gram-negative bacteria after this time period, these patients are at high risk to acquire CRI and CR-BSI (168–170). A prospective study by Franceschi and colleagues demonstrated that the risk for CRI correlated inversely with the distance of the catheter insertion site from the burn wound (171). Therefore, a catheter should be placed as far as possible from the burned skin, 2 to 3 days after the accident. *P. aeruginosa* is the most frequently isolated microorganism from catheters in burned patients (168,171,172). In future, the use of coated catheters may become routine for this patient population (72,102). The International Society for Burn Injuries (ISBI) and the WHO still recommend to change intravascular catheters every 72 hours (173). For pediatric patients, this interval was extended to 7 days (174). In the author's opinion, this recommendation is no longer appropriate if the insertion site is remote from the burned skin area or/and a coated catheter is used.

B. HIV-Infected Patients

AIDS patients were considered to be at higher risk to develop CRI or CR-BSI than non-AIDS patients. Raviglione and colleagues reviewed 46 AIDS patients with Hickman catheters: CRI and CR-BSI occurred in 23% and 10%, respectively (175). In another study, the catheter was the source of infection in 73% of bacteremic episodes in HIV-positive patients (176). *S. aureus* is one of the most frequently isolated microorganism from catheters of AIDS patients (175,177), probably because of the high proportion of *S. aureus* carriers in this group (55%) and the host's inability to control the infection/colonization locally (178,179). Infection-free survival of central venous catheter was significantly prolonged with tunneled catheters compared to percutaneously placed central catheters ($P < 0.05$) (180). Therefore, a tunneled or a totally implanted catheter is recommended in AIDS patients with diseases requiring lifelong IV treatment (see Chapter 11).

XI. SUMMARY

Diagnosis of CRI and CR-BSI is difficult. Clinical signs of infection are frequently absent, making laboratory diagnosis very important. However, the optimal microbiologic method to confirm a diagnosis of CRI or CR-BSI is still controversial. Removal of the catheter, quantitative culture of the catheter segment and empirical antimicrobial treatment is recommended for episodes of suspected CR-BSIs. As an exception, most episodes due to CoNS can be treated with antimicrobial agents without catheter removal. Many different approaches are necessary to prevent these serious nosocomial infections. In the future, commercially available, coated catheters will help to further reduce the incidence of CRI and CR-BSI. The CDC guideline for prevention of intravascular device–related infections may help to adapt the current science to hospital practice (34). However, much remains to be learned about the pathogenesis, prevention, and treatment of CRI and CR-BSI.

REFERENCES

1. Maki DG. Pathogenesis, prevention, and management of infections due to intravascular devices used for infusion therapy. In: Bisno AL, Waldvogel FA, eds. Infections Associated With Indwelling Medical Devices. 2nd ed. Washington, DC: American Society for Microbiology, 1994:155–212.
2. Nyström B, Larsen SO, Dankert J, et al. Bacteraemia in surgical patients with intravenous devices: a European multicentre incidence study. The European Working Party on Control of Hospital Infections. J Hosp Infect 1983; 4:338–349.
3. Neuhof H, Seley GP. Acute suppurative phlebitis complicated by septicemia. Surgery 1947; 21:831–842.
4. Elliott TSJ, Faroqui MH, Tebbs SE, Armstrong RF, Hanson GC. An audit programme for central venous catheter-associated infections. J Hosp Infect 1995; 30: 181–191.
5. Jarvis WR, Edwards JR, Culver DH, et al. Nosocomial infection rates in adult and pediatric intensive care units in the United States. National Nosocomial Infections Surveillance System. Am J Med 1991; 91:185S–191S.
6. Norwood S, Ruby A, Civetta J, Cortes V. Catheter-related infections and associated septicemia. Chest 1991; 99:968–975.
7. Pittet D, Tarara D, Wenzel RP. Nosocomial bloodstream infection in critically ill patients. Excess length of stay, extra costs, and attributable mortality. JAMA 1994; 271:1598–1601.
8. Smith RL, Meixler SM, Simberkoff MS. Excess mortality in critically ill patients with nosocomial bloodstream infections. Chest 1991; 100:164–167.
9. Arnow PM, Quimosing EM, Beach M. Consequences of intravascular catheter sepsis. Clin Infect Dis 1993; 16:778–784.

10. Rüden H, Gastmeier P, Daschner F, Schumacher M. First national prevalence survey of nosocomial infections in German hospitals in 1994. Interscience Conference on Antimicrobial Agents and Chemotherapy, San Francisco, 1995. Abstract.

11. Vincent JL, Bihari DJ, Suter PM, et al. The prevalence of nosocomial infection in intensive care units in Europe. Results of the European Prevalence of Infection in Intensive Care (EPIC) Study. EPIC International Advisory Committee. JAMA 1995; 274:639–644.

12. Maki DG, Botticelli JT, LeRoy ML, Thielke TS. Prospective study of replacing administration sets for intravenous therapy at 48- vs 72-hour intervals. 72 hours is safe and cost-effective. JAMA 1987; 258:1777–1781.

13. Haley RP, Schaberg DR, Crossley KB, Von Allmen S, McGowan JEJ. Extra charges and prolongation of stay attributable to nosocomial infections: a prospective inter-hospital comparison. Am J Med 1981; 70:51–58.

14. Maki DG. Nosocomial bacteremia. An epidemiologic overview. Am J Med 1981; 70:719–732.

15. Pittet D, Wenzel RP. Nosocomial bloodstream infections. Secular trends in rates, mortality, and contribution to total hospital deaths. Arch Intern Med 1995; 155: 1177–1184.

16. Pittet D, Hulliger S, Auckenthaler R. Intravascular device-related infections in critically ill patients. J Chemother 1995; 7(suppl 3):55–66.

17. National Nosocomial Infection Surveillance (NNIS). A report from the national nosocomial infections surveillance (NNIS) system. Am J Infect Control 1995; 23: 377–385.

18. Garner JS, Jarvis WR, Emori TG, Horan TC, Hughes JM. CDC definitions for nosocomial infections, 1988. Am J Infect Control 1988; 16:128–140.

19. Maki DG, Ringer M, Alvarado CJ. Prospective randomised trial of povidone-iodine, alcohol, and chlorhexidine for prevention of infection associated with central venous and arterial catheters. Lancet 1991; 338:339–343.

20. Michel LA, Bradpiece HA, Randour P, Pouthier R. Safety of central venous catheter change over guidewire for suspected catheter-related sepsis. A prospective randomized trial. Int Surg 1988; 73:180–186.

21. Cheesbrough JS, Finch RG, Burden RP. A prospective study of the mechanisms of infection associated with hemodialysis catheters. J Infect Dis 1986; 154:579–589.

22. Kelly CS, Ligas JR, Smith CA, Madden GM, Ross KA, Becker DR. Sepsis due to triple lumen central venous catheters. Surg Gynecol Obstet 1986; 163:14–16.

23. Lee RB, Buckner M, Sharp KW. Do multi-lumen catheters increase central venous catheter sepsis compared to single-lumen catheters? J Trauma 1988; 28:1472–1475.

24. Segura M, Alvarez Lerma F, Tellado JM, et al. Clinical trial of the effect of a new catheter hub on the prevention of central venous catheter-related sepsis. Interscience Conference on Antimicrobial Agents and Chemotherapy, San Francisco, 1995. Abstract 258.

25. Vincent JL, Bihari DJ, Suter PM, et al. The prevalence of nosocomial infection in intensive care units in Europe. JAMA 1995; 274:639–644.

26. Flowers RH, Schwenzer KJ, Kopel RF, Fisch MJ, Tucker SI, Farr BM. Efficacy of an attachable subcutaneous cuff for the prevention of intravascular catheter-related infection. A randomized, controlled trial. JAMA 1989; 261:878–883.

27. Maki DG, Cobb L, Garman JK, Shapiro JM, Ringer M, Helgerson RB. An attachable silver-impregnated cuff for prevention of infection with central venous catheters: a prospective randomized multicenter trial. Am J Med 1988; 85:307–314.

28. Richet H, Hubert B, Nitemberg G, et al. Prospective multicenter study of vascular-catheter-related complications and risk factors for positive central-catheter cultures in intensive care unit patients. J Clin Microbiol 1990; 28:2520–2525.

29. Pittet D, Chuard C, Rae AC, Auckenthaler R. Clinical diagnosis of central venous catheter line infections: a difficult job. Interscience Conference on Antimicrobial Agents and Chemotherapy 1991; 31:174. Abstract.

30. Eyer S, Brummitt C, Crossley K, Siegel R, Cerra F. Catheter-related sepsis: prospective, randomized study of three methods of long-term catheter maintenance. Crit Care Med 1990; 18:1073–1079.

31. Snyder RH, Archer FJ, Endy T, et al. Catheter infection. A comparison of two catheter maintenance techniques. Ann Surg 1988; 208:651–653.

32. Cobb DK, High KP, Sawyer RG, et al. A controlled trial of scheduled replacement of central venous and pulmonary-artery catheters. N Engl J Med 1992; 327:1062–1068.

33. Centers for Disease Control Working Group. Guidelines for prevention of intravenous therapy-related infections. Infect Control 1981; 3:62–79.

34. Pearson ML. The hospital infection control practices advisory committee. Guideline for prevention of intravascular device-related infections. Infect Control Hosp Epidemiol 1996; 17:438–473.

35. Garrison RN, Wilson MA. Intravenous and central catheter infections. Surg Clin North Am 1994; 74:557–570.

36. Maki DG, Stolz SS, Wheeler S, Mermel LA. A prospective, randomized trial of gauze and two polyurethane dressings for site care of pulmonary artery catheters: implications for catheter management. Crit Care Med 1994; 22:1729–1737.

37. Mermel LA, Maki DG. Infectious complications of Swan-Ganz pulmonary artery catheters. Pathogenesis, epidemiology, prevention, and management. Am J Respir Crit Care Med 1994; 149:1020–1036.

38. Raad II, Hohn DC, Gilbreath BJ, et al. Prevention of central venous catheter-related infections by using maximal sterile barrier precautions during insertion. Infect Control Hosp Epidemiol 1994; 15:231–238.

39. Low DE, Willey BM, McGeer AJ. Multidrug-resistant enterococci: a threat to the surgical patient. Am J Surg 1995; 169:8S–12S.

40. Linnemann CC Jr, Moore P, Staneck JL, Pfaller MA. Reemergence of epidemic methicillin-resistant Staphylococcus aureus in a general hospital associated with changing staphylococcal strains. Am J Med 1991; 91:238S–244S.

41. Anonymous. Recommendations for preventing the spread of vancomycin resistance. Recommendations of the Hospital Infection Control Practices Advisory Committee (HICPAC). MMWR 1995; 44:1–13.

42. Anonymous. From the Centers for Disease Control and Prevention. Nosocomial enterococci resistant to vancomycin—United States, 1989–1993. JAMA 1993; 270:1796.

43. Rupp ME, Archer GL. Coagulase-negative staphylococci: pathogens associated with medical progress. Clin Infect Dis 1994; 19:231–243.

44. Voss A, Milatovic D, Wallrauch Schwarz C, Rosdahl VT, Braveny I. Methicillin-resistant *Staphylococcus aureus* in Europe. Eur J Clin Microbiol Infect Dis 1994; 13:50–55.

45. Maki DG, Weise CE, Sarafin HW. A semiquantitative culture method for identifying intravenous-catheter-related infection. N Engl J Med 1977; 296:1305–1309.

46. Bone RC. Let's agree on terminology: definitions of sepsis. Crit Care Med 1991; 19: 973–976.

47. Bone RC. Sepsis, sepsis syndrome, and the systemic inflammatory response syndrome (SIRS). JAMA 1995; 273:155–156.

48. Rangel Frausto MS, Pittet D, Costigan M, Hwang T, Davis CS, Wenzel RP. The natural history of the systemic inflammatory response syndrome (SIRS). A prospective study. JAMA 1995; 273:117–123.

49. Hall G, Hedstrom SA, Heimdahl A, Nord CE. Prophylactic administration of penicillins for endocarditis does not reduce the incidence of postextraction bacteremia. Clin Infect Dis 1993; 17:188–194.

50. Siegman-Igra Y, Anglim AM, Adal K, Strain BA, Farr BM. Diagnosis of vascular catheter related bloodstream infections (CRBSI). Interscience Conference on Antimicrobial Agents and Chemotherapy, 1994. Abstract J53.

51. Markus S, Buday S. Culturing indwelling central venous catheter in situ. Infect Surg 1989; 157–162.

52. Raad II, Baba M, Bodey GP. Diagnosis of catheter-related infections: the role of surveillance and targeted quantitative skin cultures. Clin Infect Dis 1995; 20:593–597.

53. Cercenado E, Ena J, Rodriguez Creixems M, Romero I, Bouza E. A conservative procedure for the diagnosis of catheter-related infections. Arch Intern Med 1990; 150:1417–1420.

54. Groeger JS, Lucas AB, Thaler HT, et al. Infectious morbidity associated with long-term use of venous access devices in patients with cancer. Ann Intern Med 1993; 119:1168–1174.

55. Sherertz RJ, Raad II, Belani A, et al. Three-year experience with sonicated vascular catheter cultures in a clinical microbiology laboratory. J Clin Microbiol 1990; 28:76–82.

56. Cleri DJ, Corrado ML, Seligman SJ. Quantitative culture of intravenous catheters and other intravascular inserts. J Infect Dis 1980; 141:781–786.

57. Mitchell A, Atkins S, Royle GT, Kettlewell MG. Reduced catheter sepsis and prolonged catheter life using a tunnelled silicone rubber catheter for total parenteral nutrition. Br J Surg 1982; 69:420–422.

58. Elam JH, Elam M. Surface modification of intravenous catheters to reduce local tissue reactions. Biomaterials 1993; 14:861–864.

59. Tebbs SE, Elliott TS. Modification of central venous catheter polymers to prevent in vitro microbial colonisation. Eur J Clin Microbiol Infect Dis 1994; 13:111–117.

60. Herrmann M, Vaudaux PE, Pittet D, et al. Fibronectin, fibrinogen, and laminin act as mediators of adherence of clinical staphylococcal isolates to foreign material. J Infect Dis 1988; 158:693–701.

61. Widmer AF, Frei R, Rajacic Z, Zimmerli W. Correlation between in vivo and in vitro efficacy of antimicrobial agents against foreign body infections. J Infect Dis 1990; 162:96–102.

62. Zimmerli W, Frei R, Widmer AF, Rajacic Z. Microbiological tests to predict treatment outcome in experimental device-related infections due to *Staphylococcus aureus*. J Antimicrob Chemother 1994; 33:959–967.

63. Widmer AF, Gaechter A, Ochsner PE, Zimmerli W. Antimicrobial treatment of orthopedic implant-related infections with rifampin combinations. Clin Infect Dis 1992; 14:1251–1253.

64. Sherertz RJ, Forman DM, Solomon DD. Efficacy of dicloxacillin-coated polyurethane catheters in preventing subcutaneous *Staphylococcus aureus* infection in mice. Antimicrob Agents Chemother 1989; 33:1174–1178.

65. Sherertz RJ, Carruth WA, Hampton AA, Byron MP, Solomon DD. Efficacy of antibiotic-coated catheters in preventing subcutaneous *Staphylococcus aureus* infection in rabbits. J Infect Dis 1993; 167:98–106.

66. Cooper GL, Schiller AL, Hopkins CC. Possible role of capillary action in pathogenesis of experimental catheter-associated dermal tunnel infections. J Clin Microbiol 1988; 26:8–12.

67. Groeger JS, Lucas AB, Coit D, et al. A prospective, randomized evaluation of the effect of silver impregnated subcutaneous cuffs for preventing tunneled chronic venous access catheter infections in cancer patients. Ann Surg 1993; 218:206–210.

68. Greenfeld JI, Sampath L, Popilskis SJ, Brunnert SR, Stylianos S, Modak S. Decreased bacterial adherence and biofilm formation on chlorhexidine and silver sulfadiazine-impregnated central venous catheters implanted in swine. Crit Care Med 1995; 23:894–900.

69. Farber BF, Wolff AG. The use of nonsteroidal antiinflammatory drugs to prevent adherence of *Staphylococcus epidermidis* to medical polymers. J Infect Dis 1992; 166:861–865.

70. Mermel LA, Stolz SM, Maki DG. Surface antimicrobial activity of heparin-bonded and antiseptic-impregnated vascular catheters. J Infect Dis 1993; 167:920–924.

71. Kamal GD, Pfaller MA, Rempe LE, Jebson PJ. Reduced intravascular catheter infection by antibiotic bonding. A prospective, randomized, controlled trial. JAMA 1991; 265:2364–2368.

72. Maki DG, Wheeler SJ, Stolz SM, Mermel LA. Clinical trial of a novel antiseptic central venous catheter. Interscience Conference on Antimicrobial Agents and Chemotherapy, 1991; 31:174. Abstract.

73. Raad I, Costerton W, Sabharwal U, Sacilowski M, Anaissie E, Bodey GP. Ultrastructural analysis of indwelling vascular catheters: a quantitative relationship between luminal colonization and duration of placement. J Infect Dis 1993; 168:400–407.

74. Lederle FA, Parenti CM, Berskow LC, Ellingson KJ. The idle intravenous catheter. Ann Intern Med 1992; 116:737–738.

75. Raad I, Darouiche R. Central venous catheters coated with Minocycline and Rifampin for the prevention of catheter-related bacteremia. Interscience Conference on Antimicrobial Agents and Chemotherapy, San Francisco, 1995; 258. Abstract.

76. Darouiche R, Raad I, Morck D. Scanning electron microscopy studies and antimicrobial durability of indwelling central venous catheters coated with Minocycline and Rifampin. Interscience Conference on Antimicrobial Agents and Chemotherapy, San Francisco, 1995. Abstract 258.

77. Costerton JW, Ellis B, Lam K, Johnson F, Khoury AE. Mechanism of electrical enhancement of efficacy of antibiotics in killing biofilm bacteria. Antimicrob Agents Chemother 1994; 38:2803–2809.

78. Bodey GP, Zermeno A, Raad I. Novel approach for the prevention of catheter infections: iontophoretic catheter using silver wire. Interscience Conference on Antimicrobial Agents and Chemotherapy, Orlando, FL 1994. Abstract.

79. Brun-Buisson C, Abrouk F, Legrand P, Huet Y, Larabi S, Rapin M. Diagnosis of central venous catheter-related sepsis. Critical level of quantitative tip cultures. Arch Intern Med 1987; 147:873–877.

80. Collignon PJ. Diagnosis of central vein catheter-related sepsis (letter). Arch Intern Med 1987; 147:2214, 2216–2214, 2217.

81. Gil RT, Kruse JA, Thill-Baharozian MC, Carlson RW. Triple- vs single-lumen central venous catheters. A prospective study in a critically ill population. Arch Intern Med 1989; 149:1139–1143.

82. Pinilla JC, Ross DF, Martin T, Crump H. Study of the incidence of intravascular catheter infection and associated bacteremia in critically ill patients. Crit Care Med 1983; 11:21–25.

83. Mermel LA, McCormick RD, Springman SR, Maki DG. The pathogenesis and epidemiology of catheter-related infection with pulmonary artery Swan-Ganz catheters: a prospective study utilizing molecular subtyping. Am J Med 1991; 91(suppl 3B):3B-197S–3B-205S.

84. Prager RL, Silva J Jr. Colonization of central venous catheters. South Med J 1984; 77:458–461.

85. Michel L, McMichan JC, Bachy JL. Microbial colonization of indwelling central venous catheters: statistical evaluation of potential contaminating factors. Am J Surg 1979; 137:745–748.

86. Lazarus HM, Creger RJ, Bloom AD, Shenk R. Percutaneous placement of femoral central venous catheter in patients undergoing transplantation of bone marrow. Surg Gynecol Obstet 1990; 170:403–406.

87. Williams JF, Seneff MG, Friedman BC, et al. Use of femoral venous catheters in critically ill adults: prospective study. Crit Care Med 1991; 19:550–553.

88. Brawley RL, Weber DJ, Samsa GP, Rutala WA. Multiple nosocomial infections. An incidence study. Am J Epidemiol 1989; 130:769–780.

89. Trottier SJ, Veremakis C, O Brien J, Auer AI. Femoral deep vein thrombosis associated with central venous catheterization: results from a prospective, randomized trial. Crit Care Med 1995; 23:52–59.

90. Pettigrew RA, Lang SD, Haydock DA, Parry BR, Bremner DA, Hill GL. Catheter-related sepsis in patients on intravenous nutrition: a prospective study of quantitative catheter cultures and guidewire changes for suspected sepsis. Br J Surg 1985; 72: 52–55.

91. Ryan JA Jr, Abel RM, Abbott WM, et al. Catheter complications in total parenteral nutrition. A prospective study of 200 consecutive patients. N Engl J Med 1974; 290: 757–761.

92. Raad I, Davis S, Khan A, Tarrand J, Elting L, Bodey GP. Impact of central venous catheter removal on the recurrence of catheter-related coagulase-negative staphylococcal bacteremia. Infect Control Hosp Epidemiol 1992; 13:215–221.

93. Elliott TS, Faroqui MH, Armstrong RF, Hanson GC. Guidelines for good practice in central venous catheterization. Hospital Infection Society and the Research Unit of the Royal College of Physicians. J Hosp Infect 1994; 28:163–176.

94. Burgert SJ, Classen DC, Burke JP, Blatter DD. Candidal brain abscess associated with vascular invasion: a devastating complication of vascular catheter-related candidemia. Clin Infect Dis 1995; 21:202–205.

95. Lecciones JA, Lee JW, Navarro EE, et al. Vascular catheter-associated fungemia in patients with cancer: analysis of 155 episodes. Clin Infect Dis 1992; 14:875–883.

96. Raad II, Sabbagh MF. Optimal duration of therapy for catheter-related *Staphylococcus aureus* bacteremia: a study of 55 cases and review (see comments). Clin Infect Dis 1992; 14:75–82.

97. Malanoski GJ, Samore MH, Pefanis A, Karchmer AW. *Staphylococcus aureus* catheter-associated bacteremia. Minimal effective therapy and unusual infectious complications associated with arterial sheath catheters. Arch Intern Med 1995; 155:1161–1166.

98. Jernigan JA, Farr BM. Short-course therapy of catheter-related *Staphylococcus aureus* bacteremia: a meta-analysis. Ann Intern Med 1993; 119:304–311.

99. Benoit JL, Carandang G, Sitrin M, Arnow PM. Intraluminal antibiotic treatment of central venous catheter infections in patients receiving parenteral nutrition at home. Clin Infect Dis 1995; 21:1286–1288.

100. Farber BF, Kaplan H, Clogston AG. *Staphylococcus epidermidis* extracted slime inhibits the antimicrobial action of glycopeptide antibiotics. J Infect Dis 1990; 161:37–40.

101. Darouiche RO, Dhir A, Miller AJ, Landon GC, Raad II, Musher DM. Vancomycin penetration into biofilm covering infected prostheses and effect on bacteria. J Infect Dis 1994; 170:720–723.

102. Raad I, Darouiche R, Hachem R, Mansouri M, Bodey GP. The broad-spectrum activity and efficacy of catheters coated with minocycline and rifampin. J Infect Dis 1996; 173:418–424.

103. Widmer AF, Pittet D. Optimal duration of therapy for catheter-related *Staphylococcus aureus* bacteremia. Clin Infect Dis 1992; 14:1259–1260.

104. Raad I, Narro J, Khan A, Tarrand J, Vartivarian S, Bodey GP. Serious complications of vascular catheter-related *Staphylococcus aureus* bacteremia in cancer patients. Eur J Clin Microbiol Infect Dis 1992; 11:675–682.

105. Hilf M, Yu VL, Sharp J. Antibiotic therapy for *Pseudomonas aeruginosa* bacteremia: outcome corellation in a prospective study of 200 patients. Am J Med 1989; 87:540–547.

106. Hyatt JM, Nix DE, Stratton CW, Schentag JJ. In vitro pharmacodynamics of piperacillin, piperacillin-tazobactam, and ciprofloxacin alone and in combination against *Staphylococcus aureus, Klebsiella pneumoniae, Enterobacter cloacea,* and *Pseudomonas aeruginosa.* Antimicrob Agents Chemother 1995; 39:1711–1716.

107. O'Keefe SJ, Burnes JU, Thompson RL. Recurrent sepsis in home parenteral nutrition patients: an analysis of risk factors. J Parenter Enteral Nutr 1994; 18:256–263.

108. Rex JH, Bennett JE, Sugar AM, Edwards JE, Washburn RG. Intravascular catheter exchange and duration of candidemia. Clin Infect Dis 1995; 21:994–996.

109. Iwen PC, Kelly DM, Reed EC, Hinrichs SH. Invasive infection due to *Candida kru-sei* in immunocompromised patients not treated with fluconazole. Clin Infect Dis 1995; 20:342–347.

110. Anaissie E. Opportunistic mycoses in the immunocompromised host: experience at a cancer center and review. Clin Infect Dis 1992; 14(suppl 1):S43–53.

111. Goldmann DA, Martin WT, Worthington JW. Growth of bacteria and fungi in total parenteral nutrition solutions. Am J Surg 1973; 126:314–318.

112. D'Angio R, Quercia RA, Treiber NK, McLaughlin JC, Klimek JJ. The growth of microorganisms in total parenteral nutrition admixtures. J Parenter Enteral Nutr 1987; 11:394–397.

113. Gilbert M, Gallagher SC, Eads M, Elmore MF. Microbial growth patterns in a total parenteral nutrition formulation containing lipid emulsion. J Parenter Enteral Nutr 1986; 10:494–497.

114. Maki DG, McCormack KN. Defatting catheter insertion sites in total parenteral nutrition is of no value as an infection control measure. Controlled clinical trial. Am J Med 1987; 83:833–840.

115. Maki DG, Goldmann DA, Rhame FS. Infection control in intravenous therapy. Ann Intern Med 1973; 79:867–887.

116. Linares J, Sitges-Serra A, Garau J, Perez JL, Martin R. Pathogenesis of catheter sepsis: a prospective study with quantitative and semiquantitative cultures of catheter hub and segments. J Clin Microbiol 1985; 21:357–360.

117. McCarthy MC, Shives JK, Robison RJ, Broadie TA. Prospective evaluation of single and triple lumen catheters in total parenteral nutrition. J Parenter Enteral Nutr 1987; 11:259–262.

118. Faubion WC, Wesley JR, Khalidi N, Silva J. Total parenteral nutrition catheter sepsis: impact of the team approach. J Parenter Enteral Nutr 1986; 10:642–645.

119. Armstrong CW, Mayhall CG, Miller KB, et al. Clinical predictors of infection of central venous catheters used for total parenteral nutrition. Infect Control Hosp Epidemiol 1990; 11:71–78.

120. Snydman DR, Murray SA, Kornfeld SJ, Majka JA, Ellis CA. Total parenteral nutrition-related infections. Prospective epidemiologic study using semiquantitative methods. Am J Med 1982; 73:695–699.

121. Bonadimani B, Sperti C, Stevanin A, et al. Central venous catheter guidewire replacement according to the Seldinger technique: usefulness in the management of patients on total parenteral nutrition. J Parenter Enteral Nutr 1987; 11:267–270.

122. Dankner WM, Spector SA, Fierer J, Davis CE. *Malassezia* fungemia in neonates and adults: complication of hyperalimentation. Rev Infect Dis 1987; 9:743–753.

123. Garcia CR, Johnston BL, Corvi G, Walker LJ, George WL. Intravenous catheter-associated *Malassezia furfur* fungemia. Am J Med 1987; 83:790–792.

124. Halpin TC Jr, Dahms BB. Complications associated with intravenous lipids in infants and children. Acta Chir Scand Suppl 1983; 517:169–177.

125. Wey SB, Mori M, Pfaller MA, Woolson RF, Wenzel RP. Risk factors for hospital-acquired candidemia. A matched case-control study. Arch Intern Med 1989; 149:2349–2353.

126. Sitzmann JV, Townsend TR, Siler MC, Bartlett JG. Septic and technical complica-

tions of central venous catheterization. A prospective study of 200 consecutive patients. Ann Surg 1985; 202:766–770.

127. Fan ST, Teoh-Chan CH, Lau KF, Chu KW, Kwan AK, Wong KK. Predictive value of surveillance skin and hub cultures in central venous catheters sepsis. J Hosp Infect 1988; 12:191–198.

128. Flynn PM, Shenep JL, Stokes DC, Barrett FF. In situ management of confirmed central venous catheter-related bacteremia. Pediatr Infect Dis J 1987; 6:729–734.

129. Raucher HS, Hyatt AC, Barzilai A, et al. Quantitative blood cultures in the evaluation of septicemia in children with Broviac catheters. J Pediatr 1984; 104:29–33.

130. Yeung C, May J, Hughes R. Infection rate for single lumen v triple lumen subclavian catheters. Infect Control Hosp Epidemiol 1988; 9:154–158.

131. Armstrong CW, Mayhall CG, Miller KB, et al. Prospective study of catheter replacement and other risk factors for infection of hyperalimentation catheters. J Infect Dis 1986; 154:808–816.

132. Howard L, Claunch C, McDowell R, Timchalk M. Five years of experience in patients receiving home nutrition support with the implanted reservoir: a comparison with the external catheter. J Parenter Enteral Nutr 1989; 13:478–483.

133. Danzig LE, Short LJ, Collins K, et al. Bloodstream infections associated with a needleless intravenous infusion system in patients receiving home infusion therapy. JAMA 1995; 273:1862–1864.

134. Graham DR, Molnar VL, Tolan VL, Loscher DM. Nosohusial bacteremia. Interscience Conference on Antimicrobial Agents and Chemotherapy, Orlando, FL, 1994; J58.

135. Mermel LA, Parenteau S, Tow SM. The risk of midline catheterization in hospitalized patients. A prospective study. Ann Intern Med 1995; 123:841–844.

136. Vanhuynegem L, Parmentier P, Potvliege C. In situ bacteriologic diagnosis of total parenteral nutrition catheter infection. Surgery 1988; 103:174–177.

137. Maki DG, Band JD. A comparative study of polyantibiotic and iodophor ointments in prevention of vascular catheter-related infection. Am J Med 1981; 70:739–744.

138. Widmer AF, Orth B, Uhr M, Rinaldi M, Frei R. Contaminated skin lotion: the source for an outbreak of *Paecilomyces lilacinus* infection at a BMT unit. Interscience Conference on Antimicrobial Agents and Chemotherapy, 1994. Abstract J245.

139. Doebbeling BN, Stanley GL, Sheetz CT, et al. Comparative efficacy of alternative hand-washing agents in reducing nosocomial infections in intensive care units. N Engl J Med 1992; 327:88–93.

140. Widmer AF, Perschmann M, Gasser TC, Frei R. Alcohol (ALC) vs chlorhexidinegluconate (CHG) for preoperative hand scrub: a randomized cross-over clinical trial. Interscience Conference on Antimicrobial Agents and Chemotherapy, Orlando, FL, 1994. Abstract.

141. Shapiro JM, Bond EL, Garman JK. Use of a chlorhexidine dressing to reduce microbial colonization of epidural catheters. Anesthesiology 1990; 73:625–631.

142. Conly JM, Grieves K, Peters B. A prospective, randomized study comparing transparent and dry gauze dressings for central venous catheters. J Infect Dis 1989; 159:310–319.

143. Maki DG, Ringer M. Evaluation of dressing regimens for prevention of infection

with peripheral intravenous catheters. Gauze, a transparent polyurethane dressing, and an iodophor-transparent dressing. JAMA 1987; 258:2396–2403.

144. Ricard P, Martin R, Marcoux JA. Protection of indwelling vascular catheters: incidence of bacterial contamination and catheter-related sepsis. Crit Care Med 1985; 13:541–543.

145. Young GP, Alexeyeff M, Russell DM, Thomas RJ. Catheter sepsis during parenteral nutrition: the safety of long-term OpSite dressings. J Parenter Enteral Nutr 1988; 12: 365–370.

146. Vazquez RM, Jarrard MM. Care of the central venous catheterization site: the use of a transparent polyurethane film. J Parenter Enteral Nutr 1984; 8:181–186.

147. Hoffmann KK, Weber DJ, Samsa GP, Rutala WA. Transparent polyurethane film as an intravenous catheter dressing. JAMA 1992; 267:2072–2076.

148. Moro ML, Vigano EF, Cozzi Lepri A. Risk factors for central venous catheter-related infections in surgical and intensive care units. The Central Venous Catheter-Related Infections Study Group. Infect Control Hosp Epidemiol 1994; 15:253–264.

149. Gantz NM, Presswood GM, Goldberg R, Doern G. Effects of dressing type and change interval on intravenous therapy complications rates. Diagn Microbiol Infect Dis 1984; 2:325–332.

150. Bregenzer T, Widmer AF, Conen D. Routine replacement of peripheral catheters is not necessary: a prospective study. Can J Infect Dis 1995; 6(suppl C):247C. Abstract.

151. Widmer AF, Nettleman M, Flint K, Wenzel RP. The clinical impact of culturing central venous catheters. A prospective study. Arch Intern Med 1992; 152:1299–1302.

152. Widmer AF. IV-related infections. In: Wenzel RP, ed. Prevention and Control of Nosocomial Infections. 2nd ed. Baltimore: Williams & Wilkins, 1993:556–579.

153. Puntis JW, Holden CE, Smallman S, Finkel Y, George RH, Booth IW. Staff training: a key factor in reducing intravascular catheter sepsis. Arch Dis Child 1991; 66: 335–337.

154. Armstrong CW, Mayhall CG, Miller KB, et al. Clinical predictors of infection on central venous catheters used for total parenteral nutrition. Infect Control Hosp Epidemiol 1991; 12:407–411.

155. Snyder RH, Archer FJ, Endy T, et al. Catheter infection. A comparison of two catheter maintenance techniques. Ann Surg 1988; 208:651–653.

156. Tomford JW, Hershey CO, McLaren CE, Porter DK, Cohen DI. Intravenous therapy team and peripheral venous catheter-associated complications: a prospective controlled study. Arch Intern Med 1984; 144:1191–1194.

157. Hershey CO, Tomford JW, McLaren CE, Porter DK, Cohen DI. The natural history of intravenous catheter-associated phlebitis. Arch Intern Med 1984; 144:1373–1375.

158. Hamory BH, Pearson SK, Duff KR. Efficacy of professional IV therapy team in reducing complication of IV cannulae. American Meeting of the American Society for Microbiology, 1984. Abstract L2.

159. Lim SH, Smith MP, Machin SJ, Goldstone AH. A prospective randomized study of prophylactic teicoplanin to prevent early Hickman catheter-related sepsis in patients receiving intensive chemotherapy for haematological malignancies. Eur J Haematol Suppl 1993; 54:10–13.

160. Lim SH, Smith MP, Machin SJ, Goldstone AH. Teicoplanin and prophylaxis of Hickman catheter insertions. Eur J Surg Suppl 1992; 39–42.

161. Lim SH, Smith MP, Salooja N, Machin SJ, Goldstone AH. A prospective randomized study of prophylactic teicoplanin to prevent early Hickman catheter-related sepsis in patients receiving intensive chemotherapy for haematological malignancies. J Antimicrob Chemother 1991; 28:109–116.

162. Bock SN, Lee RE, Fisher B, et al. A prospective randomized trial evaluating prophylactic antibiotics to prevent triple-lumen catheter-related sepsis in patients treated with immunotherapy. J Clin Oncol 1990; 8:161–169.

163. Ranson MR, Oppenheim BA, Jackson A, Kamthan AG, Scarffe JH. Double-blind placebo controlled study of vancomycin prophylaxis for central venous catheter insertion in cancer patients. J Hosp Infect 1990; 15:95–102.

164. McKee R, Dunsmuir R, Shitby M, Garden OJ. Does antibiotic prophylaxis at the time of catheter insertion reduce the incidence of catheter-related sepsis in intravenous nutrition. J Hosp Infect 1985; 6:419–425.

165. Vassilomanolakis M, Plataniotis G, Koumakis G, et al. Central venous catheter-related infections after bone marrow transplantation in patients with malignancies: a prospective study with short-course vancomycin prophylaxis. Bone Marrow Transplant 1995; 15:77–80.

166. Anonymous. Recommendations for preventing the spread of vancomycin resistance. Hospital Infection Control Practices Advisory Committee (HICPAC). Infect Control Hosp Epidemiol 1995; 16:105–113.

167. Neu HC. The crisis in antibiotic resistance. Science 1992; 257:1064–1073.

168. Gregory JA, Schiller WR. Subclavian catheter changes every third day in high risk patients. Am Surg 1985; 51:534–536.

169. Pruitt BA Jr, Stein JM, Foley FD, Moncrief JA, O'Neill JA Jr. Intravenous therapy in burn patients. Suppurative thrombophlebitis and other life-threatening complications. Arch Surg 1970; 100:399–404.

170. Maki DG, Jarrett F, Sarafin HW. A semiquantitative culture method for identification of catheter-related infection in the burn patient. J Surg Res 1977; 22:513–520.

171. Franceschi D, Gerding RL, Phillips G, Fratianne RB. Risk factors associated with intravascular catheter infections in burned patients: a prospective, randomized study. J Trauma 1989; 29:811–816.

172. Husain MT, Karim QN, Tajuri S. Analysis of infection in a burn ward. Burns 1989; 15:299–302.

173. Latarjet J. A simple guide to burn treatment. International Society for Burn Injuries in collaboration with the World Health Organization. Burns 1995; 21:221–225.

174. Sheridan RL, Weber JM, Peterson HF, Tompkins RG. Central venous catheter sepsis with weekly catheter change in paediatric burn patients: an analysis of 221 catheters. Burns 1995; 21:127–129.

175. Raviglione MC, Battan R, Pablos-Mendez A, Aceves-Casillas P, Mullen MP, Taranta A. Infections associated with Hickman catheters in patients with the acquired immunodeficiency virus. Am J Med 1989; 86:780–786.

176. Jacobson MA, Gellermann H, Chambers H. *Staphylococcus aureus* bacteremia and recurrent staphylococcal infection in patients with acquired immunodeficiency syndrome and AIDS-related complex. Am J Med 1988; 85:172–176.

177. Buchman AL, Guss W, Ament ME. *Staphylococcus aureus* Hickman catheter infections. Am J Med 1991; 91:103–104.
178. Raviglione MC, Mariuz P, Pablos-Mendez A, Battan R, Ottuso P, Taranta A. High *Staphylococcus aureus* nasal carriage rate in patients with acquired immunodeficiency syndrome or AIDS-related complex. Am J Infect Control 1990; 18:64–69.
179. Battan R, Raviglione MC, Wallace J, Cort S, Boyle JF, Taranta A. *S. aureus* nasal carriage among homosexual men with and without HIV infection. Am J Infect Control 1991; 19:98–100.
180. Stanley HD, Charlebois E, Harb G, Jacobson MA. Central venous catheter infections in AIDS patients receiving treatment for cytomegalovirus disease. J Acquir Immune Defic Syndr 1994; 7:272–278.
181. Groeger JS, Lucas AB, Thaler HT, et al. Infectious morbidity associated with long-term use of venous access devices in patients with cancer. Ann Intern Med 1993; 119:1168–1174.
182. Collignon PJ, Munro R. Limitations of semiquantitative method for catheter culture. J Clin Microbiol 1988; 26:1075–1076.
183. Collignon PJ, Soni N, Pearson I, Sorrell T, Woods P. Sepsis associated with central vein catheters in critically ill patients. Intens Care Med 1988; 14:227–231.
184. Collignon PJ, Chan R, Munro R. Rapid diagnosis of intravascular catheter-related sepsis. Arch Intern Med 1987; 147:1609–1612.
185. Collignon PJ, Soni N, Pearson IY, Woods WP, Munro R, Sorrell TC. Is semiquantitative culture of central vein catheter tips usefuls in the diagnosis of catheter-associated bacteremia? J Clin Microbiol 1986; 24:532–535.
186. Cooper GL, Hopkins CC. Rapid diagnosis of intravascular catheter-associated infection by direct Gram staining of catheter segments. N Engl J Med 1985; 312:1142–1147.
187. Haslett TM, Isenberg HD, Hilton E, Tucci V, Kay BG, Vellozzi AM. Microbiology of indwelling central intravascular catheters. J Clin Microbiol 1988; 26:696–701.
188. Maki DG, Ringer M. Risk factors for infusion-related phlebitis with small peripheral venous catheters. A randomized controlled trial. Ann Intern Med 1991; 114:845–854.
189. Rushforth JA, Hoy CM, Kite P, Puntis JWL. Rapid diagnosis of central venous catheter sepsis. Lancet 1993; 342:402–403.

9

Peripheral Venous Catheters

C. Glen Mayhall

University of Texas Medical Branch at Galveston, Galveston, Texas

I. INTRODUCTION

Intravascular cannulae are among the most commonly used devices in the delivery of modern healthcare. It has been estimated that 150 million intravascular devices are purchased by hospitals and clinics each year in the United States (1). The overwhelming majority of these cannulae are peripheral venous catheters (PVCs) and needles. Approximately 25 million patients per year in the United States receive infusion therapy through peripheral intravenous cannulae (2). Phlebitis or inflammation at the site of vessel cannulation occurs commonly, ranging between 15% and 70% in adults (2–6) and between 10% and 13% in children (7,8). However, the great majority of instances of phlebitis are aseptic (not related to infection), and the phenomenon appears most closely related to the physicochemical characteristics of the materials from which catheters are constructed and the type of infusate administered through the catheters (2–8). Few PVCs removed from patients with phlebitis are found to be colonized on semi-quantitative culture (2,4,7,9–12).

Because inflammation at the catheter site raises the suspicion of infection, because infection cannot be ruled out without removal and culture of the catheter, and because there is a statistically significant relationship between phlebitis and catheter-related infection (2), aseptic phlebitis will be discussed as well as catheter-related colonization and infection.

II. PATHOGENESIS OF PERIPHERAL VENOUS CATHETER-RELATED PHLEBITIS, COLONIZATION, AND INFECTION

A. Phlebitis

The pathogenesis of phlebitis is related to the effects of various physical and chemical factors on the cannulated blood vessel.

1. Physical Factors

Physical factors related to the development of aseptic phlebitis include cannula composition, cannula length, cannula bore, distortion of the cannula tip, anatomical location of the cannula tip, trauma at venipuncture, rate of flow of infusate, duration of cannulation, and manipulation of the cannula in situ (2,5–8,10, 11,13–19). The effect of catheter composition is related to both the direct irritant effect of the material used (polyvinyl chloride and polyethylene are more irritating than Teflon and polyurethane) and the stiffness of the catheter (the relatively stiffer Teflon cannula is more irritating than the more flexible silicone catheter) (6,11,13,14).

While certain plastics are less likely than others to cause phlebitis, the surface characteristics and etching of the catheter surface during the manufacturing process are probably more important than the type of plastic (6,15). Longer cannulae are more often associated with thrombophlebitis than shorter catheters, perhaps owing to the greater difficulty of insertion of longer catheters, resulting in more trauma (16). Large-bore catheters are more often associated with phlebitis than small-bore catheters, probably owing to the decreased blood flow around large-bore catheters, particularly when they are inserted into small veins (6). Distortion or damage to the catheter tip has been shown to be significantly related to phlebitis (Fig. 1) (5). Cannulae inserted in the dorsum of the hand, the wrist, the lower extremities, or over the joints without joint immobilization have been associated with phlebitis (2,6), but studies attempting to relate location of cannula insertion in the upper extremity to phlebitis have yielded inconsistent results (13).

Trauma at the time of insertion has been associated with phlebitis. Thus, phlebitis may be more likely to occur when cannulae are inserted as a sheath around the venipuncture needle than when they are inserted through a needle (17). The rate of flow of infusates may be important, with slower infusion rates, particularly with more irritant solutions, leading to more irritation of the vein (18). The duration of cannulation is an established risk factor for development of phlebitis in both adults and children (2,6–8,16–18). However, the duration of can-

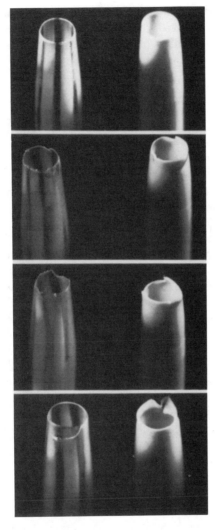

Figure 1   Photomicrographs showing damage to the tips of Vialon and Teflon catheters. The Vialon catheter is shown on the left and the Teflon catheter on the right of each panel. The top two panels show damage gradings of 0 and 1, and the lower two panels show damage gradings of 2 and 3.

nulation is less important in children, and catheters may be left in place up to 144 hours without much risk of phlebitis (8). Manipulation of the cannula in situ by more frequent dressing changes (daily versus every other day) has been found to be significantly related to the development of phlebitis (10).

2. Chemical Factors

Several chemical factors predispose to the development of phlebitis, including pH and osmolarity of the infusate, inherent irritating properties of certain infusates, and particulate matter in the infusate.

Low pH of infusates is associated with phlebitis (6,13,17,19–22). Thus, glucose solutions have a pH of 3.4 to 5 to prevent caramelization during autoclaving, and it has been shown that neutralization of the acidic pH of glucose solutions results in reduced rates of phlebitis (19–21). Solutions with high osmolarity (> 600 mOsm/L) are also associated with phlebitis (23). Certain chemicals in infusates are inherently irritating to venous endothelium including benzodiazepines, barbiturates and other anesthetic agents, and cephalosporin antibiotics (13). Other antibiotics that may cause phlebitis when given intravenously are vancomycin, metronidazole, erythromycin, and amphotericin B. Particulate matter (extraneous, mobile, undissolved substances) including rubber, chemicals, glass, cellulose fibers, and fungi may be present in parenteral solutions (13). Particulates may irritate the venous endothelium and cause inflammation. That particulates may induce phlebitis is supported by two randomized controlled studies of in-line filtration of parenteral fluids which showed either that in-line filtration prolonged the phlebitis-free survival of infusions (24) or reduced the per-day incidence of phlebitis with a significant reduction on day 3 ($P < 0.001$) (25). However, not all studies of in-line filtration have demonstrated a protective effect against phlebitis (26).

3. Plastic Catheters vs. Steel Needles

Steel needles have frequently been used as the cannula of first choice for short-term infusions because of the belief that they present a lower risk of phlebitis and infection. In the only randomized clinical trial of steel needles versus a plastic (Teflon) catheter by Tully and colleagues, there was no significant difference between the two types of cannula with respect to colonization/infection (27). However, phlebitis was significantly more likely to occur with Teflon catheters, and infiltration significantly more likely to occur with steel needles. In a study of the complications of steel needles used for infusion therapy in patients with hematologic malignancy, Band and Maki noted higher rates of aseptic phlebitis with steel needles than Tully and colleagues (33.8% vs. 8.8%) and higher rates of catheter-related infection (5.4% vs. 1.5%) and catheter-related bacteremia (2.1%

vs. 0%) (28). Thus, steel needles may pose a higher risk of infectious and noninfectious complications in patients with underlying malignancies.

B.   Catheter-Related Colonization and Infection

1.   *Microbial Adherence*

Microorganisms may cause cannula-related infection by migrating into the subcutaneous catheter tract, by entering the lumen of the cannula after catheter hub contamination, or by colonizing (seeding) the cannula hematogenously with microorganisms from some other site in the body. However, one of the most important factors determining whether a microorganism can cause catheter colonization or catheter-related infection is its ability to adhere to catheter surfaces.

The degree of adherence of microorganisms to catheters is determined by the materials from which catheters are manufactured, physical characteristics of catheter surfaces, deposition of host proteins on catheter surfaces, and certain characteristics of microorganisms that allow them to attach to surfaces including elaboration of an extracellular polysaccharide substance known as glycocalyx or slime. Using scanning electron microscopy, Locci and colleagues demonstrated irregularities on the internal and external surfaces of unused intravenous catheters (29). These authors suggested that such defects might provide sites of attachment for bacteria that came into contact with catheter surfaces. Ashkenazi and coworkers showed by scanning electron microscopy that bacteria adhered initially to irregularities on the inner and outer surfaces of the catheters (30). Other undefined characteristics of various catheter materials appear to play a role in binding of microorganisms to these surfaces as well. Thus, bacteria adhered least to siliconized steel needles and Teflon catheters, and most to polyethylene and polyvinyl chloride catheters (30,31).

Host proteins including fibronectin, fibrinogen, and laminin are deposited onto the surface of catheters after their insertion. Bacteria, particularly *S. aureus* and coagulase-negative staphylococci, adhere to these proteins (32,33). *S. aureus* binds most strongly to fibronectin and fibrinogen, and coagulase-negative staphylococci most strongly to fibronectin.

The surface characteristic of bacteria most important in binding to a catheter surface is hydrophobicity (30). Thus, hydrophobic bacteria such as *S. aureus* and *Serratia marcescens* bind better to catheter surfaces than do less hydrophobic species like *Escherichia coli*.

Some strains of bacteria, particularly strains of coagulase-negative staphylococci, produce an extracellular glycocalyx composed of either polysaccharide or glycoprotein that is purported to provide a mechanism for adherence to surfaces (34). While slime may protect microorganisms from host phagocytic cells and antimicrobial agents, initial attachment does not appear to be mediated by slime (32). However, slime has an adverse effect on the host response which appears to ated by interference with induction of normal T-cell proliferation and a ytic effect on some of these cells (35). Slime also interferes with the antimicrobial activity of vancomycin and teicoplanin (36). When slime was added to wells containing vancomycin and an inoculum of *S. epidermidis*, the minimum inhibitory concentration (MIC) was increased fourfold when compared with wells containing the same concentration of antibiotic and inoculum but without slime. Slime also reversed the synergistic effect of vancomycin with gentamicin against *S. epidermidis*. Addition of slime had no effect on the MICs of cefazolin, clindamycin, rifampin, or LY146032.

2. Colonization of the Subcutaneous Catheter Tract

The most important pathogenetic mechanism by which microorganisms cause catheter colonization and catheter-related infection is migration of microorganisms from the skin surface around the point at which the catheter penetrates the skin into the subcutaneous catheter tract (Fig. 2). Maki lists nine categories of evidence that support this pathogenetic mechanism as the most important mechanism (37). Some of this evidence will be discussed below.

There are several studies demonstrating that microorganisms recovered from skin at the catheter site are the etiologic agents of catheter colonization and catheter-related infections. These studies show a correlation between a high density of microorganisms on the skin at the catheter site and the occurrence of catheter colonization or catheter-related infection (38–40), and in two of these studies the species recovered from the skin was usually the causative agent of the catheter colonization or catheter-related infection (38,39). While the latter studies assessed only central venous catheters used for total parenteral nutrition, there is no reason to believe that the mechanism of colonization/infection would be different for PVCs.

Patients with burns have a higher density of microorganisms on the surface of the burn wound than is found on normal skin, and these patients have a higher incidence of catheter-related infections than patients without burns (41–43). In addition cutaneous colonization at the catheter insertion site at the time of catheter removal was a risk factor for catheter-related infection (relative risk = 6.16), and the incidence of catheter-related infection correlated inversely with the distance of the catheter insertion site from the burn wound (43).

Further support for the skin as a source of microorganisms that cause catheter-related infections is provided by reports of outbreaks of catheter-related infections associated with application of contaminated antiseptics to the skin prior to insertion of intravascular devices (44–46).

As a corollary to the above observations, the more effective removal of microorganisms from the skin around the site at which the catheter is inserted results in a lower catheter-related infection rate. Thus, Maki and associates observed that preparation of the skin with chlorhexidine prior to catheter inser-

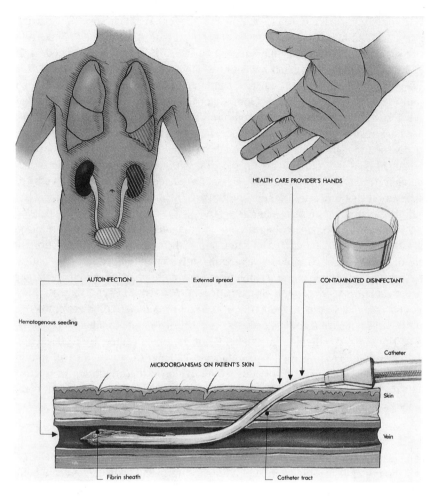

Figure 2 Sources of peripheral venous catheter infection. Microorganisms that contaminate the skin at the catheter insertion site may migrate into the subcutaneous catheter tract, multiply to high concentrations, and eventually colonize the fibrin sheath present on the intravascular portion of the catheter.

tion was associated with a significantly lower rate of catheter-related infection and bacteremia than when povidone-iodine or 70% alcohol was used for skin preparation (47).

Additional evidence for migration of microorganisms from the skin surface into the subcutaneous catheter tract as the most important pathogenetic mechanism for development of catheter-related infections includes the observations that

(1) microorganisms are found mainly on the external surfaces of colonized catheters when they are examined microscopically on removal, and (2) the presence of microorganisms on the external surfaces of catheters is related to the occurrence of catheter-related bacteremia. Thus, on removal, Cooper and Hopkins cultured intravascular catheters semiquantitatively and then Gram-stained them (48). The direct catheter Gram stain technique was 100% sensitive and 96.9% specific for catheter colonization as defined by semiquantitative culture. Microorganisms were observed on the external surface of all 41 catheters with a positive semiquantitative culture but on the internal (luminal) surface of only four catheters. That microorganisms on the external surface of the catheter are the source for microorganisms that cause catheter-related bacteremia is shown by the observation that a positive semiquantitative catheter culture is highly correlated with the occurrence of bacteremia (48–50).

Finally, when bovine collagen cuffs impregnated with silver ions are placed subcutaneously at the catheter insertion site at the time of catheter insertion, the rate of catheter-related infection is significantly decreased. Thus, Maki and coworkers observed a decrease in infection rates of from 28.9% with control noncuffed catheters to 9.1% with cuffed catheters ($P = 0.002$) (51). Likewise, Flowers and associates noted a reduction in the rate of catheter colonization of from 34.5% with noncuffed control catheters to 7.7% with cuffed catheters ($P = 0.02$) (50). The marked reduction in catheter colonization or catheter-related infection by blocking the entrance to the subcutaneous catheter tract with a silver-impregnated bovine collagen cuff provides strong evidence that migration of microorganisms from the skin surface into the catheter tract is the most important pathogenetic mechanism for development of catheter-related infections.

3. Hub Contamination

The data for hub contamination as a mechanism for development of catheter colonization or catheter-related infection for short-term catheters are less convincing than the data for migration of microorganisms into the subcutaneous catheter tract. Contamination of the hub may be the most important mechanism for colonization and catheter-related infection involving long-term catheters (> 30 days) (52), but the evidence for hub contamination as an important mechanism in short-term catheters (< 30 days) is much less convincing. First, there is no validated standardized technique for culturing catheter hubs, and the meaning of positive qualitative cultures is unclear. Second, in some of the studies, when isolates of the same species were recovered from both hub and catheter tip, they were considered to be the same strain if they had the same antibiogram. The development of molecular typing has shown that antibiograms may be nonspecific markers for determining when two isolates are from the same clone. Third, most of the studies implicating contamination of the hub as the pathogenetic mechanism for development of catheter colonization and catheter-related infection are flawed by using historic controls (53), by failing to explain why the majority of catheters with contaminated hubs also have positive semiquantitative catheter (external surface) cultures (54), and by combining short-term and long-term catheters in the same study (55). The most convincing data supporting hub contamination as an important mechanism for catheter-related infection are those published by deCicco and colleagues (56).

After migrating down the subcutaneous catheter tract or, less commonly, down the luminal surface of the catheter, microorganisms may reach and adhere to the fibrin sheath which forms around the intravascular portion of all catheters as early as 24 hours after their insertion (57). Multiplication in the fibrin sheath may lead to shedding of microorganisms into the bloodstream, giving rise to catheter-related bacteremia. Thrombus formation at the catheter tip may perpetuate the multiplication of microorganisms (42,58). If multiplication takes place to the extent that microorganisms invade the venous wall or an intraluminal abscess develops, the patient has a life-threatening infection termed septic or suppurative thrombophlebitis (42).

4. Hematogenous Seeding

Another mechanism by which catheter-related infection develops is hematogenous seeding (53,54). Microorganisms that enter the bloodstream from another source may adhere to the fibrin sheath surrounding the intravascular portion of the catheter. Catheter-related infection develops much less commonly by hematogenous seeding than by migration of microorganisms down the external or internal surfaces of catheters. Likewise, contaminated infusion fluids are uncommonly the source of microorganisms that cause catheter-related infection (2,12,28).

III.   CLINICAL MANIFESTATIONS

A.   Phlebitis

The presence of fever is not necessary for the diagnosis of aseptic phlebitis. Phlebitis is diagnosed by the presence of local signs of inflammation without evidence of infection, i.e., without the presence of purulent drainage from the catheter insertion site. The local signs of phlebitis include erythema, palpable venous cord, tenderness, pain, increased warmth, induration, swelling, and lymphangitis (2–4,9,12,59).

B.   Catheter-Related Infection

Catheter-related infection may also be manifested by the same local signs of inflammation observed to occur with aseptic phlebitis, as noted above. Patients with catheter-related infection may have fever; in some cases, a purulent discharge may be noted at the site of catheter insertion (10,60).

Septic thrombophlebitis may occur in any patient with an intravenous catheter, but burn patients are at a particularly high risk of this complication (42). Septic thrombophlebitis may complicate both central and peripheral venous cannulation (42,61). Most patients with septic thrombophlebitis have fever and signs of sepsis, and 72% to 100% have bacteremia (42,61). Baker and associates reported on a series of cases of septic thrombophlebitis in a population of patients with intravenous catheters and persons in the community who abused drugs (61). Local signs of septic thrombophlebitis included local pain in 83% of patients, swelling in 37%, erythema and edema in 62%, abscess in 43%, a palpable cord in 20%, lymphadenopathy in 13%, and spontaneous drainage of pus in 9% (61). Local signs of septic thrombophlebitis in burn patients may occur in less than 50% of cases (42). It must also be kept in mind that signs and symptoms of septic thrombophlebitis may not appear for days after the intravenous cannula is removed (62). The most common systemic complication of septic thrombophlebitis is septic embolism, usually to the lungs (61).

IV. ETIOLOGY OF INFECTIONS ASSOCIATED WITH PERIPHERAL VENOUS CATHETERS

A. Catheter Colonization and Catheter Site Infections

Catheter colonization (>15 cfu on semiquantitative culture without local signs of infection) and catheter-related site infection [purulent drainage from the point at which the catheter penetrates the skin (see below)] may occur and be limited to the catheter tract or may also give rise to bacteremia.

1. Adults

There is no national database that compiles data on the etiology of colonization or catheter-related infection for PVCs. The only data available are from published studies from individual institutions. Maki and Ringer observed that for Teflon catheters 4.7% were colonized with coagulase-negative staphylococci, 0.2% with *S. aureus*, and none with gram-negative bacilli or yeasts. For polyurethane catheters 6.7% were colonized by coagulase-negative staphylococci, none by *S. aureus* or gram-negative bacilli, and 0.2% by yeasts (2). In a second study, Maki and Ringer found that 4.9% of 2088 PVCs were colonized by coagulase-negative staphylococci, 0.1% by *S. aureus*, and none by gram-negative bacilli or yeasts (12). The most common microorganism colonizing PVCs in the series of Righter and co-workers was *S. epidermidis*. *S. aureus* accounted for only 2 of 59 isolates, and gram-negative bacilli for 2 of 59 isolates (4).

2. Children

In a study of 50 PVCs in neonates, Wilkins and colleagues found 13 cannulae (26%) to be positive on semiquantitative culture. Of 22 isolates from these catheters, 19 were *S. epidermidis*, one was *S. haemolyticus*, one was *S. warneri*, and one was *S. aureus* (62). In their study of intravenous catheters in neonates, Cronin and colleagues recovered 43 isolates at a colony count of ≥15 cfu on semi-quantitative culture of 531 PVCs (63). Thirty-four of 43 (79%) were coagulase-negative staphylococci. Only one (2.3%) was *S. aureus;* the remaining isolates were *Enterococcus* 5 (11.6%), *E. coli* 2 (4.7%), and *Candida parapsilosis* 1 (2.3%).

In older children from general medical wards in a children's hospital, Garland and associates found 12 of 115 (10.4%) PVCs to be colonized (64). Eleven of the 12 (91.6%) were colonized by *S. epidermidis*, and one (8.4%) was colonized by an α-hemolytic *Streptococcus*. In a later study of critically ill children, Garland and associates found 54 (11.8%) of 459 PVCs to be colonized (8). Coagulase-negative staphylococci were recovered from 51 of 54 (94.4%) catheters. *Enterococcus faecalis* and β-hemolytic *Streptococcus* were each recovered from two catheters, and yeasts were recovered from four catheters.

It would appear, from the limited data available, that the overwhelming majority of catheter colonizations and local catheter-related infections of PVCs in both adults and children are caused by gram-positive cocci. Most of the gram-positive coccal isolates are coagulase-negative staphylococci. There are rare isolates of *S. aureus*, gram-negative bacilli, and yeasts.

B.   Catheter-Related Bacteremia

Catheter-related bacteremia uncommonly complicates the use of PVCs in adults or children.

1.   Adults

No cases of bacteremia were identified in either of the two studies of PVCs by Maki and Ringer (2,12), and Righter and co-workers observed no cases of bacteremia in their series (4). The best data on the etiology of catheter-related bacteremias that complicate the use of PVCs in adults are from a multicenter study in Australia (65). Collignon and his co-workers found that *S. aureus* was most often the cause of bacteremia associated with PVCs. Gram-positive cocci were the cause in 181 (75.4%) of 240 episodes, and *S. aureus* was the cause in 149 (62.1%) episodes. Gram-negative bacilli accounted for 55 (22.9%) of 240 episodes, and fungi for only 4 (1.7%) episodes.

2.   Children

There are also few data on the cause of catheter-related bacteremias in children. The seven bacteremias in neonates in the study of Cronin and colleagues were all caused by coagulase-negative staphylococci, and *Enterococcus* was also isolated from the blood of one of these patients (63). Systemic *Candida* infections in neonates may also be associated with the use of PVCs (66). In their study on the complications of PVCs in critically ill children, Garland and associates observed a single case of catheter-related bacteremia caused by group A, β-hemolytic *Streptococcus* (8).

3. Patients With Human Immunodeficiency Virus (HIV) Infection

Unpublished data from a cohort study of HIV-infected patients at five Veterans Hospitals revealed that *S. aureus* (41%) was the most common cause of peripheral intravenous catheter-related bacteremia in this population (R Gaynes, Hospital Infections Program, Centers for Disease Control and Prevention, personal communication, 1995). Fifteen (27.3%) of the 55 cases of peripheral venous catheter-related bacteremia had coagulase-negative staphylococci isolated from blood followed by *Klebsiella pneumoniae* (7.3%), *Pseudomonas aeurginosa* (7.3%), *E. coli* (3.6%), *Candida albicans* (3.6%) and other microorganisms (12.7%). The etiologies of catheter-related colonization and infection are shown in Table 1

C.   Catheter-Related Septic Thrombophlebitis

As with catheter-related infection and catheter-related bacteremia, the most common causes of septic thrombophlebitis are gram-positive cocci (42,61,67). *S. aureus* is by far the most frequently isolated gram-positive coccus (42,61,67). Gram-negative bacilli make up approximately 20% of isolates (61,67). Yeasts do not appear to be a common cause of septic thrombophlebitis except in burn patients (42,61,67).

Gram-positive cocci cause most of the cases of catheter-related infection, catheter-related bacteremia, and catheter-related septic thrombophlebitis. In adults most cases of catheter colonization and catheter site infection are caused by coagulase-negative staphylococci, whereas *S. aureus* is the most common cause of catheter-related bacteremia and septic thrombophlebitis. On the other hand, coagulase-negative staphylococci are the most common cause of both catheter site infection and catheter-related bacteremia in children.

V.   EPIDEMIOLOGY OF PERIPHERAL VENOUS CATHETER-RELATED PHLEBITIS AND COLONIZATION/INFECTION

A.   Rates of Catheter-Related Phlebitis and Colonization/Infection

1.   Phlebitis

a.   Adults

Rates of aseptic phlebitis range between 2.3% and 51.9% (2,4,5,10–12,16, 27,28,68,69). The high variability of rates cannot be accounted for by differences in definitions of phlebitis or by differences in materials from which the catheters are constructed. In the overwhelming majority of published reports the rates of phlebitis range between 16.7% and 51.9% (2,4,5,10–12,16,28,68). It is of interest that the most carefully performed study found the lowest rate of phlebitis (2.3%) (69).

b. Children
Only two studies in children report rates of aseptic phlebitis (7,8). They reported rates of 10.4% in one study and 13% in the other. It is unclear why children have lower rates of phlebitis than adults. The differences in rates between children and adults cannot be accounted for by differences in definitions of phlebitis or differences in the materials from which catheters were manufactured.

2. Catheter Site Colonization

a. Adults
Catheter-related colonization in PVCs has been reported to occur at a much lower rate than aseptic phlebitis. In six studies in which the semiquantitative catheter culture technique of Maki and co-workers (9) was used to culture peripheral intravenous cannulae on removal, the colonization rates ranged between 1.4% and 6.9% (2,4,10,12,27,28). Differences in colonization rates could not be accounted for by differences in catheter materials or time in situ. However, the study that yielded a cannula colonization rate of 5.4% for steel needles was carried out in a population of patients with hematologic malignancies (28).

b. Children
In three studies of PVCs in children in which catheters were cultured semiquantitatively on removal (9), rates of catheter colonization ranged between 10.4% and 11.8% (7,8,64). In two studies in neonates in which catheters were cultured semiquantitatively (9), rates were 26% and 13% (62,63). The differences between the rates in children and adults could not be accounted for by differences in culture techniques, catheter materials, or time in situ.

B. Rates of Catheter-Related Bacteremia

1. Adults
In five of eight studies of PVCs, no cases of catheter-related bacteremia were identified (2,4,10,12,27). In the other three studies catheter-related bacteremia occurred at a rate of 0.08% to 1.9% (28,68,69). In the multicenter study by Collignon and co-workers from Australia, peripheral intravenous catheter-related bacteremia occurred at a rate of between 0 and 1.28 cases per 1000 catheters purchased; this translated to a rate of ≤0.1% (65). In the unpublished cohort study of HIV-infected patients at five Veterans Hospitals, there were 66 PVC-related bloodstream infections (BSI) for a rate of 1.5 bloodstream infections per 1000

Table 1 Etiologies of Peripheral Venous Catheter-Related Infections

References	Microorganisms	Number of isolates	Percentage of total isolates (%)
Adults			
Maki and Ringer (2) (catheter isolates ≥15 cfu)	Coagulase-negative staphylococci	59	96.7
	Staphylococcus aureus	1	1.6
	Yeast	1	1.6
Righter et al. (4) (catheter isolates ≥15 cfu)	*S. epidermidis*	26	44.1
	Streptococcus species	13	22.0
	Neisseria species	4	6.8
	Yeast	4	6.8
	Micrococcus species	3	5.1
	Diphtheroids	3	5.1
	S. aureus	2	3.4
	Bacillus species	2	3.4
	Serratia marcescens	1	1.7
	Acinetobacter species	1	1.7
Maki and Ringer (12) (catheter isolates ≥15 cfu)	Coagulase-negative staphylococci	103	98.1
	S. aureus	2	1.9
Collignon et al. (66) (blood isolates)	*S. aureus*	149	62.1
	Coagulase-negative staphylococci	26	10.8
	Streptococcus species	3	1.3
	Enterococcus species	2	0.8
	Corynebacterium species	1	0.4
	Escherichia coli	3	1.3
	Klebsiella species	15	6.3
	Enterobacter species	12	5.0
	Serratia species	4	1.7
	Other enterobacteriaceae	5	2.1
	Pseudomonas species	7	2.9
	Other gram-negative microorganisms	9	3.8
	Candida albicans	4	1.7

Gaynes (personal communication) (blood isolates, HIV-positive patients)		
S. aureus	21	38.2
Coagulase-negative staphylococci	15	27.3
K. pneumoniae	4	7.3
P. aeruginosa	4	7.3
E. coli	2	3.6
C. albicans	2	3.6
Other microorganisms	7	12.7
Children		
Wilkins et al. (62) (catheter isolates ≥15 cfu)		
S. epidermidis	19	86.4
S. aureus	1	4.5
S. haemolyticus	1	4.5
S. warneri	1	4.5
Cronin et al. (63) (catheter isolates ≥15 cfu)		
Coagulase-negative staphylococci[a]	34	79.1
S. aureus	1	2.3
Enterococcus[a]	5	11.6
E. coli	2	4.7
C. parapsilosis	1	2.3
Garland et al. (64) (catheter isolates ≥15 cfu)		
S. epidermidis	11	91.7
Streptococcus species	1	8.3
Garland et al. (8) (catheter isolates ≥15 cfu)[b]		
Coagulase-negative staphylococci	78	86.7
Streptococcus pyogenes	2	2.2
Enterococcus faecalis	2	2.2
Yeasts	4	4.4
C. parapsilosis	3	3.3
Malassezia furfur	1	1.1

[a]Some of these catheter isolates may have caused bacteremia.
[b]Catheters cultured by both semiquantitative and quantitative techniques.

catheter-days (R. Gaynes, personal communication, 1995). Fifty-five of these patients had only PVCs (i.e., did not have a central line as well) for a rate of 1.2 BSI per 1000 catheter-days.

2. Children

Peripheral venous catheter-related bacteremia rates are also very low in children. In three published studies there were no cases of bacteremia (7,62,64), and in one report the bacteremia rate was 0.15% (8).

Taken together, these data indicate that both adult and pediatric patients with PVCs are at very low risk for catheter-related bacteremia.

C. Rates of Catheter-Related Septic Thrombophlebitis

No cohort studies of septic thrombophlebitis that complicates the use of PVCs have been published, so rates for this complication are unknown. However, since bacteremia is a prominent manifestation of septic thrombophlebitis and the rate of peripheral intravenous cannula-related bacteremia is very low, the rate of septic thrombophlebitis complicating the insertion of PVCs would also be expected to be very low.

D. Risk Factors for Phlebitis and Catheter Site Colonization and Infection

1. Phlebitis

a. Adults

Risk factors for phlebitis have been identified in three prospective studies of PVCs using similar definitions for phlebitis and multivariable analysis of the data (2,5,69). All three studies identified duration of cannulation as a risk factor. Risk factors identified by two of the three studies included infusion of antibiotics and use of Teflon rather than polyurethane catheters (2,5). All three studies identified a risk factor in some way related to female gender: having a cesarean section (5), being hospitalized in an obstetrics and gynecology hospital (69), or simply being female (2). Other risk factors included cannula tip damage (5), having a high risk diagnosis (cancer, immunodeficiency diseases), catheter order (higher rates of phlebitis for catheters inserted after the first catheter), and an interaction of length and order (length of catheterization increased the risk of phlebitis only for first catheters) (69). In a second analysis, Maki and Ringer identified risk factors for severe phlebitis, which was defined as having a phlebitis score higher than the 77th percentile of all phlebitis scores (2). Catheter duration, female gender, infusion of antibiotics, and use of Teflon rather than polyurethane catheters were important predictors of severe phlebitis. Having had phlebitis with a previous catheter and having catheter-related infection were also risk factors for severe phlebitis.

b. Children

Only one prospective study using a standard definition of phlebitis and multivariable techniques for analysis of data has been published in the pediatric literature (7). Using multiple linear regression, Nelson and Garland identified parenteral nutrition, infusion of nafcillin and aminoglycosides, and older age (those who developed phlebitis had a mean age of about 6 years while those without phlebitis had a mean age of about 4 years) as independent risk factors for phlebitis in children.

2. *Catheter Site Colonization and Local Infection*

a. Adults

Only three prospective studies of peripheral catheter colonization and/or local catheter-related infection have been published (12,28,70). In only two of these studies were catheters (steel needles) cultured semiquantitatively on removal (12,28). In one of these publications Band and Maki assessed risk factors for colonization of steel needles in patients with hematologic malignancy (28). Using only univariate statistical analytical techniques, they identified local inflammation and needle placements exceeding 72 hours as risk factors. In the only study using semiquantitative cultures of catheters and multivariable statistical analysis, Maki and Ringer found colonization of the catheter site, colonization of the hub, moisture or blood beneath the dressing, and longer duration of catheter placement (3.8 ± 1.8 days vs. 2.7 ± 1.6 days) to be risk factors for local catheter-related infection (12). They identified systemic antimicrobial therapy as protective (relative risk 0.47, 95% confidence interval 0.31–0.73).

Ena and associates carried out a cross-sectional study of phlebitis and catheter-related infection in a university-affiliated hospital in Madrid, Spain (70). Catheters were not cultured, and local catheter-related infection was diagnosed by local signs of inflammation and/or fever not attributable to other causes. Of 353 intravascular catheters 273 (77.3%) were peripheral intravenous catheters. Risk factors identified by logistic regression analysis were infection at any other body site, inappropriate catheter care (defined as any deviation from Centers for Disease Control and Prevention guidelines for catheter care), and inappropriate length of catheter use (not defined). A hospital stay of longer than 14 days had a borderline relationship with catheter-related infection. The data on risk factors from this study have to be interpreted with caution, because catheters were not cultured and because 22.7% of the catheters were not PVCs.

b. Children

There have been no prospective studies published in the pediatric literature that used standard culture techniques to identify colonized catheters or local catheter-related infection and multivariable analysis of the data to identify risk factors for catheter colonization. Garland and associates conducted a prospective study of complications of PVCs in critically ill children and analyzed their data using multivariable techniques, but cultured catheters with unvalidated modifications of a semiquantitative culture technique (9) and a quantitative culture technique (71). They found infusion of diazepam, infusion of lipids, catheter duration greater than 144 hours, and age ≤1 year to be independent risk factors for catheter colonization (8).

Cronin and co-workers performed a prospective study and assessed risk factors for colonization of multiple types of catheters, but stratified their analysis by catheter type (63). Using only univariate analytical techniques, they identified duration of catheterization (longer than 3 days), absence of antibiotic therapy in the 4 days prior to catheter removal, use of the catheter for infusion of hyperalimentation solution, and low birth weight (<1500 g) as risk factors for PVC colonization.

In a prospective study in which only 40% of the catheters were cultured and data were analyzed only by univariate techniques, Garland and associates were unable to find a significant relationship between catheter colonization and age, gender, race, conditions of catheter placement (elective versus emergency situation, site, catheter size, number of catheters), local complications including extravasation and phlebitis, and duration of catheterization (64). There was a borderline relationship between absence of antibiotic infusion through the catheter and catheter colonization.

There is little agreement among these studies with respect to risk factors for catheter colonization, and the data should be interpreted cautiously because of differences in study populations and deficiencies in study design and data analysis.

E. Risk Factors for Peripheral Venous Catheter-Related Bacteremia

No studies have been published that assess risk factors for peripheral venous catheter-related bacteremia. Bacteremias associated with PVCs are so uncommon that huge numbers of patients would have to be enrolled in a multicenter study. Given the low morbidity and mortality attributed to such bacteremias, it is unlikely that such a study will ever be done.

VI. DIAGNOSIS OF CATHETER COLONIZATION, LOCAL CATHETER-RELATED INFECTION, AND CATHETER-RELATED BACTEREMIA

A. Clinical Manifestations

Although local signs of inflammation (palpable cord, erythema, tenderness, swelling) may be associated with positive catheter cultures (see below) (9,40), it is clear that local signs of inflammation occur most often with negative catheter cultures (aseptic phlebitis) (2,4,10). The only local sign that is diagnostic of local catheter-related infection is drainage of purulent fluid from the site at which the catheter penetrates the skin (10,60,71). Thus, in the absence of purulent drainage, local signs of inflammation alone are an indication to remove the catheter and submit it for appropriate culture (see below), but without purulent drainage, local signs of inflammation alone are not diagnostic of catheter-related infection. On the other hand, the absence of signs of inflammation at the catheter site does not rule out catheter colonization/catheter-related infection, i.e., does not predict that catheter cultures will be negative (4,9,10,72).

Septic thrombophlebitis should be considered in patients who have fever and a positive blood culture without an obvious source and who have a PVC in place or who have had a PVC recently removed (42,61). Local signs of infection may occur in less than half of these patients (42,73). When local signs of inflammation are present, they may include pain, swelling, erythema, palpable cord, lymphadenopathy, purulent drainage, and local abscess (61).

Septic thrombophlebitis should be considered in the absence of local signs at presently or recently cannulated venous sites in patients with persistent fever and bacteremia with no identifiable source. This may be particularly important in burn patients (42,73). All currently and recently cannulated veins should be examined for signs of inflammation and purulent drainage. An attempt should be made to express purulent fluid from previously cannulated sites. In patients with continuing fever and bacteremia with no identifiable source and negative findings on examination of current and previously cannulated venous sites, it may be necessary to surgically explore these sites starting in the area of the vein where the tip of the previous cannula was likely to have been positioned (42,73). For patients with ongoing fever and bacteremia with an unknown source who have an intravascular catheter(s) in place, the catheter(s) should be removed and submitted for appropriate cultures (see below). Any purulent drainage should be cultured and a gram-stained smear examined microscopically.

B.   Application of Microbiologic Techniques for Diagnosis of Catheter Colonization and Catheter-Related Infections

1.   Cultures

The three types of specimens that may be cultured to establish the diagnosis of catheter colonization/catheter-related infection are purulent drainage from a site of venous cannulation, the cannula, and the patient's blood.

a.   Purulent Drainage from the Catheter Site

When local catheter-related infection is suspected, the cannulated site should be carefully assessed for the presence of purulent drainage and any purulent fluid sampled carefully with a sterile swab so as to avoid contamination from skin around the cannula site. The swab should be promptly submitted for culture.

b. Catheters

Culture of a catheter in broth has a high sensitivity but low specificity, because even a single bacterial cell from the surrounding skin that contaminates the catheter on removal will give rise to a positive broth culture after overnight incubation. Thus, a negative broth culture indicates that the catheter is not colonized or that there is not local cannula-related infection, but a positive culture in broth is difficult to interpret.

To improve on the diagnostic accuracy of catheter cultures, Maki and co-workers developed a semiquantitative culture technique in which catheter segments were rolled across the surface of an agar plate using a flamed forceps (9). They found that cultures yielding ≥ 15 cfu were significantly associated with local inflammation and septicemia. Maki and co-workers considered that a positive catheter culture (≥ 15 cfu) indicated catheter-related infection. However, since Maki and co-workers' description of this culture technique, it has become clear that many catheters removed from inflamed sites are culture-negative (2,4,10,12) and that catheters that yield ≥ 15 cfu on semiquantitative culture may be from sites with no signs of local inflammation (7,8). Thus, a positive semiquantitative catheter culture is currently considered to represent catheter colonization rather than catheter-related infection. However, because catheter colonization is considered to be a precursor of catheter-related infection, and because colonized catheters may give rise to bacteremia (72), catheter colonization is considered an adverse event.

Collignon and colleagues reevaluated the semiquantitative catheter culture technique of Maki and co-workers (9) and found that the technique was still a useful indicator of central vein catheter-related bacteremia (49). However, they noted that a threshold of ≥ 5 cfu improved the sensitivity of the technique with no change in specificity. Since these authors cultured only the tips of central venous catheters, it is unclear how their observations might apply to PVCs.

Because the semiquantitative catheter culture technique cultures only the outside of the catheter and has relatively low positive predictive value, quantitative culture techniques were developed to overcome these deficiencies in the semiquantitative culture technique (71,72,74). Catheters were immersed in broth and the lumina were flushed with broth followed by quantitative culture of the broth (74), or catheters were sonicated in broth followed by quantitative culture of the broth (71,72). The sensitivity, specificity, and positive and negative predictive values for the quantitative broth sonication technique were 93%, 95%, 76% and 99%, respectively (72). However, only the study by Cleri and associates clearly included PVCs and they considered $>10^3$ cfu as the threshold for infection, because counts of $\geq 10^3$ cfu were associated with bacteremia (74). Since 111 of 149 catheters in this study were PVCs, it would appear that this diagnostic technique could be applied to PVCs. In the reports of the quantitative sonication technique either the types of catheters studied were not reported (71) or only central venous catheters were included (72). Thus, it is unclear whether or not the broth sonication technique can be applied to PVCs.

Another quantitative culture technique that has been used to diagnose catheter-related infection is quantitative culture of blood samples obtained simultaneously from the intravascular cannula and from a peripheral vein (40,75–77). When the quantity of microorganisms in blood obtained from the catheter exceeds the quantity of microorganisms in peripheral venous blood by ≥ fourfold (77), ≥ sevenfold (76) or ≥ tenfold (40), catheter-related infection is diagnosed. None of the studies have included PVCs. This culture technique is particularly useful for central venous catheters because it permits catheter-related infection to be ruled out without removing the catheter. This is important for central venous catheters, because they are more expensive to insert than PVCs and because insertion may be associated with serious complications. Given the relatively low cost and low risk for insertion of PVCs, it is likely that simply removing a suspect PVC and inserting a new one at another site would be more cost effective than differential quantitative blood cultures.

2. Microscopic Examination of Stained Catheter Segments

In 1985, Cooper and Hopkins reported on a technique that involved direct gram staining of catheter segments immediately after removal (48). They cultured the catheter segments by the semiquantitative technique of Maki and co-workers (9) prior to Gram staining and compared the semiquantitative culture results with the results of microscopic examination of Gram-stained catheter segments. Sensitivity of the Gram stain technique was 100%, specificity was 96.9%, positive predictive value was 83.9%, and negative predictive value was 100%. All bacteremias were associated with catheters considered positive by the Gram stain technique. Unfortunately, only 8 (2.4%) of the catheters were PVCs, making conclusions about application of this technique to PVCs tenuous.

Zufferey and co-workers developed a technique for microscopical examination of catheters stained directly by acridine orange (78). These authors also cultured the catheters using the semiquantitative method of Maki and co-workers (9) prior to staining them with acridine orange. Compared to the semiquantitative cultures, the direct acridine orange staining technique had a sensitivity of 84%, a specificity of 100%, a positive predictive value of 86%, and a negative predictive value of 99%. The overall agreement with semiquantitative culture was 98%. Four hundred ninety-eight of the 710 (70%) catheters studied were PVCs. Thus, it would appear that this technique could be applied to PVCs.

Coutlée and colleagues (79) also compared direct staining of catheter segments with Gram stain and acridine orange with the semiquantitative culture method (9). These investigators found lower sensitivity, specificity, positive predictive value, and negative predictive value for direct Gram staining and direct acridine orange staining than did Cooper and Hopkins (48) and Zufferey and coworkers (78), respectively. Except for fungal infections, Coutlée and colleagues did not consider either of these direct staining techniques very useful for diagnosis of catheter-related infections. However, unlike the studies of Cooper and Hopkins (48) and Zufferey and co-workers (78), the study of Coutlée and colleagues (79) was retrospective and included only 99 catheters. Twenty-three percent of the catheters in the latter study were PVCs. While microscopical examination of directly stained catheters may be laborious, it would appear that such techniques provide valid data for diagnosing or excluding catheter-related infection. Since only eight PVCs were studied by Cooper and Hopkins (48), more data are needed on the application of the direct gram staining technique to PVCs.

C. Definitions of Catheter Colonization, Local Catheter-Related Infection, and Catheter-Related Bacteremia

1. Catheter colonization. Recovery of ≥ 15 cfu from the catheter on semiquantitative (9), or $>10^3$ cfu from the catheter using the quantitative culture technique of Cleri and associates (74) in the absence of purulent drainage from the point at which the catheter penetrates the skin.

2. Local catheter-related infection. Purulent drainage from the point at which the catheter penetrates the skin, or signs of local inflammation and a positive semiquantitative catheter segment culture.

3. Septic thrombophlebitis. Presence of purulent fluid in the lumen of a vein or histopathologic evidence of invasion of the venous wall by microorganisms on venous wall biopsy.

4. Catheter-related bacteremia. Same species of microorganism recovered from blood cultures and either culture of purulent drainage from the point at which the catheter penetrates the skin or from a positive semiquantitative (9) or quantitative (74) culture of the catheter and no other identifiable source for the bacteremia. (For coagulase-negative staphylococci, there must be at least two positive blood cultures, and the isolates from blood must have the same antibiogram as the isolate from the catheter.)

VII. SPECIAL TYPES OF PERIPHERAL VENOUS CATHETERS

A. Heparin Lock Cannulae

Heparin lock cannulae were developed by Stern and colleagues to permit intermittent dosing of intravenous antibiotics in patients with cystic fibrosis and complicating pulmonary infections (80). Since that time, heparin locks have been used extensively, but few studies have been published on the infectious complications encountered with use of these devices.

1. Adults

The only study of heparin lock cannulae in adults was published by Ferguson and associates in 1976 (81). They noted a phlebitis rate of 12%. Cultures were performed on 119 heparin lock needles on removal. Qualitative cultures were taken by first flushing the heparin lock with brain heart infusion broth and then removing the needle tip and placing it in the same type of broth. Fifty-three percent of cannulae associated with phlebitis had a positive flush culture versus 1% positive flush cultures in cannulae not related with phlebitis ($P = 2.3 \times 10^{-8}$). On the other hand, positive needle tip cultures were not significantly related to phlebitis ($P > 0.50$). None of the patients with heparin locks developed bacteremia. Microorganisms isolated from heparin lock flush cultures and needle tip cultures included *S. epidermidis*, *Micrococcus* spp., and aerobic diphtheroids.

Risk factors for a positive flush culture included duration of usage (> 96 hours), number of different drugs infused or injected through the heparin lock, and number of manipulations of the device. The only risk factor for a positive needle tip culture was the number of manipulations. Only two episodes of phlebitis occurred prior to 96 hours of heparin lock needle dwell time.

The only report in the literature on bacteremia associated with the use of heparin lock needles is a letter to the editor by Agger and Maki (82). They described two cases of bacteremia in two patients with leukemia and heparin locks in place. They suggested that needle-related septicemia may occur more frequently in patients with cancer and other immunocompromising conditions.

2. Children

Taylor and co-workers have published the only study on heparin locks in children (83). They randomized 39 newborn infants in an intermediate care nursery to receive parenteral medications by a heparin lock catheter or by an intravenous line kept patent by a continuous low infusion rate. None of the patients in the study developed thrombophlebitis, local catheter-related infection, or bacteremia. The only significant difference in the two groups was that patients with the continuous infusion had more episodes of subcutaneous infiltration.

B. Midline Catheters

Midline catheters are 3- to 8-inch PVCs made of silicone or polyurethane and inserted into larger peripheral veins in the vicinity of the antecubital fossa with the tip lying distal to the central veins (84,85). One of these devices is made of a novel composite polymer, an elastomeric hydrogel that softens and expands in length and diameter after insertion (85).

There are only two published studies that assess the risk of infection associated with the use of midline catheters (84,86). Both are prospective observational studies. Haywood and colleagues studied 41 catheters in 27 children and young adults with cystic fibrosis (86). They observed no phlebitis and no infections, but neither condition was defined by the authors.

Mermel and associates studied 251 midline catheters in 238 patients (84). Infections were well defined, and both catheter hubs and catheter segments were cultured on removal. They were able to obtain 140 catheters for culture. The rate of phlebitis was 15.7%, or 18.3 per 1000 catheter-days. Catheter colonization occurred at a rate of 4.2%, or 5 per 1000 catheter-days, and bacteremia at a rate of 0.7%, or 0.8 per 1000 catheters-days. Significant growth was noted from 3% of the hubs and 0.7% of infusate specimens. Microorganisms recovered from colonized catheters included coagulase-negative staphylococci, *Klebsiella pneumoniae*, and *S. aureus*. The one case of bacteremia was caused by *S. aureus*.

Although the number of catheter colonizations was small, Mermel and associates used Poisson regression to show that catheter colonization occurred at a significantly higher rate in catheters in place for less than 8 days compared to those in place for 8 to 14 days. They interpreted this to mean that midline catheters do not need to be changed on a regular basis if the patient has no unexplained fever or purulent drainage at the insertion site.

Another uncommon but important complication has been observed in association with use of the elastomeric hydrogel composite catheter (Landmark, Menlo Care, Inc., Menlo Park, CA). Several reports have been published describing a type B, unpredictable, nonallergic anaphylactoid reaction triggered by insertion and use of these catheters (84,87–89). Reactions in patients have been characterized by dyspnea, urticaria, abdominal or back pain, and hypotension (85). Some pregnant women had spontaneous abortions and three patients had temporally related cardiac arrest (85). It has been speculated that a toxin or allergen such as a toxic plasticizer may be present on the luminal surface of these catheters and released by flushing (84). The mechanism of this untoward effect remains to be elucidated.

C.   Peripherally Inserted Central Venous Catheters (PICCs)

Insertion of catheters into central veins by way of a peripheral vein rather than a subclavian or jugular vein was first introduced by Bottino and colleagues for administration of chemotherapeutic agents and blood products to patients with malignant neoplasms (90). These catheters are silicone elastomer (Silastic) catheters inserted through large veins in the antecubital fossa. Although these catheters have been in use for more than 15 years, few studies have been published on the infectious complications of these devices.

Rates of phlebitis have ranged between 2.2% and 9.7% (91–93). Local catheter site infections have been assessed in only two studies. Giuffrida and associates noted a 0.4% cumulative incidence of suppurative thrombophlebitis in their patients with PICCs (94), and Pauley and co-workers observed a 5% catheter colonization rate using a semiquantitative culture technique (95). Rates of catheter-related bacteremia have been reported in three studies and range between 2.2% and 0.6% (91,93) or 0.48 and 0.8 infections per 1000 catheter days, respectively (92,93). Rates of local catheter-related infection are similar to those for short PVCs. Catheter-related bacteremia rates for PICCs are about the same as those associated with short PVCs and are much lower than those for centrally inserted central venous catheters. Raad and colleagues found higher rates of catheter-related infections for PICCs inserted into cancer patients (96). Local catheter-related colonization and infection occurred at a rate of 12.3%; the PICC-related bacteremia rate was 3.9%. More studies are needed to determine whether use of PICCs in cancer patients is associated with higher infection rates.

In patients without cancer, most catheter-related infections were caused by coagulase-negative staphylococci (91,92,95); *S. aureus*, α-hemolytic streptococci and *Candida albicans* were each reported once (95). Raad and colleagues found the same microorganisms in cancer patients with PICC-related bloodstream infections, but also noted *Serratia marcescens*, *Mycobacterium chelonei*, *Enterococcus faecalis*, and *Acinetobacter anitratus* (96).

The data on risk factors for PICC colonization/infection are scant. The only attempt to elucidate risk factors for infections that complicate the use of PICCs was in the study published by Raad and colleagues (96). In a univariate analysis, these investigators identified therapy for acute lymphocytic or acute myelocytic leukemia as the only factor significantly associated with PICC-related infections. Treatment with corticosteroids, neutropenia, thrombocytopenia, renal insufficiency, and bone marrow transplantation were not identified as risk factors for catheter-related infection in patients with PICCs. There was no difference in catheter colonization rates between those patients who received antibiotics and those who did not. Raad and colleagues also noted that site inflammation with negative catheter cultures occurred in 40 of 154 (26%) PICCs but in only 5 of 188 (2.7%) subclavian central venous catheters.

D. Peripheral Parenteral Nutrition

Although peripheral intravenous catheters have been used to administer parenteral nutrition fluids (peripheral parenteral nutrition [PPN]), there are few data on infection rates, microbial etiologies, or risk factors for infections that complicate this type of therapy. In a study of only nine patients receiving PPN, Stokes and Hill observed no infections and no thrombophlebitis (97). Nordenström and associates prospectively studied 142 surgical patients receiving PPN and recorded the incidence and severity of infusion phlebitis but did not assess the incidence, etiology, or risk factors for infections that complicate the administration of parenteral nutrition fluids by this route (98). They noted an overall incidence of phlebitis of 18% but showed that the incidence of phlebitis was significantly lower when a compounded mixture of fluids was administered compared to infusion of fluids from separate bottles. These studies show that delivery of parenteral nutrition fluids via a peripheral vein is very effective in meeting the nutritional needs of patients (97,98). However, prospective, randomized controlled trials and prospective cohort studies analyzed using multivariable techniques are needed to define the infectious risks associated with delivery of parenteral nutrition fluids by this route.

VIII. PREVENTION OF PHLEBITIS AND PERIPHERAL VENOUS CATHETER-RELATED INFECTIONS

A. Phlebitis

1. Catheter Materials

In three prospective controlled studies (two randomized), the rate of aseptic phlebitis for polyurethane catheters versus Teflon catheters was lower by 27% to 46% (2,5,11). Thus it would appear that, when all other factors are equal, use of polyurethane catheters would provide the lowest risk of phlebitis.

2. Rotation of Catheter Sites

Previous recommendations that PVCs be rotated to a new site every 48 to 72 hours were based on an increase in risk of catheter-related infections when these devices remained in situ for longer than 48 to 72 hours. However, catheter-related infection rates for PVCs are currently so low that recommendations for rotation of sites at 48 to 72 hours in adults are now based on reducing the incidence of phlebitis (12,69,99). Phlebitis is less of a problem in pediatric patients, and it does not appear necessary to rotate PVC sites in children (7,8).

3. Buffering Acidic Solutions

As noted above, acidic solutions are associated with aseptic phlebitis. Several studies have shown that buffering acidic solutions substantially reduces the occurrence of phlebitis (17,21,100).

4. Avoiding Use of Solutions With High Osmolarity

As noted above, solutions with an osmolarity > 600 mOsm/L are associated with a significant increase in phlebitis. This was noted to be particularly associated with infusion of amino acids and solutions with a high potassium content infused into small veins (23). It has been recommended that osmolarity be maintained below 600 mOsm/L, that very high concentrations of potassium be avoided, that infusions of such fluids not be administered by small veins, and that catheter insertion sites be rotated daily (23).

5. Use of Transdermal Glyceryl Trinitrate

It has been postulated that irritation of the endothelium of veins by insertion of cannulae causes venoconstriction and that this contributes to phlebitis. It has been further postulated that application of an agent close to the insertion site that would keep the vein dilated might reduce the incidence of phlebitis (101). Two randomized clinical trials in which glyceryl trinitrate, a vasodilator, was applied near the cannula insertion site showed a significant reduction in phlebitis compared to placebo (101,102). O'Brien and co-workers studied the cost effectiveness of transdermal glyceryl trinitrate prophylaxis using a Markov process and concluded that such prophylaxis would be cost-effective for cannulae that remained in place >50 hours (103). The only side effect noted with transdermal glyceryl trinitrate was headache easily managed with simple analgesics (102). While transdermal glyceryl trinitrate appears promising for prophylaxis of infusion phlebitis, more studies on efficacy, safety, and cost-effectiveness are needed before recommending that such prophylaxis be widely adopted.

6. Inline Filtration of Infusion Fluids

It has been postulated that particulate contamination of infusion fluids is an important cause of infusion phlebitis (24–26). However, randomized controlled clinical trials of inline filters have yielded conflicting results (24–26,104). Given that inline filters have not been shown to be efficacious in the prevention of infusion phlebitis or infections associated with intravenous infusions, that certain drugs given in low doses may suffer a loss in potency as a result of filtration (105), and that inline filters add to the cost of infusion therapy, their routine use in infusion therapy cannot be recommended. Filters may be required for infusion of certain drugs, and filters should be used in accordance with pharmaceutical manufacturers' recommendations.

B.   Catheter-Related Colonization and Infection

Detailed recommendations for the prevention of PVC-related infections are provided in Table 2. Some of the most important aspects of prevention of infections that complicate the use of PVCs are discussed in more detail below.

1. Catheter Selection

Microorganisms adhere more avidly to polyethylene and polyvinyl chloride, and catheters constructed from these materials are associated with a higher rate of catheter colonization than are catheters made from Teflon and polyurethane (2,30,31). Thus, it would appear that use of polyurethane catheters in adults would provide the lowest rates of aseptic phlebitis (as noted above) and catheter colonization (2,5,11). Data are insufficient on which catheters are most appropriate for use in children.

Table 2   Recommendations for the Prevention of Peripheral Venous
Catheter-Related Infections

Recommendation	Category[a]
I. General recommendations for intravascular-device use	
A. Healthcare worker education and training	
Conduct ongoing education and training of healthcare workers regarding indications for the use of and procedures for the insertion and maintenance of intravascular devices, and appropriate infection control measures to prevent intravascular device-related infections.	IA
B. Surveillance	
1. Conduct surveillance for intravascular device-related infections to determine device-specific infection rates, monitor trends in those rates, and assist in identifying lapses in infection control practices within one's own institution. Express data as the number of catheter-related infections or catheter-related bloodstream infections per 1000 catheter-days to facilitate comparisons with national trends.	II
2. Palpate the catheter insertion site for tenderness daily through the intact dressing.	IB
3. Visually inspect the catheter site if the patient develops tenderness at the insertion site, fever without obvious source, or symptoms of local or bloodstream infection.	IB
4. In patients who have large, bulky dressings that prevent palpation or direct visualization of the catheter insertion site, remove the dressing, visually inspect the catheter site at least daily and apply a new dressing.	II
5. Record the date and time of catheter insertion in an obvious location near the catheter insertion site (e.g., on the dressing or on the bed).	IB
6. Do not routinely perform surveillance cultures of patients or of devices used for intravascular access.	IB
C. Hand washing	
Wash hands using an antiseptic-containing product before palpating, inserting, changing, or dressing any intravascular device.	II
D. Barrier precautions during catheter insertion and care	
1. Wear vinyl or latex gloves when inserting an intravascular catheter, as required by the Occupational Safety and Health Administration (OSHA) Bloodborne Pathogens Standard.	IB
2. Wear vinyl or latex gloves when changing the dressings on intravascular catheters.	IB
3. NO RECOMMENDATION for the use of sterile vs. nonsterile gloves during dressing changes.	Unresolved issue
E. Catheter site care	
1. Cutaneous antisepsis and antimicrobial ointmeps. Cleanse the skin with an appropriate antiseptic including 70% alcohol, 10% povidone-iodine, or 2% tincture of iodine before catheter insertion.	IA

Table 2 Continued

Recommendation	Category[a]
2. Catheter site dressing regimens	
a. Use either a sterile gauze or transparent dressing to cover the catheter site.	IA
b. Leave dressings in place until the catheter is removed or changed, or the dressing becomes damp, loosened, or soiled. Change dressings more frequently in diaphoretic patients.	IB
F. Changing intravenous catheters and administration sets	
1. Remove an intravascular device as soon as its use is no longer clinically indicated.	IA
2. Change intravenous tubing, including "piggyback" tubing no more frequently than at 72-hour intervals, unless clinically indicated.	IA
3. NO RECOMMENDATION for intravenous tubing changes beyond 72-hour intervals.	Unresolved issue
4. Change tubing used to administer blood, blood products, or lipid emulsions within 24 hours of completing the infusion.	IB
G. Preparation and quality control of intravenous admixtures	
1. Admix all parenteral fluids in the pharmacy in a laminar-flow hood using aseptic technique.	II
2. Check all containers of parenteral fluid for visible turbidity, leaks, cracks, particulate matter, and the manufacturer's expiration date before use.	IA
3. Use single-dose vials for parenteral additives or medications whenever possible.	II
4. If multidose vials are used:	
a. Refrigerate multidose vials after they are opened unless otherwise specified by the manufacturer.	II
b. Cleanse the rubber diaphragm of multidose vials with alcohol before inserting needle into the vial.	IA
c. Use a sterile needle and syringe each time a multidose vial is accessed, and avoid touch contamination of the needle prior to penetrating the rubber diaphragm.	IA
d. Discard multidose vials when empty, when suspected or visible contamination occurs, or when the manufacturer's stated expiration date is reached.	IA
H. "Hang time" for parenteral fluids	
1. Do not leave parenteral nutrition fluids hanging for longer than 24 hours.	IA
2. NO RECOMMENDATION for the "hang time" of intravenous fluids other than parenteral nutrition fluids.	Unresolved issue
I. In-line filters	
Do not routinely use filters for infection control purposes.	IA
J. Intravenous therapy personnel	
Designate trained personnel for the insertion and maintenance of intravascular devices.	IB

Table 2 Continued

Recommendation	Category[a]
K. Needleless intravascular devices	
NO RECOMMENDATION for use, maintenance, or frequency of change of needleless intravenous devices.	Unresolved issue
L. Prophylactic antimicrobials	
Do not routinely administer antimicrobials for prophylaxis of catheter colonization or bloodstream infection before insertion or during use of an intravascular device.	IB
II. Peripheral venous catheters	
A. Selection of catheter	
1. Select catheters based on the intended purpose and duration of use, known complications (e.g., phlebitis and infiltration), and experience at the institution. Use a Teflon catheter, a polyurethane catheter, or a steel needle.	IB
2. Avoid the use of steel needles for the administration of fluids/medications, which may cause tissue necrosis if extravasation occurs.	IA
3. NO RECOMMENDATION for the use of antimicrobial-impregnated peripheral venous catheters.	Unresolved issue
B. Selection of catheter insertion site	
1. In adults, use an upper-extremity site in preference to one on a lower extremity for catheter insertion. Transfer a catheter inserted in a lower-extremity site to an upper-extremity site as soon as the latter is available.	IA
2. In pediatric patients, insert catheters into a scalp, hand, or foot site in preference to a leg, arm, or antecubital fossa site.	II
C. Catheter changes	
1. In adults, change peripheral venous catheters and rotate peripheral venous sites every 48–72 hours to minimize the risk of phlebitis.	IB
2. In adults, remove catheters inserted under emergency conditions, where breaks in aseptic technique are likely to have occurred. Insert a new catheter at a different site within 24 hours.	IB
3. In pediatric patients, NO RECOMMENDATION for the frequency of change of peripheral venous catheters.	Unresolved issue
4. In pediatric patients, NO RECOMMENDATION for removal of catheters inserted under emergency conditions, where breaks in aseptic technique are likely to have occurred.	Unresolved issue
5. NO RECOMMENDATION for the frequency of change of midline catheters.	Unresolved issue
6. Remove peripheral venous catheters when the patient develops signs of phlebitis (i.e., warmth, tenderness, erythema, palpable venous cord) at the insertion site.	IA
D. Catheter and catheter site care	
1. Flush solutions, anticoagulants, and other intravenous additives	
a. Routinely flush peripheral venous heparin locks with normal saline unless they are used for obtaining blood specimens in which case a dilute heparin (10 units/ml) flush solution should be used.	IB
b. NO RECOMMENDATION for the routine application of topical nitrates near the insertion site of peripheral venous catheters.	Unresolved issue

Table 2   Continued

Recommendation	Category[a]
2. Cutaneous antiseptics and antimicrobial ointments	
NO RECOMMENDATION for the routine application of topical antimicrobial ointment to the insertion site of peripheral venous catheters.	Unresolved issue
E. Peripherally inserted central venous catheters	
1. Change peripherally inserted central venous catheters at least every 6 weeks.	IB
2. NO RECOMMENDATION for the frequency of change of peripherally inserted central venous catheters when the duration of therapy is expected to exceed 6 weeks.	Unresolved issue

[a]As in previous CDC guidelines, each recommendation is categorized on the basis of existing scientific data, theoretical rationale, applicability, and economic impact. However, the previous CDC system for categorizing recommendations has been modified as follows:

   Category IA. Strongly recommended for all hospitals and strongly supported by well-designed experimental or epidemiologic studies.

   Category IB. Strongly recommended for all hospitals and viewed as effective by experts in the field and a consensus of the Hospital Infection Control Practices Advisory Committee (HICPAC) based on strong rationale and suggestive evidence, even though definitive scientific studies may not have been done.

   Category II. Suggested for implementation in many hospitals. Recommendations may be supported by suggestive clinical or epidemiologic studies, a strong theoretical rationale, or definitive studies applicable to some, but not all, hospitals.

   NO RECOMMENDATION. Unresolved issue. Practices for which insufficient evidence or consensus regarding efficacy exists.

Source: Modified from Ref. 99.

2.   Catheter Insertion

a.   Site of Insertion

For many years it has been taught that PVCs should not be inserted into veins in the lower extremity because PVCs in the lower extremity are at a higher risk of infection than those inserted into the upper extremity. It would appear that concern for a higher risk of infection for PVCs inserted into the lower extremity is based on anecdotal reports published between 35 and 40 years ago (106–108). There are no prospective observational cohort studies or randomized clinical trials to support a higher risk of infection for PVCs inserted into the lower extremity. As will be noted in Table 2, the CDC's new guideline on prevention of intravascular device-related infections still recommends the upper extremity as the preferred site for insertion of PVCs.

b. Antiseptic Preparation of the Site

Short peripheral venous catheters should be inserted using aseptic no-touch technique after application of an antiseptic to the skin overlying the vein to be cannulated. There are few published data on which to base selection of an antiseptic for preparation of the skin prior to insertion of the catheter. It would appear that tincture of iodine is more effective than an iodophor for skin preparation prior to venipuncture to obtain blood for culture (109), but this does not necessarily translate to greater effectiveness than an iodophor for skin preparation prior to cannulation of a vein. The only randomized controlled trial of antiseptics used for skin preparation prior to insertion of an intravascular catheter was published by Maki and colleagues (47). However, this was a study of central venous and arterial catheters, and it may not be possible to extrapolate these findings to PVCs. The authors showed that 2% aqueous chlorhexidine gluconate was significantly more effective than 70% isopropyl alcohol and 10% povidone-iodine solution in preventing catheter-related infection and catheter-related bacteremias. In the absence of studies on antisepsis for the insertion of PVCs in adults, it is reasonable to conclude that 2% aqueous chlorhexidine gluconate may be the antiseptic of choice pending publication of randomized clinical trials on antiseptics for preparation of PVC insertion sites.

Garland and associates carried out a prospective, nonrandomized study of successive cohorts of neonates. During the first 6 months, 10% povidone-iodine was used for skin preparation at PVC insertion sites, followed by use of 0.5% chlorhexidine gluconate in 70% isopropyl alcohol for the next 6 months (110). The rate of catheter colonization was 9.3% with povidone-iodine and 4.7% with 0.5% chlorhexidine gluconate in 70% isopropyl alcohol ($P = 0.01$). Using logistic regression, the authors showed that 0.5% chlorhexidine gluconate in 70% isopropyl alcohol was significantly better than 10% povidone-iodine and that heavy skin colonization before catheter insertion was a significant risk factor for catheter colonization.

There are no published data on the efficacy of procedures for insertion of midline catheters or PICCs. For insertion of midline catheters, Mermel and coworkers cleansed the insertion site with povidone-iodine followed by 70% ethyl alcohol and then povidone-iodine again. The insertion site was draped with large sterile sheet drapes, and the operator wore a mask and sterile gloves (84).

The procedure for insertion of PICCs varies from center to center. The site has usually been prepped with povidone-iodine (92,96), and masks may be worn (92,94). All reports mentioned that the operator wore sterile gloves (92–94,96).

3. Application of Topical Antimicrobial Ointments to the Insertion Site

Application of an antimicrobial ointment to the site where the catheter penetrates the skin is based on the most important pathogenetic mechanism for catheter site colonization and infection. Thus, theoretically, it would be expected that a topical antimicrobial agent applied at the entrance to the subcutaneous catheter tract might block the migration of microorganisms into the tract and reduce the risk of colonization and infection. However, this approach to prevention of infection has generally been disappointing. Moran and co-workers conducted the first randomized controlled trial of topical antibiotic prophylaxis 30 years ago (111). They observed a significant protective effect of a topical preparation containing neomycin, polymyxin, and bacitracin applied to venous cutdown sites. Two randomized controlled trials of percutaneously inserted catheters by Norden (112) and Zinner and associates (113) in the 1960s using a topical preparation of polymyxin B, neomycin, and bacitracin yielded equivocal results. Colonization/ infection rates with "pathogens" were the same for the topical antibiotic and placebo groups, but colonization/infection with "pathogens" developed more slowly in the antibiotic group (112) or catheters in the antibiotic group were colonized with fewer "pathogens" (113). In both studies yeasts were recovered only from catheters to which the topical antibiotics had been applied.

In a randomized clinical trial, Maki and Band compared the prophylactic effects of polymyxin, neomycin, bacitracin (PNB) ointment, and an iodophor ointment with no ointment (114). These authors observed a significant (but what they interpreted as a marginal effect) reduction in catheter-related infections in the PNB group compared to the group who received no ointment. The iodophor ointment did not provide a significant protective effect compared to the group without ointment, and neither PNB nor the iodophor ointment reduced the incidence of catheter-related bacteremia. The maximum protective effect of PNB was seen with catheters that remained in place for > 4 days. Three of four *Candida* infections, including one septicemia, occurred in the PNB group.

Topical antimicrobial agents applied to catheter insertion sites appear to provide only marginal protection and may increase the risk of infections due to yeasts. If topical antimicrobial agents have any role in the prevention of PVC colonization or catheter-related infection, it may be for catheters that remain in place for more than 4 days.

4. Catheter Site Dressings

The catheter insertion site should be covered with a sterile dressing after catheter placement. The dressings applied usually consist of sterile gauze covered with adhesive tape or a polyurethane film. Gauze and tape dressings act as a partial barrier to contamination and permit escape of moisture so that the catheter site remains dry. However, gauze and tape dressings are not impermeable to external moisture and require removal for inspection of the catheter insertion site. On the other hand, polyurethane film dressings are impermeable to moisture from external sources and permit patients to shower without removing the dressing or risking contamination of the site, and they allow for inspection of the catheter site without removing the dressing because they are transparent. A potential disadvantage of polyurethane film dressings is that, owing to their impermeability, they may trap moisture under the dressing at the catheter insertion site and provide a moist, occluded environment conducive to multiplication of microorganisms.

Two controlled trials, one randomized (115) and one nonrandomized (116), from the mid-1980s showed a significantly increased rate of catheter colonization for PVCs covered with a polyurethane dressing when compared to gauze dressings. In neither study did catheter colonization correlate with phlebitis, and Craven and colleagues observed no difference in the incidence of bacteremia between patients with gauze dressings and those with polyurethane dressings (115). In a meta-analysis that included seven studies, Hoffmann and associates found a significant increase in catheter colonization for PVCs dressed with polyurethane film when compared with those dressed with gauze, but there was no difference in the incidence of bacteremia related to the type of dressing used (117).

Other studies have shown no difference in catheter colonization between polyurethane film and gauze dressings. Hoffmann and co-workers performed a randomized controlled trial of polyurethane film versus gauze dressings applied to PVC sites (118). They randomized 300 patients to the polyurethane group and 298 to the gauze group. No differences in catheter colonization or catheter-related bacteremia were observed. In the largest randomized clinical trial of dressings applied to PVC sites published to date, Maki and Ringer randomized 2088 patients to one of four groups: (1) sterile gauze replaced every other day; (2) gauze left in place for the duration of catheterization; (3) polyurethane film left on for the lifetime of the catheter; and (4) an iodophor-transparent dressing also left on for the lifetime of the catheter (12). There was no difference in rates of catheter colonization among the dressing groups. None of these catheters were associated with bacteremia. This very large, well-designed and well-executed controlled trial offers convincing evidence that polyurethane film dressings are as safe as gauze and tape dressings and that none of these dressings need to be routinely replaced during the lifetime of the catheter. This will likely hold true for the future with the introduction of new polyurethane films that are more permeable to moisture and that reduce the accumulation of moisture under the dressing (119).

5.   Maintenance of the Catheter and Infusion System

Given the findings of Maki and Ringer noted above and the absence of data to support routine dressing changes as an infection control measure for PVCs, it would appear that such routine changes need not be done. In accordance with the CDC Guideline on Intravascular Device-Related Infections Prevention (99), the catheter site should be assessed every day by palpating the catheter insertion site for tenderness through the intact dressing. The site should be visually inspected if the patient develops tenderness at the insertion site, fever without an obvious source, or symptoms of local or bloodstream infection. If the dressing is so bulky that palpation through the dressing is not possible, the dressing should be removed and the site inspected visually followed by placement of a new sterile dressing. Otherwise, the dressing should be left in place until the catheter is removed, or changed, or the dressing becomes damp, loosened, or soiled. It may be necessary to change dressings more frequently in diaphoretic patients.

PVCs should be removed and inserted at a new site every 48 to 72 hours, not to prevent catheter colonization or catheter-related infection, but to reduce the incidence of phlebitis (99). Since intravenous administration sets may be left in place at least 72 hours (120–122), it may be convenient to change the catheter and administration set at the same time.

6. Specialized Intravenous Therapy Personnel

Two nonrandomized studies using historical controls have shown that when specially trained personnel were used to maintain central venous catheter sites, there was a substantially lower rate of catheter-related infections than when catheter sites were maintained by personnel without special training (123,124). One nonrandomized controlled trial using an intravenous therapy team versus residents and ward nurses to insert and care for PVCs has been published (3). There was a significantly reduced rate of phlebitis, and the rates of cellulitis and septic thrombophlebitis were reduced tenfold for catheters inserted and maintained by the intravenous therapy team. However, before intravenous therapy teams can be recommended for prevention of catheter-related infections, randomized controlled clinical trials that assess both the efficacy and cost of such programs must be carried out.

REFERENCES

1. Maki DG. Infections due to infusion therapy. In: Bennett JV, Brachman PS, eds. Hospital Infections. Boston: Little, Brown, 1992:849.
2. Maki DG, Ringer M. Risk factors for infusion-related phlebitis with small peripheral venous catheters. A randomized controlled trial. Ann Intern Med 1991; 114:845–854.
3. Tomford JW, Hershey CO, McLaren CE, Porter DK, Cohen DI. Intravenous therapy team and peripheral venous catheter-associated complications. Arch Intern Med 1984; 144:1191–1194.
4. Righter J, Bishop LA, Hill B. Infection and peripheral venous catheterization. Diagn Microbiol Infect Dis 1983; 1:89–93.
5. Gaukroger PD, Roberts JG, Manners TA. Infusion thrombophlebitis: a prospective comparison of 645 Vialon and Teflon cannulae in anaesthetic and postoperative use. Anaesth Intens Care 1988; 16:265–271.
6. Turnidge J. Hazards of peripheral intravenous lines. Med J Aust 1984; 141:37–40.

7. Nelson DB, Garland JS. The natural history of Teflon catheter-associated phlebitis in children. Am J Dis Child 1987; 141:1090–1092.
8. Garland JS, Dunne WM Jr, Havens P, et al. Peripheral intravenous catheter complications in critically ill children: a prospective study. Pediatrics 1992; 89:1145–1150.
9. Maki DG, Weise CE, Sarafin HW. A semiquantitative culture method for identifying intravenous-catheter-related infection. N Engl J Med 1977; 296:1305–1309.
10. Gantz NM, Presswood GM, Goldberg R, Doern G. Effects of dressing type and change interval on intravenous therapy complication rates. Diagn Microbiol Infect Dis 1984; 2:325–332.
11. McKee JM, Shell JA, Warren TA, Campbell VP. Complications of intravenous therapy: a randomized prospective study—Vialon vs. Teflon. J Intraven Nurs 1989; 12:288–295.
12. Maki DG, Ringer M. Evaluation of dressing regimens for prevention of infection with peripheral intravenous catheters. Gauze, a transparent polyurethane dressing, and an iodophor-transparent dressing. JAMA 1987; 258:2396–2403.
13. Lewis GBH, Hecker JF. Infusion thrombophlebitis. Br J Anaesth 1985; 57:220–233.
14. Madan M, Alexander DJ, McMahon MJ. Influence of catheter type on occurrence of thrombophlebitis during peripheral intravenous nutrition. Lancet 1992; 339:101–103.
15. Bair JN, Peterson RV. Surface characteristics of plastic intravenous catheters. Am J Hosp Pharm 1979; 36:1707–1711.
16. Collin J, Collin C, Constable FL, Johnston IDA. Infusion thrombophlebitis and infection with various cannulas. Lancet 1975; ii:150–152.
17. Eremin O, Marshall V. Complications of intravenous therapy: reduction by buffering of intravenous fluid preparation. Med J Aust 1977; 2:528–531.
18. Ross SA. Infusion phlebitis. Selected factors. Nurs Res 1972; 21:313–318.
19. Hessov I, Bojsen-Møller M. Experimental infusion thrombophlebitis. Importance of the pH of glucose solutions. Eur J Intens Care Med 1976; 2:97–101.
20. Tse RL, Lee MW. pH of infusion fluids: a predisposing factor in thrombophlebitis. JAMA 1971; 215:642.
21. Fonkalsrud EW, Pederson BM, Murphy J, Beckerman JH. Reduction of infusion thrombophlebitis with buffered glucose solutions. Surgery 1968; 63:280–284.
22. Elfving G, Saikku K. Effect of pH on the incidence of infusion thrombophlebitis. Lancet 1966; i:953.
23. Gazitua R, Wilson K, Bistrian BR, Blackburn GL. Factors determining peripheral vein tolerance to amino acid infusions. Arch Surg 1979; 114:897–900.
24. Allcutt DA, Lort D, McCollum CN. Final inline filtration for intravenous infusions: a prospective hospital study. Br J Surg 1983; 70:111–113.
25. Falchuk KH, Peterson L, McNeil BJ. Microparticulate-induced phlebitis. Its prevention by in-line filtration. N Engl J Med 1985; 312:78–82.
26. Maddox RR, John JF Jr, Brown LL, Smith CE. Effect of inline filtration on postinfusion phlebitis. Clin Pharm 1983; 2:58–61.
27. Tully JL, Friedland GH, Baldini LM, Goldmann DA. Complications of intravenous therapy with steel needles and Teflon catheters. Am J Med 1981; 70:702–706.
28. Band JD, Maki DG. Steel needles used for intravenous therapy. Morbidity in patients with hematologic malignancy. Arch Intern Med 1980; 140:31–34.

29. Locci R, Peters G, Pulverer G. Microbial colonization of prosthetic devices. I. Microtopographical characteristics of intravenous catheters as detected by scanning electron microscopy. Zbl Bakt Hyg. I. Abt Orig B 1981; 173:285–292.

30. Ashkenazi S, Weiss E, Drucker MM. Bacterial adherence to intravenous catheters and needles and its influence by cannula type and bacterial surface hydrophobicity. J Lab Clin Med 1986; 107:136–140.

31. Sheth NK, Franson TR, Rose HD, Buckmire FLA, Cooper JA, Sohnle PG. Colonization of bacteria on polyvinyl chloride and Teflon intravascular catheters in hospitalized patients. J Clin Microbiol 1983; 18:1061–1063.

32. Herrmann M, Vaudaux PE, Pittet D, et al. Fibronectin, fibrinogen, and laminin act as mediators of adherence of clinical staphylococcal isolates to foreign material. J Infect Dis 1988; 158:693–701.

33. Vaudaux P, Suzuki R, Waldvogel FA, Morgenthaler JJ, Nydegger UE. Foreign body infection: role of fibronectin as a ligand for the adherence of *Staphylococcus aureus*. J Infect Dis 1984; 150:546–553.

34. Peters G, Locci R, Pulverer G. Microbial colonization of prosthetic devices. II. Scanning electron microscopy of naturally infected intravenous catheters. Zbl Bakt Hyg. I. Abt Orig B 1981; 173:293–299.

35. Gray ED, Peters G, Verstegen M, Regelmann WE. Effect of extracellular slime substance from *Staphylococcus epidermidis* on the human cellular immune response. Lancet 1984; i:365–367.

36. Farber BF, Kaplan MH, Clogston AG. *Staphylococcus epidermidis* extracted slime inhibits the antimicrobial action of glycopeptide antibiotics. J Infect Dis 1990; 161:37–40.

37. Maki DG. Infections due to infusion therapy. In: Bennett JV, Brachman PS, eds. Hospital Infections. Boston: Little, Brown, 1992:862.

38. Bjornson HS, Colley R, Bower RH, Duty VP, Schwartz-Fulton JT, Fischer JE. Association between microorganism growth at the catheter insertion site and colonization of the catheter in patients receiving total parenteral nutrition. Surgery 1982; 92:720–727.

39. Snydman DR, Gorbea HF, Pober BR, Majka JA, Murray SA, Perry LK. Predictive value of surveillance skin cultures in total-parenteral-nutrition-related infection. Lancet 1982; ii:1385–1388.

40. Armstrong CW, Mayhall CG, Miller KB, et al. Clinical predictors of infection of central venous catheters used for total parenteral nutrition. Infect Control Hosp Epidemiol 1990; 11:71–78.

41. Maki DG, Jarrett F, Sarafin HW. A semiquantitative culture method for identification of catheter-related infection in the burn patient. J Surg Res 1977; 22:513–520.

42. Pruitt BA Jr, McManus WF, Kim SH, Treat RC. Diagnosis and treatment of cannula-related intravenous sepsis in burn patients. Ann Surg 1980; 191:546–554.

43. Franceschi D, Gerding RL, Phillips G, Fratianne RB. Risk factors associated with intravascular catheter infections in burned patients: a prospective, randomized study. J Trauma 1989; 29:811–815.

44. Dixon RE, Kaslow RA, Mackel DC, Fulkerson CC, Mallison GF. Aqueous quaternary ammonium antiseptics and disinfectants. Use and misuse. JAMA 1976; 236:2415–2417.

45. Frank MJ, Schaffner W. Contaminated aqueous benzalkonium chloride. An unnecessary hospital infection hazard. JAMA 1976; 236:2418–2419.
46. Kahan A, Philippon A, Paul G, et al. Nosocomial infections by chlorhexidine solution contaminated with *Pseudomonas pickettii* (biovar VA-1). J Infect 1983; 7:256–263.
47. Maki DG, Ringer M, Alvarado CJ. Prospective randomised trial of povidone-iodine, alcohol, and chlorhexidine for prevention of infection associated with central venous and arterial catheters. Lancet 1991; 338:339–343.
48. Cooper GL, Hopkins CC. Rapid diagnosis of intravascular catheter-associated infection by direct Gram staining of catheter segments. N Engl J Med 1985; 312:1142–1147.
49. Collignon PJ, Soni N, Pearson IY, Woods WP, Munro R, Sorrell TC. Is semiquantitative culture of central vein catheter tips useful in the diagnosis of catheter-associated bacteremia? J Clin Microbiol 1986; 24:532–535.
50. Flowers RH III, Schwenzer KJ, Kopel RF, Fisch MJ, Tucker SI, Farr BM. Efficacy of an attachable subcutaneous cuff for the prevention of intravascular catheter-related infection. A randomized, controlled trial. JAMA 1989; 261:878–883.
51. Maki DG, Cobb L, Garman JK, Shapiro JM, Ringer M, Helgerson RB. An attachable silver-impregnated cuff for prevention of infection with central venous catheters: a prospective randomized multicenter trial. Am J Med 1988; 85:307–314.
52. Raad I, Costerton W, Sabharwal U, Sacilowski M, Anaissie E, Bodey GP. Ultrastructural analysis of indwelling vascular catheters: a quantitative relationship between luminal colonization and duration of placement. J Infect Dis 1993; 168:400–407.
53. Sitges-Serra A, Liñares J, Pécrez JL, Jaurrieta E, Lorente L. A randomized trial on the effect of tubing changes on hub contamination and catheter sepsis during parenteral nutrition. J Parenter Enter Nutr 1985; 9:322–325.
54. Liñares J, Sitges-Serra A, Garau J, Pérez JL, Martín R. Pathogenesis of catheter sepsis: a prospective study with quantitative and semiquantitative cultures of catheter hub and segments. J Clin Microbiol 1985; 21:357–360.
55. Salzman MB, Isenberg HD, Shapiro JF, Lipsitz PJ, Rubin LG. A prospective study of the catheter hub as the portal of entry for microorganisms causing catheter-related sepsis in neonates. J Infect Dis 1993; 167:487–490.
56. deCicco M, Panarello G, Chiaradia V, et al. Source and route of microbial colonisation of parenteral nutrition catheters. Lancet 1989; ii:1258–1261.
57. Hoshal VL Jr, Ause RG, Hoskins PA. Fibrin sleeve formation on indwelling subclavian central venous catheters. Arch Surg 1971; 102:353–358.
58. Stillman RM, Soliman F, Garcia L, Sawyer PN. Etiology of catheter-associated sepsis. Correlation with thrombogenicity. Arch Surg 1977; 112:1497–1499.
59. Hershey CO, Tomford JW, McLaren CE, Porter DK, Cohen DI. The natural history of intravenous catheter-associated phlebitis. Arch Intern Med 1984; 144:1373–1375.
60. Hampton AA, Sherertz RJ. Vascular-access infections in hospitalized patients. Surg Clin North Am 1988; 68:57–71.
61. Baker CC, Petersen SR, Sheldon GF. Septic phlebitis: a neglected disease. Am J Surg 1979; 138:97–103.
62. Wilkins EGL, Manning D, Roberts C, Davidson DC. Quantitative bacteriology of peripheral venous cannulae in neonates. J Hosp Infect 1985; 6:209–217.

63. Cronin WA, Germanson TP, Donowitz LG. Intravascular catheter colonization and related bloodstream infection in critically ill neonates. Infect Control Hosp Epidemiol 1990; 11:301–308.

64. Garland JS, Nelson DB, Cheah T, Hennes HH, Johnson TM. Infections complications during peripheral intravenous therapy with Teflon catheters: a prospective study. Pediatr Infect Dis J 1987; 6:918–921.

65. Collignon PJ. Intravascular catheter associated sepsis: a common problem. Med J Aust 1994; 161:374–378.

66. Leibovitz E, Iuster-Reicher A, Amitai M, Mogilner B. Systemic candidal infections associated with use of peripheral venous catheters in neonates: a 9-year experience. Clin Infect Dis 1992; 14:485–491.

67. Fry DE, Fry RV, Borzotta AP. Nosocomial blood-borne infection secondary to intravascular devices. Am J Surg 1994; 167:268–272.

68. Collins RN, Braun PA, Zinner SH, Kass EH. Risk of local and systemic infection with polyethylene intravenous catheters. A prospective study of 213 catheterizations. N Engl J Med 1968; 279:340–343.

69. Tager IB, Ginsberg MB, Ellis SE, et al. An epidemiologic study of the risks associated with peripheral intravenous catheters. Am J Epidemiol 1983; 118:839–851.

70. Ena J, Cercenado E, Martinez D, Bouza E. Cross-sectional epidemiology of phlebitis and catheter-related infections. Infect Control Hosp Epidemiol 1992; 13:15–20.

71. Sherertz, RJ, Raad II, Belani A, et al. Three-year experience with sonicated vascular catheter cultures in a clinical microbiology laboratory. J Clin Microbiol 1990; 28:76–82.

72. Raad II, Sabbagh MF, Rand KH, Sherertz RJ. Quantitative tip culture methods and the diagnosis of central venous catheter-related infections. Diag Microbiol Infect Dis 1992; 15:13–20.

73. O'Neill JA Jr, Pruitt BA Jr, Foley FD, Moncrief JA. Suppurative thrombophlebitis— a lethal complication of intravenous therapy. J Trauma 1968; 8:256–267.

74. Cleri DJ, Corrado ML, Seligman SJ. Quantitative culture of intravenous catheters and other intravascular inserts. J Infect Dis 1980; 141:781–786.

75. Wing EJ, Norden CW, Shadduck RK, Winkelstein A. Use of quantitative bacteriologic techniques to diagnose catheter-related sepsis. Arch Intern Med 1979; 139:482–483.

76. Fan ST, Teoh-Chan CH, Lau KF. Evaluation of central venous catheter sepsis by differential quantitative blood culture. Eur J Clin Microbiol Infect Dis 1989; 8:142–144.

77. Capdevila JA, Planes AM, Palomar M, et al. Value of differential quantitative blood cultures in the diagnosis of catheter-related sepsis. Eur J Clin Microbiol Infect Dis 1992; 11:403–407.

78. Zufferey J, Rime B, Francioli P, Bille J. Simple method for rapid diagnosis of catheter-associated infection by direct acridine orange staining of catheter tips. J Clin Microbiol 1988; 26:175–177.

79. Coutlée F, Lemieux C, Paradis J. Value of direct catheter staining in the diagnosis of intravascular-catheter-related infection. J Clin Microbiol 1988; 26:1088–1090.

80. Stern RC, Pittman S, Doershuk CF, Matthews LW. Use of a "heparin lock" in the

intermittent administration of intravenous drugs. A technical advance in intravenous therapy. Clin Pediatr 1972; 11:521–523.

81. Ferguson RL, Rosett W, Hodges GR, Barnes WG. Complications with heparin-lock needles. A prospective evaluation. Ann Intern Med 1976; 85:583–586.

82. Agger WA, Maki DG. Septicemia from heparin-lock needles. Ann Intern Med 1977; 86:657.

83. Taylor J, Shannon R, Kilbride HW. Heparin lock intravenous line. Use in newborn infants. A controlled trial. Clin Pediatr 1989; 28:237–240.

84. Mermel LA, Parenteau S, Tow SM. The risk of midline catheterization in hospitalized patients. A prospective study. Ann Intern Med 1995; 123:841–844.

85. Maki DG. Reactions associated with midline catheters for intravenous access. Ann Intern Med 1995; 123:884–886.

86. Harwood IR, Greene LM, Kozakowski-Koch JA, Rasor JS. New peripherally inserted midline catheter: a better alternative for intravenous antibiotic therapy in patients with cystic fibrosis. Pediatr Pulmonol 1992; 12:233–239.

87. Rogan DH. Allergic-type reaction to a Landmark catheter. (Letter.) J Intraven Nurs 1993; 16:118.

88. Briars G. Adverse reactions to elastomeric intravenous catheters in adolescents with cystic fibrosis. (Letter.) Lancet 1993; 342:118.

89. Blum DY. Untoward events associated with use of midterm IV devices. J Intraven Nurs 1995; 18:116–119.

90. Bottino J, McCredie KB, Groschel DHM, Lawson M. Long-term intravenous therapy with peripherally inserted silicone elastomer central venous catheters in patients with malignant diseases. Cancer 1979; 43:1937–1943.

91. Lam S, Scannell R, Roessler D, Smith MA. Peripherally inserted central catheters in an acute-care hospital. Arch Intern Med 1994; 154:1833–1837.

92. Abi-Nader JA. Peripherally inserted central venous catheters in critical care patients. Heart Lung 1993; 22:428–434.

93. Loughran SC, Borzatta M. Peripherally inserted central catheters: a report of 2506 catheter days. J Parenter Enter Nutr 1995; 19:133–136.

94. Giuffrida DJ, Bryan-Brown CW, Lumb PD, Kwun K, Rhoades HM. Central vs peripheral venous catheters in critically ill patients. Chest 1986; 90:806–809.

95. Pauley SY, Vallande NC, Riley EN, Jenner NM, Gulbinas DG. Catheter-related colonization associated with percutaneous inserted central catheters. J Intraven Nurs 1993; 16:50–54.

96. Raad I, Davis S, Becker M, et al. Low infection rate and long durability of nontunneled silastic catheters. A safe and cost-effective alternative for long-term venous access. Arch Intern Med 1993; 153:1791–1796.

97. Stokes MA, Hill GL. Peripheral parenteral nutrition: a preliminary report on its efficacy and safety. J Parenter Enter Nutr 1993; 17:145–147.

98. Nordenström J, Jeppsson B, Lovén L, Larsson J. Peripheral parenteral nutrition: effect of a standardized compounded mixture on infusion phlebitis. Br J Surg 1991; 78:1391–1394.

99. Intravascular device-related infections prevention; guideline availability; notice. Fed Register 1995; 60:49978–50006.

100. Fonkalsrud EW, Carpenter K, Masuda JY, Beckerman JH. Prophylaxis against postinfusion phlebitis. Surg Gynecol Obstet 1971; 133:253–256.
101. Khawaja HT, Campbell MJ, Weaver PC. Effect of transdermal glyceryl trinitrate on the survival of peripheral intravenous infusions: a double-blind prospective clinical study. Br J Surg 1988; 75:1212–1215.
102. Wright A, Hecker JF, Lewis GBH. Use of transdermal glyceryl trinitrate to reduce failure of intravenous infusion due to phlebitis and extravasation. Lancet 1985; ii:1148–1150.
103. O'Brien BJ, Buxton MJ, Khawaja HT. An economic evaluation of transdermal glyceryl trinitrate in the prevention of intravenous infusion failure. J Clin Epidemiol 1990; 43:757–763.
104. Rusho WJ, Bair JN. Effect of filtration on complications of postoperative intravenous therapy. Am J Hosp Pharm 1979; 36:1355–1356.
105. Butler LD, Munson JM, DeLuca PP. Effect of inline filtration on the potency of low-dose drugs. Am J Hosp Pharm 1980; 37:935–941.
106. Bansmer G, Keith D, Tesluk H. Complications following use of indwelling catheters of inferior vena cava. JAMA 1958; 167:1606–1611.
107. McNair TJ, Dudley HAF. The local complications of intravenous therapy. Lancet 1959; ii:365–368.
108. Crane C. Venous interruption for septic thrombophlebitis. N Engl J Med 1960; 262:947–951.
109. Strand CL, Wajsbort RR, Sturmann K. Effect of iodophor vs iodine tincture skin preparation on blood culture contamination rate. JAMA 1993; 269:1004–1006.
110. Garland JS, Buck RK, Maloney P, et al. Comparison of 10% povidone-iodine and 0.5% chlorhexidine gluconate for the prevention of peripheral intravenous catheter colonization in neonates: a prospective trial. Pediatr Infect Dis J 1995; 14:510–516.
111. Moran JM, Atwood RP, Rowe MI. A clinical and bacteriologic study of infections associated with venous cutdowns. N Engl J Med 1965; 272:554–560.
112. Norden CW. Application of antibiotic ointment to the site of venous catheterization—a controlled trial. J Infect Dis 1969; 120:611–615.
113. Zinner SH, Denny-Brown BC, Braun P, Burke JP, Toala P, Kass EH. Risk of infection with intravenous indwelling catheters: effect of application of antibiotic ointment. J Infect Dis 1969; 120:616–619.
114. Maki DG, Band JD. A comparative study of polyantibiotic and iodophor ointments in prevention of vascular catheter-related infection. Am J Med 1981; 70:739–744.
115. Craven DE, Lichtenberg DA, Kunches LM, et al. A randomized study comparing a transparent polyurethane dressing to a dry gauze dressing for peripheral intravenous catheter sizes. Infect Control 1985; 6:361–366.
116. Kelsey MC, Gosling M. A comparison of the morbidity associated with occlusive and nonocclusive dressings applied to peripheral intravenous devices. J Hosp Infect 1984; 5:313–321.
117. Hoffmann KK, Weber DJ, Samsa GP, Rutala WA. Transparent polyurethane film as an intravenous catheter dressing. A meta-analysis of the infection risks. JAMA 1992; 267:2072–2076.

118. Hoffmann KK, Western SA, Kaiser DL, Wenzel RP, Groschel DHM. Bacterial colonization and phlebitis-associated risk with transparent polyurethane film for peripheral intravenous site dressings. Am J Infect Control 1988; 16:101–106.

119. Maki DG, Stolz S, Wheeler S. A prospective, randomized, three-way clinical comparison of a novel, highly permeable, polyurethane dressing with 206 Swan-Ganz pulmonary artery catheters: OpSite IV3000 vs Tegaderm vs gauze and tape. I. Cutaneous colonization under the dressing, catheter-related infection. In: Maki DG, ed. Improving Catheter Site Care. London: Royal Society of Medicine, 1991:61–66.

120. Josephson A, Gombert ME, Sierra MF, Karanfil LV, Tansino GF. The relationship between intravenous fluid contamination and the frequency of tubing replacement. Infect Control 1985; 6:367–370.

121. Snydman DR, Donnelly-Reidy M, Perry LK, Martin WJ. Intravenous tubing containing burettes can be safely changed at 72 hour intervals. Infect Control 1987; 8:113–116.

122. Maki DG, Botticelli JT, LeRoy ML, Thielke TS. Prospective study of replacing administration sets for intravenous therapy at 48- vs 72-hour intervals. JAMA 1987; 258:1777–1781.

123. Nelson DB, Kien CL, Mohr B, Frank S, Davis SD. Dressing changes by specialized personnel reduce infection rates in patients receiving central venous parenteral nutrition. J Parenter Enter Nutr 1986; 10:220–222.

124. Faubion WC, Wesley JR, Khalidi N, Silva J. Total parenteral nutrition catheter sepsis: impact of the team approach. J Parenter Enter Nutr 1986; 10:642–645.

10

Infectious Complications of Swan-Ganz Pulmonary Artery Catheters and Peripheral Arterial Catheters

Leonard A. Mermel

Brown University School of Medicine and Rhode Island Hospital, Providence, Rhode Island

Dennis G. Maki

University of Wisconsin Hospital and Clinics, Madison, Wisconsin

I. SWAN-GANZ PULMONARY ARTERY CATHETERS

A. Introduction

Balloon-tipped Swan-Ganz pulmonary artery (PA) catheters have come into widespread use since their inception in the early 1970s (1). For example, a recent month-long survey of all intensive care units in one hospital demonstrated that the number of PA catheter days/total patient days was 0.24 (2); PA catheter use was greatest in the cardiothoracic ICU and least in the pediatric ICU—0.47 and 0 catheter-days/patient-days, respectively. In recent years, PA catheters have been used to guide therapeutic measures aimed at achieving supranormal levels of oxygen delivery, with conflicting results regarding mortality in critically ill patients (3–6).

The complex and unique features of the PA catheter present challenges to the user of this device unlike any other catheter used in caring for critically ill patients (7). A recent survey of academic medical centers found that nearly half of physicians and nurses using PA catheters have major gaps in their understanding of when to use this device and how to interpret data derived from it (8–10). A clear understanding of the indications and potential complications of PA catheterization is essential. Proper training, ideally intramural certification (8,9), in the

259

insertion, maintenance, and appropriate use of these catheters is imperative. Similar to other central venous catheters, PA catheter use is associated with potential life-threatening iatrogenic complications besides catheter-related bloodstream infection, such as bleeding associated with vascular injury, pneumothorax, arrhythmias, and thromboembolism (11). However, the most frequent life-threatening complication is bloodstream infection, which carries an attributable mortality of 14% to 28% (12–14).

In this chapter we review the incidence and pathogenesis of PA catheter-related infections, risk factors associated with their occurrence, and recommendations for the treatment and prevention of such infections.

B.   Features of the Catheter

PA catheters are among the most complex intravascular devices used in clinical medicine, consisting of a polyvinyl chloride or polyurethane catheter which is placed through a percutaneous, indwelling Teflon introducer sheath into a central great vein, through the right side of the heart, and into the pulmonary artery (Fig. 1). Most PA catheters are inserted into the subclavian or internal jugular vein and, far less frequently, into a femoral vein. One of the catheter lumens is used to inflate a balloon on the catheter tip. This allows the catheter to float in the bloodstream and occlude a small pulmonary artery for measurement of a "wedged" PA or left-atrial pressure. Two additional lumina of the catheter are attached to transducers, permitting continuous pressure monitoring within the pulmonary artery (PA lumen) and the cannulated central vein (CVP lumen) and measurement of the PA occlusive (wedge) pressure when the balloon is inflated. A protective plastic sleeve is usually attached to the end of the introducer sheath covering the extravascular portion of the catheter, allowing the PA catheter to be advanced or pulled back without incurring touch contamination. Pressurized bags of heparin-containing flush solution are attached to the PA and CVP lumens and each are connected to a chamber dome, which interfaces with an electromechanical transducer and a continuous-flow device.

C.   Incidence of Infection

Many prospective studies have addressed the risk of PA catheter-related infection (15–42). Cultures of introducers, in addition to PA catheter segments, were performed in four large studies (36,38,40,43). In two of these studies (38,43), cultures of all potential sources of infection were done and molecular subtyping techniques were used to reliably determine concordance among the isolates. Table 1 summarizes the 16 prospective studies in which cultures of at least 75 PA catheters were done on removal and rates of catheter-related bloodstream infections were reported. In those prospective studies using semiquantitative (28,31–33,35–40,43) or quantitative catheter culture methods (34), 2.3% to

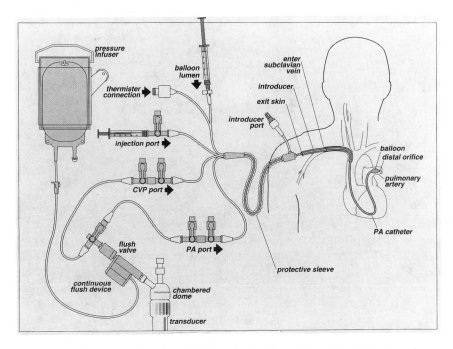

Figure 1 Schematic of a Swan-Ganz catheter placed through a Teflon introducer sheath, with an external protective plastic sleeve over the extravascular portion of the pulmonary artery (PA) catheter. *Note:* Some PA catheters do not have the injection port depicted. Adapted with permission from Ref. 7.

47.3% of Swan-Ganz catheters showed colonization of the PA catheter or introducer (median 12.4%). Overall, the median incidence of Swan-Ganz catheter-related bloodstream infection is 1.1% (range 0% to 5.3%) or a median of 3.0 (range 0% to 13.2%) bloodstream infections per 1000 catheter-days. The incidence of PA catheter-related bloodstream infection is substantially lower than that reported for other types of short-term, noncuffed central venous catheters used in the same patient population (44). Many of the prospective studies of PA catheters may have underestimated the true incidence of PA catheter-related bloodstream infection since routine cultures of introducers, hubs, and infusate were not done.

D. Microbial Profile

Coagulase-negative staphylococci, predominantly *Staphylococcus epidermidis*, are the most common pathogens associated with PA catheter infection. Of the

Table 1 Incidence of Swan-Ganz Pulmonary Artery Catheter-Related Infection

Study	Catheter (n)	Where most catheters inserted	Catheterization (mean days)	Catheter culture method	Catheter colonized (%)	Catheter-related bloodstream infection (%)	Catheter-related bloodstream infection (Per 1000 catheter-days)
Elliot et al. (16)	116	ICU	4	Broth	63.7	1.7	3.9
Michel et al. (27)	153	OR	4	Broth	19.0	0	0
Kaye et al. (28)	133	ICU	NR	SQ	9.8	2.3	NR
Groeger et al. (29)	76	ICU	3	NR[a]	26.3	3.9	13.2
Ricard et al. (30)	109	OR	2	SQ	8.3	0	0
Parsa et al. (31)	90	ICU	NR	SQ	NR	1.1	NR
Damen et al. (32)	794	OR	1	SQ	2.3	0	0
Damen et al. (33)	123	OR	1	SQ	10.6	0	0
Heard et al. (34)	87	ICU	NR	Q	18.0	5.3	NR
Fisher et al. (35)	169	NR	4	SQ	14.2	2.3	8.4
Eyer et al. (36)	156	ICU	6	SQ[a]	5.9	4.6	6.9
Horowitz et al. (37)	158	ICU	3	SQ	29.1	2.5	8.0
Mermel et al. (38)	297	OR	3	SQ[a]	21.9	0.7	2.3
Bach (39)	159	OR	2	SQ	5.0	0	0
Bull (40)	241	OR	2	SQ[a]	47.3	0.8	NR
Maki et al. (43)	442	OR	3	SQ[a]	21.7	1.1	3.6

[a]Introducer sheaths and the catheters were cultured. Hubs and infusate from each lumen of the introducer sheath and PA catheter were cultured, and molecular subtyping was done to confirm true device-related bloodstream infection.

Abbreviations: Broth = qualitatively, by immersion in liquid medium; SQ = semiquantitative roll plate; Q = quantitative by sonication; ICU = intensive care unit; OR = operating room; NR = not reported.

Source: Adapted with permission from Ref. 7.

episodes of Swan-Ganz catheter colonization and bloodstream infection reported in the literature, 56% and 37%, respectively, were due to coagulase-negative staphylococci; 19% and 11%, respectively, were due to enteric gram-negative bacilli; 7% and 16%, respectively, were due to *Candida*; and 5% and 26%, respectively, were due to *Staphylococcus aureus*. *Candida* and *S. aureus* each account for a higher percentage of PA catheter-related bloodstream infections than catheter colonization, reflecting their greater pathogenicity (Fig. 2).

E.   Risk Factors

Multivariate analysis has been used to identify independent risk factors exclusively for PA catheter-associated infection (33,38,41). Use of these catheters in patients under 1 year of age and for 3 or more days in children, placement with lesser barrier precautions [relative risk (RR) 2.1], placement in internal jugular rather than subclavian vein (RR 4.3), heavy cutaneous colonization of the insertion site (RR 5.5), and catheterization longer than 3 days (RR 3.8) or 5 days [odds ratio (OR) 14.4], have each been found to be independent predictors of an increased risk of catheter colonization. Antibiotic use is associated with reduced

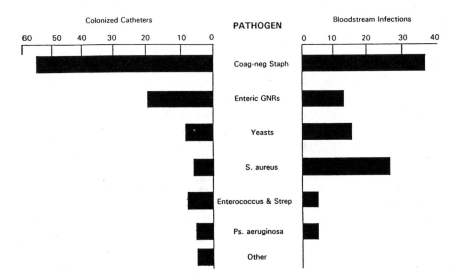

Figure 2   Microbial profile of Swan-Ganz catheter-related infection—local (catheter colonization) and bloodstream infection-based on pooled data from 14 prospective studies providing complete microbiologic data on all infected catheters. Used with permission from Ref. 7.

risk (OR 4.3). In combined studies of central venous and PA catheters using multivariate analysis (45–47), the following risk factors were associated with catheter-related infection: bacteremia or candidemia originating from another site of infection; heavy colonization of the insertion site or hub; catheterization exceeding 4 or 7 days; difficult catheter insertion; second catheterization; internal jugular vein cannulation; use of polyurethane transparent dressing; patients in a coronary care unit or on the surgery service.

1. Colonization of the Insertion Site

A number of prospective studies of PA and central venous catheters have found heavy colonization of the insertion site to be an independent risk factor of catheter-related infection (38,45,47–49). Therefore, prevention of PA catheter-related infection requires interventions which reduce cutaneous colonization of the insertion site.

2. Site of Insertion

Insertion of a PA catheter in an internal jugular vein, rather than a subclavian vein, is independently associated with a significantly increased risk of infection (38). This may be due to heavier cutaneous colonization (50), greater potential for contamination by respiratory secretions (51), and greater difficulty maintaining a catheter dressing on an internal jugular vein insertion site. Thus, placement of central venous and PA catheters in a subclavian vein, rather than an internal jugular vein, is preferable in patients who are not at increased risk of bleeding.

3. Skill of the Inserter

The experience of the inserter has not been found to be a risk factor for PA catheter-related infection, but few studies have adequately examined this risk factor (41,52). Difficult catheter insertion requiring three or more punctures has been associated with a 15-fold increased risk of central venous and PA catheter infection (45). After three unsuccessful attempts, we believe that another, more experienced individual should try to insert the catheter.

4. Barrier Precautions

Use of maximal barrier precautions—sterile gloves, a long-sleeved surgical gown, a surgical mask and hat, and a large sterile sheet drape—in contrast to using only sterile gloves, a surgical mask, and a small fenestrated drape—is associated with a twofold lower risk of PA catheter-related colonization (38). In another prospective study, wearing a sterile gown, in addition to a mask, hat, and gloves, and applying a cutaneous antiseptic for 5 minutes, led to a threefold reduction in PA catheter colonization compared to catheters inserted by clinicians not wearing a gown and spending less time preparing the insertion site (40). Maximal barrier precautions during central venous catheter insertion has been shown to reduce the incidence of catheter-related bloodstream infection fivefold (53,54).

Based on these findings, maximal barrier precautions should be considered the standard during insertion of all central venous, including PA catheters.

5. Guide Wires

In one prospective study including PA catheters, patients were randomized to one of three groups: catheter exchange every 7 days over a guide wire; catheter removal and insertion of a new catheter every 7 days; or no routine catheter change (36). There was no significant difference in the incidence of catheter-related bloodstream infection or colonization among the three groups. A more recent prospective, randomized trial of central venous and PA catheters found nearly a twofold increased incidence of catheter-related bloodstream infection with catheters placed at an old site over a guide wire (55); however, guide wire exchange reduced the risk of mechanical complications. We believe that PA catheters should not be routinely replaced over a guide wire, but that if it is considered necessary to do so because of limited sites for access, the inserter should don a new set of sterile gloves after removing the old catheter and inserting the new one over a guide wire, and cultures of the old catheter should always be done.

6. Duration of Catheterization

Most prospective studies of PA catheters using univariate analysis have shown that the risk of infection increases with the duration of catheterization (15,27,28, 34,38,42,45,56,57), but not all investigations have found such an association (16,17,22,24,36). Three studies using multivariate analysis found a strong association between prolonged catheterization and an increased risk of PA catheter colonization (33,38,41). The actuarial risk of PA catheter-related bloodstream infection is very low during the first 4 days, but rises sharply thereafter (16,28,38,43) (Fig. 3). These data suggest that a PA catheter should ideally be removed on or before the fifth day unless there are extenuating circumstances. In two prospective studies, central venous and PA catheters were randomized to regularly scheduled replacement at 3 days (55) or 7 days (36) versus no routine replacement. In both studies the incidence of catheter colonization and bloodstream infection was not significantly different in the two populations.

7. Dressings

The importance of the cutaneous microflora in the pathogenesis of vascular catheter-related infection (7) suggests that the dressing applied to the insertion site could have an important effect on the risk of infection. There have been three large prospective, randomized trials of polyurethane dressings compared with gauze dressings used to cover PA catheter insertion sites (30,43,58); none found a significant difference in the incidence of catheter-related infection. The largest trial found no increased risk of catheter colonization or bloodstream infection when two types of polyurethane dressings, changed every 5 days, were compared

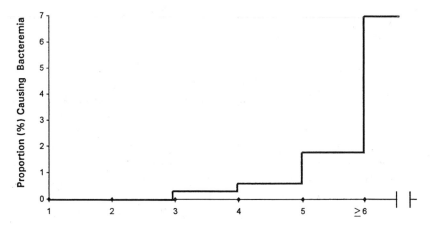

Figure 3 Relationship between the duration of Swan-Ganz catheterization and the actuarial risk of catheter-related bloodstream infection, based on pooled data (988 catheters) from four prospective studies (16,28,38,43). Adapted with permission from Ref. 7.

to gauze dressing changed every other day (43). These data suggest that polyurethane dressings may be used safely to cover the site of PA catheter insertion.

8. Heparin-Bonded Catheters

Heparin is bonded to the external surface of PA catheters in an effort to reduce thrombosis on a catheter surface during the early period after insertion (59). Because the benzalkonium chloride used to bond heparin has intrinsic antimicrobial activity, heparin-bonded PA catheters exhibit surface activity against a wide range of microbial pathogens, including *Candida albicans* (60). An analysis of prospective studies of PA catheter-related infection suggests that heparin bonding reduces the risk of infection (Table 2).

9. Other Risk Factors

Three studies have found an increased risk of PA catheter-related infection in patients with a remote focus of infection during catheterization (22,27,34). Two studies found that administration of total parenteral nutrition through PA catheters did not increase the risk of catheter-related infection (37,38), and in one study steroid use was associated with PA catheter-related infection (34).

F. Sources of Infection

There are numerous microbial reservoirs from which pathogens may gain access to a catheterized patient's bloodstream (Fig. 1): skin flora at the insertion site can

Table 2 Rates of Catheter-Related Bloodstream Infection Found in Prospective Studies of Heparin-Bonded and Non-Heparin-Bonded Pulmonary Artery Catheters

	Heparin-bonded catheters	Nonbonded catheters
Studies (n)	3	3
Total catheters studied (n)	1260	341
Catheter-related bacteremia per 100 catheters		
Mean	1.0	2.8
Range	0–2.3	0–4.6
Per 1000 catheter-days		
Mean	3.6	6.7
Range	0–8.4	0–13.2

Source: Adapted with permission from Ref. 60.

invade the transcutaneous tract and colonize the introducer sheath and PA catheter extraluminally; microbes colonizing any of the three PA catheter hubs or the introducer sheath hub can enter the catheter lumen during hub manipulation and contaminate the infusate or infusate may become contaminated by the manufacturer or during preparation in the hospital prior to use; microbes from the hands of health care workers can also contaminate the extravascular portion of the PA catheter and gain access when the catheter is advanced through the introducer sheath when repositioned; and the intravascular portion of the introducer sheath or PA catheter may become colonized hematogenously from a distant focus of infection.

Two small studies have demonstrated concordance among isolates from the introducer sheath and PA catheter tip (23,29). This concordance was demonstrated in all three cases of PA catheter-related bloodstream infection in one of the studies (29). Two studies found occasional low-level contamination of injectate used for cardiac output measurements, usually with coagulase-negative staphylococci (20,24). This was not associated with PA catheter colonization or bloodstream infection.

A number of investigators (23,24,29,34,38,43,61–64) have demonstrated low-level contamination of the extravascular portion of the PA catheter inside the external protective plastic sleeve (mean frequency of contamination, 9%). Concordance with colonized PA catheters, however, was uncommon, and concordance with bloodstream infection was rare (29,62). One randomized trial of these sleeves paradoxically found a slightly higher rate of catheter-related bloodstream infection among patients whose catheters were maintained with a sleeve rather than without one (29). This may have been due to greater manipulation of the catheters with protective sleeves. Another study found no significant difference in colonization of PA catheters protected or unprotected by a sleeve (52); however, the mean duration of catheterization was only 1 day, and there were no bloodstream infections. In the most recent prospective, randomized clinical trial (65), a dramatic reduction in bloodstream infections was associated with the use of protective sleeves in PA catheters left in situ for an average of 3.5 days. Protective sleeves are used almost universally in the United States, and, based on the available data, they may reduce the risk of PA catheter-related infection.

There are conflicting data regarding the risk of seeding an introducer sheath or PA catheter hematogenously from a distant focus of infection. Hematogenous seeding of PA catheters or introducer sheaths was demonstrated in all seven exposed catheters in one study (20) and in seven of nine exposed catheters in another (29). However, most investigators have found hematogenous seeding of introducer sheaths or PA catheters to be infrequent (17,24,25,38,43). This variability may reflect differences in the pathogens involved and types of infection seen in these investigations.

Conclusively demonstrating the source of microbes causing PA catheter-related bloodstream infection requires obtaining cultures from all potential sources of infection and utilizing molecular fingerprinting techniques to unequivocally determine concordance among isolates. In a prospective study of 297 PA catheters (38), colonization was found among 58 introducers and 20 PA catheters, and there were two cases of catheter-related bloodstream infection. Seventeen of the 20 colonized PA catheters had concordant growth on the introducer. Using molecular subtyping, 80% of colonized catheters had concordant growth with organisms isolated from the insertion site, 17% with contaminated hubs, and 19% with organisms found on the extravascular portion of the PA catheter within the protective sleeve. Isolates from colonized PA catheters were most likely to show concordance with colonized introducer sheaths (71%). Only two of the 38 catheters exposed to bloodstream infection originating from a remote focus of infection became colonized hematogenously. In another study using molecular subtyping of clinical isolates, five of 442 PA catheters were associated with bloodstream infection (43).

All seven cases of PA catheter-associated bloodstream infections in which molecular fingerprinting was employed were associated with concordant growth of the introducer, whereas only three had concordant growth of the PA catheter segment itself (38,43). In each case, the introducer sheath had been in place for at least 5 days. Since most clinicians use an introducer sheath, it is the only point of contact between a catheter segment and skin at the insertion site. Based on the above information, microbial pathogens appear to migrate extraluminally along the transcutaneous tract of the introducer, but in only an occasional case do they migrate distally to the PA catheter itself and cause bloodstream infection. Contamination of the introducer with skin flora during insertion may also be responsible for the strong association between introducer colonization and bloodstream infection. Frequent manipulation of the introducer hub may also contribute to the association between introducer colonization and Swan-Ganz catheter-related bloodstream infection. Four of the seven bloodstream infections were associated with concordant growth at the insertion site, and an equal number involved concordant growth at the catheter hub. Two of the seven PA catheter-related bloodstream infections involved contaminated infusate; however, infusate specimens were obtained only at the time of catheter removal, and this may underestimate the incidence of infusate contamination and the potential importance of this source of bloodstream infection. The extravascular portion of the PA catheter under the protective sleeve was colonized with concordant growth of organisms in one case of Swan-Ganz catheter-related bloodstream infection. Therefore, despite the advent of this technologic advance, PA catheter colonization underneath the protective sleeve may still occur, with serious consequences. Hematogenous seeding of the Swan-Ganz catheter was demonstrated in only one of the seven cases of Swan-Ganz catheter-related bloodstream infections. Although this supports most of the earlier studies, which did not employ molecular fingerprinting, lower thresholds to collect blood cultures by some clinicians may have led to an underestimation of this association.

In summary, it appears that the insertion site and the catheter hub are equally important sources of the microbes causing most serious Swan-Ganz catheter-related infections. The introducer, rather than the PA catheter itself, is the throughway for most pathogens invading the bloodstream. This likely reflects the fact that the introducer, not the PA catheter, is in direct contact with the skin. The association of introducer hub colonization with the increased risk of introducer-associated bloodstream infection requires further study.

G. Epidemics

Although there have been 28 epidemics of nosocomial sepsis associated with arterial pressure monitoring (66–69), few were traced to hemodynamic monitoring with PA catheters. In one outbreak, five cases of PA catheter-related *Enterobacter* bacteremia were traced to failure of chemical disinfection involving reusable plastic chamber domes in the monitoring circuit (70). The essential steps in dealing with a nosocomial epidemic of bloodstream infection have been outlined elsewhere (71) and should be followed if this is suspected.

H. Pathogenesis

After PA catheter insertion, microbial pathogens colonizing the insertion site or hub can quickly migrate toward the catheter tip and into the bloodstream (72,73). In some instances, extensive biofilm can be seen covering the PA catheter surface 24 hours after insertion and, in half of PA catheters, at the time of removal (25). The biofilm consists of a bacterial polysaccharide glycocalyx slime substance, host-derived proteins, and platelets. Bacterial adhesins promote attachment to intravascular catheters (74,75). Catheter-associated thrombus is associated with an increased risk of infection (76,77) since platelets and host-derived proteins—fibronectin, thrombospondin, and vitronectin—enhance binding of microbial pathogens, such as *S. aureus*, to the catheter surface (78–80). Once microbes are bound to a catheter, they may be difficult to eradicate for various reasons: the protective nature of the polysaccharide glycocalyx slime substance (81); the inability of neutrophils to kill these adherent bacteria (82); and reduced antibiotic susceptibility of these sessile bacteria, compared to planktonic ones (83).

I. Types of Infection

The animal model of infective endocarditis involves placing a vascular catheter into the internal jugular vein of a laboratory animal and passing the catheter into the right ventricle, producing a sterile vegetation. Bacteria are then introduced into the bloodstream which infect the vegetation, producing a syndrome similar to infective endocarditis in humans (84–86). To function properly, PA catheters must be passed through the right atrium and ventricle, leaving patients particularly vulnerable to developing endocarditis. Noninfective endocardial lesions (endocardial hemorrhage, thrombi, valvular thickening, or overt vegetations) are quite common after Swan-Ganz catheterization (16,87–95) and are found in as many as 91% of autopsies (94). These lesions would seem likely to predispose patients to infective endocarditis. Approximately 2% of patients who had undergone Swan-Ganz catheterization shortly before death have autopsy findings consistent with infective endocarditis (87–89,96–101). Most cases of PA catheter-related endocarditis occurred after prolonged catheterization, usually more than 3 days (89,96,101), and involved the right atrium or ventricular endocardium or the tricuspid or pulmonic valves, as single or multiple lesions (89). Pulmonic valve vegetations appear to derive almost exclusively from Swan-Ganz catheters.

Septic thrombophlebitis is an occasional complication of central venous catheter use (102–105). Local signs of venous occlusion may be seen, such as ipsilateral neck, chest wall, or arm swelling, yet the insertion site is often devoid of inflammation. Persistent high-grade bacteremia or fungemia despite removal of an infected PA catheter usually indicates septic thrombophlebitis or infective endocarditis, particularly when it involves staphylococci or *Candida* (102–105). Only a single case of great central vein septic thrombophlebitis associated with

Swan-Ganz catheterization has been reported (104). This may reflect the fact that the duration of catheterization is generally shorter with Swan-Ganz catheters than other central venous catheters. Underreporting of this catastrophic form of catheter-related bloodstream infection events is also very likely.

Septic pulmonary emboli and infarction can also be seen in patients with PA catheter-related bloodstream infection, secondary to septic thrombophlebitis (97) or infective endocarditis (87,89,96–99). Rarely, pulmonary artery mycotic aneurysm may complicate PA catheterization (106) or lung abscess and empyema, deriving from secondary infection of a coexistent pulmonary infarct (107,108).

J. Diagnosis of Infection

The signs and symptoms of patients with intravascular catheter-related bloodstream infection are indistinguishable from bloodstream infection due to other etiologies. Nevertheless, there are certain clinical findings which significantly increase the likelihood that bloodstream infection is secondary to a central venous or pulmonary artery catheter: bloodstream infection in a nonsurgical patient; bacteremia due to *S. aureus*, coagulase-negative staphylococci, or *Candida*; central venous catheter in situ; and no identifiable localized infection (109). Available techniques to diagnose catheter-related infection without catheter removal include quantitative cultures (49,110) or simply Gram stain (111) of the insertion site, and/or quantitative catheter hub cultures (112). All of these methods have relatively high positive and negative predictive values if done in the context of a febrile patient without an obvious source of infection. However, most clinicians remove a suspect device and culture it by one of the following methods: semiquantitative roll-plate culture on solid media (113); quantitative culture in liquid media by sonication (109), vortexing (114), or flushing the catheter lumen (115). The sensitivity of PA catheter cultures may be increased by culturing at least two catheter segments, such as the intradermal segment and tip (116). Using a combination of two culture techniques increases the yield (117) but may be impractical for routine cultures in the clinical microbiology laboratory. Performing central venous and Swan-Ganz catheter cultures at the bedside using the roll-plate technique also increases the yield of catheter cultures (118). Gram stain and acridine orange stain of catheter segments (119,120) or of blood drawn through the catheter (121,122) all appear to be sensitive and specific rapid diagnostic techniques. The latter methodology has the advantage of being able to diagnose catheter infection without removing the catheter.

Catheter-related bloodstream infection can also be diagnosed without catheter removal by using quantitative blood cultures using a commercial lysis centrifugation method (Isolator; Wampole Laboratories, Cranburg, NJ), or pourplate technique (123–125). With true catheter-related bloodstream infection, there is a marked step up in the concentration of organisms, usually five- to tenfold, in catheter-drawn, as compared with percutaneously drawn, blood cultures. Use of both Isolator and standard, nonquantitative radiometric blood cultures (BACTEC; Becton-Dickinson, Cokeysville, MD) appears to improve the yield of blood cultures when striving to diagnose intravascular catheter-related bloodstream infection (124).

When using standard (qualitative) blood cultures, collection of an adequate volume of blood for culture is critically important (126). However, in a recent study of adult patients (127), collection of only 1.5 ml of blood and inoculation into pediatric Isolator tubes for lysis centrifugation (E.I. Du Pont de Nemours, Wilmington, DE) was surprisingly sensitive (83%) and specific (100%) for the diagnosis of catheter-related bloodstream infection.

K.   Management of Infection

Unexplained fever in a patient without severe sepsis—hypotension, mental status changes, or decreased urine output—should prompt the patient's physician to obtain blood cultures. If quantitative blood cultures are available, one set of blood cultures can be obtained through the catheter and the other set from a peripheral vein. If quantitative blood cultures are unavailable, two sets of percutaneously drawn blood cultures should be obtained, and consideration should be made for removing the catheter. If an intravascular catheter is still necessary for optimal patient care, a new catheter can be inserted in another site or in the original site over a guide wire. However, the second catheter should be removed if the original one is found to be heavily colonized. Rapid diagnostic tests, such as Gram stain or acridine orange stain of blood obtained through the catheter, may also be used. Gram stain of the insertion site may also be helpful in this setting.

In the case of a septic patient with a PA catheter in place and in whom (1) there is no obvious other source of infection or purulence at the insertion site, (2) bloodstream infection has already been documented with staphylococci or *Candida*, or (3) the catheter has been in situ for more than 4 days, the catheter should be removed in its entirety, including the introducer sheath and PA catheter. Both should be sent for culture, in addition to obtaining blood cultures and rapid staining procedures where available. Failure to remove a colonized Swan-Ganz catheter associated with bacteremia or candidemia places the patient at undue risk of developing septic great central vein thrombophlebitis or infective endocarditis. If continued hemodynamic monitoring is necessary, this can be accomplished with insertion of a PA catheter into a new site or by noninvasive means (128). If the original catheter remained in place but quantitative blood cultures revealed a marked step up in the number of organisms that grew from the catheter-drawn, as compared to the percutaneously drawn, blood cultures, or if Gram stain or acridine orange stain of blood drawn through the catheter reveal bacteria or fungi, then the catheter should also be removed. Lastly, if the insertion site or catheter hub have significant numbers of pathogens found on quantitative culture or Gram stain, then consideration should be made for removal of the Swan-Ganz catheter in its entirety.

Removal of a heavily colonized intravenous catheter will often lead to resolution of a patient's fever (129). However, a parenteral course of antibiotics should be considered in the clinical setting of a febrile patient with negative blood cultures in whom the removed PA catheter is heavily colonized, especially by *S. aureus* or *Candida*. This is because the catheter was in close proximity to the tricuspid and pulmonic valves, which may be more susceptible to becoming secondarily infected due to catheter-induced endocardial and valvular lesions (88–90, 92,130). This recommendation may be especially important if the patient is known to have underlying valvular heart disease, especially a prosthetic valve (131). There are no available data to dictate the appropriate duration of antibiotic therapy in a febrile patient whose Swan-Ganz catheter tip reveals significant growth in the absence of another identifiable source of infection and in the face of negative blood cultures, but, a brief, 5- to 7-day course of antimicrobial therapy is reasonable in this setting.

If empiric antimicrobial therapy is used, pending the results of blood and catheter cultures, a glycopeptide antibiotic, such as vancomycin or teicoplanin, where available, should be used initially to cover methicillin-resistant staphylococci. Addition of an antibiotic effective against nosocomial gram-negative bacilli may be reasonable based on the clinical setting. Definitive therapy of PA catheter-related bloodstream infection should be based on microbiologic identification and susceptibility of the pathogens involved. The appropriate duration of antibiotic therapy for PA catheter-related bloodstream infection should be determined by a number of factors: the presence of underlying valvular heart disease or evidence of an endovascular infection—endocarditis or septic thrombophlebitis; evidence of a distant metastatic infection; or persistent, high-grade bacteremia after catheter withdrawal and initiation of appropriate antimicrobial therapy (132). If endocarditis is suspected, transesophageal echocardiography has greater sensitivity than transthoracic echocardiography for detecting vegetations—especially small vegetations, those involving prosthetic valves, or those in the right side of the heart (133,134).

Septic thrombophlebitis of the central great veins should be suspected, in the setting of persistent bacteremia or fungemia without evidence of endocarditis. The diagnosis can often be made by noninvasive techniques, such as ultrasonography (135), computerized tomography (135–137), or magnetic resonance imaging (137); however, venography remains the diagnostic standard (102–104). If bacteremia due to pathogens other than *S. aureus* clears within 3 days and the patient is without underlying valvular heart disease or clinical evidence of endocarditis, septic thrombophlebitis, or metastatic infection, then parenteral antimicrobial therapy should be administered for 7 to 14 days. However, with uncomplicated catheter-related *S. aureus* bacteremia, 14 days of parenteral antimicrobial therapy should be used (133,138–143), although some controversy remains regarding this recommendation (144). All patients with catheter-related candidemia should receive antimicrobial therapy, even if the patient's fever resolves after catheter withdrawal and subsequent blood cultures are negative (145–147). Candidemia that rapidly clears should be treated with 3 to 5 mg/kg of intravenous amphotericin B administered over 14 days (145,147,149,150), or with intravenous fluconazole (150).

Infective endocarditis originating from a colonized Swan-Ganz catheter should be treated similar to endocarditis unrelated to a catheter, with prolonged parenteral bactericidal antimicrobial therapy, using a dosage regimen appropriate for endocarditis (151). However, for patients with right-sided catheter-related bacterial endocarditis, a corollary may be drawn between these patients and those who have acquired right-sided endocarditis secondary to IV drug use, in whom 2 weeks of parenteral antibiotic therapy may be effective, especially with rapid resolution of bacteremia and in the absence of septic pulmonary emboli (140,142).

Swan-Ganz catheter-related septic thrombophlebitis of the central great veins can be reliably treated in most instances, without surgical intervention. With bacterial infection, a 4-week course of parenteral antimicrobial therapy is recommended (102–104). If *Candida* is the pathogen involved, 0.5 to 0.7 mg/kg/day of amphotericin B should be administered for a total dose of approximately 20 mg/kg (103). The efficacy of intravenous fluconazole in this clinical setting is unknown; however, it is more likely to be useful in patients initially treated with amphotericin B and in whom high-grade candidemia has resolved. Anticoagulation should also be considered unless contraindicated (102–104). Thrombolytic therapy used in the setting of central great vein septic thrombophlebitis does not appear to improve outcome and is not recommended (152).

All patients with Swan-Ganz catheter-related bloodstream infection should be monitored closely for several weeks after completing therapy, especially patients with prolonged bloodstream infection, to detect late-appearing metastatic infection or relapse of the original endovascular infection.

L. Prevention of Infection

Preventive strategies aimed at reducing the risk of intravascular catheter-related infection have been reviewed in detail elsewhere (153). The risk of catheter-related infection can be reduced by placement of the catheter in the subclavian vein rather than the internal jugular vein (Table 3). However, the reduced risk of infection at the subclavian insertion site should be weighted against the other risks, such as bleeding secondary to vascular injury (157), which is more easily managed when the catheter has been inserted in the internal jugular vein. The latter insertion site may be preferred for patients with coagulopathy or significant thrombocytopenia.

Table 3 Catheter-Related Infections: Internal Jugular vs. Subclavian Approach

Colonization		Bloodstream infection		
IJ (%)	SC (%)	IJ (%)	SC (%)	Ref.
19	7	—	—	18
16	37[a]	—	—	154
21	10[a]	—	—	114
28	15[a]	—	—	155
22	10[a]	—	—	156
35	14[a]	—	—	46
		10	3[a]	37
27	4[a]	1	0	38

[a]$P < 0.05$.
Abbreviations: IJ = internal jugular vein; SC = subclavian vein.
Source: Adapted with permission from Ref. 153.

To reduce the risk of Swan-Ganz catheter-related infection (38,40,50) and exposure to bloodborne pathogens (158), a long-sleeved, sterile surgical gown, sterile gloves, mask, eye protection, and hat should be worn during catheter insertion, and the site should be covered by a large sterile sheet drape. These same precautions should be undertaken if the catheter is exchanged over a guide wire. In this latter setting, after vigorously cleansing the insertion site with a cutaneous antiseptic, inserting the guide wire, removing the catheter, and cleansing the site once again with an antiseptic agent, the operator should reglove and ideally redrape the site, as the original gloves and drapes may have become contaminated from manipulation of the original catheter.

Povidone-iodine is the antiseptic used most frequently in the United States for cleansing intravascular catheter insertion sites (159). However, three clinical trials have found aqueous chlorhexidine to be superior to povidone-iodine at reducing the risk of catheter-related infection (160–162); aqueous chlorhexidine also appears to be superior to alcohol in this regard (160). Tincture of iodine is superior to povidone-iodine as a cutaneous antiseptic (163) and may be preferred for this reason. After tincture of iodine is used to cleanse an insertion site, it may need to be removed from the skin with alcohol to reduce the potential for irritation. Unfortunately, there are yet no commercially available preparations of chlorhexidine approved in the United States for use at intravascular catheter insertion sites. Therefore, iodine tincture may be the disinfectant of choice in the United States at the present time, whereas aqueous or, preferably, alcoholic chlorhexidine preparations should be used in countries where it is available and approved for this purpose. For institutions using povidone-iodine, a 3- to 5-min skin preparation should be used (164).

The efficacy of antibiotic prophylaxis during Swan-Ganz catheter insertion has not been studied in a prospective fashion; however, this practice is probably unwarranted based on prospective studies with central venous catheters (165) and because the risk of promoting microbial resistance with routine prophylactic antibiotic use outweighs the potential benefits (166,167).

Use of an external protective plastic sleeve may reduce the risk of PA catheter-related infection by minimizing touch contamination during manipulation of the PA catheter (65). Use of heparin-bonded Swan-Ganz catheters is associated with a reduced risk of catheter-related infection because benzalkonium chloride is used on the catheter surface as a cationic surfactant to bond the anionic heparin to the catheter (60). Therefore, we believe heparin-bonded catheters should be used rather than non-heparin-bonded catheters unless there are clinical contraindications, such as heparin-induced thrombocytopenia (168,169).

A biodegradable silver-impregnated collagen cuff (Vitacuff; Vitaphore, San Carlos, CA) attached to a central venous catheter or Swan-Ganz introducer just prior to insertion acts as a tissue interface barrier, similar to the Dacron cuffs of Hickman and Broviac catheters. In three prospective, randomized trials in which catheters were left in place for less than 2 to 3 weeks, the silver-impregnated cuff reduced the risk of catheter colonization and bloodstream infection (170–172); favorable results were seen in the study that included Swan-Ganz catheters (170). In one study of a similar duration of catheterization, the cuff was associated with an increased incidence of catheter-related bloodstream infection (173). Since the cuff is on the outside of the catheter, it does not prevent intraluminal transmission of pathogens from contaminated hubs or infusate. Similarly, the cuff does not appear to prevent catheter-related infection when a catheter is exchanged over a guide wire if the initial catheter was colonized (170).

A recent meta-analysis concluded that the use of transparent, semipermeable polyurethane dressings are associated with a threefold increased risk of catheter sepsis, compared with gauze dressings (174). However, in a recent large, prospective trial of 442 Swan-Ganz catheters, there was no difference in the incidence of catheter colonization or catheter-related bloodstream infection between gauze and transparent dressing groups (43). For this reason, either standard sterile gauze and tape or polyurethane transparent dressings are acceptable for use on the insertion site of Swan-Ganz catheters. Additionally, transparent dressings may be left in place up to 5 days between dressing changes, without increased risk of Swan-Ganz catheter-related infection (43). Newer, more permeable transparent dressings do not appear to reduce the risk of Swan-Ganz catheter-related infection, compared to standard transparent dressings (43).

Although the application of topical antimicrobial agents to the catheter insertion site may confer some protection against microbial invasion, the efficacy of this intervention remains surprisingly controversial in light of the importance of the insertion site as a reservoir of potential pathogens. There are no published studies utilizing this preventive strategy with Swan-Ganz catheters; however, it is reasonable to believe that the findings of investigations with other short-term central venous catheters are applicable. Although triple antibiotic ointments (Polymyxin, Neosporin, and Bacitracin) may reduce the incidence of bacterial catheter-related infection, use of this ointment may increase the risk of *Candida* infection (55,175). For this reason, triple antibiotic ointments are not recommended for use on central venous catheter insertion sites, especially for patients at increased risk of fungal infection. Mupirocin (Bactroban; SmithKline Beecham, Philadelphia) applied to insertion sites has been demonstrated to significantly reduce the incidence of catheter colonization (176,177). However, it is not recommended for this purpose because widespread use of this important topical agent may lead to greater resistance (178,179) and negate its utility for decolonizing patients and healthcare workers who are nasal carriers of Methicillin-resistant *S. aureus.*

Two prospective, randomized trials of topical povidone-iodine ointment applied to insertion sites have had conflicting results. Although one investigation carried out in a surgical intensive care unit found no benefit (154), in a more recent trial of patients with hemodialysis catheters there was a fourfold reduction in the incidence of catheter-related bloodstream infection (180). In a recent, non-randomized clinical trial using historical controls, the use of a chlorhexidine-impregnated urethane sponge composite (Biopatch; Johnson & Johnson, Arlington, TX) led to a reduction in central venous catheter-related bloodstream infections, from 21 to 13 per 1000 catheter-days (181).

The use of topical antimicrobial agents should be considered as an optional adjunctive measure and may be useful in instances in which the incidence of Swan-Ganz catheter-related infection remains high despite other interventions. If a topical agent is used, 10% povidone-iodine ointment is recommended. Although promising, the value of the Biopatch on the site of intravascular catheter insertion, including Swan-Ganz catheters, awaits confirmation in prospective randomized trials.

There are a number of measures aimed at reducing the risk of in-use contamination of Swan-Ganz catheter infusate and components. The delivery system should be manipulated as little as possible. No one should handle or especially enter the system without first washing their hands. Entering the monitoring circuit for the purpose of blood drawing should be limited as much as possible.

The number of stopcocks in the system should be minimized. Stopcocks should be wiped with a cutaneous antiseptic, such as using an alcohol pledget, prior to manipulation (182). Closed systems used for measuring the cardiac output by thermal dilution appears to reduce the risk of injectate contamination (183). All calibration devices, heparinized solutions, and other apparatus that come in direct contact with the fluid within the monitoring circuit must be sterile (66). Dextrose-containing solutions should not be used in hemodynamic monitoring infusions (66). Totally disposable transducer assemblies are preferred and should not be reused (66). Reusable transducers should be subjected to high-level chemical disinfection or, preferably, sterilization with ethylene oxide between patients, or when the monitoring circuit (chamber dome and continuous-flow device) is replaced (66). Centralized decontamination provides more consistent quality control; however, in an emergent situation, decontamination of reusable transducers with alcohol pledgets does not appear to increase the risk of catheter-related infection (184,185). The addition of sodium metabisulfite to a heparin-containing flush solution reduced the incidence of left atrial catheter-related infections in one study (186). However, before recommending this preventive strategy, prospective randomized studies must be done to confirm these findings and to provide data regarding the safety of these infusions.

If disposable transducers and chamber domes are used with infusions for hemodynamic monitoring, there is no need to replace the transducer assembly and other components of the delivery system, including flush solutions, more frequently than every 4 days (187). In a recent prospective trial including arterial, central venous, and Swan-Ganz catheters, the pressure monitoring infusion systems were not replaced at regular intervals (188). Only 4 of 1991 cultures of infusion fluid had significant growth, and all occurred within 48 hours of a bag change. Routine replacement of the pressure-monitoring infusion system at 72-hour intervals, as was the standard of care in the institution, would not have prevented this contamination. The new policy also led to a significant cost savings to the institution. Based on this information, it appears that the pressure-monitoring infusion system—including the transducer and associated plastic ware, tubing, and flush solutions—may not need routine replacement.

Use of an innovative catheter hub incorporating an iodine tincture reservoir reduced the incidence of serious catheter-related infection (189). However, this novel hub is not approved for use with intravascular devices in the United States at the present time. Use of needle-free connectors may reduce the risk of needle-stick injuries but may increase the risk of catheter-related infection (190–193). Therefore, if a needleless system is to be brought into an institution, careful monitoring of the catheter-associated bloodstream infections should be done.

Although there remains some controversy surrounding the safe duration of Swan-Ganz catheterization, the risk of infection is low if the catheter remains in place for no longer than 4 days (Fig. 3). It behooves the user of this device to assess the need for continued catheterization on a daily basis and to remove the catheter as soon as feasible. If Swan-Ganz catheterization beyond 4 days is considered necessary, there are three options: the catheter may be left in place, accepting that the risk of infection will begin to rise sharply; a new catheter can be placed in a new site, gaining another 4 days of very low risk; or, using a guide wire, the catheter can be exchanged with a new one, cultures of the original catheter should be done, and the new catheter should be removed if colonization is found, especially with more pathogenic organisms such as *S. aureus* or *Candida*. In the future, antiseptic-coated PA catheters may become available, similar to those found to be effective in reducing the incidence of central venous catheter-related bloodstream infections (194–197).

II.   PERIPHERAL ARTERIAL CATHETERS

A.   Introduction

Peripheral arterial catheters are commonly used to monitor the blood pressure and arterial blood gases (pH, PaO_2, $PaCO_2$) and oxygenation of critically ill or unstable patients. In a recent monthlong survey of all intensive care units in one hospital, the number of arterial catheter-days/total patient-days was 0.57 (2). The use of these catheters was greatest in the cardiothoracic ICU and lowest in the pediatric ICU—0.94 and 0.16 catheter-days/patient-days, respectively. In a recent point prevalence survey of U.S. adult ICUs, 40% of patients had arterial catheters (198).

B.   Features of the Catheter

Peripheral arterial catheters are typically made of Teflon or polyurethane. Arterial catheters are complex medical devices (Fig. 4), similar to Swan-Ganz pulmonary artery catheters. Besides the arterial catheter itself, an infusion designated for arterial pressure monitoring also includes an extended length of tubing connected to a chamber that interfaces with an electromechanical transducer. A continuous-flow device is in the line and permits periodic flushes to maintain patency of the system. This device is connected to a pressurized bag of heparin-containing flush solution. The infusion system differs from many others used in clinical practice in that the infusate characteristically runs very slowly, the fluid column interfaces with an electromechanical transducer through the diaphragm of a chamber dome, the system may contain multiple stopcocks, and the chamber dome and transducer are often attached to the patient's arm, potentially vulnerable to contamination by cutaneous microflora.

During the first decade of widescale use of arterial pressure monitoring in the U.S., chamber domes were routinely reused as a cost-saving measure. When it was recognized that failure to reliably decontaminate chamber domes between patients led to many epidemics of gram-negative bacteremia, manufacturers

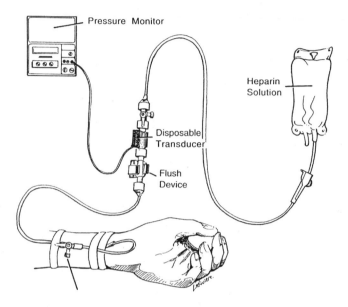

Figure 4 Schematic of a peripheral arterial catheter placed in the radial artery.

developed disposable chamber domes, which are now widely used. Despite this intervention, the permanent transducers interfacing with disposable chamber domes also became contaminated, leading to infusate contamination and epidemic bloodstream infections. Completely disposable modular systems were then developed incorporating a continuous-flow device, chamber dome, and electromechanical transducer. Increasing numbers of hospitals have moved toward the exclusive use of these disposable systems.

C. Incidence of Infection

Many prospective studies have addressed the risk of peripheral arterial catheter-related infection (17,18,28,32,33,36,40,42,199–210). However, in only one of these studies were cultures performed of all possible sources of catheter-related infection (209). Table 4 summarizes the 18 studies published after 1980, in which cultures were routinely carried out at the time of catheter withdrawal. In studies using semiquantitative or quantitative catheter culture methods, 0% to 22.6% of peripheral arterial catheters had significant growth (mean incidence of colonization 6.4%; median 4.2%). The mean incidence of arterial catheter-related blood-

Table 4   Incidence of Peripheral Arterial Catheter-Related Infection

Study	Catheters	Catheter culture method	Colonized (%)	Catheter-related bloodstream infection
Singh et al. (17)	52	SQ	11.5	0
Pinella et al. (18)	172	SQ	4.1	0
Kaye et al. (28)	102	NR	13.7	1.0
Shinozaki et al. (201)	170	NR	NR	0.6
Thomas et al. (202)	141	Q	2.8	0
Russell et al. (203)	261	NR	NR	1.1
Thomas et al. (204)	68	Q	20.5	NR
Damen et al. (32)	584	SQ	1.2	0
Sommers et al. (205)	46	SQ	2.1	0
Damen et al. (33)	349	SQ	4.3	0
Ducharme et al. (206)	70	SQ	0	0
Norwood et al. (207)	51	SQ	15.7	0
Leroy et al. (208)	164	SQ	22.6	0
Maki et al. (209)	489	SQ	3.1	0.8
Eyer et al. (36)	250	SQ	3.6	2.8
Furfaro et al. (210)	340	SQ	2.9	0
Bull et al. (40)	256	SQ	18.0	0.8
Raad et al. (42)	121	SQ	15.5	5.6

Abbreviations: SQ = semiquantitative roll-plate method; Q = quantitative by vortex method; NR = not reported.

stream infection is 0.62% (range 0% to 5.6%). It is not possible to confidently determine the incidence of arterial catheter-related bloodstream infection per 1000 catheter-days since few studies gave information regarding the number of catheter-days.

D. Microbial Profile

Coagulase-negative staphylococci, predominately *S. epidermidis*, are the most common pathogens responsible for peripheral arterial catheter colonization and bloodstream infection. Of studies delineating the pathogens involved with these infections (17,32,33,201,207,208), 59% of arterial catheters were colonized with coagulase-negative staphylococci, 17% with other gram-positive pathogens, 23%

with gram-negative bacteria, and 2% with yeast. In these prospective studies, there were only seven catheter-related bloodstream infections—four caused by coagulase-negative staphylococci, two by *Enterococcus*, and one by *Pseudomonas aeruginosa*.

E. Risk Factors

Two studies used multivariate analysis to determine independent risk factors for catheter-related infection (33,209). Heavy cutaneous colonization of the catheter insertion site (relative risk 10), age less than 1 year, prolonged dwell time in children, and insertion in an old site over a guide wire were each independent risk factors for peripheral arterial catheter-related infection. Using univariate analysis, a number of investigators have found other risk factors for peripheral arterial catheter-related infection, as described below.

1. Insertion Site

Although heavy cutaneous colonization is associated with arterial catheter-related infection (209), there are conflicting data regarding the association of inflammation with arterial catheter colonization. Some investigators (210) have found that inflammation was significantly associated with catheter colonization; others (206,208), however, have found that inflammation at the catheter insertion site was not predictive of catheter colonization. In a related study (207), cultures of the arterial catheter insertion site had a 57% and a 100% positive and negative predictive value, respectively. Based on this information, heavy arterial catheter insertion site colonization is associated with infection. However, the absence of insertion site colonization in a febrile, catheterized patient should suggest arterial catheter infection associated with a colonized catheter hub, contaminated infusate, or another site of infection.

2. Site of Insertion

Although a number of investigators have compared the incidence of infection associated with radial artery, as compared to femoral artery, insertion (17,33,202, 203), only one investigator prospectively randomized catheters to insertion at these two sites (202). Most of the studies were limited by the small number of catheters studied. Combining these investigations, there is a trend toward an increased risk of infection associated with femoral catheterization—catheter colonization and bloodstream infection 3% and 0.4%, respectively, with radial artery insertion, compared to 7% and 1.3%, respectively, for femoral artery insertion. A confounding variable in these studies is that femoral catheter insertion may be associated with more prolonged dwell time (203). Also, the number of femoral arterial catheters studied is small. Although the largest of these studies did not describe the number of patients who had radial vs. femoral arterial insertion, a significantly increased incidence of catheter colonization in the latter site was noted (33); however, using Kaplan-Meyer plots, the risk of infection associated with femoral artery insertion did not increase over time.

Drawing firm conclusions regarding the risk of infection associated with insertion in the femoral vs. the radial artery must await the results of larger prospective, randomized trials. At present, it would appear that decisions regarding which site to use for peripheral arterial catheter insertion should be based on the clinical setting.

3. Barrier Precautions

In the only prospective study of barrier precautions for arterial catheter insertion, investigators using sequential enrollment compared the incidence of catheter-related infection utilizing two different preventive strategies associated with catheter insertion (40). In the first phase, physicians inserting arterial catheters donned hat, mask, and sterile gloves. In the latter half of the study a surgical gown was also worn by the catheter inserter, and a more prolonged, 5-min skin preparation was done. The incidence of catheter colonization was 23.7% without and 14.7% with full barrier precautions and prolonged skin preparation ($P < 0.001$). It is difficult to determine the efficacy of full barrier precautions from this study since the duration of cutaneous antisepsis also varied. In many of the published studies (Table 3), sterile gloves and drapes were used, but mask, hat, and gown were not worn during arterial catheter insertion. We believe that sterile gloves and drapes are sufficient barrier precautions during insertion of these catheters.

4. Guide Wires

A single study prospectively randomized patients (1) to guide wire arterial catheter exchange every 7 days; (2) catheter insertion into a new site every 7 days; or (3) prolonged catheterization without routine guide wire exchange (36). There was no significant difference in the incidence of catheter-related infection in any of these three patient groups; however, the incidence of infection was low and the power of the analysis was very limited based on the small number of patients studied. In a nonrandomized prospective clinical trial (209), the incidence of catheter-related bloodstream infection was 3.7% in patients who had arterial catheters placed in an old site over a guide wire, as compared to 0% in patients whose arterial catheters were inserted in a new site ($P < 0.01$). All six arterial catheter-related bloodstream infections were in the guide wire exchange group. Data from these studies suggest that routine guide wire exchange of peripheral arterial catheters does not reduce the incidence of systemic catheter-related infection but rather increases the risk.

5. Duration of Catheterization

A number of investigators found that prolonged catheter insertion was associated with an increased cumulative risk of peripheral arterial catheter-related infection (28,33,40,42,202,208); however, others did not find this to be the case (17,36,210). Although the cumulative incidence of arterial catheter-related infection increases with time, the risk of infection per day of catheterization (i.e., the incidence density) does not increase with prolonged catheterization (18,208,210). In three prospective trials (201,202,210) the arterial catheter, transducer assembly, and associated plasticware were not routinely changed. The combined incidence of catheter colonization and catheter-related bloodstream infection was 2.9% and 0.2%, respectively—both comparable to median rates for all prospective clinical trials. One group of investigators (187) found that the incidence of transducer fluid contamination was not significantly different when the fluids were randomized to be changed every 2 days or every 4 days, yet, the cumulative prevalence of transducer fluid contamination was greater when the fluids were changed every 8 days compared with every 2 days. In another study (201) none of 170 transducer fluid samples were contaminated despite a policy that allowed the catheters, transducers, and associated plasticware to remain in place without routine changes. More recently, the incidence of transducer fluid contamination was found to be extremely low despite prolonged arterial and Swan-Ganz catheter dwell times, and routine replacement of the transducer fluid every 3 days would not have prevented the few cases of contamination that occurred (188).

Based on the above information, it would appear that routine replacement of peripheral arterial catheters, transducers, and associated plasticware is unnecessary so long as the insertion site is devoid of purulence or fluctuance and the patient does not have unexplained fever or other symptoms of occult infection that may be due to the catheter itself.

6. Hematogenous Seeding

In prospective studies, only 3 of 94 arterial catheters exposed to bacteremia or fungemia from a distant focus of infection had concordant growth on the catheter surface when removed (207–210). One episode of "rebound bacteremia" was observed associated with hematogenous seeding of an arterial catheter (209). Based on this information, it would appear that the risk of hematogenous seeding of arterial catheters is low, similar to the majority of studies of Swan-Ganz catheters. However, return of fever in previously treated bacteremic or fungemic patients should alert the clinician to the possibility of seeding of the catheter, prompting removal of the catheter for culture if no other source of fever is evident.

7. Dressings

A single study compared the risk of arterial catheter-related bloodstream infection in patients whose catheter insertion site was covered with transparent polyurethane film dressings vs. gauze and tape dressings (58). In this study of 400 arterial catheters, use of transparent dressing replaced every other day increased the risk of catheter-related bloodstream infection more than fivefold. Large, prospective, randomized trials are needed to definitively determine the risk of arterial catheter-associated infection when using transparent vs. gauze and tape dressings. At the present time, we believe that use of gauze and tape dressings on arterial catheter insertion sites may be preferable to transparent polyurethane dressings.

8. Antibiotic Use

Antibiotic use during catheterization has had no impact on the incidence of catheter colonization, including the use of vancomycin (42,208,210). A prospective, randomized trial of central venous catheters also found that prophylactic vancomycin did not reduce the incidence of catheter-related infection (165). Based on these findings and the increased risk of the development of antibiotic resistance with widespread use (166,167), antibiotic prophylaxis should not be used for arterial catheter insertion.

9. Cutaneous Antisepsis

In one clinical trial, patients with arterial catheters were prospectively randomized to have the insertion sites cleansed with aqueous chlorhexidine, alcohol, or povidone-iodine (160). The incidence of catheter-related infection was 0.7%, 4.3%, and 5.6% in each of these groups, respectively. None of the four arterial catheter-related bloodstream infections occurred in the group randomized to chlorhexidine, and the incidence of catheter-related infection was significantly lower than the chlorhexidine group compared to the alcohol and povidone-iodine groups combined ($P = .03$). These data suggest that chlorhexidine is the antiseptic of choice for preparation of insertion sites for arterial catheterization. In another study, arterial catheter colonization was significantly reduced using an antiseptic combining alcoholic chlorhexidine and benzalkonium chloride compared with povidone-iodine (162).

10. Other Risk Factors

In one prospective trial, patients underwent radial arteriography prior to catheter removal (208). Eight percent of the arterial catheters, mean dwell time of 6.5 days, had radiographically evident thrombus formation. However, the incidence of arterial catheter colonization was 25% and 23% in patients with and without evidence of thrombus, respectively. Despite the fact that a number of microbial pathogens, in particular S. aureus, have an avidity for binding to host-derived protein components of thrombus (78–80), the association of thrombus and arterial catheter colonization was not demonstrated in this small study.

The use of an arterial catheter with 120 cm of pressure tubing through which blood was drawn back to clear the line of heparin before sampling has been associated with an increased risk of catheter colonization compared to another arterial pressure monitoring device which had a one-way valve which did not allow blood backflow into the tubing (210).

F.   Sources of Infection

Bacteria and fungi may gain access to a catheterized patient's bloodstream from skin at the insertion site, stopcock contamination, contamination of the transducer assembly, contamination of infusate during preparation or during catheter use, or intraluminal contamination secondary to drawing blood into the line during an episode of bacteremia or fungemia. Cultures of all potential sources of arterial catheter-related infection were performed in only one study (209). Three percent and 2.9% of infusate and hub specimens had significant growth, respectively. Of the six episodes of primary catheter-related bloodstream infection, two each were due to colonization of the skin, hub, and infusate, respectively; one case of catheter-related bloodstream infection had an unidentifiable source. All six primary catheter-related bloodstream infections occurred in patients whose arterial catheters were exchanged over a guide wire and in whom the insertion site was cleansed with povidone-iodine or alcohol, as compared to chlorhexi-dine. Information gathered from this investigation supports the fact that there are myriad potential sources of bloodstream infection in patients with arterial catheters and preventive strategies should be aimed at each of these potential reservoirs.

In one study (207), the incidence of transducer fluid contamination increased significantly when the duration of catheterization was greater than 2 days. These investigators also found that 8 of 14 insertion site cultures with significant growth were associated with concordant growth on a catheter segment. Catheter colonization only occurred in the presence of microbial growth at the insertion site.

Using arterial catheters with a long stagnant column of infusate, another group of investigators found that 12 of 102 transducer fluid cultures had significant microbial growth; 4 of these 12 fluid samples were associated with concordant bacteremia (209). Investigators using arterial catheters without the stagnant column observed that 23 of 98 infusate specimens drawn through the arterial catheter stopcock had significant growth (208); however, in only 4 of the 23 instances of contamination was the arterial catheter tip found to be colonized with concordant growth of bacteria or fungi, and there were no associated bloodstream infections. Interestingly, the incidence of infusate contamination increased during the summer months. In another study (201) of arterial catheters assembled without a stagnant column of infusate, none of the 170 transducer fluids had significant growth sampled despite prolonged catheterization and no routine change of the catheter, transducer assembly, or related plasticware. However, stopcock contamination increased significantly with the duration of catheterization; 10% and 26% of stopcocks used for 4 or less days vs. 5 or more days had significant growth, respectively. In a study of peripheral arterial and PA catheters (187), contamination of transducer fluid collected through a stopcock was not significantly different when the transducers were changed every 2 days or every 4 days; however, contamination increased significantly when transducer fluids were changed every 8 days as compared to every 2 days. The single episode of transducer-related bloodstream infection occurred on the day the transducer fluid was initially contaminated and would have been unaffected by more frequently scheduled replacement of the transducer assembly. In another combined study, infusate contamination was exceedingly rare, 0.1%, despite no routinely scheduled component changes (188). The contamination that occurred would not have been avoided had the institution maintained a policy for changing pressure monitoring components every 3 days.

In some of the studies cited above, the investigators found that the cumulative rate of microbial colonization increased with the duration of catheterization; however, in those prospective studies performed without routinely changing the catheter, transducer, or associated plasticware (201,202,210), the combined incidence of arterial catheter-associated bloodstream infection was very low—0.15%, despite prolonged dwell time. Thus, routine replacement of pressure-monitoring components does not appear to be necessary.

G. Epidemics

Physicians using arterial catheters must remain vigilant in regard to the risk of epidemic bloodstream infection associated with this device. The insidious nature of epidemic arterial catheter-related bloodstream infection is reflected by the fact that these epidemics last on average 11 months before being recognized, compared to 3 months with epidemics of bacteremia deriving from other sources (211). There have been 28 epidemics associated with arterial pressure monitoring published between 1971 and 1990 (66–69; Table 5). Nearly 75% of these epidemics were due to faulty decontamination of the transducer components. This was often the result of using a dilute quaternary ammonium solution, which fostered contamination by resistant nosocomial gram-negative bacilli. Eleven of the 28 epidemics occurred despite using disposable chamber domes with reusable transducer heads. Nine of the epidemics were associated with carriage of the epidemic strain on the hands of healthcare providers. Contamination of fluids that come in contact with the pressure monitoring device, such as heparinized saline flush solutions or contaminated disinfectant solutions, contaminated calibration systems, and contaminated ice used to chill syringes, have all been associated with epidemics.

Table 5 Epidemiology of Epidemic Bloodstream Infections Traced to Arterial Pressure Monitoring

Epidemiology[a]	Epidemics (n)
Faulty decontamination of transducer components	18
Reusable transducer heads used with disposable chamber domes	11
Reusable chamber domes	6
Reuse of disposable chamber domes	3
Carriage of epidemic organisms on hands of users	9
Contaminated heparinized saline solutions	3
Use of dextrose-containing fluids instead of saline	3
Contaminated disinfectant solution	3
Contaminated calibration system	2
Contaminated ice used to chill syringes for blood-gas specimens	1

[a]In many of the outbreaks, more than one source or probable mechanism of contamination was implicated.

Source: Adapted with permission from Ref. 66.

Although manufacturers state that disposable equipment should not be reused, reuse of disposable chamber domes has been associated with epidemic bloodstream infections traced to arterial pressure monitoring. To our knowledge, there have been no large epidemics of arterial catheter-related bloodstream infection traced to contaminated infusions used for pressure monitoring in hospitals exclusively using disposable transducers. However, two unusual cases of arterial catheter-related bloodstream infection due to *Achromobacter xylosoxidans* in one patient and *Flavobacterium meningosepticum* and *Comamonas acidovorans* in another patient, occurred in a hospital using disposable transducers (212). These two unusual cases may have been related to preparation of heparinized saline solutions used for pressure monitoring in a nonsterile environment over a sink. However, environmental cultures of this area failed to grow the bacteria found in the blood of these two patients.

Many of the outbreaks associated with arterial pressure monitoring were caused by unusual nosocomial, gram-negative bacilli, such as *Serratia*, non-*aeruginosa Pseudomonas*, *Burkholderia cepacia*, and *Enterobacter* species, which are able to proliferate in fluids with minimal nutritional support (Table 6). Finding such bacteria in blood cultures of patients with arterial pressure moni-

Table 6   Microbial Profile of Epidemic Nosocomial Bloodstream Infections Deriving From Contamination of Arterial Pressure-Monitoring Systems

	Epidemics (n)	
Pathogen	Single pathogen	Multiple-organism outbreaks
Serratia marcescens	6	—
Burkholderia cepacia	4	—
Comamonas acidovorans	—	2
Pseudomonas fluorescens	—	2
Pseudomonas aeruginosa	1	—
Stenotrophomonas maltophilia	1	—
Pseudomonas spp.	—	1
Enterobacter cloacae	2	2
Enterobacter aerogenes	1	—
Enterobacter spp.	—	1
Achromobacter xylosoxidans	1	—
Acinetobacter calcoaceticus	1	—
Acinetobacter spp.	—	1
Klebsiella oxytoca	1	—
Citrobacter diversus	—	1
Flavobacterium sp.	2	—
Candida parapsilosis	2	—
Candida spp.	1	—

Source: Adapted with permission from Ref. 66.

toring, or blood cultures growing other unusual gram-negative pathogens such as *Achromobacter, Acinetobacter,* or *Flavobacterium,* should alert the clinician to the possibility of an epidemic deriving from contamination of arterial pressure monitoring systems. A single bacteremia may reflect a sporadic endemic case. However, two or more bacteremias should prompt an immediate investigation to determine the etiology and, if due to arterial pressure monitoring, to identify the reservoir and mechanism of introduction of these pathogens into the patients' monitoring systems.

H. Pathogenesis

The pathogenesis of peripheral arterial catheter-related infection is similar to that of Swan-Ganz pulmonary artery catheters. Using electron microscopy, biofilms containing bacteria have been observed on the surface of radial and femoral arterial catheters after 1 day in situ (213). Thus, microbial pathogens may colonize arterial catheters during or shortly after insertion, although early invasion of the bloodstream appears to be uncommon. The reason for the very low incidence of bloodstream infections associated with peripheral arterial catheters may be due in part to the fact that the catheter is made of Teflon or polyurethane. There is less bacterial adherence to Teflon (214) or polyurethane (215) than catheters made of other materials such as polyvinychloride. There is also less avid binding of host-derived proteins, such as fibronectin, to polyurethane catheters, compared to catheters made of other materials (215). The bioburden of microbes at the radial artery insertion site is also significantly less than insertion sites of central venous catheters, and the radial artery site also is less likely to be colonized with microbes other than coagulase-negative staphylococci (50).

In conclusion, although microbes are commonly found on arterial catheter segments, the catheter material and host immune response appear to act together to limit their proliferation and bloodstream infection.

I. Types of Infection

Infective endocarditis associated with arterial pressure monitoring is extremely rare. More commonly reported is localized suppurative infection involving the cannulated artery. In one prospective evaluation of arterial catheters (209), a single case of endarteritis was described involving thrombus formation in the artery that contained *Candida*.

Infected radial artery pseudoaneurysms associated with arterial pressure monitoring has recently been reviewed (216). Six cases occurred at one hospital over 6 years. The duration of radial artery catheterization was significantly longer in patients who developed infected pseudoaneurysms than in patients who had radial arterial catheters in place without this complication—12.5 vs. 4.3 days, respectively ($P < 0.05$). Patients with this complication were older than noninfected patients admitted to the same intensive care units—72 vs. 54 years, respectively ($P < 0.05$). The infected patients also appeared to have had more prolonged stays in the intensive care unit prior to the development of this infection. Most of these patients presented with an expanding or fluctuant pulsatile mass at the radial artery insertion site. Some of these symptoms developed as late as 6 weeks after the catheter had been removed. Five of the six cases of infected radial artery pseudoaneurysms were caused by *S. aureus*. All four infected pseudoaneurysms secondary to radial artery catheterization previously reported in the literature (217–219) were due to infection with *S. aureus*. Infected pseudoaneurysms, predominantly caused by *S. aureus*, have also been reported in association with femoral arterial pressure monitoring (220). Some of the infections involving the radial artery, as well as those associated with brachial artery catheters, have also been associated with Osler's nodes, Janeway lesions, and splinter hemorrhages in the extremity (217–219,221) and, in some cases, surrounding erythema, cellulitis, or, rarely, purulent drainage from the catheter insertion site.

J. Diagnosis of Infection

The microbiologic methods available for the diagnosis of peripheral arterial catheter-related infection are no different from those available for other intravascular devices; unfortunately, there are no systematic investigations comparing the sensitivity and specificity of different methodologies with arterial catheters.

Inflammation surrounding the catheter insertion site does not appear to be sensitive or specific for arterial catheter-related infection (206,208,210). Insertion site cultures had positive and negative predictive values of 57% and 100%, respectively, in one study (207) and may be of some value in accessing the febrile patients with arterial catheters.

K. Management of Infection

In general, the management of peripheral artery catheter-related infection is similar to that of Swan-Ganz catheters. Finding a pulsatile mass around the insertion site while the catheter is in situ, or after catheter withdrawal, should prompt surgical exploration with Gram stain and cultures, and debridement, possibly en bloc resection, if an infected pseudoaneurysm is found. In this setting, intravenous antibiotic therapy should be initiated to cover resistant staphylococci with vancomycin (or teicoplanin where available), pending the results of microbiologic sensitivity testing.

L. Prevention of Infection

As previously mentioned, there appears to be a trend toward greater risk of infection when the femoral artery insertion site is used, but the limitations of these studies make it impossible to draw firm conclusions with regard to the preferred site of peripheral arterial catheterization based on the current literature. What can be said, is that the risk of serious infection appears to be quite low when the catheters are inserted in either the radial or femoral artery.

Although sterile gloves and drapes are likely to be adequate barrier precautions during arterial catheter insertion, a long-sleeved, sterile surgical gown, mask, and eye protection should also be worn to reduce the risk of exposure to potential bloodborne pathogens. Similar to Swan-Ganz catheters, chlorhexidine is the cutaneous antiseptic of choice for insertion site preparation (209). In countries where chlorhexidine is not approved for this purpose, tincture of iodine should be used (163).

There have been no prospective, randomized clinical trials exclusively assessing the risk of arterial catheter-related infection with or without the use of topical antimicrobial agents or comparing gauze and tape to transparent poly-urethane dressings. In one study (33), insertion of peripheral arterial catheters in young children under the age of 1 year and prolonged dwell time in children were found to be independent risk factors of infection. It is not known if the use of an antimicrobial ointment, such as povidone-iodine ointment, on the arterial catheter insertion site in these patients will lead to reduced the risk of infection. Until this issue is resolved, the use of topical antimicrobial agents should be considered optional. Regarding dressings used to cover arterial catheter insertion sites, gauze and tape may be preferable to transparent dressings.

Based on the available data from prospective studies, routine replacement of the arterial catheter, transducer, chamber dome assembly, and associated plas-ticware at scheduled intervals appears to be unnecessary. Because of the epidemics associated with faulty decontamination of reusable transducers, dis-posable, single-use transducer assemblies should be used and discarded after a single use. Other precautions regarding the monitoring equipment are similar to those discussed above in the section on prevention of Swan-Ganz catheter-related infections.

There are no prospective studies of innovative arterial catheter hubs or anti-septic-coated arterial catheters. Because of the low incidence of peripheral arteri-al catheter-related bloodstream infection, it will be difficult to show an impact of any new strategy unless very large numbers of patients are studied. Any new pre-ventive strategy must be shown to be cost-effective, especially since the incidence of infection is so low at the current time. It is important, however, for clinicians using peripheral arterial catheters to assess the need for continued arterial pressure monitoring on a daily basis and remove the catheter as soon as feasible. It is hoped that future technologic advances will permit hemodynamic monitoring of patients noninvasively (128), further reducing their risk of hospital-acquired infection.

REFERENCES

1. Swan HJC, Ganz W, Forrester J, Marcus H, Diamond G, Chonette D. Catheterization of the heart in man with use of a flow-directed balloon-tipped catheter. N Engl J Med 1970; 283:447–451.
2. Tuchschmidt J, Sharma OP. Impact of hemodynamic monitoring in a medical intensive care unit. Crit Care Med 1987; 15:840–843.
3. Shoemaker WC, Appel PL, Kram HB, Waxman K, Lee T-S. Prospective trial of supranormal values of survivors as therapeutic goals in high-risk surgical patients. Chest 1988; 94:1176–1186.

4. Tuchschmidt J, Fried J, Astiz M, et al. Elevation of cardiac output and oxygen delivery improves outcome in septic shock. Chest 1992; 102:216–220.

5. Fleming A, Bishop M, Shoemaker W, et al. Prospective trial of supranormal values as goals of resuscitation in severe trauma. Arch Surg 1992; 127:1175–1181.

6. Gattinoni L, Brazzi L, Pelosi P, et al. A trial of goal-oriented hemodynamic therapy in critically ill patients. N Engl J Med 1995; 333:1025–1032.

7. Mermel LA, Maki DG. Infectious complications of Swan-Ganz pulmonary artery catheters. Am J Respir Crit Care Med 1994; 149:1020–1036.

8. Iberti TJ, Fischer EP, Leibowitz AB, et al. A multicenter study of physicians' knowledge of the pulmonary artery catheter. JAMA 1990; 264:2928–2932.

9. Bone RC. High-tech predicament: pulmonary artery catheters. JAMA 1990; 264: 2933.

10. Iberti TJ, Daily EK, Leibowitz AB, Schecter CB, Fischer EP, Silverstein JH. Assessment of critical care nurses' knowledge of the pulmonary artery catheter. Crit Care Med 1994; 22:1674–1678.

11. Matthay MA, Chatterjee K. Bedside catheterization of the pulmonary artery: risks compared with benefits. Ann Intern Med 1988; 109:826–834.

12. Martin MA, Pfaller MA, Wenzel RP. Coagulase-negative staphylococcal bacteremia. Mortality hospital stay. Ann Intern Med 1989; 110:9–16.

13. Smith RL, Meixler SM, Simberkoff MS. Excess mortality in critically ill patients with nosocomial bloodstream infections. Chest 1991; 100:164–167.

14. Pittet D, Wenzel RP. Nosocomial bloodstream infection in the critically ill. JAMA 1994; 272:1820.

15. Applefeld JJ, Caruthers TE, Reno DJ, Civetta JM. Assessment of the sterility of long-term cardiac catheterization using thermodilution Swan-Ganz catheter. Chest 1978; 74:377–380.

16. Elliott CG, Zimmerman GA, Clemmer TP. Complications of pulmonary artery catheterization in the care of critically ill patients. Chest 1979; 76:647–652.

17. Singh S, Nelson N, Acosta I, Check FE, Puri VK. Catheter colonization and bacteremia with pulmonary and arterial catheters. Crit Care Med 1982; 10:736–739.

18. Pinilla JC, Ross DF, Martin T, Crump H. Study of the incidence of intravascular catheter infection and associated septicemia in critically ill patients. Crit Care Med 1983; 11:21–25.

19. Boyd KD, Thomas SJ, Gold J, Boyd AD. A prospective study of complications of pulmonary artery catheterizations in 500 consecutive patients. Chest 1983; 84:245–249.

20. Miller JJ, Venus B, Mathru M. Comparison of the sterility of long-term central venous catheterization using single lumen, triple lumen, and pulmonary artery catheters. Crit Care Med 1984; 12:634–637.

21. Samsoondar W, Freeman JB, Coultish I, Oxley C. Colonization of intravascular catheters in the intensive care unit. Am J Surg 1985; 149:730–732.

22. Myers ML, Austin TW, Sibbald WJ. Pulmonary artery catheter infections. A prospective study. Ann Surg 1985; 201:237–241.

23. Senagore A, Waller JD, Bonnell BW, Bursch LR, Scholten DJ. Pulmonary artery catheterization: A prospective study of internal jugular and subclavian approaches. Crit Care Med 1987; 15:35–37.

24. Hudson-Civetta JA. Civetta JM, Martinez OV, Hoffman TA. Risk and detection of pulmonary artery catheter-related infection in septic surgical patients. Crit Care Med 1987; 15:29–34.

25. Passerini L, Phang PT, Jackson FL, Lam K, Costerton JW, King EG. Biofilms on right heart flow-directed catheters. Chest 1987; 92:440–446.

26. Levy JH, Nagle DM, Curling PE, Waller JL, Kopel M, Tobia V. Contamination reduction during central venous catheterization. Crit Care Med 1988; 16:165–167.

27. Michel L, Marsh HM, McMichan JC, Southorn PA, Brewer NS. Infection of pulmonary artery catheters in critically ill patients. JAMA 1981; 245:1032–1036.

28. Kaye W, Wheaton M, Potter-Bynoe G. Radial and pulmonary artery catheter-related sepsis. Crit Care Med 1983; 11:249. Abstract.

29. Groeger J, Carlon GC, Howland WS. Contamination shields for pulmonary artery catheters. Crit Care Med 1983; 11:230. Abstract.

30. Ricard P, Martin R, Marcoux JA. Protection of indwelling vascular catheters: Incidence of bacterial contamination and catheter-related sepsis. Crit Care Med 1985; 13:541–543.

31. Parsa MH, Al-Sawwaf M, Shoemaker WC. Complications of pulmonary artery catheterization. Prob Gen Surg 1985; 2:133–144.

32. Damen J, Verhoef J, Bolton DT, et al. Microbiologic risk of invasive hemodynamic monitoring in patients undergoing open-heart operations. Crit Care Med 1985; 13:548–555.

33. Damen J, Ver Der Twell I. Positive tip cultures and related risk factors associated with intravascular catheterization in pediatric cardiac patients. Crit Care Med 1988; 16:221–228.

34. Heard SO, Davis RF, Sherertz RJ, et al. Influence of sterile protective sleeves on the sterility of pulmonary artery catheters. Crit Care Med 1987; 15:499–502.

35. Fisher MA, Maxwell LP, Teba L. Pulmonary artery catheters: risk factors for infection (abstract). In: Program and Abstracts of the Twenty-eighth Interscience Conference on Antimicrobial Agents and Chemotherapy, October, 1988, Los Angeles, CA. Washington, D.C.: American Society for Microbiology, 1988:273.

36. Eyer S, Brummitt C, Crossley K, Siegel R, Cerra F. Catheter-related sepsis: Prospective, randomized study of three methods of long-term catheter maintenance. Crit Care Med 1990; 18:1073–1079.

37. Horowitz HW, Dworkin BM, Savino JA, Byrne DW, Pecora NA. Central catheter-related infections: comparison of pulmonary artery catheters and triple lumen catheters for the delivery of hyperalimentation in a critical care setting. J Parenter Enteral Nutr 1990; 14:588–592.

38. Mermel LA, McCormick RD, Springman SR, Maki DG. The pathogenesis and epidemiology of catheter-related infection with pulmonary artery Swan-Ganz catheters. A prospective study using molecular subtyping. Am J Med 1991; 38:197S–205S.

39. Bach A, Stubbig K, Geiss HK. Infectious risk of replacing venous catheters by the guide-wire technique. Zbl Hyg 1992; 193:150–159.

40. Bull DA, Neumayer LA, Hunter GC, et al. Improved sterile technique diminishes the incidence of positive line cultures in cardiovascular patients. J Surg Res 1992; 52:106–110.

41. Rello J, Coll P, Net A, Prats G. Infection of pulmonary artery catheters. Epidemiologic characteristics and multivariate analysis of risk factors. Chest 1993; 103:132–136.

42. Raad I, Umphrey J, Khan A, Truett LJ, Bodey GP. The duration of placement as a predictor of peripheral and pulmonary artery catheter infections. J Hosp Infect 1993; 23:17–26.

43. Maki DG, Stolz SS, Wheeler S, Mermel LA. A prospective, randomized trial of gauze and two polyurethane dressings for site care of pulmonary artery catheters: implications for catheter management. Crit Care Med 1994; 22:1729–1737.

44. Hulliger S, Pittet D. Incidence and morbidity of central venous catheter-related infections in intensive care units. In: Abstracts of The Infectious Diseases Society of America Annual Meeting, October, 1994, Orlando, FL. Washington, D.C., Infectious Diseases Society of America, 1994:162. Abstract.

45. Maki DG, Will L. Risk factors for central venous catheter-related infection within the ICU. A prospective study of 345 catheters. In: Program and Abstracts of the Third International Conference of Nosocomial Infections, August, 1990, Atlanta, GA. Atlanta: Centers for Disease Control, National Foundation for Infectious Diseases; 1990:54. Abstract.

46. Richet H, Hubert B, Nitemberg G, et al. Prospective multicenter study of vascular-catheter-related complications and risk factors for positive central-catheter cultures in intensive care unit patients. J Clin Microbiol 1990; 28:2520–2525.

47. Moro ML, Vigano EF, Lepri AC. Risk factors for central venous catheter-related infections in surgical and intensive care units. Infect Control Hosp Epidemiol 1994; 15:253–264.

48. Conly JM, Grieves K, Peters B. A prospective, randomized study comparing transparent and dry gauze dressings for central venous catheters. J Infect Dis 1989; 159: 310–319.

49. Armstrong CW, Mayhall CG, Miller KB, et al. Clinical predictors of infection of central venous catheters used for total parenteral nutrition. Infect Control Hosp Epidemiol 1990; 11:71–78.

50. Maki DG. Marked difference in skin colonization of insertion sites for central venous, arterial and peripheral IV catheters. The major reason for differing risks of catheter-related infection? In: Program and Abstracts of the Thirtieth Interscience Conference on Antimicrobial Agents and Chemotherapy, October, 1990, Atlanta, GA. Washington, D.C.: American Society for Microbiology, 1990:712. Abstract.

51. Michel L, McMichan JC, Bachy JI. Microbial colonization of indwelling central venous catheters: statistical evaluation of potential contaminating factors. Am J Surg 1979; 137:745–748.

52. Damen J, Bolton D. A prospective analysis of 1400 pulmonary artery catheterizations in patients undergoing cardiac surgery. Acta Anaesthesiol Scand 1986; 30:386–392.

53. Raad II, Hohn DC, Gilbreath J, et al. Prevention of central venous catheter-related infections by using maximal sterile barrier precautions during insertion. Infect Control Hosp Epidemiol 1994; 15:231–238.

54. Maki DG. Yes, Virginia, aseptic technique is very important: maximal barrier precautions during insertion reduce the risk of central venous catheter-related bacteremia. Infect Control Hosp Epidemiol 1994; 15:227–230.

55. Cobb DK, High KP, Sawyer RG, et al. A controlled trial of scheduled replacement

of central venous and pulmonary-artery catheters. N Engl J Med 1992; 327:1062–1068.

56. Sise MJ, Hollingsworth P, Brimm JE, Peters RM, Virgilio RW, Shackford SR. Complications of the flow-directed pulmonary-artery catheter: A prospective analysis in 219 patients. Crit Care Med 1981; 9:315–318.

57. Civetta JM, Hudson-Civetta JA, Dion L, Ghows MB, Angood PB, Martinez O. Duration of illness effects catheter related infection and bacteremia. In: Program and Abstracts of the Twenty-seventh Interscience Conference on Antimicrobial Agents and Chemotherapy, October, 1987, New York, NY. Washington, D.C.: American Society for Microbiology, 1987:1141. Abstract.

58. Maki DG, Will L. Colonization and infection associated with transparent dressings for central venous, arterial, and hickman catheters. In: Program and Abstracts of the Twenty-fourth Interscience Conference on Antimicrobial Agents and Chemotherapy, October, 1984, Washington, D.C. Washington, D.C.: American Society for Microbiology, 1984:933. Abstract.

59. Hoar PF, Wilson RM, Mangano DT, Avery GJ, Szarnicki RJ, Hill JD. Heparin bonding reduces thrombogenicity of pulmonary artery catheters. N Engl J Med 1981; 305:993–995.

60. Mermel LA, Stolz SM, Maki DG. Surface antimicrobial activity of heparin-bonded and antiseptic-impregnated vascular catheters. J Infect Dis 1993; 167:920–924.

61. Johnston WE, Prough DS, Royster RL, et al. Short-term sterility of the pulmonary artery catheter inserted through an external plastic shield. Anesthesiology 1984; 61:461–464.

62. Baele P, Pedemonte O. Zech F, Kestens-Servaye Y. Clinical use and bacteriological studies of catheter contamination sleeves. Intens Care Med 1984; 10:297–300.

63. Murray MJ, Wignes M, McMichan JC. Assessment of sterility of pulmonary artery catheter sheaths. Anesth Analg 1986; 65:1218–1221.

64. Kopman EA, Sandza JG. Manipulation of the pulmonary-artery catheter after placement: maintenance of sterility. Anesthesiology 1978; 48:373–374.

65. Cohen Y, Fosse JP, Karoubi JL, et al. Prospective assessment of the value of the Arrow "hands off" catheter in the prevention of systemic infections associated with pulmonary-artery catheters. In: Program and Abstracts of the Thirty-fifth Interscience Conference on Antimicrobial Agents and Chemotherapy, September, 1995, San Francisco, CA. Washington, D.C.: American Society for Microbiology, 1995:J9. Abstract.

66. Mermel LA, Maki DG. Epidemic bloodstream infections from hemodynamic pressure monitoring: signs of the times. Infect Control Hosp Epidemiol 1989; 10:47–53.

67. Hekker TAM, Overhage WV, Schneider AJ. Pressure transducers: an overlooked source of sepsis in the intensive care unit. Intens Care Med 1990; 16:511–512.

68. Gahrn-Hansen B, Alstrup P, Dessau R, et al. Outbreak of infection with *Achromobacter xylosoxidans* from contaminated intravascular pressure transducers. J Hosp Infect 1988; 12:1–6.

69. Thomas A, Lalitha MK, Jesudason MV, John S. Transducer related *Enterobacter cloacae* sepsis in post-operative cardiothoracic patients. J Hosp Infect 1993; 25:211–215.

70. Weinstein RA, Emori TG, Anderson RL, Stamm WE. Pressure transducers as source

of bacteremia after open heart surgery. Report of an outbreak and guidelines for prevention. Chest 1976; 69:338–44.

71. Maki DG. Infections due to infusion therapy. In: Bennett JV, Brachman PS, eds. Hospital Infections. Boston: Little, Brown, 1992:849–898.

72. Cooper GL, Schiller AL, Hopkins CC. Possible role of capillary action in pathogenesis of experimental catheter-associated dermal tunnel infections. J Clin Microbiol 1988; 26:8–12.

73. Pittet D, Lew PD, Auckenthaler R, Waldvogel FA. Bacterial spread as a pathogenic factor in catheter-related infections. In: Program and Abstracts of the Thirtieth Interscience Conference on Antimicrobial Agents and Chemotherapy, October, 1990, Atlanta, GA. Washington, D.C.: American Society for Microbiology, 1990:26. Abstract.

74. Tojo M, Yamasita N, Goldmann DA, Pier GB. Isolation and characterization of a capsular polysaccharide adhesin from *Staphylococcus epidermidis*. J Infect Dis 1988; 157:713–722.

75. Timmerman CP, Fleer A, Besnier JM, et al. Characterization of a proteinaceous adhesin of *Staphylococcus epidermidis* which mediates attachment to polystyrene. Infect Immunol 1991; 59:4187–4192.

76. Stillman RM, Seligman F, Garcia L, Sawyer PN. Etiology of catheter-associated sepsis. Correlation with thrombogenicity. Arch Surg 1977; 112:1496–1499.

77. Raad II, Luna M, Khalil SAM, Costerton JW, Lam C, Bodey GP. The relationship between the thrombotic and infectious complications of central venous catheters. JAMA 1994; 271:1014–1016.

78. Herrmann M, Vaudaux PE, Pittet D, et al. Fibronectin, fibrinogen, laminin act as mediators of adherence of clinical staphylococcal isolates to foreign material. J Infect Dis 1988; 158:693–701.

79. Herrmann M, Suchard SJ, Boxer LA, et al. Thrombospondin binds to *Staphylococcus aureus* and promotes staphylococcal adherence to surfaces. Infect Immunol 1991; 59:279–288.

80. Herrmann M, Lai QJ, Albrecht RM, et al. Adhesion of *Staphylococcus aureus* to surface-bound platelets: role of fibrinogen/fibrin and platelet integrins. J Infect Dis 1993; 167:312–322.

81. Hoyle BD, Jass J, Costerton JW. The biofilm glycocalyx as a resistance factor. J Antimicrob Chemother 1990; 26:1–6.

82. Zimmerli W, Lew PD, Waldvogel FA. Pathogenesis of foreign body infection. Evidence for a local granulocyte defect. J Clin Invest 1984; 73:1191–1200.

83. Sheth NK, Franson TR, Sohnle PG. Influence of bacterial adherence to intravascular catheters on in-vitro antibiotic susceptibioity. Lancet 1985; 2:1266–1268.

84. Garrison PK, Freedman LR. Experimental endocarditis I. Staphylococcal endocarditis in rabbits resulting from placement of a polyethylene catheter in the right side of the heart. Yale J Biol Med 1970; 42:394–410.

85. Durack DT, Beeson PB. Experimental bacterial endocarditis I. Colonization of a sterile vegetation. Br J Exp Pathol 1972; 53:44–49.

86. Tsao MMP, Katz D. Central venous catheter-induced endocarditis: human correlate of the animal experimental model of endocarditis. Rev Infect Dis 1984; 6:783–790.

87. Greene JF Jr, Fitzwater JE, Clemmer TP. Septic endocarditis and indwelling pulmonary artery catheters. JAMA 1975; 233:891–892.

88. Ford SE, Manley PN. Indwelling cardiac catheters. An autopsy study of associated endocardial lesions. Arch Pathol Lab Med 1982; 106:314–317.

89. Rowley KM, Clubb KS, Walker Smith GJ, Cabin HS. Right-sided infective endocarditis as a consequence of flow-directed pulmonary-artery catheterization. A clinicopathological study of 55 autopsied patients. N Engl J Med 1984; 311:1152–1156.

90. Pace NL, Horton W. Indwelling pulmonary artery catheters. JAMA 1975; 233:893–894.

91. Katz JD, Cronau LH, Barash PG, Mandel SD. Pulmonary artery flow-guided catheters in the perioperative period. Indications and complications. JAMA 1977; 237:2832–2834.

92. Lange HW, Galliani CA, Edwards JE. Local complications associated with indwelling Swan-Ganz catheters: autopsy study of 36 cases. Am J Cardiol 1983; 52: 1108–1111.

93. Horst HM, Obeid FN, Vij D, Bivins BA. The risks of pulmonary arterial catheterization. Surg Gynecol Obstet 1984; 159:229–232.

94. Connors AF Jr, Castele RJ, Farhat NZ, Tomashefski JF Jr. Complications of right heart catheterization. A prospective autopsy study. Chest 1985; 88:567–572.

95. Becker RC, Martin RG, Underwood DA. Right-sided endocardial lesions and flow-directed pulmonary artery catheters. Cleve Clin J Med 1987; 54:384–388.

96. Ehrie M, Morgan AP, Moore FD, O'Connor NE. Endocarditis with the indwelling balloon-tipped pulmonary artery catheter in burn patients. J Trauma 1978; 18:664–666.

97. Sasaki TM, Panke TW, Dorethy JF, Lindberg RB, Pruitt BA. The relationship of central venous and pulmonary artery catheter position to acute right-sided endocarditis in severe thermal injury. J Trauma 1979; 19:740–743.

98. Powell DC, Bivins BA, Bell RM, Sachatello CR, Griffen WO Jr. Bacterial endocarditis in the critically ill surgical patient. Arch Surg 1981; 116:311–314.

99. Iqbal SM, Hehir RL, Ehrich DA. Right sided endocarditis following Swan-Ganz catheterization: detection by two-dimensional echocardiography. Ultrasound Med Biol 1982; 8:701–704.

100. Van Der Bel-Kahn J, Fowler NO, Doerger P. Right heart catheter lesions: any significance? Am J Clin Pathol 1984; 82:137–147.

101. Ducatman BS, McMichan JC, Edwards WD. Catheter-induced lesions of the right side of the heart. JAMA 1985; 253:791–795.

102. Verghese A, Widrich WC, Arbeit RD. Central venous septic thrombophlebitis—the role of medical therapy. Medicine 1985; 64:394–400.

103. Strinden WD, Helgerson RB, Maki DG. Candida septic thrombosis of the great veins associated with central catheters. Clinical features and management. Ann Surg 1985; 202:653–658.

104. Kaufman J, Demas C, Stark K, Flancbaum L. Catheter-related septic central venous thrombosis current therapeutic options. West J Med 1986; 145:200–203.

105. Topiel MS, Bryan RT, Kessler CM, Simon GL. Case report: treatment of silastic catheter-induced central vein septic thrombophlebitis. Am J Med Sci 1986; 291:425–428.

106. Roush K, Scala-Barnett DM, Donabedian H, Freimer EH. Rupture of a pulmonary

artery mycotic aneurysm associated with *Candida* endocarditis. Am J Med 1988; 84: 142–144.

107. Shin MS, Ho K-J. Cavitary pulmonary lesions complicating use of flow-directed balloon-tipped catheters in two cases. AJR 1979; 132:650–652.

108. McLoud TC, Putman CE. Radiology of the Swan-Ganz catheter and associated pulmonary complications. Radiology 1975; 116:19–22.

109. Mermel LA, Velez LA, Zilz MA, Maki DG. Epidemiologic and microbiologic features of nosocomial bloodstream infection (NBSI) implicating a vascular catheter source: a case-control study of 85 vascular catheter-related and 101 secondary NBSIs. In: Program and Abstracts of the Thirty-first Interscience Conference on Antimicrobial Agents and Chemotherapy, October, 1991, Chicago, IL. Washington, D.C.: American Society for Microbiology, 1991:454. Abstract.

110. Raad II, Baba Bodey GP. Diagnosis of catheter related infections: role of surveillance and targeted quantitative skin cultures. Clin Infect Dis 1995; 20:593–597.

111. McGeer A, Righter J. Improving our ability to diagnose infections associated with central venous catheters: value of Gram's staining and culture of entry site swabs. Can Med Assoc J 1987; 137:1009–1021.

112. Segura M, Llado L, Guirao X, et al. A prospective study of a new protocol for 'in situ' diagnosis of central venous catheter related bacteraemia. Clin Nutr 1993; 12: 103–107.

113. Armstrong CW, Mayhall CG, Miller KB, et al. Clinical predictors of infection of central venous catheters used for total parenteral nutrition. Infect Control Hosp Epidemiol 1990; 11:71–78.

114. Brun-Buisson C, Abrouk F, Legrand P, Huet Y, Larabi S, Rapin M. Diagnosis of central venous catheter-related sepsis. Critical level of quantitative tip cultures. Arch Intern Med 147:873–877.

115. Cleri DJ, Corrado ML, Seligman SJ. Quantitative culture of intravenous catheters and other intravascular inserts. J Infect Dis 1980; 141:781–786.

116. Rello J, Coll P, Net A, Prats G. Evaluation of different catheters' parts for identification of pulmonary artery catheter colonisation. Scand J Infect Dis 1991; 23:655–656.

117. Sherertz R, Heard S, Raad I. Diagnosis of triple-lumen catheter infection: Comparison of roll-plate, sonication and flushing methodologies. J Clin Micro 1997; in press.

118. Hnatiuk OW, Pike J, Stoltzfus D, Lane W. Value of bedside plating of semiquantitative cultures for diagnosis of central venous catheter-related infections in ICU patients. Chest 1993; 103:896–899.

119. Cooper GL, Hopkins CC. Rapid diagnosis of intravascular catheter-associated infection by direct gram staining of catheter segments. N Engl J Med 1985; 18:1142–1147.

120. Linares J, Sitges-Serra A, Garau J, Perz JL, Martin R. Pathogenesis of catheter sepsis: a prospective study with quantitative and semiquantitation of catheter hub and segments. J Clin Microbiol 1985; 21:357–360.

121. Rushforth JA, Hoy CM, Kite P, Puntis JWL. Rapid diagnosis of central venous catheter sepsis. Lancet 1993; 342:402–403.

122. Moonens F, Alami SE, Van Gossum A, Struelens M, Serruys E. Usefulness of Gram staining of blood collected from total parenteral nutrition catheter for rapid diagnosis of catheter-related sepsis. J Clin Microbiol 1994; 1578–1579.

123. Mosca R, Curtas S, Forbes B, Meguid MM. The benefits of isolator cultures in the management of suspected catheter sepsis. Surgery 1987; 102:718–723.

124. Ascher DP, Shoupe BA, Robb M, Maybee DA, Fischer GW. Comparison of standard and quantitative blood cultures in the evaluation of children with suspected central venous line sepsis. Diagn Microbiol Infect Dis 1992; 15:499–503.

125. Capedevila JA, Planes AM, Palomar M, et al. Value of differential quantitative blood cultures in the diagnosis of catheter-related sepsis. Eur J Clin Microbiol Infect Dis 1992; 11:403–407.

126. Mermel LA, Maki DG. Detection of bacteremia in adults: consequences of culturing an inadequate volume of blood. An Intern Med 1993; 119:270–272.

127. Douard MC, Clementi E, Arlet G, et al. Negative catheter-tip culture and diagnosis of catheter-related bacteremia. Nutrition 1994; 10:397–404.

128. McIntyre KM, Vita JA, Lambrew CT, Freman J, Loscalzo J. A noninvasive method of predicting pulmonary-capillary wedge pressure. N Engl J Med 1992; 327:1715–1720.

129. Sattler FR, Foderaro JB, Aber RC. *Staphylococcus epidermidis* bacteremia associated with vascular catheters: an important cause of febrile morbidity in hospitalized patients. Infect Control 1984; 5:279–283.

130. Greene JF Jr, Cummings KC. Aseptic thrombotic endocardial vegetations. A complication of indwelling pulmonary artery catheters. JAMA 1973; 225:1525–1526.

131. Terpenning MS, Buggy BP, Kauffman CA. Hospital-acquired infective endocarditis. Arch Intern Med 1988; 148:1601–1603.

132. Raad II, Sabbagh MF. Optimal duration of therapy for catheter-related *Staphylococcus aureus* bacteremia: a study of 55 cases and review. Clin Infect Dis 1992; 14:75–82.

133. Shapiro SM, Young E, De Guzman S, et al. Transesophageal echocardiography. N Engl J Med 1995; 332:1268–1275.

134. Winslow T, Foster E, Adams JR, Schiller NB. Pulmonary valve endocarditis: improved diagnosis with biplane transesophageal echocardiography. J Am Soc Echocardiogr 1992; 5:206–210.

135. Albertyn LE, Alcock MK. Diagnosis of internal jugular vein thrombosis. Radiology 1987; 162:505–508.

136. Mori H, Fukua T, Isomoto I, Maeda H, Hayashi. CT diagnosis of catheter-induced septic thrombus of vena cava. J Comp Assist Tomogr 1990; 14:236–238.

137. Braun IF, Haffman JC, Malko JA, Petigrew RI, Danniels W, Davis PC. Jugular venous thrombosis: MR imaging. Radiology 1985; 157:357–360.

138. Mylotte JM, McDermott C. *Staphylococcus aureus* bacteremia caused by infected intravenous catheters. Am J Infect Control 1987; 15:1–6.

139. Ehni WF, Reller LB. Short-course therapy for catheter-associated *Staphylococcus aureus* bacteremia. Arch Intern Med 1989; 149:533–536.

140. Chambers HF, Miller RT, Newman MD. Right-sided *Staphylococcus aureus* endocarditis in intravenous drug abusers: two-week combination therapy. Ann Intern Med 1988; 109:619–624.

141. Bowler I, Conlon C, Crook D, Peto KT. Optimum duration of therapy for catheter related *Staphylococcus aureus* bacteremia: a cohort study of 75 patients. In: Program and Abstracts of the Thirty-second Interscience Conference on Antimicrobial Agents

and Chemotherapy, October, 1992, Anaheim, CA. Washington, D.C.: American Society for Microbiology, 1992:833. Abstract.

142. Torres-Tortosa M, deCueto M, Vergara A, et al. Prospective evaluation of a two-week course of intravenous antibiotics in intravenous drug addicts with infective endocarditis. Eur J Clin Microbiol Infect Dis 1994; 7:559–564.

143. Malanoski GJ, Samore MH, Pefanis A, Karchmer AW. *Staphylococcus aureus* catheter-associated bacteremia. Minimal effective therapy and unusual infectious complications associated with arterial sheath catheters. Arch Intern Med 1995; 155:1161–1166.

144. Jernigan JA, Farr BM. Short-course therapy of catheter-related *Staphylococcus aureus* bacteremia: a meta-analysis. Ann Intern Med 1993; 119:304–311.

145. Rose HD. Venous catheter-associated candidemia. Am J Med Sci 1978; 275:265–269.

146. Beutler SM, Young LS, Linquist LB, Montomerie JZ, Edwards JE Jr. Delayed complications of candidemia. In: Program and Abstracts of the Twenty-second Interscience Conference on Antimicrobial Agents and Chemotherapy, October, 1982, Miami, FL. Washington, D.C.: American Society for Microbiology, 1982:496. Abstract.

147. Leccoines JA, Lee JW, Navarro EE, et al. Vascular catheter-associated fungemia in patients with cancer: analysis of 155 episodes. Clin Infect Dis 1992; 14:875–883.

148. Edwards JE. Should all patients with candidemia be treated with antifungal agents? Clin Infect Dis 1992; 15:422–423.

149. Marsh PK, Tally FP, Kellum J, Callow J, Gorbach SL. *Candida* infections in surgical patients. Ann Surg 1983; 198:42–47.

150. Rex JH, Bennett JE, Sugar AM, et al. A randomized trial comparing fluconazole with amphotericin B for the treatment of candidemia in patients without neutropenia. N Engl J Med 1994; 331:1325–1330.

151. Scheld WM, Sande MA. Endocarditis and intravascular infections. In: Mandell GL, Douglas RG, Bennett JE, eds. Principles and Practices of Infectious Diseases. 4th ed. New York: Churchill Livingstone, 1995:740–782.

152. LaQuaglia MP, Caldwell C, Lucas A, et al. A prospective randomized double-blind trial of bolus urokinase in the treatment of established Hickman catheter sepsis in children. J Pediatr Surg 1994; 29:742–745.

153. Mermel LA. Prevention of intravascular catheter-related infections. Infect Dis Clin Pract 1994; 3:391–398.

154. Prager RL, Silva J. Colonization of central venous catheters. South Med J 1984; 77:458–461.

155. Collignon P, Soni N, Pearson I, et al. Sepsis associated with central vein catheters in critically ill patients. Intens Care Med 1988; 14:227–231.

156. Gil RT, Kruse JA, Thili-Baharozian MC, Carlson RW. Triple- vs. single-lumen central venous catheters. A prospective study in a critically ill population. Arch Intern Med 1989; 149:1139–1143.

157. Robinson JF, Robinson WA, Cohn A, Garg K, Armstrong JD. Perforation of the great vessels during central venous line placement. Arch Intern Med 1995; 155:1225–1228.

158. Centers for Disease Control. Recommendations for prevention of HIV transmission in health-care settings. MMWR 1987; 36:1S–18S.

159. Clemence MA, Walker D, Farr BM. Central venous catheter practices: results of a survey. Am J Infect Control 1995; 23:5–12.

160. Maki DG, Ringer M, Alvarado CJ. Prospective randomized trial of povidone-iodine, alcohol, and chlorhexidine for prevention of infection associated with central venous and arterial catheters. Lancet 1991; 338:339–343.

161. Sheehan G, Leicht K, O'Brien M, et al. Chlorhexidine vs. povidone-iodine as cutaneous antisepsis for prevention of vascularcatheter infection. In: Programs and Abstracts of the Thirty-third Interscience Conference on Antimicrobial Agents and Chemotherapy, October 1993, New Orleans, LA. Washington, D.C.: American Society for Microbiology, 1993:1616. Abstract.

162. Mimoz O, Pieroni L, Lawrence C, et al. Prospective, randomized trial of two antiseptic solutions for prevention of central venous or arterial catheter colonization and infection in intensive care units. Crit Care Med 1996; 24:1818–1823.

163. Strand CL, Wajsbort RR, Sturmann K. Effect of iodophor vs iodine tincture skin preparation on blood culture contamination rate. JAMA 1993; 269:1004–1006.

164. Fauerbach LL, Schoppman MJ, Singh VR, et al. A comparison of the efficacy of different antiseptics for intravascular site preparation. In: Program and Abstracts of the Thirty-first Interscience Conference on Antimicrobial Agents and Chemotherapy, October 1991, Chicago, IL. Washington, D.C.: American Society for Microbiology, 1991:1269. Abstract.

165. McKee R, Dunsmuir R, Whitby M, Garden OJ. Does antibiotic prophylaxis at the time of catheter insertion reduce the incidence of catheter-related sepsis in intravenous nutrition? J Hosp Infect 1985; 6:419–425.

166. Neu HC. The crisis in antibiotic resistance. Science. 1992; 257:1064–1072.

167. Levy SB. Confronting multidrug resistance. A role for each of us. JAMA 1993; 269:1840–1842.

168. Laster J, Silver D. Heparin-coated catheters and heparin-induced thrombocytopenia. J Vasc Surg 1988; 7:667–672.

169. Moberg PQ, Geary VM, Sheikh FM. Heparin-induced thrombocytopenia: a possible complication of heparin-coated pulmonary artery catheters. J Cardiothorac Anesth 1990; 4:226–228.

170. Maki DG, Cobb L, Garman JK, Shapiro J, Ringer M. An attachable silver-impregnated cuff for prevention of infection with central venous catheters. Am J Med 1988; 85:307–315.

171. Flowers RH III, Schwenzer KJ, Kopel RF, Fisch MJ, Tucker SI, Farr BM. Efficacy of attachable subcutaneous cuff for the prevention of intravascular catheter-related infection. JAMA 1989; 261:878–883.

172. Rafkin HS, Hoyt JW, Crippen DW. Prevention of certified venous catheter-related infection with a silver-impregnated cuff (abstract). Chest 1990; 98:117S.

173. Bonawitz SC, Hammell EJ, Kirkpatrick JR. Prevention of central venous catheter sepsis: a prospective randomized trial. Am Surg 1991; 57:618–623.

174. Hoffmann KK, Weber DJ, Samsa GP, Rutala WA. Transparent polyurethane film as an intravenous catheter dressing. A meta-analysis of the infection risks. JAMA 1992; 267:2072–2076.

175. Maki DG, Band JD. A comparative study of polyantibiotic and iodophor ointments in prevention of vascular catheter-related infection. Am J Med 1981; 70:739–744.

176. Hill RLR, Fisher AP, Ware RJ, Wilson S, Casewell MW. Mupirocin for the reduction of colonization of internal jugular cannulae—a randomized controlled trial. J Hosp Infect 1990; 15:311–321.

177. Hill R, Ben Salem R, Casewell MW. Topical calcium mupirocin for the prevention of colonization of intravascular cannulae—a randomised double-blind controlled trial. In: Program and Abstracts of the Thirty-third Interscience Conference on Antimicrobial Agents and Chemotherapy, October 1993, New Orleans, LA. Washington, D.C.: American Society for Microbiology, 1993: 1212. Abstract.

178. Kauffman CA, Terpenning MS, He X, et al. Attempts to eradicate methicillin-resistant *Staphylococcus aureus* from a long-term-care facility with the use of mupirocin ointment. Am J Med 1993; 94:371–378.

179. Zakrzewska-Bode A, Mujtjens ML, Liem KD, Hoogkamp-Korstanje JAA. Mupirocin resistance in coagulase negative staphylococci, after topical prophylaxis for the reduction of colonization of central venous catheters. J Hosp Infect 1995; 31: 189–193.

180. Levin A, Mason AJ, Jindal KK, Fong IW, Goldstein MB. Prevention of hemodialysis subclavian vein catheter infections with topical povidone-iodine. Kidney Int 1991; 40:934–938.

181. Keyserling H, Dykes F, Newsome P, Trotochaurd K. Pilot study of a chlorhexidine disc catheter dressing in a neonatal unit. NAVAN 1995; 1:12–13. Abstract.

182. Salzman MB, Isenberg HD, Rubin LG. Use of disinfectants to reduce microbial contamination of hubs of vascular catheters. J Clin Microbiol 1993; 31:475–479.

183. Yonkman CA, Hamory BH. Comparison of three methods of maintaining a sterile injectate system during cardiac output determinations. Am J Infect Control 1984; 12: 276–281.

184. Talbot GH, Skros M, Provencher M. 70% alcohol disinfection of transducer heads: experimental trials. Infect Control 1985; 6:237–239.

185. Platt R, Lehr JL, Marion S, et al. Safe and cost-effective cleaning of pressure-monitoring transducers. Infect Control Hosp Epidemiol 1988; 9:409–416.

186. Freeman R, Holden MP, Lyon R, Hjersing N. Addition of sodium metabisulphite to left atrial catheter infusates as a means of preventing bacterial colonisation of the catheter tip. Thorax 1982; 37:142–144.

187. Luskin RL, Weinstein RA, Natan C, Chamberlin WH, Kabsin SA. Extended use of disposable pressure transducers: a bacteriologic evaluation. JAMA 1986; 255:916–920.

188. O'Malley MK, Rhame FS, Cerra FB, McComb RC. Value of routine pressure monitoring system changes after 72 hours of continuous use. Crit Care Med 1994; 22:1424–1430.

189. Segura M, Alvarez-Lerma F, Tellado JM, et al. A clinical trial on the prevention of catheter-related sepsis using a new hub model. Ann Surg 1996; 223:363–369.

190. Maki DG, Stolz S, McCormick, Spiegel C. Possible association of a commercial needleless system with central venous catheter-related bacteremia. In: Program and Abstracts of the Thirty-fourth Interscience Conference on Antimicrobial Agents and Chemotherapy, October 1994, Orlando, FL. Washington, D.C.: American Society for Microbiology, 1994:J201. Abstract.

191. Danzig LE, Short LJ, Collins K, et al. Bloodstream infections associated with a

needleless intravenous infusion system in patients receiving home infusion therapy. JAMA 1995; 273:1862–1864.

192. Vassallo D, Blanc-Jouvan M, Bret M, et al. *Staphylococcus aureus* septicemia and a needleless system of infusion. In: Program and Abstracts of the Thirty-fifth Interscience Conference on Antimicrobial Agents and Chemotherapy, September 1995, San Francisco, CA. Washington, D.C.: American Society for Microbiology, 1995: J12. Abstract.

193. Kellerman S, Shay D, Howard J, Feusner J, Goes CI, Jarvis W. Bloodstream infections associated with needleless devices used for central venous catheter access in children receiving home health care. In: Program and Abstracts of the Thirty-fifth Interscience Conference on Antimicrobial Agents and Chemotherapy, September 1995, San Francisco, CA. Washington, D.C.: American Society for Microbiology, 1995:J11. Abstract.

194. Maki DG, Stolz SM, Wheeler SJ, Mermel LA. Clinical trial of a novel antiseptic central venous catheter. In: Program and Abstracts of the Thirty-first Interscience Conference on Antimicrobial Agents and Chemotherapy, October 1991, Chicago, IL. Washington, DC: American Society for Microbiology, 1991:461. Abstract.

195. Bach A, Schmidt H, Böttiger B, et al. Retention of antibacterial activity and bacterial colonization of antiseptic-bonded central venous catheters. J Antimicrob Chemother 1996; 37:315–322.

196. Clemence MA, Anglim AM, Jernigan JA, et al. A study of prevention of cather related bloodstream infection with an antiseptic impregnated catheter. In: Program and Abstracts of the Thirty-fourth Interscience Conference on Antimicrobial Agents and Chemotherapy, October 1994, Orlando, FL. Washington, D.C.: American Society for Microbiology, 1994:J199. Abstract.

197. Goldschmidt H, Hahn U, Salwender H-J, et al. Prevention of catheter-related infections by silver coated central venous catheters in oncological patients. Zbl Bakt 1995; 283:215–223.

198. Brown RB, Colodny SM, Drapkin MS, et al. One-day prevalence study of 118 intensive care units. Infect Control Hosp Epidemiol 1995; 16:438. Abstract.

199. Band JD, Maki DG. Infections caused by arterial catheters used for hemodynamic monitoring. Am J Med 1979; 67:735–741.

200. Maki DG, Hassemer CA. Endemic rate of fluid contamination and related septicemia in arterial pressure monitoring. Am J Med 1981; 70:733–738.

201. Shinozaki T, Deane RS, Mazuzan JE Jr, et al. Bacterial contamination of arterial lines. JAMA 1983; 249:223–225.

202. Thomas F, Burke JP, Parker J, et al. The risk of infection related to radial vs femoral sites for arterial catheterization. Crit Care Med 1983; 11:807–812.

203. Russell JA, Joel M, Hudson RJ, Mangano DT, Schlobohm M. Prospective evaluation of radial and femoral artery catheterization sites in critically ill adults. Crit Care Med 1983; 11:936–939.

204. Thomas F, Orme JF, Clemmer TP, Burke JP, Elliott CG, Gardner RM. A prospective comparison of arterial catheter blood and catheter-tip cultures in critically ill patients. Crit Care Med 1984; 12:860–862.

205. Sommers M, Baas LS, Beiting AM. Nosocomial infections related to four methods of hemodynamic monitoring. Heart Lung 1987; 16:13–19.

206. Ducharme FM, Gauthier M, Lacroix J, Lafleur L. Incidence of infection related to

arterial catheterization in children: a prospective study. Crit Care Med 1988; 16:272–276.

207. Norwood SH, Cormier B, McMahon NG, Moss A, Moore V. Prospective study of catheter-related infection during prolonged arterial catheterization. Crit Care Med 1988; 16:836–839.

208. Leroy O, Billiau V, Beuscart C, et al. Nosocomial infections associated with long-term radial artery cannulation. Intens Care Med 1989; 15:241–246.

209. Maki DG, Ringer M. Prospective study of arterial catheter-related infection: incidence, sources of infection and risk factors. In: Program and Abstracts of the Twenty-ninth Interscience Conference on Antimicrobial Agents and Chemotherapy September 1989, Houston, TX. Washington, D.C.: American Society for Microbiology, 1989:1075. Abstract.

210. Furfaro S, Gauthier M, Lacroix J, Nadeau D, Lafleur L, Mathews S. Arterial catheter-related infections in children: a 1-year cohort analysis. Am J Dis Child 1991; 145:1037–1043.

211. Beck-Sague CM, Jarvis WR. Epidemic bloodstream infections associated with pressure transducers: a persistent problem. Infect Control Hosp Epidemiol 1989; 10:54–59.

212. Leggiadro RJ, Luedtke GS, Anderson MS, Storgion SA, Bugnitz MC, Barrett FF. Persistent, unusual gram-negative bacteremia associated with arterial pressure monitoring in a pediatric intensive care unit. Infect Control Hosp Epidemiol 1992; 13:556–558.

213. Passerini L, Lam K, Costerton W, King EG. Biofilms on indwelling vascular catheters. Crit Care Med 1992; 20:665–673.

214. Sheth NK, Franson TR, Rose HD, Buckmire FLA, Cooper JA, Sohne PG. Colonization of bacteria on polyvinyl chloride and Teflon intravascular catheters in hospitalized patients. J Clin Microbiol 1983; 18:1061–1063.

215. Vaudaux P, Pittet D, Haeberli A, et al. Fibronectin is more active than fibrin or fibrinogen in promoting *Staphylococcus aureus* adherence to inserted intravascular catheters. J Infect Dis 1993; 167:633–641.

216. Falk PS, Scuderi PE, Sheretz RJ, Motsinger SM. Infected radial artery pseudoaneurysms occurring after percutaneous cannulation. Chest 1992; 101:490–495.

217. Fanning WL, Aronson M. Osler node, janeway lesions and splinter hemorrhages. Arch Dermatol 1977; 113:648–649.

218. Cohen A, Reyes R, Kirk M. Fulks RM. Osler's nodes, pseudoaneurysm formation, and sepsis complicating percutaneous radial artery cannulation. Crit Care Med 1984; 12:1078–1079.

219. Arnow PM, Costas CO. Delayed rupture of the radial artery caused by catheter-related sepsis. Rev Infect Dis 1988; 10:1035–1037.

220. Soderstrom CA, Wasserman DH, Ransom KJ, Caplan ES, Cowley RA. Infected false femoral artery aneurysms secondary to monitoring catheters. J Cardiovasc Surg 1983; 24:63–68.

221. Maki DG, McCormick RD, Wirtnen GW. Septic endarteritis due to intraarterial catheters for cancer chemotherapy. I. Clinical features. II. Risk factors. III. Guidelines for prevention. Cancer 1979; 44:1228–1240.

11

Long-Term Central Venous Catheters
Infectious Complications and Cost

Issam I. Raad and Hossam Safar*

University of Texas M. D. Anderson Cancer Center, Houston, Texas

I. INTRODUCTION

A. Evaluation of Central Venous Catheters

Long-term venous access devices have revolutionized the medical care of chronically ill patients. Clinicians who treated such patients 30 or 40 years ago can particularly appreciate the impact of these devices. Using small peripheral venous catheters, the treatment of cancer patients was once complicated by extravasation of toxic agents and thrombosis of peripheral veins, which often limited intravenous therapy. The introduction of long-term silicone venous devices allowed the safe administration of chemotherapy drugs, blood products, total parenteral nutrition (TPN), fluids, antibiotics, and other substances over an extended period of time. There is no doubt that such devices helped improve morbidity and mortality and minimized human suffering.

B. Types of Central Venous Catheters

Four general types of long-term catheters are available (Fig. 1): tunneled catheters, nontunneled catheters, implantable ports, and peripherally inserted central catheters (PICCs).

**Current affiliation:* Univerisity of Texas Health Science Center.

1. Tunneled Catheters

The first tunneled catheter was developed by Broviac in the early 1970s for patients who required long-term TPN (1). Subsequently, Hickman developed another long-term tunneled catheter for patients undergoing bone marrow transplantation (2). In contrast with the thick-walled Hickman and Broviac catheters, Groshong developed a thin-walled catheter characterized by a two-slit valve adjacent to a rounded, closed end that remains closed unless fluids are being infused or blood is being withdrawn. This eliminates the need to clamp the catheter and decreases the risk of intraluminal blood clotting or infusion of air when the catheter is not in use. Tunneled catheters usually exit the body midway between the nipple and sternum and are tunneled for several inches to the cannulated vein. All tunneled catheters have a Dacron cuff that is located in the proximal subcutaneous segment 5 cm from the exit site. The Dacron cuff becomes enmeshed with fibrous tissue, anchoring the catheter and creating a tissue interface barrier against the migration of skin organisms. Tunneled catheters are available in single-, double-, or triple-lumen cannulae.

2. Nontunneled Catheters

Nontunneled subclavian silicone catheters have the smallest lumen and external diameter. They can be maintained for extended periods up to 400 days (3). They can be inserted percutaneously in the subclavian vein in outpatient nonsurgical settings. If a nontunneled catheter becomes displaced or a catheter-related infection (CRI) occurs, it can be exchanged over a guide wire.

3. Implantable Ports

Implantable ports consist of a metal or plastic port inserted completely beneath the skin and connected to a catheter tube (4). Ports are usually placed in a subcutaneous pocket of the upper chest wall (central subclavian ports) or in the antecubital area of the arm (peripheral ports). Ports are available as single or double lumen catheters with or without the Groshong's valve.

4. Peripherally Inserted Central Catheters

During the last decade, the use of PICCs has gained acceptance as a method for long-term venous access. A PICC is a type of catheter that is inserted peripherally at or above the antecubital space in the cephalic vein, the basilic vein, the medial cephalic vein, or the medial basilic vein and advanced into the central venous system. This catheter is usually inserted percutaneously in the outpatient nonsurgical setting by a trained infusion therapy nurse. It has been shown at our center that these catheters are safe and have a mean duration of placement of 87 days. PICCs are associated with a low infection rate and low cost (3). Generally, the

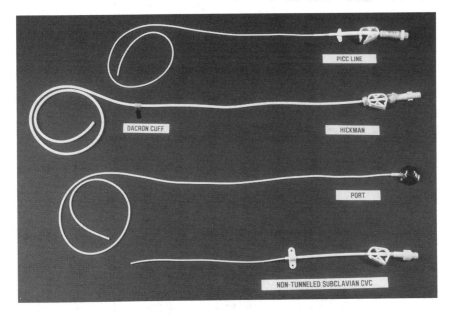

Figure 1 Four types of long-term silicone catheters: PICC line, Hickman (with Dacron cuff), port, and nontunneled subclavian central venous catheters.

catheters are composed of silicone elastomers or polyurethane material and may or may not have a Groshong valve. PICC placement requires only local anesthesia and minimal surgery.

II. EPIDEMIOLOGY OF INFECTIOUS COMPLICATIONS

Uncomplicated, long-term intravenous access contributes significantly to the comfort of patients with a variety of conditions, such as hematologic malignancies, solid tumors, sickle cell anemia, aplastic anemia, endocarditis, burns, Crohn's disease, osteomyelitis, and other cases in which a large vessel is required for safe infusion. Infection remains a significant cause of morbidity for patients with long-term central venous catheters (CVCs). Catheter-related infections can be classified as exit site infections, tunnel tract infections, port pocket infections, and catheter-related bacteremia or fungemia. Catheter-related sepsis and exit site infections are common to all types of catheters; however, port pocket infections and tunnel infections are specific of implantable devices and tunneled catheters, respectively. Phlebitis is more common with PICC.

It is difficult to interpret and compare reports of CRIs because of differences in populations, catheter use, length of catheterization, and methods of diagnosing true CRI. Several factors have been reported to correlate with the incidence of infection: type of fluid infused, therapy with interleukin-2, the patient's neutrophil count, and occurrence of catheter thrombosis.

In one study, patients with tunneled catheters that had been placed primarily for TPN experienced a higher rate of infection (22.9%) than patients whose catheters were placed for antibiotic management of infection (12.7%) or patients who received chemotherapy only (4.9%) (5). Patients receiving biologic modifiers such as interleukin-2 have also been shown to have a higher risk for catheter infection caused by staphylococcal organisms (6–9).

In a study conducted by Howell and colleagues of patients with long-term indwelling tunneled CVCs who were followed for a total of 12,410 catheter-days, neutropenia of <500 neutrophils per mm^3 of blood was the only independent risk for catheter-related infection ($P = 0.018$) (10). Catheter infections were significantly more likely to occur during the first week of neutropenia than during the remaining neutropenic days. However, in a study conducted at our center (3) neither neutropenia, bone marrow transplantation, use of high-dose steroids, nor infusion of vesicant chemotherapy agents through the CVC predisposed patients to catheter infection. The only statistically significant risk factor for catheter infection was hematologic malignancy (acute lymphocytic leukemia or acute myelocytic leukemia).

The same was observed by Groeger and colleagues (11) in a study of patients with leukemia who had shorter infection-free periods compared with patients with lymphomas or myeloma ($P = 0.02$), but neutropenia was not evaluated as a risk factor except at the time of catheter insertion. In addition, patients with solid tumors who had catheters had longer infection-free periods than those who had hematologic diseases ($P = 0.005$) (11). Independent of neutropenia, patients with hematologic malignancies may be at a higher risk of infection because of excessive manipulation of catheters resulting from the high frequency of blood transfusions and blood withdrawals done through the catheter.

A recent postmortem study on long-term CVC use conducted at our center demonstrated that 38% of catheterized veins have evidence of mural thrombosis and that vascular mural thrombosis of the catheterized veins was significantly associated with catheter-related septicemia (12). This relationship was independent of other host or catheter variables such as underlying disease, thrombocytopenia, and site and duration of catheterization. It has been previously demonstrated at the subclinical microscopic level that the fibrin sheath, which engulfs most indwelling catheters, promotes the adherence of staphylococci and *Candida* species. Our postmortem study offers evidence that the pathology of mural thrombosis of catheterized veins is associated with clinical catheter-related sepsis. Two other studies evaluating a related question failed to document an association between clotting of the catheter and risk of infection (10,11).

III. PATHOGENESIS AND MICROBIOLOGY OF CATHETER-RELATED INFECTION

A. Adherence Factors

In prospective studies, the most common organisms causing catheter infection have been coagulase-negative *Staphylococcus*, *S. aureus*, and yeasts. Extensive reviews of cases of long-term CVC sepsis implicated coagulase-negative staphylococci in more than 50% of the infections. Adherence of the bacteria to the catheter surface depends on the interaction of the host, the microbial factors, and the catheter material (13–15).

First, the host considers the catheter a foreign body and reacts by forming a thrombin sleeve around it (16,17). This thrombin layer is rich in fibrin and fibronectin (substances that *S. aureus* and *Candida* adhere to tightly). Both *S. aureus* and *C. albicans* are coagulase-producing organisms that benefit from the process of thrombogenesis by adhering tightly to the fibrin-rich layer of the biofilm (18,19). Coagulase-negative staphylococci adhere to fibronectin but not to fibrin (19).

Second, the microbial factors consist of the production of fibrous glycocalyx. Microbial organisms, particularly slime-producing coagulase-negative staphylococci, enhance adherence by producing a fibrous glycocalyx, also known as extracellular slime, that constitutes the microbial substance of the biofilm (20–23). The biofilm layer, which is made of microbial and host substances, is conducive not only to the continued adherence of the organisms, but also to their maintenance, because it acts as a barrier that protects embedded organisms from antibiotics, phagocytic neutrophils, macrophages, and antibodies (24–27).

The third factor that plays a role in the adherence process is the catheter material. Several investigators have shown, for example, that *S. aureus* and *Candida* species adhere better to polyvinyl chloride catheters than to Teflon catheters (28,29). Several prospective studies in which quantitative catheter cultures were used have shown that the most common organisms causing CRIs are coagulase-negative staphylococci, *S. aureus*, and *Candida* species (30–37). *C. albicans* and *C. parapsilosis* account for most of the *Candida* species causing CRIs.

B. Bacterial Colonization

The source of catheter colonization remains a controversial issue. For short-term polyurethane catheters, Maki (38) showed that the skin is the most common source for catheter colonization and catheter-related bacteremia. Sitges-Serra et al. (39–41) have emphasized the hub as the most common source of catheter-related septicemia. To assess the degree of luminal and extraluminal colonization of long-term CVCs, we prospectively studied 359 indwelling silicone CVCs from a cohort of 340 consecutive cancer patients. All CVCs were cultured by the roll-plate and sonication quantitative culture techniques. Semiquantitative electron microscopy was done on all CVCs associated with catheter infection and on matched culture-negative controls. External surface colonization, most likely originating from the skin, was predominant in the first 10 days of the catheter placement; luminal colonization, probably originating from the hub, became predominant after 30 days of catheter placement. Luminal colonization increased progressively with duration of catheterization in both premortem and postmortem catheters, supporting the notion that prolonged excessive use of catheters would lead to contaminated hubs and in turn to increased luminal colonization (42).

Port pocket infection, usually caused by gram-positive cocci, often follow direct inoculation or migration of organisms along the accessing needle. While coagulase-negative staphylococci and *S. aureus* are introduced through the skin and contaminated hubs (38–41), many of the *Candida* infections are thought to seed hematogenously from the gastrointestinal tract and adhere to the fibrin and fibronectin on the surface of the catheter (43). Infusion-related sepsis caused by contaminated infusate is often caused by gram-negative bacilli such as *Enterobacter*, *Pseudomonas*, *Citrobacter*, and *Serratia* species (13).

IV.   COMPARISON OF CATHETERS

A.   Infection Rates

No prospective randomized study in the literature has compared the complications related to the different types of catheters including nontunneled subclavian catheters. The available studies published to date are controversial. Reporting catheter infections according to the percentage of catheters that become infected without considering the duration of catheter use is inappropriate. Many institutions now report catheter infection rates on the number of infection episodes per 100 or 1000 patient-days of catheter use. Using this new concept, the incidence of catheter-related infection with both tunneled and nontunneled long-term silicone catheters ranges from 1.0 to 1.9 episodes per 1000 catheter-days. In 13 studies reviewed by Clarke and Raffin (44), 17 studies reviewed by Press et al. (45), and 21 studies reviewed by Decker and Edwards (46), the incidence of long-term CVC infection was found to be in the range of 1.4 per 1000 catheter-days. The review by Howell et al. included 26 studies of 3948 catheters in 3478 adult cancer patients and found a CVC infection rate of 1.9 per 1000 catheter-days (10).

The study of 108 catheters conducted by Pasqual et al. (47) comparing Groshong and Hickman catheters indicated that there was no significant difference in septic complications resulting from the use of these devices. Keung et al. (48) conducted a retrospective, comparative study of infectious complications associated with 111 long-term CVCs of different types. Using the log rank test and Cox's multivariate analysis, they also found no significant difference in catheter-related infections between Hickman and Groshong catheters or between subcutaneous ports and tunneled catheters. Likewise, Mueller et al. (49), in a prospective randomized trial comparing complications in external tunneled catheters and subcutaneous ports in 100 children and adults, found no significant difference in the incidence of infection between the two types of devices.

Conversely, Gleeson et al. (50) conducted a study on 104 catheters and found that catheter sepsis occurred with 32% of Groshong catheters versus 16.2% of Hickman ports ($P = 0.04$). Carde and colleagues reported a trial of 100 patients with solid tumors who were randomly assigned to implanted ports or tunneled catheter treatment; the rates of infection were 2% and 11%, respectively (51).

Because of the contradiction in the literature associated with comparing the rates of infection of different types of catheters, Sariego and colleagues (52) retrospectively reviewed a total of 1422 catheters including 730 single-lumen Hickman catheters, 368 double-lumen Hickman catheters, and 307 single-lumen ports. Overall, 60 catheters were removed, replaced, or both prior to completion of the intended therapy (4%). Reasons for removal were infection in 1% of cases and catheter malfunction in 3%. The percentage of ports removed was significantly greater than the percentage of Hickman catheters removed ($P < 0.001$). Another study conducted by Mirro and colleagues (53) involving 120 Hickman catheters, 146 Broviac catheters, and 93 implantable ports in children with malignancy showed that, when all causes of catheter failure were considered, such as infection, obstruction, or dislodgment, indwelling ports had a significantly longer duration of use than percutaneous Hickman or Broviac catheters ($P = 0.0009$). In a prospective, observational study conducted on 1630 long-term venous catheters (788 percutaneous catheters and 680 ports), Groeger and colleagues found that the incidence of infection per device per day was 12 times greater with externalized tunneled catheters than with ports (11).

The number of lumina was thought to play a role in catheter-related infections, but in several studies the rate was not statistically significant. One study conducted by Early et al. (54) showed that infection rate was significantly less in the single-lumen catheter than in the double-lumen catheter (one infection per 1210 days versus one infection per 496 days, respectively; $P \leq 0.02$); however, this study is retrospective and therefore subject to various elements of bias.

Unfortunately, the results obtained from studies comparing ports and tunneled catheters are limited by the small number of patients and poor study design. We are not aware of a single prospective randomized study where the risk factors for catheter infection (such as underlying diseases, neutropenia, thrombosis, duration of placement, and the various uses of the catheter) were matched among the patients undergoing such comparative evaluation. In the absence of such a study, comparisons are subject to selection bias in this very complicated patient population. However, after reviewing the current literature, one may conclude that ports may be associated with the lowest infection rates.

B. Durability, Life Style, and Cost

Creating the tunneled catheter was thought to be a means of preventing migration of microorganisms from skin along the intercutaneous surface of the catheter. However, analysis of data from The University of Texas M. D. Anderson Cancer Center (3,55) in comparison with published data on tunneled catheters revealed that tunneled cuffed catheters had no distinct advantage over percutaneous non-tunneled subclavian silicone catheters. One advantage of percutaneous nontunneled subclavian silicone catheters such as the Hohn catheters (Davol, Inc., Bard Access System, Salt Lake City, UT) is that they can be inserted in the outpatient setting. These devices can also be removed easily if a catheter-related complication occurs, and they are associated with long durability (mean duration of placement is 136 days), low infection rate (0.9 infections per 1000 catheter-days), and significant cost savings when compared to surgically implantable catheters (ports and Hickman and Broviac) (Table 1) (9). However, percutaneous nontunneled subclavian silicone catheters require daily heparin injection and weekly dressing changes, which are disadvantages.

There are several disadvantages to using tunneled catheters. The procedures involved in inserting and removing these devices are more invasive and more costly than some other catheter placement procedures. Daily heparin injections are also required, except for Groshong tunneled CVCs. Because it is an external catheter, the patient's body image can be affected, and this serves as a constant reminder of their disease. The daily to weekly site care, cost of maintenance (including dressing materials, dressings cost, frequency of flushing, and cap changing), and surgery to insert the device (which necessitates postoperative care for 7 to 10 days) are other disadvantages of tunneled catheter use. However, one advantage of tunneled catheters is that breaks or tears in the device can be repaired easily (56). They can be easily maintained in a home setting and can be removed in an outpatient or inpatient setting (57).

Implantable ports carry less risk of infection and less interference with the patient's body image and life style. Maintenance is minimal, and there is no visible reminder of the patient's illness. The presence of this device is revealed only by a small bump under the skin, allowing the patient freedom of activity (58). Implantable ports are preferred in children and patients with active life styles, especially those who enjoy water sports. However, disadvantages to the use of implantable catheters are their high cost, the 7- to 10-day postoperative care period after insertion, and the objection of some patients to the needlestick required to access the port. Removal of the port also requires a minor surgical procedure.

PICCs offer inexpensive outpatient placement that does not require surgery and can usually be performed by a specialized nurse. They are easily removed in an outpatient setting. Their major disadvantages are that daily care is required and that they do affect the patient's body image and activity. Because the catheter is not tunneled and may not be sutured, an occlusive dressing over the exit site is

Table 1 Estimated Insertion Cost (to the Patient) of Catheters at M. D. Anderson Cancer Center

Cost items	Nontunneled		Hickman Tunneled CVC	Ports
	PICC	Subclavian		
Physician	$116[a]	$374	$953	$953
Clinic	90	90	90	90
Catheter	65	88	95	730
Supplies	149	94	799	799
X-ray	115	115	96	96
Fluoroscopic imaging	—	—	81	81
Coagulation study	47	47	47	47
Anesthesia	—	—	274	274
Operating room	—	—	635	635
Recovery room	—	—	236	236
Hospital room	—	—	—	375
Total	$582	$808	$3306	$4316

[a]PICCs are inserted by nurses. The $116 is the nurse's insertion fee.

required at all times. In addition, because of their small lumen size, some PICCs are not recommended for blood withdrawal because they tend to collapse when aspirated (59).

The PICC is gaining acceptance as a long-term venous access device. A review of the literature indicates no detailed description of the complications resulting from the use of this type of catheter. PICC-associated phlebitis is reported in 3.8% to 18% of cases (60–62). This phlebitis is mostly aseptic and has been reported to resolve within 24 to 48 hours without the need to remove the catheter (63). Sepsis associated with this type of catheter is low. In published literature of 296 inserted PICCs, there were only two documented cases of bacteremia (0.7%) (60–65). In a prospective observational study of 154 PICCs at our institution, we have demonstrated that such catheters have a mean duration of placement of 87 days with an infection rate of 1.9/1000 catheter-days (3). Of the PICC devices inserted, 3.9% were associated with catheter-related bacteremia, and 26% were associated with aseptic phlebitis. Hence, this aseptic phlebitis represents one of the major disadvantages of PICC devices.

In conclusion, given the high cost of surgically inserted catheters (ports and tunneled devices) and the long durability of nontunneled percutaneous catheters (such as nontunneled subclavian catheters and PICCs), the primary physician should consider the percutaneous nontunneled silicone catheter as the first option when long-term venous access is required in the chronically ill patient. Ports should be considered in children and in patients who have an active life style or are concerned about cosmetic appearance. The role of the externalized tunneled catheter (Hickman or Broviac) devices should be critically reevaluated given the high cost of their insertion and lack of significant advantages (infection-free durability) over the PICC and nontunneled silicone subclavian catheters.

V.   PREVENTIVE STRATEGIES

A.   Tunneling and Ports

The surgically implantable CVCs represent one of the earliest attempts to prevent the migration of skin organisms along the intercutaneous segment of the catheter. Indeed, the Dacron cuff incorporated into the subcutaneous segment of the tunneled Hickman and Broviac devices does create a tissue interface mechanical barrier against the migration of skin organisms (1,2). The completely implanted subcutaneous ports have been developed in the 1980s with the same intention of avoiding the migration of organisms from the skin along the intercutaneous pathway into the bloodstream (4). However, although the septicemia rate of surgically implantable intravascular devices is low, these devices continue to be associated with serious septicemia episodes as well as tunnel or port site infections (11,66). Given the high cost of inserting and removing such devices, which is in the range of $3000 to $4000 per device, one has to ask the question (3), "Could the same end point of a long durability and low infection rate be achieved by using safe nontunneled silicone catheters?"

Recently, two prospective randomized studies evaluated the effect of catheter tunneling on catheter-related infections (67,68). One study evaluated long-term CVCs (mostly silicone catheters) placed in immunocompromised patients. The risk of catheter-related bacteremia associated with tunneled and nontunneled CVCs were 2% and 5%, respectively. The difference was not significant, most likely due to the relatively small number of patients in each group (107 and 105 patients in each group.) In another study, involving short-term polyurethane catheters placed in the internal jugular vein of critically ill patients, tunneled CVCs were associated with a significantly lower rate of catheter-related bacteremia than nontunneled CVCs. Therefore, tunneling of CVCs may decrease the risk of catheter-related bacteremia. But is the additional cost of tunneling justified by this risk reduction?

B.   Maximal Sterile Barriers

At M. D. Anderson Cancer Center, we recently showed that nontunneled silicone CVCs inserted in the subclavian vein could be maintained for a long period of time (mean duration of stay of 100 days) with a very low infection rate (1.3 per 1000 catheter-days). This is particularly true if these catheters are cared for by a specialized infusion therapy team and are inserted under maximal sterile barrier precautions. We recently conducted a randomized prospective controlled trial comparing maximal sterile barrier precautions (which involves wearing sterile gloves, a mask, a gown, and a cap and using a large drape) during the insertion of a nontunneled subclavian silicone CVC versus control normal procedures (which involves wearing only gloves and using a small drape) as the control (67). The catheter-related sepsis rate was 6.3 times higher in the control group compared to maximal sterile barrier ($P = 0.03$). Most (67%) of the catheter infections in the control group occurred during the first week postinsertion, whereas all the infections in the sterile barrier group occurred more than 2 months following insertion ($P = <0.01$). Cost benefit analysis of these data showed the use of such precautions as highly cost-effective. Such data are compelling in favor of using maximal sterile barriers during the insertion of nontunneled silicone catheters, particularly in the outpatient nonsurgical setting. What was remarkable about that study, however, was that the catheter-related septicemia rate in the control arm was 0.5 per 1000 catheter-days whereas in the maximal sterile barrier arm the catheter-related septicemia rate was reduced to 0.08 per 1000 catheter-days. The mean duration of stay was 67 to 70 days, and these long-term catheters were followed up to 100 days. Hence, one can conclude that nontunneled silicone catheters (inserted in the subclavian vein or as PICC lines) are associated with a very low infection rate if inserted in an aseptic manner and cared for meticulously (3,69).

C. Flushing With Antimicrobials

Because the catheter hub and catheter lumen could be a major source of colonization, prevention of catheter infection has been attempted through the use of antimicrobial or anticoagulant flush solutions. Schwartz et al. used a solution consisting of heparin/vancomycin to flush tunneled CVCs and compared its efficacy to that of heparin alone (70). Daily flushing with a heparin/vancomycin solution decreased the frequency of catheter-related bacteremia caused by vancomycin-susceptible gram positive organisms colonizing the lumen. However, the impact on the overall incidence of catheter-related bacteremia was not assessed, and the authors concentrated only on gram-positive infections. Irrespective of its efficacy, there are at least three factors that can potentially limit the use of heparin/vancomycin catheter flush solutions: (1) the incompatibility of heparin and vancomycin; (2) the limitation of the activity of vancomycin against gram-positive bacteria that might lead to superinfection with gram-negative bacilli and *Candida;* and (3) the concern over the development of vancomycin-resistant gram-positive cocci given the fact that vancomycin is the only therapeutic drug of choice for the treatment of established infections caused by methicillin-resistant staphylococci and penicillin-resistant enterococci. This concern is particularly heightened during this era of emerging vancomycin-resistant enterococci.

Recently, Raad et al. developed a new flush solution consisting of a new combination of low concentration minocycline and EDTA (71). EDTA has been shown to have an anticoagulant activity equal to or even stronger than heparin, and this anticoagulant activity is not diminished by the addition of minocycline. Hence, there is no incompatibility between EDTA and minocycline. In contrast, this combination was found to have a broad spectrum and often synergistic activity against methicillin-resistant staphylococci, gram-negative bacilli (such as *E. aerogenes* and *Stenotrophomonas maltophilia*), and *C. albicans*. In addition, neither minocycline nor EDTA is used in the treatment of bloodstream infections; hence, the risk of the emergence of organisms resistant to this microbicidal combination is low and should not result in a therapeutic dilemma. In a rabbit model of vascular catheter-related infection, this combination was found to be highly efficacious in preventing *S. epidermidis* bacteremia, catheter-related septic phlebitis, and right-sided endocarditis when compared with heparin. This flush solution was also found to prevent the recurrence of catheter infections in several patients who were prone to infection and other complications.

D.   Silver Iontophoresis

Several studies have shown that the attachable silver-impregnated cuff can reduce the incidence of CRIs among critically ill patients with short-term CVCs (mean duration of placement 5.6 to 9.1 days) (72,73). Given the biodegradable nature of the collagen in which the silver ions are chelated, the antimicrobial activity of the collagen cuff is short-lived and hence does not prevent long-term CVC-related infections. This was demonstrated in at least two studies whereby the silver cuff failed to protect against infections and the longer-term CVC (72) (mean duration of placement 20 days) or in the long-term tunneled Hickman catheters (74,75). We recently developed a silver iontophoretic catheter (Fig. 2) in which silver ions are electrically generated at the subcutaneous segment of the device, thereby preventing the migration of organisms from the skin along the transcutaneous pathway into the intravascular compartment (76,77). This catheter allows the release of silver ions over a period of several months and has been shown to have a broad spectrum in vitro inhibitory activity against bacteria and *Candida*. This catheter was also shown in vitro to have a long durability in preventing the migration of organisms and maintaining antimicrobial activity against *S. epidermidis* (76). In a rabbit model, the silver iontophoretic catheter was safe and significantly more efficacious than catheters coated with chlorhexidine and silver sulfadiazine in preventing colonization with *S. aureus* ($P < 0.05$) (77).

E.   Long-Term Coating of Silicone Catheters

In the concluding statement of the study on silver-impregnated attachable cuffs published in the *American Journal of Medicine* 1988, Dennis Maki made the fol-

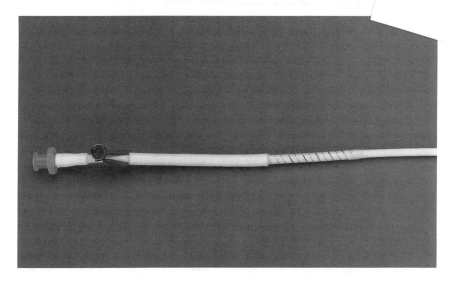

Figure 2 The silver iontophoretic catheter (SIC). A silicone catheter with a 1.5-volt battery near the hub connected to two parallel silver wires helically wrapped around the proximal segment.

lowing comment: "Binding of a nontoxic antiseptic or antimicrobial to the entire catheter surface or incorporation of such a substance into the catheter material itself may ultimately prove to be the most effective technologic innovation for reducing the risk of device-related infections" (72).

In the early 1990s, significant progress has been made in demonstrating that short-term polyurethane catheters could be coated with various antiseptics and antimicrobial agents resulting in a significant decrease in catheter-related bacteremia. Kamal and colleagues demonstrated the protective efficacy of bonding short-term CVCs with cefazolin using a cationic bonding surfactant, the tridodecyl methylammonium chloride (TDMAC) (78). Maki and colleagues coated CVCs with silver sulfadiazine chlorhexidine and demonstrated that such catheters were twofold less likely to become colonized and were at least fourfold less likely to produce bacteremia (79). More recently, we coated polyurethane triple-lumen catheters with a combination of minocycline and rifampin, also using TDMAC, and demonstrated that such catheters have broad-spectrum in vitro inhibitory activity against gram-positive bacteria, gram-negative bacteria, and *C. albicans* (80). These catheters were also found to be highly efficacious in preventing colonization in a rabbit model and in a multicenter prospective randomized clinical trial (81,82). Unfortunately, TDMAC does not bind well to silicone surfaces, where the long-term antimicrobial effect is most desired. Impregnating antimicrobial or antiseptic agents into the silicone catheters in a system that will provide a slow release of these antimicrobials through the external and internal surface over the prolonged placement of such long-term nontunneled silicone catheters would be the challenge of the future. This new development would represent a major technological advance for the prevention of long-term catheter-related infections and would represent a cost-effective alternative to the surgically implantable catheters.

REFERENCES

1. Broviac JW, Cole JJ, Scribner GH. A silicone rubber atrial catheter for prolonged parenteral alimentation. Surg Gynecol Obstet 1973; 136:602.
2. Hickman RO, Buckner CD, Clift RA, et al. A modified right atrial catheter for access to the venous system in marrow transplant recipients. Surg Gynecol Obstet 1979; 148:871.
3. Raad I, Davis S, Becker M, et al. Low infection rate and long durability of nontunneled silastic catheters: a safe and cost-effective alternative for long-term venous access. Arch Intern Med 1993; 153:1791–1796.
4. Goodman MS, Wickman R. Venous access devices: an overview. Oncol Nurs Forum 1984; 11:16–23.
5. Fuchs PC, Gustafson ME, King JT, et al. Assessment of catheter-associated infection risk with the Hickman right atrial catheter. Infect Control 1984; 5:226.
6. Siegel J, Puri RK. Interleukin-2 toxicity. J Clin Oncol 1991; 9:694–701.
7. Bock SN, Lee RE, Fisher B, et al. A prospective randomized trial evaluating prophylactic antibiotics to prevent triple lumen catheter-related sepsis in patients treated with immunotherapy. J Clin Oncol 1990; 8:161–169.
8. Murphy PM, Lane HC, Gollin JI, Fauci AS. Marked disparity in incidence of receiving interleukin-2 or interferon-gamma. Ann Intern Med 1988; 108:36–41.
9. Syndman DR, Sullivan B, Gill M, Gould JA, Parkinson DR, Atkins DB. Nosocomial sepsis with interleukin-2. Ann Intern Med 1990; 112:102–107.
10. Howell PB, Walters PE, Donowitz GR, Farr BM. Risk factors for infection of adult patients with cancer who have tunnelled central venous catheters. Cancer 1995; 75(6):1367–1374.
11. Groeger JS, Lucas AB, Thaler HT, et al. Infectious morbidity associated with long-term use of venous access devices in patients with cancer. Ann Intern Med 1993; 119:1168–1174.
12. Raad II, Luna M, Khalil S-A M, Costerton JW, Lam C, Bodey GP. The relationship between the thrombotic and infectious complications of central venous catheters. JAMA 1994; 271(13):1014–1016.
13. Hampton AA, Sherertz RJ. Vascular-access infections in hospitalized patients. Surg Clin North Am 1988; 68:57–71.
14. Elliott TSJ. Intravascular-device infections. J Med Microbiol 1988; 27:161–167.
15. Maki DG. Risk factors for nosocoial infection in intensive care: 'devices vs nature' and goals for the next decade. Arch Intern Med 1989; 149:30–35.
16. Brismar R, Hardstedt C, Jacobson S. Diagnosis of thrombosis by catheter phlebography after prolonged central venous catheterization. Ann Surg 1981; 194:779–783.

17. Ahmed N, Payne RF. Thrombosis after central venous cannulation. Med J Aust 1976; 1:217.

18. Herrmann M, Vaudaux PE, Pittet D, et al. Fibronectin, fibrinogen, and laminin act as mediators of adherence of clinical staphylococcal isolates to foreign material. J Infect Dis 1988; 158:693–701.

19. Vaudaux P, Pittet D, Haeberli A, et al. Host factors selectively increase staphylococcal adherence on inserted catheters: a role for fibronectin and fibrinogen or fibrin. J Infect Dis 1989; 160:865–875.

20. Christensen GD, Simpson WA, Bisno AL, Beachey EH. Adherence of slime-producing strains of *Staphylococcus epidermidis* to smooth surfaces. Infect Immun 1982; 37:318–326.

21. Christensen GD, Simpson WA, Younger JJ, et al. Adherence of coagulase-negative staphylococci to plastic tissue culture plates: a quantitative model for the adherence of staphylococci to medical devices. J Clin Microbiol 1985; 22:996–1006.

22. Falcieri E, Vaudaux P, Huggler E, Lew D, Waldvogel F. Role of bacterial exopolymers and host factors on adherence and phagocytosis of *Staphylococcus aureus* in foreign body infection. J Infect Dis 1987; 155:524–531.

23. Costerton JW, Irvin RT, Cheng KJ. The bacterial glycocalyx in nature and disease. Annu Rev Microbiol 1981; 35:299–324.

24. Davenport DS, Massanari RM, Pfaller MA, et al. Usefulness of a test for slime production as a marker for clinically significant infections with coagulase-negative staphylococci. J Infect Dis 1986; 153:332–339.

25. Sheth NK, Franson TR, Sohnle PG. Influence of bacterial adherence to intravascular catheters on in vitro antibiotic susceptibility. Lancet 1985; 2:1266–1268.

26. Farber BF, Kaplan MH, Clogstron AG. *Staphylococcus epidermidis* extracted slime inhibits the antimicrobial action of glycopeptide antibiotics. J Infect Dis 1990; 161:37–40.

27. Costerton JW, Lappin-Scott HM. Behavior of bacteria in biofilms. Am Soc Microbiol News 1989; 55:650–654.

28. Sheth NK, Franson TR, Rose HD, et al. Colonization of bacteria on polyvinyl chloride and Teflon intravascular catheter in hospitalized patients. J Clin Microbiol 1983; 18:1061–1063.

29. Rotrosen D, Calderone RA, Edwards JE Jr. Adherence of *Candida* species to host tissues and plastic surfaces. Rev Infect Dis 1986; 8:73–85.

30. Collignon PG, Soni N, Pearson IY, Woods WP, Munro R, Sorrell TC. Is semiquantitative culture of central vein catheter tips useful in the diagnosis of catheter-associated bacteremia? J Clin Microbiol 1986; 24:532–535.

31. Moyer MA, Edwards LD, Farley L. Comparative culture methods on 101 intravenous catheters. Arch Intern Med 1983; 143:66–69.

32. Snydman DR, Murray SA, Kornfeld SJ, Majka JA, Ellis Ca. Total parenteral nutrition-related infections: prospective epidemiologic study using semiquantitative methods. Am J Med 1982; 73:695–699.

33. Cleri DJ, Corrado ML, Seligman SJ. Quantitative culture of intravenous catheters and other intravascular inserts. J Infect Dis 1980; 141:781–786.

34. Bjornson HS, Colley R, Bower RH, Duty VP, Schwartz-Fulton JT, Fisher JE. Association between microorganism growth at the catheter insertion site and colonization of the catheter in patients receiving total parenteral nutrition. Surgery 1982; 92:720–726.

35. Brun-Buisson C, Abrouk F, Legrand P, Huet Y, Larabi S, Rapin M. Diagnosis of central venous catheter-related sepsis: critical level of quantitative tip cultures. Arch Intern Med 1987; 147:873–877.

36. Sherertz RJ, Raad II, Balani A, Koo L, Rand K. Three-year experience with sonicated vascular catheter cultures in a clinical microbiology laboratory. J Clin Microbiol 1990; 28:76–82.

37. Raad II, Sabbagh MF, Rand KH, Sherertz RJ. Quantitative tip culture methods and the diagnosis of central venous catheter-related infections. Diagn Microbiol Infect Dis 1991; 15:13–20.

38. Maki DG. Sources of infection with central venous catheters in an ICU: a prospective study. In: Program and Abstracts of the 28th Interscience Conference on Antimicrobial Agents and Chemotherapy, Los Angeles, 1988; 157. Abstract 269.

39. Sitges-Serra A, Puig P, Linares J, et al. Hub colonization as the initial step in an outbreak of catheter-related sepsis due to coagulase negative staphylococci during parenteral nutrition. JPEN 1984; 8:668–672.

40. Sitges-Serra A, Linares J, Perez JL, Jaurrieta E, Lorente L. A randomized trial on the effect of tubing changes on hub contamination and catheter sepsis during parenteral nutrition. JPEN 1985; 9:322–325.

41. Linares J, Sitges-Serra A, Garau J, Perez JL, Martin R. Pathogenesis of catheter sepsis: a prospective study with quantitative and semiquantitative cultures of catheter hub and segments. J Clin Microbiol 1985; 21:357–360.

42. Raad I, Costerton W, Sabbarwal U, Sacilowski M, Anaissie E, Bodey GP. Ultrastructural analysis of indwelling catheters: a quantitative relationship between luminal colonization and duration of placement. J Infect Dis 1993; 168:400–407.

43. Maki DG. Pathogenesis, prevention, and management of infections due to intravascular devices used for infusion therapy. In: Bisno AL, Waldvogel FA, eds. Infections Associated With Indwelling Medical Devices. Washington: American Society for Microbiology, 1989:161–77.

44. Clarke DE, Raffin TA. Infectious complications of indwelling long-term central venous catheters. Chest 1990; 97(4):966–972.

45. Press OW, Ramsey PG, Larson EB, Fefer A, Hickman RO. Hickman catheter infections in patients with malignancies. Medicine 1984; 63(4):189–200.

46. Decker MD, Edwards KM. Central venous catheter infections. Pediatr Clin North Am 1988; 35(3):579–612.

47. Pasquale MD, Campbell JM, Magnant CM. Groshong versus Hickman catheters. Surgery 1992; 174:408–410.

48. Keung Y-K, Watkins K, Chen S-C, Groshen S, Silberman H, Douer D. Comparative study of infectious complications of different types of chronic central venous access devices. Cancer 1994; 73(11):2832–2837.

49. Mueller BU, Skelton J, Callender DPE, et al. A prospective randomized trial comparing the infectious complications of the externalized catheters versus a subcutaneously implanted device in cancer patients. J Clin Oncol 1992; 10:1943–1948.

50. Gleeson NC, Fiorica JV, Mark JE, et al. Externalized Groshong catheters and Hickman ports for central venous access in gynecologic oncology patients. Gynecol Oncol 1993; 51:372–376.

51. Carde P, Cossett-Delaigue MF, LaPlanche A, Chareau I. Classical external

indwelling central venous catheter versus totally implanted venous access systems for chemotherapy administration: a randomized trial in 100 patients with solid tumors. Eur J Cancer Clin Oncol 1989; 6:939–944.

52. Sariego J, Bootorabi B, Matsumoto T, Kerstein M. Major long-term complications in 1,422 permanent venous access devices. Am J Surg 1993; 165:249–251.

53. Mirro J, Rao BN, Kumar M, et al. A comparison of placement techniques and complications of externalized catheters and implantable port use in children with cancer. J Pediatr Surg 1990; 25(1):122–124.

54. Early TF, Gregory RT, Wheeler JR, Snyder SO, Gayle RG. Increased infection rate in double-lumen versus single-lumen Hickman catheters in cancer patients. South Med J 1990; 83(1):34–36.

55. Broadwater JR, Henderson MA, Bell JL, et al. Outpatient percutaneous central venous access in cancer patients. Am J Surg 1990; 160:676–680.

56. Anderson MA, Aker SN, Hickman RO. The double-lumen Hickman catheter. Am J Nurs 1982; 82:272–277.

57. Goodman MS, Wickman R. Venous access devices: an overview. Oncol Nurs Forum 1984; 11:16–23.

58. Bagnall H, Ruccione K. Experience with a totally implanted venous access device in children with malignant disease. Oncol Nurs Forum 1987; 14:51–56.

59. Slater H, Goldfarb IW, Jacob HE, et al. Experience with long-term outpatient venous access utilizing percutaneously placed silicone elastomer catheters. Cancer 1985; 56:2074–2077.

60. Markel S, Reynen K. Impact on patient care: 2652 PIC catheter days in the alternative setting. J Intravenous Nur 1990; 13(6):347–351.

61. Rutherford C. Insertion and care of multiple lumen peripherally inserted central line catheters. J Intravenous Nurs 1988; 11(1):16–19.

62. Borwn JM. Peripherally inserted central catheters: use in homecare. J Intravenous Nurs 1989; 12(3):144–147.

63. Chathas MK. Percutaneous central venous catheters in neonates. JOGNN 1986; 144(11):324–332.

64. Rutherford C. A study of single lumen peripherally inserted central line catheter dwelling time and complications. J Intravenous Nurs 1988; 11(3):169–173.

65. Nakamura RT, Sato Y, Erenberg A. Evaluation of a percutaneously placed 27-gauge central venous catheter in neonates weighing <1200 grams. JPEN 1990; 14(3):295–299.

66. Benezra D, Kiehn TE, Gold GWM, Brown AE, Turnbull ADM, Armstrong D. Prospective study of infections in indwelling central venous catheters using quantitative blood cultures. Am J Med 1988; 85:495–498.

67. Andrivet P, Bacquer A, Vu Ngoc C, et al. Lack of clinical benefit from subcutaneous tunnel insertion of central venous catheters in immunocompromised patients. CID 1994; 18:199–206.

68. Timsit JF, Sebille V, Farkas JC, et al. Effect of subcutaneous tunneling on internal jugular catheter-related sepsis in critically ill patients. JAMA 1996; 276:1416–1420.

69. Raad II, Hohn DC, Gilbreath BJ, et al. Prevention of catheter-related infections by using maximal sterile barrier precautions during insertion. Infect Control Hosp Epidemiol 1994; 15(4):231–238.

70. Schwartz C, Henrickson KJ, Roghmann K, Powell K. Prevention of bacteremia attributed to luminal colonization of tunneled central venous catheters with vancomycin-susceptible organism. J Clin Oncol 1990; 8:1591–1597.

71. Raad I, Hachem R, Sherertz R. Minocycline-EDTA (M-EDTA) flush solution for the prevention of vascular catheter infection. In: Proceedings of the 34th Interscience Conference on Antimicrobial Agents and Chemotherapy, Orlando; 1994:69. Abstract J57.

72. Maki DG, Garman JK, Shapiro JM, Ringer M, Helgerson RB. An attachable silver-impregnated cuff for prevention of infection with central venous catheters: a prospective randomized multicenter trial. Am J Med 1988; 85:307–314.

73. Flowers RH III, Shwenzer KJ, Kopel RF, Fisch MJ, Tucker SI, Farr BM. Efficacy of an attachable subcutaneous cuff for the prevention of intravascular catheter-related infection: a randomized, controlled trial. JAMA 1989; 261:878–883.

74. Clementi E, Mario O, Arlet G, et al. Usefulness of an attachable silver-impregnated cuff for prevention of catheter-related sepsis (CRS). In: Program and Abstracts of the 31st Interscience Conference on Antimicrobial Agents and Chemotherapy, Chicago; 1991:175. Abstract 460.

75. Groeger JS, Lucas AB, Coit D, et al. A prospective randomized evaluation of silver-impregnated subcutaneous cuffs for preventing tunneled chronic venous access catheter infections in cancer patients. Ann Surg 1993; 218:206–210.

76. Raad I, Hachem R, Zermeno A, Dumo M, Bodey GP. In vitro antimicrobial efficacy of silver iontophoretic catheter. Biomaterials. In press.

77. Raad I, Hachem R, Zermeno A, et al. Silver iontophoretic catheter: a prototype of long-term antiinfective vascular access device. J Infect Dis. In press.

78. Kamal GD, Pfaller MA, Rempe LE, Jebson PJR. Reduced intravascular catheter infection by antibiotic bonding. JAMA 1991; 265:2364–2368.

79. Maki DG, Wheller SJ, Stolz SM, Mermel LA. Clinical trial of a novel antiseptic central venous catheter. In: Program and Abstracts of the 31st Interscience Conference on Antimicrobial Agents and Chemotherapy, Chicago; 1991:176. Abstract 461.

80. Raad I, Darouiche R, Hachem R, Bodey GP. The broad spectrum activity of catheters coated with minocycline and rifampin (M/R) against bacteria and fungi. In: Program and Abstracts of the 34th Interscience Conference on Antimicrobial Agents and Chemotherapy, Orlando; 1994:194. Abstract J195.

81. Raad I, Hachem R, Darouiche R, Bodey G. Efficacy of minocycline/rifampin (M/R) in preventing staphylococcal infections: in vitro and in vivo correlation. In: Program and Abstracts of the 33rd Interscience Conference on Antimicrobial Agents and Chemotherapy, New Orleans; 1993:258. Abstract 758.

82. Raad I, Darouiche R. Central venous catheters (CVC) coated with minocycline and rifampin (M/R) for the prevention of catheter-related bacteremia (CRB). In: Program and Abstracts of the 35th Interscience Conference on Antimicrobial Agents and Chemotherapy, San Francisco; 1995:258. Abstract J7.

12

Infections Associated with Central Nervous System Implants

Roger Bayston

City Hospital, Nottingham, England

I. INTRODUCTION

Hydrocephalus is caused by the accumulation of cerebrospinal fluid (CSF) within the ventricular system, almost always due to inadequate reabsorption. This in turn can be due to fetal maldevelopment; infections such as congenital toxoplasmosis or meningitis (including tuberculous); periventricular hemorrhage in premature neonates; or hemorrhage, trauma, or malignancy later in life. It therefore affects all age groups and arises from a variety of underlying pathologies.

A. Development of CSF Shunts

Though attempts have been made to treat raised intracranial pressure through the ages, successful treatment became possible only after the introduction of the silicone shunt by Holter and Pudenz in the 1950s. This led to the development of a variety of silicone devices of basically similar design for the controlled drainage of fluids. The Holter shunt consists of two matched silicone slit valves in metal housing, connected to a ventricular catheter and a distal catheter (Fig. 1). The two valves must ensure that flow is neither too fast nor too slow, and that it is unidirectional. There is usually an integrated reservoir in the system. Later shunts differ in appearance but incorporate the same features and functions. Recent advances have brought valve systems that employ different mechanisms (e.g., Orbis-Sigma, Cordis, USA) or which can be adjusted noninvasively by electromagnetic means after implantation (e.g., Sophy, Sophysa, France; Medos, Johnson & Johnson Professional, USA).

B. Routes of Shunting

Currently the preference is to drain CSF from the lateral cerebral ventricle using a parietal, frontal, or occipital burr hole to the peritoneal cavity (ventriculoperitoneal or VP; Fig. 2), though the original ventriculoatrial (VA) route draining into the right atrium via the jugular vein is still used in approximately 8% to 10% of cases worldwide. Drainage of CSF from the lumbar theca to the peritoneal cavity is sometimes undertaken, though it is suitable only for cases in which there is free communication between the ventricular system and the spinal theca. This is not the case in spina bifida, where there is a Chiari II malformation. Other routes, such as drainage to the pleural space or the gallbladder, are used less commonly.

C. External Ventricular Drains, Reservoirs, and Similar Devices

1. External Ventricular Drainage

For short-term control of intracranial pressure, or in the presence of infection, an external ventricular drain (EVD) can be used. This exteriorizes through a scalp incision usually tunneled away from the burr hole, and the CSF drains into a sterile bag in a closed system. There is some means of pressure regulation, either hydrostatically or by means of a valve (Fig. 3).

2. Ventricular Reservoirs

Ommaya reservoirs (Heyer Schulte, USA), consisting of a ventricular catheter connecting extradurally to a silicone or metal-silicone reservoir "button" (Fig. 4) are inserted to allow frequent ventricular access without repeated cerebral puncture. They are used for injection of antibiotics or oncologic drugs and for pressure monitoring or withdrawal of CSF for pressure control or analysis.

3. Ascites Shunts

A shunt system very similar to those used for hydrocephalus is used in cases of hepatic cirrhosis or malignancy to drain ascitic fluid from the peritoneal cavity to the venous system (Fig. 5). An example in common use is the LeVeen shunt.

4. Intraspinal Drug Delivery Devices

While drugs such as morphine, for intractable pain, or baclophen, for relief of spasticity, can be administered intravenously, there is no doubt that their effects are greater, more immediate, and more easily controlled if they are administered intrathecally. The most efficient way of doing this is by means of a catheter insert-

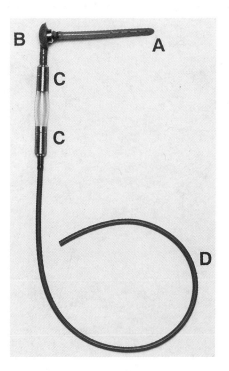

Figure 1 The Holter valve and shunt for control of hydrocephalus. (A) Ventricular catheter; (B) Rickham reservoir for sampling, pressure measurement, etc; (C) unidirectional flow-control valves in a steel housing; (D) distal catheter to right atrium VA shunt or peritoneal cavity (VP shunt). Apart from the valve housings and the base of the reservoir, all parts are silicone.

ed into the spinal theca and connected via a pump to a reservoir. The whole system is implanted and the reservoir can be recharged percutaneously (Fig. 6).

Infection is an important cause of morbidity associated with the use of all of these devices, contributing significantly to treatment failure and deterioration of the primary illness.

II. INFECTIONS ASSOCIATED WITH HYDROCEPHALUS SHUNTS

A.   Etiology of Shunt Infections

1. Incidence of Infection

The incidence of CSF shunt infection is similar whether the VA or the VP route is used (1). Rates varying from less than 1% to more than 20% of operations have

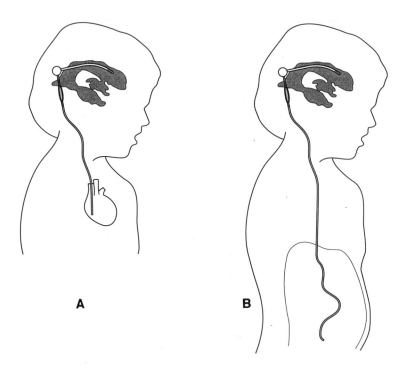

Figure 2 (A) Route of ventriculoatrial shunt for hydrocephalus; (B) route of ventriculoperitoneal shunt.

been reported (2–5), and an average of 10% is often quoted. However, this conceals a number of variables. Firstly, there is often confusion between (1) internal shunt infection where the lumen of the shunt is colonized, and (2) external infection involving the tissue surrounding the shunt, which is usually secondary to a postoperative wound infection, though some external infections develop later owing to trauma or skin erosion over the shunt. Internal shunt infections constitute the majority. Also, incidences are cited from different types of study. Retrospective surveys probably give the most accurate figure, as prospective surveys are usually associated with a fall in infection rate due to the conduction of the study (6). In addition there is a considerably higher incidence in the newborn period than in later years. While approximately 3% to 5% of shunts placed in older children and adults become infected, the incidence can be as high as 25% in those inserted in premature neonates (7,8). While certain components of the neonatal immune system are immature, this is unlikely to be relevant in view of the way in which shunt infections arise, by mainly cutaneous bacteria entering the incision at insertion. A recent study has shown that neonates who have very high

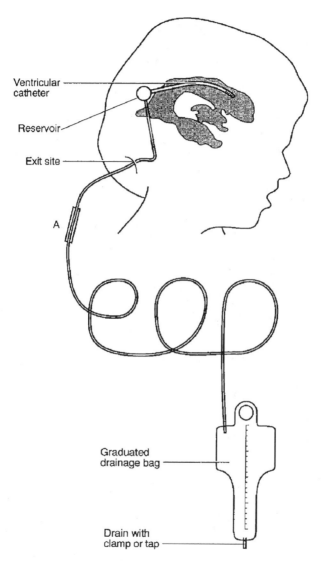

Figure 3 External ventricular drainage for raised intracranial pressure. (A) Either a drip chamber or a unidirectional valve to prevent reflux of fluid. Other designs may have an integral manometer for pressure measurement, three-way taps, injection ports, etc. The drainage bag is usually designed to be discarded when full, but some have a drain so that the bag can be emptied and reused without disconnection.

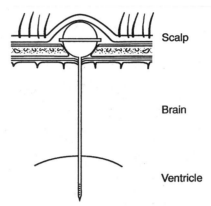

Figure 4 Ommaya reservoir for ventricular access. This is made from silicone, but other designs, such as the Rickham reservoir, also have steel parts.

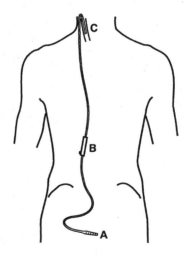

Figure 5 Peritoneovenous shunt for control of intractable ascites. (A) Peritoneal catheter with inlet holes; (B) unidirectional valve to prevent reflux; (C) distal catheter to jugular vein. Alternatively, the distal catheter may drain ascitic fluid to the portal vein. The shunt is made from silicone.

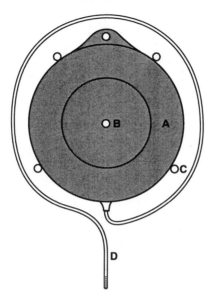

Figure 6 Totally implantable intraspinal drug delivery device. (A) Housing for reservoir, battery, and pump; (B) injection port for recharging reservoir; (C) loops for tissue fixation; (D) catheter to spinal theca.

numbers of normal flora on their skins preoperatively are particularly likely to develop a shunt infection. Moreover, there is a higher incidence of multiresistant, highly adherent strains of coagulase-negative staphylococci (CoNS) in this group (9).

2. Mechanisms of CSF Shunt Infection: Causative Organisms

There is now little doubt that almost all internal shunt infections arise from organisms gaining access to the CSF or shunt at operation. The causative organisms have been shown in many cases to be derived from the patient's skin (9–11). In centers where the incidence is abnormally high, there may be other contributing factors such as contamination of the air in the operating theater and this could explain the fall in infection rate in one study to 8%, still considered to be unacceptable, following the introduction of surgical isolators (7). The majority are caused by CoNS, and particularly *Staphylococcus epidermidis*. Some are caused by *Staphylococcus aureus*, coryneforms, or other gram-positive bacteria, while in most studies gram-negative bacilli are involved in a minority of cases (Table 1).

External infections, on the other hand, are usually caused by *S. aureus* or gram-negative bacilli, and only rarely by CoNS. Occasionally, polymicrobial

Table 1 Bacteria Causing CSF Shunt Infections

Study	No. of cases	Percent				
		S. epidermidis	S. aureus	Enterococcus	Coryneforms	GNB[a]
Shapiro et al. (10)	20	55	20	0	5	20
Pople et al. (9)	46	70	4	2	8	4
Renier et al. (7)	80	50	24	0	0	18
Schoenbaum et al. (3)	68	62	25	3	1	6
George et al. (106)	123	40	20	0	0	20
Total	337	55	19	1	3	14

[a]GNB = enteric gram-negative bacilli.

infections are seen in patients with VP shunts. The organisms are usually representative of the colonic flora and their presence indicates perforation of the intestine by the distal catheter. *Candida* shunt infections are usually contracted at operation and, while rare, are associated particularly with long preoperative hospitalization and exposure to antibiotics (12).

3. Virulence Factors

The predominance of *S. epidermidis*, also seen in other implant-related infections, is due not only to its frequency as a member of the skin flora, but also to the ability of many strains to adhere to silicone elastomer and then to produce exopolymer ("slime") which facilitates microcolony formation (13–16). Coryneforms causing shunt infections have also been shown to produce exopolysaccharide (17).

4. Community-Acquired Meningitis

Patients with shunts appear to be equally at risk from community-acquired meningitis due to *Haemophilus influenzae*, *Neisseria meningitidis*, or *Streptococcus pneumoniae* as those without shunts. However, these organisms are unable to adhere to silicone elastomer and to colonize the shunts, and these cases should be distinguished from shunt infections.

B. Diagnosis

1. Presenting Symptoms

Infection in VA and VP shunts presents differently. In patients with VA shunts, symptoms worthy of medical attention often do not appear for many months or years after operation, even though retrospective review will often show sporadic positive blood cultures and pyrexial episodes. Early cases are characterized by fever, tachycardia, and rigors, and the clinical diagnosis is usually not difficult. However, in cases in which the presentation is delayed, fever may be rare or intermittent, sometimes occurring as episodes of pyrexia and chills several days or weeks apart. Secondary immune phenomena appear, giving rise to transient rashes, arthralgia, muscular aches, and other vague symptoms. Anemia is a universal finding. Eventually, immune complex disease results in glomerulonephritis with blood, protein, and casts in the urine; loin pain; hypertension; uremia; and low creatinine clearance (18–21). The immune complexes are deposited along with complement and immunoglobulins on the glomerular basement membranes, precipitating an acute inflammatory response with destruction of glomeruli. First described in 1965 by Black et al. (18), the condition was later termed "shunt nephritis" by Stauffer (19). Shunt nephritis can be associated with shunt infections due to organisms other than CoNS, and coryneforms (22,23) and propionibacteria (24,25) have also been implicated. Immune vasculitis, appearing as ulcerative and hemorrhagic skin lesions, has also been reported (1). There are many published and anecdotal reports of incorrect diagnosis based on such symptoms (1,26,27), some resulting in tragedy.

VP shunt infections usually present within a few months of operation. Fever is less common and there is usually return of the features of hydrocephalus with headache, vomiting, and visual disturbance. Abdominal signs and symptoms may be absent, or there may be pain or bloating. In rare cases the abdominal pain may present as an acute emergency, sometimes resulting in inappropriate surgical intervention (28). Erythema can often be seen over the track of the lower catheter, and in cases due to *S. aureus* the catheter tip may protrude from the old incision site. Radiological examination often shows a cystic collection of fluid around the tip of the distal catheter (29,30). This explains the earlier presentation than that seen in VA infections: the peritoneal inflammation resulting from the infection causes adhesions and omental occlusion of the shunt, while obstruction due to infection is rarely seen in VA shunts. Anemia and immune complex disease are not seen in VP shunt infections.

Lumboperitoneal shunt infections present in a similar way to VP shunt infections, though spinal arachnoiditis may develop, giving rise to back pain. Ventriculopleural shunts often present with obstruction as in VP shunts but with respiratory distress due to large collections of CSF in the pleural space.

In all types of shunt, ventriculitis is common but not universal, and there is often only a feeble intracranial inflammatory response.

2. Diagnostic Tests

Blood culture is almost always undertaken in the investigation of suspected shunt infection. In early VA infections culture is usually positive, but in later cases a positive culture might never be obtained even though infection is later proved by shunt examination on removal (21). Alternatively, a culture contaminated with CoNS or "diphtheroids" can lead to an incorrect false-positive diagnosis. To further complicate matters, coryneforms commonly grow only in the aerobic bottle of a blood culture set, further suggesting contamination (31). Blood culture is rarely positive in VP shunt infection by CoNS. Consecutively isolated strains of CoNS can be compared by identification using a system such as API Staph (bio-Mérieux; France) and antibiogram, but further discrimination is always needed, and a variety of molecular typing methods are available. Tests for "pathogenicity" based on exopolymer ("slime") production are not useful (16,32,33).

CSF can be aspirated aseptically from the shunt reservoir, and if organisms are seen on microscopy, the diagnosis is confirmed irrespective of CSF neutrophil count. However, the design of some shunts in common use allows aspiration of normal CSF from the reservoir where infection is confined to the shunt tubing and ventriculitis is absent (29,34), and negative results should be interpreted with caution.

Hematological investigations including peripheral white blood cell counts are generally not helpful, with the exception of hemoglobin determination in suspected VA infection. Erythrocyte sedimentation rate (ESR) is affected by many factors and is slow to react, making it less useful than C-reactive protein (CRP) determination. This can be carried out rapidly and accurately in modern laboratories and is a useful though nonspecific indicator of inflammatory response. The test has been found to be useful in detection of VP shunt infection though it remains normal in most cases of VA infection (35,36).

3. Serological Diagnostic Tests

As the majority of shunt infections are caused by CoNS, measurement of antibody to these organisms can be useful in diagnosis. Different antigens are used to detect VA and VP shunt infections, probably because of differences in the way antigen is processed and presented in the blood and the peritoneal cavity. An agglutination test employing a heat-treated whole-cell "antigen," the anti-*Staphylococcus epidermidis* titer (ASET), has been in use for many years with VA shunts (37,38). Healthy individuals have no antibody to this antigen until about 6 months of age, and no maternal antibody appears to be transmitted. The titer then rises through 160 to about 320 to 640 in adulthood. In CoNS VA shunt infections titers rise to at least four or five times the age-normal and in older children and adults can reach >40,000. Those with CoNS VP shunt infections show no significant change in titer using this test though immunoblotting against whole-cell proteins has shown that in these cases antibody is produced against proteins of 29 kDa to 97 kDa. Antibody also reacts with polysaccharide B from the bacterial cell wall (39,40) in VP and VA shunt infections; an ELISA diagnostic test has shown promising results (41) which are being evaluated clinically. Until such tests are brought into use, infective and noninfective obstruction in VP shunts must be distinguished by clinical examination and CRP determination. Symptoms of distal catheter obstruction appearing within 6 months of operation and a positive CRP test strongly suggest infection.

In VA shunt infections becoming apparent more than 1 year after operation, immune complex disease can be detected by determination of serum C3c and C4 complement levels. Renal biopsy is rarely indicated.

4. Consequences of Shunt Infection

VA shunt infection may give rise to longstanding low-grade illness with debility, anorexia, poor sleep patterns, loss of school or employment time, and possible renal failure. VP shunt infections can result in peritoneal adhesions, intraperitoneal abscesses, repeated operation for obstruction, and recurrence of raised intracranial pressure. Ventriculitis occurs with both types of shunt. Shunt infection is an important cause of loss of IQ points (42,43). The more serious consequences in each type of shunt can be avoided by early, accurate diagnosis.

5. External Infections in Shunts

In external infections there is usually erythema over the valve or catheter, often associated with a dehisced surgical incision or trauma. There may also be frank suppuration. Though there may be fever and general toxicity, many patients remain well. In the early stages there is no ventriculitis or peritonitis, but infection eventually spreads along the catheter track.

6. Visceral Perforation

Perforation of a hollow abdominal viscus, usually the intestine, by the distal catheter is accompanied by surprisingly few symptoms in most cases (11,44,45) and may be suspected only when the tip of the catheter protrudes from the anus. The CSF usually contains several enteric organisms including anaerobes. There is usually no peritonitis.

C. Treatment

1. Problems of Treatment of CSF Shunt Infections

The problems associated with treatment of shunt infections are related to the properties of the infecting organisms and to chemotherapeutic pharmacokinetics. Many strains of CoNS and coryneforms are multiresistant, showing insusceptibility to penicillin, methicillin, cephalosporins, aminoglycosides, macrolides, and often quinolones. They are also capable of producing extensive biofilm within the shunt tubing. Organisms in the biofilm mode are slow-growing and relatively insusceptible to antimicrobials (46,47). The lack of a vigorous inflammatory response to most shunt infections means that almost all agents given systemically will fail to penetrate into the CSF in therapeutic concentrations, even for planktonic bacteria.

There is also an effective excretion pathway from the CSF space for carboxylic acids such as β-lactams (48). For these reasons, attempts to treat shunt infections without shunt removal have usually failed. Cohen et al. (49) gave intravenous methicillin for more than 50 days, without effect, before administering the drug intraventricularly for a similar period. The infection persisted and was eradicated only on shunt removal. This early experience has been repeated many times since using a variety of agents.

2.   Shunt Removal

A useful randomized comparison of three methods of treatment was carried out by James et al. (50) (Table 2). In group A the shunt was removed and intravenous, and intraventricular antimicrobials were given for 7 days. In group B the infected shunt was immediately replaced with a new one, and antimicrobials were injected into it daily for 3 weeks. In group C the shunt was not removed, but both intravenous and intraventricular antimicrobials were given for 3 weeks. Various antimicrobials were used depending on susceptibility test results. Each group consisted of 10 patients. In each of the first two groups, where the infected shunt was removed, all 10 patients were cured, whereas only three patients were cured in the third group. In addition, the mean hospital stay of 24 days in the first group was exceeded by 9 and 23 days in groups B and C, respectively; two patients in group C died. This study confirmed the experience of most physicians and sur-

Table 2 Randomized Comparison of Three Methods of Treatment for CSF Shunt Infection

Group	Treatment	Mean hospital stay (days)	Outcome
A: 10 patients	Shunt removal; IV antibiotics 7 days; IVent antibiotics 7 days	24 ± 7	10 cured
B: 10 patients	Shunt removal; immediate replacement; IV antibiotics 3 weeks; ISh antibiotics 2 weeks	33 ± 8	9 cured 1 relapsed
C: 10 patients	IV antibiotics 3 weeks; ISh antibiotics 2 weeks	47 ± 37	3 cured 7 failures 2 deaths

Abbreviations: IV = intravenous; IVent = intraventricular; ISh = intrashunt.
Source: From Ref. 50.

geons involved in treating shunt infections, and clearly indicated that shunt removal must form part of the management.

3. Antimicrobials Used in Treatment of CSF Shunt Infections

A wide variety of antimicrobials have been used in the treatment of shunt infections, even when we consider only those caused by gram-positive bacteria. In view of what is known of the effect of biofilms on antimicrobial activity, one cannot be guided by susceptibility tests alone, except in the case of resistance. In addition a chosen antimicrobial must either be suitable for intraventricular administration or be capable of attaining therapeutic CSF concentrations in the absence of meningeal inflammation. The β-lactams are therefore not suitable for treatment of shunt infection due to gram-positive bacteria. Chloramphenicol was used for many years in neurosurgical infection and meningitis because of its ability to reach the CSF even after oral administration, in the absence of meningeal inflammation. However, this drug has no place in the treatment of shunt infection as its binding to the bacterial ribosome is reversible, and its action on gram-positive bacteria is bacteriostatic. Treatment failures have been reported, and in the author's early experience the drug has been uniformly ineffective, even after intraventricular administration (1). Trimethoprim also reaches the CSF after oral administration (51) and has been used in conjunction with intraventricular gentamicin to treat shunt infection (52), though the results were not encouraging.

Rifampicin is highly active against most strains of gram-positive bacteria involved in shunt infections, and it also attains therapeutic CSF concentrations in the absence of meningeal inflammation even when given orally. However, its use alone results in rapid development of resistance (53).

Gentamicin has been used to treat CoNS shunt infections and has been given both intravenously and intraventricularly, though once again results have been disappointing (1).

Of the glycopeptides, most experience has been gained with vancomycin. While this agent when given intravenously fails to give satisfactory CSF concentrations in the absence of inflammation, it has been given safely by the intraventricular route in relatively large doses (54,55). With very rare exceptions all CoNS and most other gram-positive bacteria causing shunt infection are susceptible, though strains of enterococci resistant to glycopeptides have recently appeared (56). Fortunately these have not yet posed a problem in shunt infections. Visconti and Peters (57) successfully treated a case of CoNS shunt infection with intravenous and intraventricular vancomycin, the latter in a dose of 20 mg daily, and shunt removal.

Ring et al. (58) removed the VP shunt in a CoNS infection, but the ventriculitis persisted despite treatment with chloramphenicol and nafcillin. The patient recovered rapidly following institution of oral rifampicin and intravenous vancomycin. A similar case was reported by Gombert et al. (59).

Ryan et al. (54) treated a case of enterococcal meningitis with intravenous vancomycin and intraventricular gentamicin without success, measurable CSF drug levels not having been achieved. Intraventricular vancomycin 20 mg daily was begun and the drug levels became satisfactory, but there was no clinical improvement until oral rifampicin was added, when prompt recovery occurred. As it became clear that the most successful antimicrobial therapy for CoNS shunt infection should include intraventricular vancomycin along with shunt removal, a multicenter prospective clinical trial was established to investigate this (60). In the 24 cases receiving vancomycin 20 mg daily intraventricularly along with another systemic antimicrobial (flucloxacillin or rifampicin) and shunt removal, 22 were cured without relapse, and two were lost to follow-up. In cases where the dose had been reduced or where the protocol had otherwise not been complied with, the success rate was significantly lower. It is interesting to note that in this study nine patients were inadvertently included who did not undergo shunt removal, and five relapsed on stopping treatment, a further patient dying of a secondary infection. In only three cases was the infection eradicated, and all underwent revision for distal catheter obstruction soon afterward.

Teicoplanin has also been used intraventricularly in a few cases. Venditti et al. (62) successfully treated two cases of shunt infection due to methicillin-resistant *S. aureus* with 20 mg and 40 mg daily intraventricularly; Guerrero et al. (63) used 10 mg daily in two cases. In all four cases the shunt was removed. While there would appear to be no advantage in using teicoplanin instead of vancomycin intraventricularly, in rare cases of rifampicin resistance where intravenous vancomycin might be used, teicoplanin could be substituted on the grounds that it is less toxic by the intravenous route and is easier to administer.

4. Recommended Regimen for CSF Shunt Infections

Further experience has now shown that the regimen of shunt removal and external ventricular drainage, intraventricular vancomycin 20 mg daily and rifampicin 300 mg twice daily orally or intravenously for 7 to 10 days succeeds in eradicating CoNS infection in almost 100% of cases. In patients with very small ventricles the daily dose of vancomycin can be lowered to 10 mg, but it is important to realize that the dose is based on ventricular volume—not body weight or age. CSF drug levels can be monitored, but in our hands this is no longer done routinely as high CSF concentrations (80 to 200 mg/L) of vancomycin are expected and are not associated with toxicity. The external drain is managed with scrupulous aseptic care to avoid secondary infection, though the short duration of treatment makes this less likely. Vancomycin can be diluted in 2 ml of sterile water for injection, or in 2 ml of freshly aspirated CSF, and should always be flushed into the ventricle with 0.5 to 1 ml water. The external drain should be clamped during injection and for about 1 hour afterward. The last dose of vancomycin should be given perioperatively when the new shunt is inserted, and the rifampicin should also be stopped at this time. There is no requirement for continuation of either agent postoperatively. Continuation of rifampicin alone is likely to lead to spread of resistant strains. The regimen is also satisfactory for shunt infections due to *S. aureus*, coryneforms, and susceptible enterococci. A Working Party of the British Society for Antimicrobial Chemotherapy has recently recommended the adoption of this regimen (61).

Though the recommended regimen includes shunt removal, Brown and Jones (64) have reported success with CoNS but not *S. aureus* using intraventricular vancomycin and oral rifampicin without shunt removal in selected patients. Further confirmation is awaited.

5. Infections due to Gram-Negative Bacilli

In shunt infections caused by gram-negative bacilli there is almost always sufficient meningeal inflammation to ensure penetration of β-lactams and aminoglycosides. The shunt should be removed and intravenous ceftazidime or gentamicin should be given for up to 14 days. There is no requirement to continue antibiotics postoperatively after shunt replacement.

6. Infections Due to Visceral Perforation

Polymicrobial infections, in which the lower catheter of the VP shunt has perforated the large bowel or the vagina, should be treated with shunt removal in the usual manner, using gentle traction on the lower catheter. There is usually no evidence of peritonitis, and laparotomy is not indicated, the perforation healing spontaneously (45,65,66). Broad-spectrum antimicrobials (amoxicillin-clavulanic acid or a second- or third-generation cephalosporin) including metronidazole should be given for up to 14 days or until the infection is eradicated. Reshunting, if necessary, may need to be by the VA route.

7. Infections Due to Candida

Candida shunt infection is uncommon (12) and usually leads to obstruction of both VA and VP shunts due to hyphal growth in the tubing. Intravenous amphotericin B and flucytosine should be given and the CSF monitored for eradication of the infection. Alternatively, intravenous fluconazole can be used, subject to susceptibility tests (67). There is no advantage in giving amphotericin B intraventricularly unless CSF levels are found to be low. Severe neurotoxicity has been reported when this route is used (68). Shunt removal is mandatory.

8. External Infections in Shunts

In cases of external shunt infection, intravenous antimicrobials should be given immediately. Cefuroxime is recommended for staphylococci and gram-negative bacilli, but, in case of methicillin-resistant *S. aureus*, gentamicin, vancomycin, or teicoplanin should be substituted. For *Pseudomonas aeruginosa* or other resistant gram-negative bacilli, ceftazidime or a quinolone should be used. However, unless treatment is begun early, the shunt is very unlikely to be salvaged. Signs of shunt obstruction, failure to defervesce, or persistence of erythema or purulence should prompt shunt removal and continuation of antimicrobials for 10 to 14 days before reshunting on the opposite side.

9. Community-Acquired Meningitis

Community-acquired meningitis in patients with shunts should be treated conventionally and the shunt should not be removed (1,69–72) as it is not at risk of secondary colonization from *H. influenzae, S. pneumoniae*, or *N. meningitidis*. The presence of a shunt in such cases probably helps to regulate intracranial pressure and improve the outcome (69). In *H. influenzae* infections chloramphenicol should be considered, as experience suggests that it gives better results than cephalosporins (1). Stern et al. (72) successfully treated one patient with chloramphenicol without shunt removal but failed in a second case with exteriorization of the shunt and intravenous cefuroxime. Rennels and Wald (70) also succeeded with chloramphenicol in their four cases.

D. Prevention

1. Preoperative Skin Preparation

There is now ample evidence that virtually all shunt infections due to gram-positive bacteria are introduced during insertion or revision of the device. There is also evidence that the causative organisms in most cases are derived from the patient's skin flora, surviving the skin preparation to contaminate the incision and gain access to the CSF or the shunt as it is inserted (9–11). The use of various agents for preoperative skin preparation has been reviewed (1). Aqueous povidone iodine gives disappointing results, and any alcoholic preparation is superior owing to the effect of the alcohol. Aqueous chlorhexidine gives better results in terms of skin disinfection than aqueous povidone iodine, but again alcoholic chlorhexidine is superior and is probably the best agent. However, irrespective of the agent used, the skin is disinfected but not sterilized, and bacteria reemerge from the follicles and glands to enter the incision approximately 20 min later (10,73).

In an attempt to prevent access of skin flora to the incision, gauze packs soaked in either antimicrobials or antiseptics have been used (74,75). Full-scale trials are probably impracticable, though such a system would appear to be useful.

Impervious adhesive drapes are also used to prevent contamination of the incision by skin flora, though studies have shown either no effect (73,76) or an increase in infection associated with their use (74). Nevertheless, nonimpervious cloth drapes, which rapidly become soaked in blood, CSF, and irrigating fluid, are an obvious risk, and properly applied impervious drapes probably offer an advantage.

Despite the attention to skin preparation and shaving, the use of antimicrobial incision packs and impervious drapes, the incision and instruments, clips, and gloves become contaminated by skin flora. It is easy to see that these bacteria are readily introduced into the shunt and ventricular system.

2. Antimicrobial Prophylaxis

A large number of studies have been carried out to determine the efficacy of prophylactic antimicrobials. The agents used have varied widely, but many have used intravenous flucloxacillin, methicillin, or nafcillin, given preoperatively. As stated previously, these antimicrobials and most others fail to attain measurable concentrations in the CSF in the absence of meningeal inflammation and are therefore unlikely to have any effect on the incidence of shunt infection, with the possible exception of external infections. This is also true of glycopeptides and aminoglycosides. Wang et al. (51) used cotrimoxazole in a double-blind, randomized controlled trial but failed to show an effect. Interestingly, Blomstedt et al. (77), also using cotrimoxazole and approximately the same regimen, claimed a highly significant beneficial effect of prophylaxis. This could have been due to the very high incidence (23%) in their control group, as opposed to 6% in the prophylaxis group. Such trials, which involve a very high infection rate, are the only ones to conclude that antimicrobial prophylaxis is of benefit. Brown (78) has reviewed studies of prophylaxis, assessing their validity according to whether they are controlled, are randomized, use historical controls, contain sufficient numbers of infections and patients, etc. Most trials were flawed in their design, and the data could not be used. The most common flaws were the nature of controls and the number of patients enrolled. In most centers, where infection rates of 5% to 7% in controls would be anticipated, approximately 700 patients would be needed to show a statistically significant result with satisfactory α and β errors (79,80). It is now considered unlikely that a satisfactory, properly constructed trial of sufficient size will ever be undertaken successfully. Three recent meta-analyses have been carried out in an attempt to resolve the issue. Reider et al. (81) analyzed five trials and did not detect a significant effect. Langley et al. (82) reviewed 37 studies from which they chose 12 that met their criteria for validity. In this group only one trial claimed a significant benefit, but Langley et al. considered, on meta-analysis of the group, that antimicrobial prophylaxis was beneficial. Similarly, Haines and Walters (83) evaluated nine publications (eight of which appeared in Langley's study) and found a beneficial effect after meta-analysis. These three papers have been analyzed by Brown et al. (84). It appears that the meta-analyses themselves can be criticized for poorly discriminating selection criteria. In addition, the protective effect of antimicrobial prophylaxis was limited to studies with control infection rates higher than 15%. There were also so many different antimicrobial agents and regimens used that the findings failed to guide the practitioner as to which to use, if any. The conclusion of the British Society for Antimicrobial Chemotherapy Report (84) was that there was no clearly proven benefit to be expected from the use of antimicrobial prophylaxis in shunt surgery. However, if surgeons felt that they should use prophylaxis, the report recommends that vancomycin 10 mg and gentamicin 3 mg should be instilled into the ventricular system at operation. If external shunt infections are seen to be a particular problem, a first- or second-generation cephalosporin such as cephradine or cefuroxime, or alternatively amoxicillin-clavulanic acid, should be given intravenously at induction.

3. Antimicrobial Processing of Shunts

In view of the seemingly inevitable contamination of the incision and thence the shunt and CSF in some patients, and as conventional measures such as antimicrobial prophylaxis have failed to reduce the shunt infection rate beyond an unacceptable minimum, a process has been developed that confers longlasting protection against colonization in vitro (85). Briefly, the process consists of using a volatile nonpolar solvent to expand the molecular matrix of the silicone, and to act as a vehicle for introduction of nonvolatile antimicrobials. After removal of the volatile solvent, the matrix reverts to its previous volume and the antimicrobials become incorporated throughout it. Extended duration of protective activity is created by slow release of the antimicrobials from the biomaterial surface maintained by a diffusion gradient within the material. The two agents that have been found to give superior antimicrobial activity and which are physicochemically compatible with the process are clindamycin and rifampicin. The combination is significantly more protective than each alone. Processed shunts contain less than 0.1% by weight of the antimicrobials. Extensive preclinical studies have now been carried out to determine biocompatibility for developing neural tissues and other classes of tissue through which a shunt passes, as well as the effect on the incidence of postshunt epilepsy (86) and resistance to repeated challenge for 28 days by numbers of bacteria 4 orders of magnitude greater than are normally found in an incision (87). Mechanical studies have shown no deleterious effects on valve function at the concentrations used (88). Recent studies have also shown that the presence of a conditioning film, a layer of protein and glycoprotein deposited on the surfaces of shunts during their use (89), does not affect the protective action of the process, the duration of which is in excess of 60 days (90). Conditioning films are responsible for obliterating the effects of surface modifications or antimicrobials applied as coatings.

A pilot clinical trial has been carried out in the U.S. and the U.K. to establish safety, and a definitive clinical trial is now being conducted. Experimental data suggest that protection can be expected against at least 95% of CoNS, *S. aureus*, and coryneforms (87), and hopefully the incidence of shunt infection can be driven down even further by this development.

4.   Role of Staff Training and Experience in Prevention

Many clinical trials of prevention of shunt infection have failed because the expected number of infections in the control group, based on the pretrial infection rate, has fallen on commencing the trial, necessitating an unrealistic extension of the trial to achieve statistical significance—the Hawthorn effect (6). This usually has the effect of depleting the numbers of infections in the trial so that it becomes statistically invalid. The phenomenon, now well known, is due to a general increase in awareness of the problem being addressed, and a corresponding heightening of the care taken by all personnel involved. This clearly indicates that the most powerful prophylactic measure must be continuing education and training of all staff involved in shunting to ensure constant high standards. However, it is appreciated that certain patients present special problems, and extra measures such as processed "antibacterial" shunts might be particularly useful in these cases.

III.   EXTERNAL VENTRICULAR DRAINS

A.   Factors Involved in EVD Infections

1.   Use of EVD and Incidence of Infection

EVDs are used for short-term control of CSF pressure, this being facilitated either by a valve which also helps to prevent reflux, or by raising or lowering a drip chamber (Fig. 3). Infection becomes more likely the longer the EVD is in place, and after about 10 days the incidence rises steeply. This can be due either to exit site infection or to reflux of bacteria from contamination of the collecting bag. Patients are often ambulant as they recover, and the drainage bag can become inverted or compressed. While staphylococci are encountered, many infections are due to gram-negative bacilli, especially in prolonged drainage during treatment of a shunt infection. However, there are few published data on EVD infections, perhaps reflecting the common view that management of EVD is viewed as a nursing concern rather than a medical one. Published studies are not comparable and do not assist in forming a consistent view. Mori and Raimondi (91) treated 23 cases of shunt infection with EVD for an average of 3 weeks, revising each electively after 2 weeks. They reported secondary infection, mainly due to gram-negative bacilli, but did not state the incidence. Santini et al. (92) treated 27 cases, eight with shunt infection, for an average of 13 days and encountered three secondary infections—two CoNS and one *P. aeruginosa.* Marro et al. (93) used a percutaneously inserted, nontunneled EVD in 70 infants of less than 35 weeks' gestation, keeping the tube in place for about 7 days. They had one proven infection (CoNS) and five suspected infections. Anwar et al. (94) found two secondary infections in 19 patients; Leonhardt et al. (95) found none in 13 cases. Harbaugh et al. (96), using EVD for control of CSF pressure in premature neonates after periventricular hemorrhage, also found no infections in 11 cases.

2.   Colonization of EVD Tubing

One difficulty is that the finding of organisms in CSF taken from an EVD does not necessarily indicate infection of the patient so much as colonization of the tubing, though this might eventually progress retrogradely to cause infection. Scarff et al. (97) found this in seven cases, though they could find no evidence of infection.

3.   Duration of EVD and Infection

EVDs should be used for as short a time as possible and managed with scrupulous aseptic technique. If necessary, the whole system should be replaced after 10 to 14 days. If the same site of entry on the scalp is used, this should be thoroughly cleaned with alcoholic chlorhexidine between removal of the first tube and insertion of the second.

B.   Antimicrobial Prophylaxis

Prophylactic antimicrobials are not indicated. Patients being treated for shunt infection will be receiving antimicrobials anyway, and in those with hemorrhage or undergoing pressure monitoring, prophylactic antimicrobials are likely to increase the risk of infection with a resistant organism.

C.   Treatment of EVD Infection

If secondary infection occurs, with symptoms and raised CSF neutrophil count, the EVD should be replaced and high-dose intravenous antimicrobials (second- or third-generation cephalosporin for initial treatment and for confirmed infection with gram-negative bacilli; flucloxacillin or cefuroxime for *S. aureus*) should be given immediately. If methicillin-resistant CoNS are involved, intravenous vancomycin and oral rifampicin should be given. If intraventricular therapy is considered to be required, owing either to poor clinical response or to lack of inflammatory response, as is often seen with CoNS, intraventricular vancomycin 10 to 20 mg daily for 5 days should be given into the clamped proximal EVD tubing after rigorous antisepsis. In the case of unresponsive ventriculitis due to gram-negative bacilli, intraventricular gentamicin 3 to 5 mg daily can be given, though the inflammatory response is usually sufficient to allow therapeutic CSF levels of intravenously administered drugs to be achieved. A further change of EVD may be advisable after 3 or 4 days.

IV. VENTRICULAR ACCESS RESERVOIRS

A. Use of Reservoirs and Incidence of Infection

The Ommaya reservoir is most commonly used, though others are also available. It consists of a dome-shaped chamber connected at its base to a ventricular catheter (Fig. 4). The chamber is positioned extracranially under a scalp flap well away from the incision. Ventricular CSF can be accessed by puncturing the dome percutaneously. CSF pressure can be monitored, samples can be aspirated for analysis, or antimicrobials or cytotoxic drugs can be introduced. If the scalp is carefully prepared and fine needles are used, the risk of infection is low, though in long-term reservoirs punctured daily for several months—for instance, when treating AIDS-related lymphoma—the infection rate can be 10% to 15% (98). When infection does occur it is often due to staphylococci or coryneforms.

B. Treatment of Ventricular Access Reservoir Infection

Treatment of reservoir infections is relatively simple. It is advisable to remove the reservoir and insert a new one, though some have succeeded without doing so (99). Sutherland et al. (100) were unsuccessful in treating a patient with malignant meningitis secondary to mammary carcinoma for a reservoir infection due to CoNS with intravenous vancomycin. The peak CSF vancomycin level was found to be subtherapeutic, and when the drug was given intraventricularly via the reservoir, the infection was eradicated. Lishner et al. (101) also used intraventricular vancomycin successfully. It is therefore recommended that staphylococcal infections be treated with intraventricular vancomycin 10 to 20 mg daily for 5 days given into a new reservoir. In the event of infection due to P. aeruginosa, the reservoir should be removed immediately and high-dose intravenous ceftazidime begun. Intraventricular gentamicin 3 to 5 mg daily can also be given.

V. INTRASPINAL DRUG DELIVERY DEVICES (IDDD)

A. Types of IDDD

There are two main types of intraspinal drug delivery device. One consists of an implanted intrathecal catheter and injection port, resembling the Mediport intravenous access device, and a pump and reservoir which are external and connected to the port by a needle. The second and most satisfactory from the point of view of infection is the totally implanted device, where programmable pump, reservoir, and intrathecal catheter are all internal (102).

B. Causes of IDDD Infection

The main risk of infection in totally implanted IDDDs is associated with the need for periodic percutaneous recharging of the reservoir with morphine or baclophen. Infection of the tissue pocket housing the reservoir sometimes occurs, usually due to *S. aureus*. Introduction of bacteria, usually CoNS, into the reservoir leads to colonization of the system and to meningitis.

C.   Treatment of IDDD Infection

Intravenous flucloxacillin or vancomycin should be given, and if the infection fails to resolve or if meningitis develops, the system should be removed. The IDDD can be used in such cases to administer intrathecal vancomycin via the reservoir. In one case involving CoNS, Bennett et al. (103) charged the reservoir with 50 mg/L vancomycin and programmed the pump to deliver 5 mg daily intrathecally for 30 days. Rifampicin 600 mg bid was also given orally. The infection was eradicated without removal of the IDDD. The concentration of vancomycin in the CSF was 54 mg/L, but, as in the treatment of CSF shunt infection, no toxicity resulted. Vancomycin also appeared to be chemically compatible with baclophen. The authors suggest that, in retrospect, a shorter course of treatment might have been sufficient.

D.   Antimicrobial Prophylaxis for IDDD Infection

Prophylactic antimicrobials given at the time of IDDD insertion or recharging the reservoir are probably not required, and, though no formal studies have been carried out, they have not been of benefit in the cases in which they have been used.

VI.   PERITONEOVENOUS SHUNTS FOR ASCITES

A.   Use of Ascites Shunts and Incidence of Infection

Devices resembling shunts for hydrocephalus are available for the control of ascites in cirrhosis or malignant liver disease. They drain ascitic fluid from the peritoneal cavity to the venous system via the jugular vein. Reflux of blood is prevented by a valve system. Patients with intractable ascites are in the late stages of liver failure, and shunts are intended to remain in place for only 1 or 2 years. They are required to drain a large volume of fluid with a high protein content, and obstruction is a major problem. Infection can also occur, giving rise to peritonitis, colonization of the shunt, and septicemia. *S. aureus* and enteric gram-negative bacilli have been implicated in most cases, and, while many infections appear to be introduced at insertion, some appear much later. An important factor may be the grossly impaired immunity of the ascitic peritoneal cavity.

B.   Treatment of Infected Ascites Shunts

There are few published reports of infection in ascites shunts, but those that mention its management recommend shunt removal and intravenous antimicrobials. The agents should be selected according to susceptibility tests, but gentamicin or cefuroxime should be given initially. The primary illness, the resulting impaired immunity, and presence of septicemia suggest that treatment should continue for at least 3 weeks.

C. Antimicrobial Prophylaxis

While antimicrobial prophylaxis has been used at the time of shunt insertion, the results have been disappointing. Smajda and Franco (104) used oral oxacillin, giving it for 10 days postoperatively, but 15 of 54 patients developed infection nevertheless. Hillaire et al. (105) reported similar results with ofloxacin and cefotetan. In view of the likely causative organisms, either gentamicin or cefuroxime should be given intravenously at induction of anesthesia, though there is no evidence to support this practice.

REFERENCES

1. Bayston R. Hydrocephalus Shunt Infections. London; Chapman and Hall, 1989.
2. Schimke RT, Black PH, Mark VH, Schwartz MN. Indolent *Staphylococcus albus* or *aureus* bacteremia after ventriculo-atriostomy. N Engl J Med 1961; 264:264–270.
3. Schoenbaum SC, Gardner P, Shillito J. Infections of cerebrospinal fluid shunts: epidemiology, clinical manifestations and therapy. J Infect Dis 1975; 131:543–552.
4. Walters BC, Hoffman HJ, Hendrick EB, Humphreys RP. Cerebrospinal fluid shunt infection. Influences on initial management and subsequent outcome. J Neurosurg 1984; 60:1014–1021.
5. Choux M, Genitori L, Lang D, Lena G. Shunt implantation: reducing the incidence of shunt infection. J Neurosurg 1992; 77:875–880.
6. Entwistle NJ, Nisbet JD. Educational Research in Action. London: University of London Press, 1972.
7. Renier D, Lacombe J, Pierre-Khan A, Sainte-Rose C, Hirsch JF. Factors causing acute shunt infection. J Neurosurg 1984; 61:1072–1078.
8. Ammirati M, Raimondi AJ. Cerebrospinal fluid shunt infections in children. A study of the relationship between the aetiology of hydrocephalus, age at the time of shunt placement, and infection rate. Child's Nervous System 1987; 3:106–109.
9. Pople IK, Bayston R, Hayward RD. Infection of cerebrospinal fluid shunts in infants: a study of etiological factors. J Neurosurg 1992; 77:29–36.
10. Bayston R, Lari J. A study of the sources of infection in colonised shunts. Dev Med Child Neurol 1974; 16 (suppl 32):16–22.
11. Shapiro S, Boaz J, Kleiman M, Kalsbeck J, Mealey J. Origin of organisms infecting ventricular shunts. Neurosurgery 1988; 22:868–872.
12. Sanchez-Portocarrero J, Martin-Rabadan P, Saldana CJ, Perez-Cecilia F. *Candida* cerebrospinal fluid shunt infection. Report of two new cases and review of the literature. Diagn Microbiol Infect Dis 1994; 20:33–40.
13. Bayston R, Penny SR. Excessive production of mucoid substance by *Staphylococcus* SIIA: a possible factor in colonisation of Holter shunts. Dev Med Child Neurol 1972; 27 (suppl 14):25–28.

14. Peters G, Locci R, Pulverer G. Microbial colonisation of prosthetic devices II. Scanning electron microscopy of naturally infected intravenous catheters. Zentralbl Bakteriol Mikrobiol Hyg 1981; I Abt Orig B 173:293–299.

15. Guevara JA, Zuccaro G, Trevisan A, Denoya CD. Bacterial adhesion to cerebrospinal fluid shunts. J Neurosurg 1987; 67:438–445.

16. Bayston R, Rodgers J. Production of extra-cellular slime by *Staphylococcus epidermidis* during stationary phase of growth: its association with adherence to implantable devices. J Clin Pathol 1990; 43:866–870.

17. Bayston R, Compton C, Richards K. Production of extracellular slime by coryneforms colonizing hydrocephalus shunts. J Clin Microbiol 1994; 32:1705–1709.

18. Black JA, Challacombe DN, Ockenden BG. Nephrotic syndrome associated with bacteraemia after shunt operations for hydrocephalus. Lancet 1965; ii:921–924.

19. Stauffer UG. Shunt nephritis—a complication of ventriculoatrial shunts. Dev Med Child Neurol 1970; 12(suppl 22):161–164.

20. Bayston R, Swinden J. The aetiology and prevention of shunt nephritis. Zeit Kinderchir 1979; 28:377–384.

21. Bayston R, Rodgers J. Role of serological tests in the diagnosis of immune complex disease in infection of ventriculoatrial shunts for hydrocephalus. Eur J Clin Microbiol Infect Dis 1994; 13:417–420.

22. Moss SW, Gary NE, Eissinger RP. Nephritis associated with a diphtheroid-infected cerebrospinal fluid shunt. Am J Med 1977; 63:318–319.

23. O'Regan S, Makker SP. Shunt nephritis: demonstration of diphtheroid antigen in glomeruli. Am J Med Sci 1979; 278:161–165.

24. Beeler BA, Crowder JG, Smith JW, White A. *Propionibacterium acnes:* pathogen in central nervous system shunt infection. Report of three cases including immune complex glomerulonephritis. Am J Med 1977; 61:935–938.

25. Rekate HL, Ruch T, Nulsen FE. Diphtheroid infections of cerebrospinal fluid shunts. The changing pattern of shunt infection in Cleveland. J Neurosurg 1980; 52:553–556.

26. Pinals RS, Tunnessen WW. Shunt arthritis. J Pediatr 1977; 91:681.

27. Nolan CM, Flanigan WJ, Rastogi SP, Brewer TE. Vancomycin penetration into CSF during treatment of patients receiving haemodialysis. South Med J 1980; 73:1333–1334.

28. Reynolds M, Sherman JO, Malone DG. Ventriculoperitoneal shunt infection masquerading as an acute surgical abdomen. J Pediatr Surg 1983; 18:951–954.

29. Bayston R, Spitz L. Infective and cystic causes of malfunction of ventriculoperitoneal shunts for hydrocephalus. Zeit Kinderchir 1977; 22:419–424.

30. Latchaw JP, Hahn JF. Intraperitoneal pseudocyst associated with ventriculoperitoneal shunt. Neurosurgery 1981; 8:469–472.

31. Bayston R, Higgins J. Biochemical and cultural characteristics of "JK" coryneforms. J Clin Pathol 1986; 39:654–660.

32. Needham CA, Stempsey W. Incidence, adherence and antibiotic resistance of coagulase negative *Staphylococcus* species causing human disease. Diagn Microbiol Infect Dis 1984; 2:293–299.

33. Alexander W, Rimland D. Lack of correlation of slime production with pathogenicity in continuous ambulatory peritoneal dialysis peritonitis caused by coagulase negative staphylococci. Diagn Microbiol Infect Dis 1987; 8:215–220.

34. Bayston R, Spitz L. The role of retrograde movement of bacteria in ventriculoatrial shunt colonisation. Zeit Kinderchir 1978; 25:352–356.

35. Bayston R. Serum C-reactive protein test in diagnosis of septic complications of cerebrospinal fluid shunts for hydrocephalus. Arch Dis Child 1979; 54:545–547.

36. Castro-Gago M, Sanguinedo P, Garcia C, et al. Valor de la proteina C-reactiva (PCR) en el diagnostico de las complicaciones infecciosas de los "shunts" en nos niños hidrocefalos. Ann Esp Pediatr 1982; 16:47–52.

37. Bayston R. Serological surveillance of children with CSF shunting devices. Dev Med Child Neurol 1975; 35(suppl 17):104–110.

38. Holt RJ. The early serological detection of colonisation by *Staphylococcus epidermidis* of ventriculoatrial shunts. Infection 1980; 8:8–12.

39. Losnegard N, Oeding P. Immunochemical studies on polysaccharides from *Staphylococcus epidermidis*. I. Isolation and characterisation. Acta Pathol Microbiol Scand 1963; 58:482–492.

40. Barsham S, Bayston R, Ali SY. Detection of antibodies to *Staphylococcus epidermidis* in infected total hip replacements by an enzyme linked immunosorbent assay. J Clin Pathol 1985; 38:839–840.

41. Bayston R. Hydrocephalus shunt infections. J Antimicrob Chemother 1994; 34(suppl A):75–84.

42. Luthardt TH. Bacterial infections in ventriculo-auricular shunt systems. Dev Med Child Neurol 1970; 22:105–107.

43. McClone DG, Czyzewski D, Raimondi AJ, Somers RC. Central nervous system infections as a limiting factor in the intelligence of children with meningomyelocele. Pediatrics 1982; 70:338–342.

44. Wilson CB, Pertan V. Perforation of the bowel complicating peritoneal shunt for hydrocephalus. Report of two cases. Am Surg 1966; 32:601–603.

45. Brook I, Johnson N, Overturf G, Wilkins J. Mixed bacterial meningitis: a complication of ventriculo- and lumbo-peritoneal shunts. J Neurosurg 1977; 47:961–964.

46. Brown MRW, Collier PJ, Gilbert P. Influence of growth rate on susceptibility to antimicrobial agents: modification of cell envelope and batch and continuous culture studies. Antimicrob Agents Chemother 1990; 34:1623–1628.

47. Evans RC, Holmes CJ. Effect of vancomycin hydrochloride on *Staphylococcus epidermidis* biofolm associated with silicone elastomer. Antomicrob Agents Chemother 1987; 31:889–894.

48. Spector R, Lorenzo AV. Inhibition of penicillin transport from the cerebrospinal fluid after intracisternal inoculation of bacteria. J Clin Invest 1974; 54:316–325.

49. Cohen SJ, Callaghan RP. Septicaemia due to colonisation of Spitz-Holter valves by *Staphylococcus*. Br Med J 1961; i:860–863.

50. James HE, Walsh JW, Wilson HD, et al. Prospective randomised study of therapy in cerebrospinal fluid shunt infection. Neurosurg 1980; 7:459–463.

51. Wang EEL, Prober CG, Hendrick EB, et al. Prophylactic sulphamethoxazole and trimethoprim in ventriculoperitoneal shunt surgery. A double-blind, randomised, placebo-controlled trial. JAMA 1984; 251:1174–1177.

52. Bayston R, Rickwood AMK. Factors involved in antibiotic treatment of cerebrospinal fluid shunt infections. Zeit Kinderchir 1981; 34:339–345.

53. Mandell GL, Moorman DR. Treatment of experimental staphylococcal infections: effect of rifampicin alone and in combination on development of rifampicin resistance. Antimicrob Agents Chemother 1980; 17:658–662.

54. Ryan JL, Pachner A, Andriole VT, Root RK. Enterococcal meningitis: combined vancomycin and rifampicin therapy. Am J Med 1980; 68:449–451.

55. Young EJ, Ratner RE, Clarridge JE. Staphylococcal ventriculitis treated with vancomycin. South Med J 1981; 74:1014–1015.

56. Lynn WA, Clutterbuck E, Want S, et al. Treatment of CAPD peritonitis due to glycopeptide-resistant *Enterococcus faecium* with quinopristin/dalfopristin. Lancet 1994; 344:1025–1026.

57. Visconti EB, Peters G. Vancomycin treatment of cerebrospinal fluid shunt infections. Report of two cases. J Neurosurg 1979; 51:245–246.

58. Ring JC, Cates KL, Belani KK, et al. Rifampicin for CSF shunt infections caused by coagulase negative staphylococci. J Pediatr 1979; 95:317–319.

59. Gombert ME, Landesman SH, Corrado ML, et al. Vancomycin and rifampicin therapy for *Staphylococcus epidermidis* meningitis associated with CSF shunts. J Neurosurg 1981; 55:633–636.

60. Bayston R, Hart CA, Barnicoat M. Intraventricular vancomycin in the treatment of ventriculitis associated with cerebrospinal fluid shunting and drainage. J Neurol Neurosurg Psychiatr 1987; 50:1419–1423.

61. Bayston R, de Louvois J, Brown EM, Hedges AJ, Johnston RA, Lees P. Treatment of infections associated with shunting for hydrocephalus. Br J Hosp Med 1995; 53: 368–373.

62. Venditti M, Micozzi A, Serra P, Buniva G, Palma L, Martino P. Intraventricular administration of teicoplanin in shunt associated ventriculitis caused by methicillin resistant *Staphylococcus aureus.* J Antimicrob Chemother 1988; 21:513–515.

63. Guerrero MLF, de Gorgolas M, Roblas RF, Campos JM. Treatment of cerebrospinal fluid shunt infections with teicoplanin. Eur J Clin Microbiol Infect Dis 1994; 13: 1056–1058.

64. Brown EM, Jones EM. Non-surgical management of CSF shunt infections. Eur J Pediatr Surg 1995; 5(suppl I):26.

65. Rubin RC, Ghatak NR, Visudhipan P. Asymptomatic perforated viscus and gram negative ventriculitis as a complication of valve-regulated ventriculoperitoneal shunts. J Neurosurg 1972; 37:616–618.

66. Grosfeld EL, Cooney OR, Smith J, Campbell RL. Intra-abdominal complications following ventriculoperitoneal shunt procedures. Pediatrics 1974; 54:791–796.

67. Cruciani M, Di Perri G, Molesini M, Vento S, Concia E, Bassetti D. Use of fluconazole in the treatment of *Candida albicans* hydrocephalus shunt infection. Eur J Clin Microbiol Infect Dis 1992; 11:957.

68. Fisher JF, Dewald J. Parkinsonism associated with intraventricular amphotericin B. J Antimicrob Chemother 1983; 12:97–99.

69. Shurtleff DB, Foltz EL, Christie D. Ventriculoauriculostomy-associated infections: a 12 year study. J Neurosurg 1971; 35:686–694.

70. Rennels MB, Wald ER. Treatment of *Haemophilus influenzae* type b meningitis in children with cerebrospinal fluid shunts. J Pediatr 1980; 97:424–426.

71. Leggiadro RJ, Atluru VL, Katz SP. Meningococcal meningitis associated with cerebrospinal fluid shunts. Pediatr Infect Dis 1984; 3:489–490.

72. Stern S, Bayston R, Hayward R. *Haemophilus influenzae* meningitis in the presence of cerebrospinal fluid shunts. Child's Nerv Syst 1988; 4:164–165.
73. Raahave D. Effect of plastic skin and wound drapes on the density of bacteria in operation wounds. Br J Surg 1976; 63:421–426.
74. Tabara Z, Forrest DM. Colonisation of CSF shunts: preventive measures. Zeit Kinderchir 1982; 37:156–158.
75. Fitzgerald R, Connelly B. An operative technique to reduce valve colonisation. Zeit Kinderchir 1984; 39(suppl II):107–109.
76. Jackson DW, Pollock AV, Tindall DS. The value of plastic adhesive drape in prevention of wound infection. A controlled trial. Br J Surg 1971; 58:340–342.
77. Blomstedt GC. Results of trimethoprim-sulphamethoxazole prophylaxis in ventriculostomy and shunting procedures. A double-blind randomised trial. J Neurosurg 1985; 62:694–697.
78. Brown EM. Antimicrobial prophylaxis in neurosurgery. J Antimicrob Chemother 1993; 31(suppl B):49–63.
79. Walters BC, Hoffman HJ, Hendrick EB, Humphreys RP. Decreased risk of infection in cerebrospinal fluid shunt surgery using prophylactic antibiotics: a case-control study. Zeit Kinderchir 1985; 40(suppl 1):15–18.
80. Bayston R, Bannister C, Boston V, Burman R, et al. A prospective randomised controlled trial of antimicrobial prophylaxis in hydrocephalus shunt surgery. Zeit Kinderchir 1990; 45(suppl 1):5–7.
81. Reider MJ, Frewen TC, Del Maestro RF. The effect of cephalothin prophylaxis on postoperative ventriculoperitoneal shunt infections. Can Med Assoc J 1987; 136:935–938.
82. Langley JM, LeBlanc JC, Drake JM, Milner R. Efficacy of antimicrobial prophylaxis in cerebrospinal fluid shunt placement: a meta-analysis. Clin Infect Dis 1993; 17:98–103.
83. Haines SJ, Walters BC. Antibiotic prophylaxis for cerebrospinal fluid shunts: a meta-analysis. Neurosurgery 1994; 34:87–92.
84. Brown E, de Louvois J, Bayston R, Hedges AJ, Johnston RA, Lees P. Antimicrobial prophylaxis in neurosurgery and after head injury. Lancet 1994; 344:1547–1551.
85. Bayston R, Milner RDG. Antimicrobial activity of silicone rubber used in hydrocephalus shunts, after impregnation with antimicrobial substances. J Clin Pathol 1981; 34:1057–1062.
86. Abed WT, Alavijeh MS, Bayston R, Shorvon SD, Patsalos PN. An evaluation of the epileptogenic properties of a rifampicin/clindamycin-impregnated shunt catheter. Br J Neurosurg 1994; 8:725–730.
87. Bayston R, Grove N, Siegel J, Lawellin D, Barsham S. Prevention of hydrocephalus shunt catheter colonization in vitro by impregnation with antimicrobials. J Neurol Neurosurg Psychiatr 1989; 52:605–609.
88. Bayston R. Effect of antibiotic impregnation on the function of slit valves used to control hydrocephalus. Zeit Kinderchir 1980; 31:353–359.
89. Brydon HL, Bayston R, Kier G, Thompson E, Hayward RD, Harkness W. Protein adsorption to hydrocephalus shunt catheters. Eur J Pediatr Surg 1995; 5(suppl I):34.
90. Bayston R, Lambert E. Protection of CSF shunts against infection by impregnation with antimicrobial agents. Further in-vitro studies. Eur J Pediatr Surg 1995; 5(suppl I):41–42.

91. Mori K, Raimondi AJ. An analysis of external ventricular drainage as a treatment for infected shunts. Child's Brain 1975; 1:243–250.

92. Santini J-J, Billard C, Boissonnet H, Borderon JC. Surveillance bactériologique des dérivations ventriculaires externés chez l'enfant. Neurochirurgie 1982; 28:379–382.

93. Marro PJ, Dransfield DA, Mott SH, Allan WC. Posthemorrhagic hydrocephalus. Use of an intravenous-type catheter for cerebrospinal fluid drainage. Am J Dis Child 1991; 145:1141–1146.

94. Anwar M, Doyle AJ, Kadam S, Hiatt IM, Hegyi T. Management of posthemorrhagic hydrocephalus in the preterm infant. J Pediatr Surg 1986; 21:334–337.

95. Leonhardt A, Steiner H-H, Linderkamp O. Management of posthemorrhagic hydrocephalus with a subcutaneous ventricular catheter reservoir in preterm infants. Arch Dis Child 1989; 64:24–28.

96. Harbaugh E, Saunders L, Edwards H. External ventricular drainage for control of posthemorrhagic hydrocephalus in premature infants. J Neurosurg 1981; 55:766–770.

97. Scarff TB, Nelson PB, Reigel DH. External drainage for ventricular infection following cerebrospinal fluid shunts. Child's Brain 1978; 4:129–136.

98. Chamberlain MC, Dirr L. Involved-field radiotherapy and intra-Ommaya methotrexate/cytarabine in patients with AIDS-related lymphomatous meningitis. J Clin Oncol 1993; 11:1978–1984.

99. Hirsch BE, Amodio M, Einzig AI, Halevy R, Soeiro R. Instillation of vancomycin into a cerebrospinal fluid reservoir to clear infection. Pharmacokinetic considerations. J Infect Dis 1991; 163:197–200.

100. Sutherland GE, Palitang EG, Marr JJ, Lwedke SL. Sterilisation of Ommaya reservoir by instillation of vancomycin. Am J Med 1981; 71:1068–1070.

101. Lishner M, Scheinbaum R, Messner HA. Intrathecal vancomycin in the treatment of Ommaya reservoir infection by *Staphylococcus epidermidis*. Scand J Infect Dis 1991; 23:10–14.

102. Müller H, Zierski J. Pumps in pharmacotherapy. In: Müller H, Zierski J, Penn RD. Local-Spinal Therapy of Spasticity. Berlin: Springer-Verlag, 1988.

103. Bennett MI, Tai YMA, Symonds JM. Staphylococcal meningitis following Synchromed intrathecal pump implant: a case report. Pain 1994; 56:243–244.

104. Smajda C, Franco D. The LeVeen shunt shunt in the elective treatment of intractable ascites in cirrhosis. A prospective study on 140 patients. Ann Surg 1985; 210:488–493.

105. Hillaire S, Labianca M, Borgonovo G, Smajda C, Grange D, Franco D. Peritoneovenous shunting of intractable ascites in patients with cirrhosis: improving results and predictive factors of failure. Surgery 1993; 113:373–379.

106. George R, Leibrock L, Epstein M. Long-term analysis of cerebrospinal fluid shunt infections. J Neurosurg 1979; 51:804–811.

13

Infections Associated with Chronic Peritoneal Dialysis

Henri Alexander Verbrugh
Erasmus University Hospital Rotterdam, Rotterdam, The Netherlands

I. INTRODUCTION

Chronic peritoneal dialysis (CPD) is increasingly used as the renal replacement therapy of choice in many countries. The number of patients on CPD was approximately 4000 in 1980 but reached 95,200 by the end of 1994 (1). The annual increase from 1991 to 1994 was 15%. The proportion of patients with end-stage renal disease treated by CPD (versus haemodialysis) varies considerably from country to country, being less than 10% in Italy, France, Germany, and Japan and 50% or greater in the United Kingdom, New Zealand, and Mexico. These differences are thought to be largely due to national differences in the way renal replacement therapy is organized and reimbursed. The CPD technique per se is not questioned. In contrast, CPD has been validated in many studies, and, although there are limits in dialysis adequacy, CPD has several advantages over hemodialysis (2,3). Currently, two types of CPD are practiced: continuous ambulatory peritoneal dialysis (CAPD), and continuous cyclic peritoneal dialysis (CCPD). CAPD was first introduced in the late 1970s by Popovich et al. (4) and Oreopoulos et al. (5) as a machine-free regimen that entailed the continuous presence of dialysate in the peritoneal cavity. Approximately every 6 hours dialysate is exchanged for fresh PD fluid using gravitational forces only to drain and refill the abdominal cavity. CCPD was introduced in the early 1980s to cater to patients who were incapable of performing the exchanges manually or who were unwilling to interrupt

353

their daily routines for dialysate exchanges (6). In CCPD rapid nocturnal fluid exchanges are performed through a bedside cycling machine. Miniaturization technology has now allowed such machines to become easily portable, further improving patients' freedom to schedule their own activities. By the end of 1994 approximately 25% of all CPD in the U.S. was of the CCPD variety.

From the very beginning of peritoneal dialysis in the 1960s, the technique has been plagued by infectious complications—especially, high rates of acute bacterial peritonitis. The introduction by Tenckhoff and Schechter (7) of a tunneled catheter segment with Dacron felt cuffs at either end of its track through the abdominal wall was the first major step forward in reducing the risk of infection (Fig. 1). With the popularization of CAPD in the 1980s much attention has been given to further improve aseptic techniques, especially during the exchange procedure. Many devices have been proposed, including in-line bacterial filters,

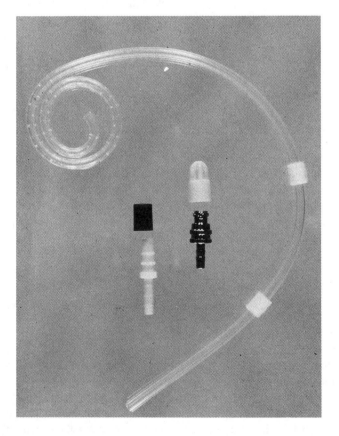

Figure 1   Classical curved Tenckhoff catheter with double Dacron felt cuffs.

ultraviolet light-based germicidal boxes, and antiseptic-containing cuffs around the external connectors. Reductions in peritonitis rates have been consistently observed only in those centers that have switched to integrated "Y systems" that flush the potentially contaminated connector with sterile dialysate before fresh dialysate enters the peritoneum (8–10). Even so, peritonitis and infection at the exit site or in the tunnel track around the Tenckhoff catheter remain prevalent problems in most CPD programs around the world.

II. EPIDEMIOLOGY

The remainder of the chapter will focus on bacterial peritonitis and exit site infections around the permanent Tenckhoff catheter. This is not to say that CAPD patients may not also suffer from other types of infections related to the uremic state or to diseases underlying their renal insufficiency. However, the incidences of peritonitis and tunnel track infections are such that they are largely responsible for the infectious morbidity seen among CPD patients. The incidence of bacterial peritonitis was high, approximately one episode per 2.5 patient-months CAPD, in the early years of CAPD. Infection rates were also high in the learning phases of most centers starting with this treatment modality in the early 1980s (rates of one episode per 3 to 6 months for European centers in 1985) (3,11). With more experience, and probably also due to changes in the vital statistics of the patients treated, most centers managed to achieve peritonitis rates of one episode per 6 to 12 patient-months prior to the introduction of the Y connector systems (see above). In this era the probability of remaining free from peritonitis after 12 months on CAPD was less than 50% (8–10). In centers using the Y sets peritonitis rates now vary from one episode per 15 to 25 months, perhaps up to one per 33 months in some centers (8–10,12–14).

The distribution of organisms causing acute peritonitis has previously been collated from the literature up to 1989 and published (15). Studies detailing the distribution of peritonitis-causing organisms published in 1991 to 1994 reveal a very similar pattern (Table 1). Thus, CAPD-causing organisms are predominantly gram-positive with staphylococcal species causing 60% of all episodes of peritonitis. Gram-negative bacilli are responsible for only 20% of the episodes, equally divided among enteric bacilli and the *Acinetobacter*, *Pseudomonas*, and other glucose-nonfermenting species. Anaerobes are rarely isolated and fungi, usually *Candida* species, cause approximately 2% of peritonitis episodes in CAPD patients. However, even the most recently published studies do not all address the effect of the introduction of the Y systems on the species distribution in their respective centers. The few studies that have evaluated this show specifically that Y sets reduce the rate of infection due to coagulase-negative staphylococci but not those of the other species listed in Table 1 (12–14). Thus, the relative contribution to the total number of peritonitis episodes caused by gram-negative bacilli and

Table 1   Species Distribution of Microbial Pathogens Causing Peritonitis in
Patients Undergoing Chronic Peritoneal Dialysis

Microbial species	Mean (range) percentage of total isolates as published in the literature	
	1980s	1990s
Gram-positive bacteria	74 (41–87)	74 (46–84)
Coagulase-negative staphylococci	44 (16–58)	46 (19–56)
S. aureus	14 (3–33)	14 (5–21)
Streptococcus, Enterococcus spp.	12 (1–16)	10 (1–20)
Corynebacterium spp.	3 (0–10)	3 (0–7)
Other[a]	1 (0–6)	1 (0–5)
Gram-negative bacilli	19 (1–36)	23 (14–36)
Enterobacteriaceae[b]	11 (0–17)	10 (7–25)
Glucose-nonfermenting[c]	8 (1–18)	13 (5–26)
Anaerobic bacteria	< 1 (0–3)	< 1 (0–1)
Fungi[d]	2 (0–9)	2 (0–9)
Miscellaneous[e]	2 (0–5)	1 (0–11)
Mixed species	2 (0–14)	< 1 (0–5)

[a]*Bacillus* spp. predominantly.
[b]*Escherichia coli, Enterobacter, Klebsiella, Citrobacter,* and *Serratia* spp. primarily.
[c]*Acinetobacter* and *Pseudomonas* spp. predominantly.
[d]Predominantly *Candida* spp.
[e]Includes *Haemophilus, Neisseria, Pasteurella, Agrobacterium, Chlamydia, Flavobacterium*
  spp., and mycobacteria and unidentified isolates.
Note: Percentages for the 1980s are from Ref. 15 and are based on 1569 episodes observed
  in adults. Data from the 1990s are pooled from Refs. 12 and 16–23 and are based on 1661
  episodes.

fungi in patients will most probably increase along with the introduction of
Y sets.

The risk of peritonitis may also be influenced by the premorbid state of the
patients. Thus, advanced age, diabetes mellitus, black race, and being HIV-positive have all been associated with higher incidences of CAPD-associated peritonitis (10,24,25). Also, *S. aureus* may cause more infections in children whereas less *Pseudomonas* and fungi may trouble HIV-positive patients on CAPD
(15,25).

Risk of peritonitis is not equally distributed among all patients on CAPD.
Patients who have had one episode of peritonitis have an increased risk of peritonitis recurring at a later date. In one recent national study in the U.S. the peritonitis rate in patients using Y sets was one episode per 20.6 patient-months for

the first episode, but this rate increased to one per 8.2 patient-months for a subsequent episode (10). Vice versa, a small minority of patients will remain free of peritonitis for many years on CAPD.

Infection of the exit site of the Tenckhoff catheter through the abdominal skin and, much less frequently, infection of the tunnel track through the abdominal wall are also observed regularly in CAPD patients. Today, incidence rates for exit site infection are on a par with those of peritonitis, usually one episode per 12 to 24 months on CAPD (14,21,25), sometimes found to be less frequent (26,27). These infections are commonly caused by *S. aureus*, coagulase-negative staphylococci, and *Pseudomonas* spp. (Table 2). Tunnel track infections occur at approximately 20% the rate of exit site infection (14) and may be associated with concurrent exit site infection and subsequent peritonitis.

III. CLINICAL PRESENTATION AND COMPLICATIONS

The signs and symptoms of CAPD peritonitis are a *cloudy dialysate effluent*, *abdominal pain* or tenderness, and *fever.* The earliest suggestive sign of peritonitis is usually cloudy fluid. However, occasionally abdominal pain may be the initial complaint, and in children an increased temperature may be the earliest finding (Table 3). Nausea, vomiting, and diarrhea may also be present, more often in patients who have gastroenteritis due to the same organisms—e.g., *Campylobacter* (28) or *Aeromonas* (29). Cloudy dialysate alone may not be due to infection and inflammation, unless cell count and differential show the increased presence of polymorphonuclear neutrophils (PMN). Other causes of cloudy effluent include retrograde blood contamination during menstruation (30) and peritoneal

Table 2 Species Distribution of Microbial Pathogens Causing Exit Site and Tunnel Track Infection in CAPD Patients

Microbial species	Mean (range) percentage of isolates
Staphylococcus aureus	42 (33–81)
Coagulase-negative staphylococci	28 (6–33)
Pseudomonas spp.	14 (6–21)
Enterobacteriaceae[a]	4 (3–8)
Others[b]	12 (0–16)

[a]*Escherichia coli, Proteus* spp., *Enterobacter* spp.
[b]*Corynebacterium, Enterococcus* spp., and fungi.
Note: Percentages computed from data pooled from Refs. 14, 21, 25, and 26 are based on 547 episodes observed in adults.

Table 3 Clinical Presentation of CAPD Peritonitis

Signs and symptoms	Number (%) of episodes
Cloudy effluent	116 (99)
Abdominal pain	99 (85)
Fever	25 (21)
Nausea and vomiting	18 (15)
Diarrhea	11 (9)
Total episodes	117

Source: From Ref. 18.

fluid eosinophilia as an allergic manifestation to plasticizers or other foreign constituents in the dialysis fluid (31). However, in bacterial or fungal peritonitis the cell count uniformly reveals more than 100 cells/mm^3 effluent, with more than 50% of these cells being PMNs. Clearly, the clinical presentation is to a large extent determined by the pathogenic potential of the infecting species and by the virulence factors carried by the invading strain of a given species. Thus, wide variations in clinical presentation may be expected. In general, however, peritonitis caused by coagulase-negative staphylococci is clinically a mild disease. In contrast, infections due to *S. aureus*, hemolytic streptococci, and gram-negative bacilli may be clinically severe and even fatal (32–34). However, mortality due to peritonitis in CAPD patients is low (2% to 3%) and may be due in part to secondary complications such as myocardial infarction and cachexia. The major complication of CAPD peritonitis and exit site infection is technique failure. Technique failure entails the need to remove the Tenckhoff catheter and to transfer the patient to hemodialysis in order to control the infection, either in the acute phase or in case of repeatedly relapsing infection (1).

Exit site infection is characterized by the presence of purulent drainage and erythema of the skin at the catheter-epidermal interface. Induration and tenderness along the tunnel track indicates tunnel infection, with or without discharge and positive culture. A positive culture from an exit site in the absence of signs of inflammation does not necessarily constitute or herald infection (27). Another important feature of CAPD-peritonitis is its tendency to relapse upon discontinuation of apparently successful therapy. Relapse rates are especially high following infections due to the *Staphylococcus, Pseudomonas* spp., and fungal species. Relapses and reinfection are also seen with exit site and tunnel track infections.

A separate entity, not of a directly infectious nature, is so-called sclerosing peritonitis that may complicate CAPD. In sclerosing peritonitis, peritoneal thickening, laminar intestinal concrescence, and diffuse hemorrhage occur, often resulting in patient death from ileus. Intestinal obstruction and loss of ultrafiltration are also features of this dreaded complication. The etiology of sclerosing peritonitis remains uncertain, but recurrent episodes of bacterial or fungal peritonitis may well be a major risk factor (35). Fortunately, this complication is rare and, if it occurs, it is a late one.

IV. PATHOGENESIS OF CAPD PERITONITIS

Different routes of bacterial invasion into the peritoneal cavity exist in CAPD patients. The most common access used by coagulase-negative staphylococci, *S. aureus*, and other gram-positive pathogens is via the Tenckhoff catheter. In contrast, enteric bacilli may reach the peritoneal cavity by direct transmigration (also known as *translocation*) from the gut across the intestinal wall (28,29,36). Intestinal pathologies including diverticulosis and ischemic or ulcerative bowel diseases may facilitate this mode of peritoneal contamination (37). A third route is hematogenous spread from a distant focus to the peritoneum; this route may be important in peritonitis due to streptococci, *Listeria*, and *Haemophilus* (34). Finally, infections ascending through the fallopian tubes may be the cause of peritonitis in women undergoing CAPD (34). Most episodes are due to organisms of the patient's own microflora. Thus, carriers of *S. aureus* are at threefold to fivefold increased risk of *S. aureus* exit site infection when compared to noncarriers (see below).

The sequence of events following peritoneal contamination in CAPD patients can be separated into three different scenarios.

1. Bacteria do not adhere to surfaces of the peritoneum or Tenckhoff catheter present in the abdominal cavity and are therefore likely to be flushed out again during subsequent fluid exchanges; no inflammation ensues. Thus, contamination does not always lead to clinical peritonitis (38,39).

2. Bacteria adhere to the surface of the plastic Tenckhoff catheter and form a biofilm on the foreign material. Biofilms per se do not necessarily induce inflammation that becomes clinically noticeable. Biofilms are found on many if not all Tenckhoff catheters removed for various (infectious and noninfectious) reasons. In many cases the presence of biofilm is not temporarily associated with the occurrence of clinical peritonitis (40,41). However, it has been proposed that biofilm-derived microorganisms may become the cause of peritonitis at some later stage even though the forces that would drive such transition are presently unknown.

3. Bacteria adhere to the peritoneal membrane, either directly upon entry into the abdominal cavity or via an intermediate residence within the biofilm on the Tenckhoff catheter (see point 2 above). Bacterial adher-

ence to the mesothelial cell monolayer of the peritoneal membrane is theoretically most probable, since these cells are the most prevalent type of cell present in the peritoneal cavity. In a relevant animal model preferential adherence to the membrane has been demonstrated (42). It is presently thought that bacterial adherence to the membrane is the crucial first step in the pathogenesis of CAPD peritonitis (43). In contrast, the role of the free-floating leukocytes (macrophages predominantly) in this phase is probably limited. It has been shown that at the prevailing densities of these cells in uninfected dialysate effluent ($<10^5$/ml), they are not likely to encounter invading bacteria (44). In addition, the levels of opsonins, needed for efficient recognition of bacteria by leukocytes, are so low that bacteria-leukocyte encounters may not be effective—i.e., result in bacterial engulfment by the leukocytes (45). Lack of leukocytes and opsonins is due to the repeated drainage and instillation of large volumes of dialysis fluid. In animal models such dilution has been shown to greatly diminish the phagocytic defense of the peritoneal cavity (46). At later stages of peritonitis, when massive numbers of leukocytes (PMN) migrate into the cavity, these cells constitute the major host response to bacterial challenge.

The subsequent cascade of the inflammatory response following bacterial adherence to the peritoneal membrane is depicted in Figure 2. Importantly, mesothelial cells become directly activated by bacteria (47), or indirectly via activated macrophages (48), to secrete chemotactic agents (IL-8 and MCP-1) in polarized fashion. These cytokines attract large numbers of leukocytes into the peritoneal cavity (43). The peritoneal membrane may further contribute to inflammation by generating prostaglandins and other cytokines (e.g., Il-6). Migration of leukocytes from peritoneal capillaries across vascular endothelium and peritoneal mesothelium is in itself a complex process involving cell/cell interactions via specific ligands in the leukocyte membrane (CR-3 and VLA-4) and receptors present on endothelial and mesothelial cells (ICAM-1 and VCAM-1) (49). Leukocyte migration is accompanied by exudation of serum proteins including opsonic molecules such as C3, IgG, and fibronectin. In this manner an intra-abdominal milieu is created that is effectively antibacterial (44). However, continued exchanges with fresh dialysis fluids that are intrinsically rather damaging for host defense cells and proteins (50–53) may partly negate the beneficial effect of the peritoneal inflammatory response.

Also, bacteria may have become sequestered at sites—e.g., within biofilm or within cells—where they cannot be attacked properly by the inflammatory cells (41,54). This feature may help explain the partial response to antibiotic therapies that do not specifically target such difficult-to-reach sites of microbial growth and survival. Patients who are further compromised—e.g., diabetics or others with immune function disorders affecting their phagocytes—are especially prone to

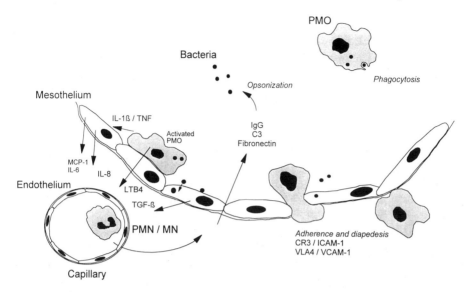

Figure 2 Schematic presentation of the inflammatory response of the peritoneal membrane. Bacteria directly or indirectly, via activation of peritoneal macrophages (PMO), stimulate mesothelial cells to excrete pro-inflammatory cytokines IL-6, IL-8, monocyte chemotactic protein-1 (MCP-1), and transforming growth factor-β (TGF-β) that attract polymorphonuclear (PMN) and mononuclear (MN) leukocytes from nearby capillaries in the submesothelial loose connective tissue. Diapedesis of PMN and MN require coordinated adhesion to mesothelial cell in which leukocyte adhesion molecules CR3 (on PMN) and VLA-4 (on MN) interact with ligands ICAM and VCAM on mesothelium. Exudation of opsonic proteins IgG, C3, and fibronectin also occurs.

experience recurrent infection (25,55,56). Also, higher rates of *S. epidermidis* peritonitis have been observed in patients whose dialysates fail to opsonize these coagulase-negative staphylococci (57).

V. DIAGNOSIS OF INFECTION

In patients with signs and symptoms laboratory evaluation of effluent dialysate should include a total white cell count with differential, a Gram-stain, and culture. In patients who have only abdominal pain with or without fever but who have clear effluents containing less than 100 PMN/mm³ the diagnosis of peritonitis is uncertain and immediate initiation of therapy is not necessary. In contrast, patients with cloudy fluid accompanied by abdominal pain or fever require prompt initiation of therapy, and diagnostic laboratory studies should be obtained expeditiously. A Gram stain is positive in up to 40% of episodes of peritonitis, and when positive it is predictive of the type of organism in 85% of cases. Since fungi may grow slowly, a Gram stain is particularly useful in the early recognition of fungal peritonitis. Many techniques have been described for the isolation of pathogens from infected CAPD effluent (15). As in blood cultures, the sensitivity of the culture increases with the volume that is sampled. Generally, enrichment broths (e.g., blood-culturing systems) are reported to have superior sensitivity compared to direct plating of sediments. The yields of the direct plating methods are significantly increased if the cell sediment is first lysed (freeing cell-associated bacteria) through the action of detergents, sonication, or osmotic shock. More than 90% of the episodes of CAPD peritonitis are culture-positive. However, routine culture of clear dialysate from uninfected patients may also grow bacteria in up to 27% of the samples (39); such growth probably reflects the intermittant entry and outflow of low numbers of bacteria in and out of the peritoneal space (see above).

Purulent exudate from inflamed exit sites may be cultured by routine swabbing and forwarding to the medical microbiology laboratory utilizing standard transport media. Culturing of an erythematous exit site in the absence of a discharge does not provide clinically useful reports, and culture results usually demonstrate commensal skin flora. Gram stains should be routinely performed on all exudate material since this will reveal the presence or absence of leukocytes and the type(s) of organism(s) present.

If catheters are removed as a consequence of infection, culturing of several sections of the catheter (intraperitoneal, tunnel track, exit site) may be helpful in establishing the etiological role of the organisms attached. New molecular techniques including PCR-mediated DNA fingerprinting and pulsed-field gel electrophoresis of bacterial DNA will allow genotyping of virtually all pathogens causing infections in CAPD patients (58). Thus, sources of strains and routes of infection can now be traced accurately.

VI. TREATMENT

The majority of CAPD-related episodes of peritonitis are initially treated empirically, or on the basis of the result of a Gram stain. Many different antimicrobial agents and combinations thereof have been used to treat CAPD peritonitis (59). Both national and international working parties have set guidelines that are regularly updated (60,61). Based on published data on the types and resistance patterns of organisms isolated (15), the empirical regimen should include vancomycin (1 to 2 g every 7 days) and either an aminoglycoside (gentamicin, tobramycin, or netilmicin, 40 mg/day), or a third-generation cephalosporin with antipseudomonal activity (e.g., ceftazidime, 1 g/day). Vancomycin is needed since many staphylococci are methicillin-resistant (15). All agents are preferentially given via the intraperitoneal route—aminoglycosides once daily, and the cephalosporin divided in equal doses/exchange (Fig. 3) (61). Oral therapies with fluoroquinolones are not recommended since their bioavailability may vary widely in these patients, and only low dialysate levels are reached that are associated with frequent relapses of peritonitis (62). A high rate of relapse (11/73; 15%) was also observed in one study, when, through intraperitoneal dosing, mean dialysate levels of 10 mg/L ciprofloxacin were achieved; 10 of 11 relapsing organisms were gram-positive organisms (63). Thus, fluoroquinolone monotherapy may not suffice. Failure may be due to inaccessibility of the organisms within intracellular sites or due to phenotypic antimicrobial resistance of sessile bacteria located within catheter-associated biofilm (see above). Also, peritoneal dialysis fluid may constitute a milieu in which bacteria display increased resistance to antibiotics (44,64). The carbapenem imipenem/cilastatin has also been used with some initial success, but high rates of gastrointestinal side effects were noted (16). In cases where methicillin-resistant staphylococci are cultured β-lactam antibiotics alone do not work well clinically. Peritonitis due to yeasts may be amendable to medical treatment alone, although catheter removal is still recommended if the

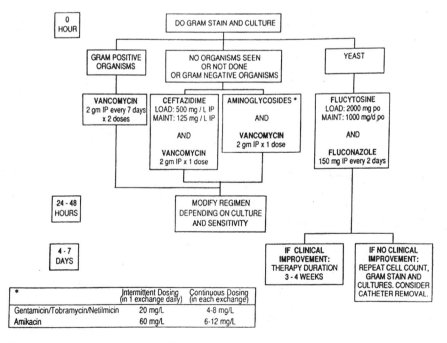

Figure 3   Flow chart for the initial, empiric therapy of CAPD-associated peritonitis. Reprinted from Ref. 61.

patient does not respond in 4 to 7 days. When culture results become available, the broad-spectrum empirical regimens should be streamlined (61). The optimal length of treatment is unknown but may be as short as 7 days, 10 to 14 days being considered sufficient by most centers.

In cases of failure to obtain resolution of signs and symptoms of infection or if the infection relapses repeatedly in the face of appropriate antimicrobial treatments, the patient needs to be reassessed carefully for the presence of occult pathologies within the abdomen or along the catheter and for the presence of unusual organisms. Patients with staphylococcal infections may have oral rifampicin added to their regimen since this agent kills biofilm-associated bacteria as well as staphylococci sequestered inside host cells (65). Fibrinolytic agents such as urokinase have also been used in this setting with some success (61,66); however, its exact mode of action remains unknown.

There are few data on the therapeutic efficacy of methods to cure exit site infections. Combination therapy including rifampicin in case of staphylococcal etiology or ciprofloxacin in case of gram-negative infection is currently recommended for 2 to 4 weeks (61). For pseudomonal or fungal exit site infection associated with peritonitis, the treatment of choice is *early* catheter removal. Shaving off the Dacron cuff at the external exit site may, in some patients, result in cure (61).

VII.   PREVENTION

Several strategies for the prevention of peritonitis and exit site infections in CAPD patients are currently pursued. One strategy is to further increase the antimicrobial barriers for entry into the peritoneal cavity. Improvements in connector technology may still lower the rate of intraluminal contamination during the exchange procedures; in-line bacterial filters, if they can be made cost-effective, would also serve this goal. In addition, the choice of catheter design and the orientation of catheter placement in the patient may all affect the likelihood of catheter contamination and the formation of progressive biofilm along its surfaces (61). Thus, catheters would ideally be made of a material that is fully biocompatible with the surrounding human tissues while also preventing the adherence of bacteria. Of course, the catheter placement procedure should be performed under strict aseptic conditions, as is done for other types of implant surgery. Design and placement should avoid as much as possible the chance that catheters are subjected to trauma and repeated or continued mechanical stress.

A second strategy is to modulate the patient's commensal flora. Most importantly, *S. aureus* nasal carriers have now been identified to be at increased risk (three- to fourfold) of infection, especially exit site infection, with their own strain (67). Elimination of nasal carriership with mupirocin has been shown to prevent such infection (68). Antimicrobial prophylaxis (e.g., with a first-generation cephalosporin) is also indicated at the time of catheter implantation and during invasive procedures known to be associated with transient bacteremia (61). Prophylaxis is *not* recommended for extended use. Such use would only contribute to the already high antibiotic pressure extended on the commensal flora of the CPD patient and his surroundings, thereby increasing the risk of emergence of resistant strains (65,69,70).

REFERENCES

1. Nolph KD. Peritoneal dialysis registry update. Proceedings of the 15th Annual Conference on Peritoneal Dialysis, Baltimore, Feb. 12–14, 1995:179–182.
2. Serkes KD, Blagg ChR, Nolph KD, Vanesh EF, Shapiro F. Comparison of patient and technique survival in continuous ambulatory peritoneal dialysis (CAPD) and haemodialysis: A multi-center study. Perit Dial Int 1990; 10:15–19.
3. Gokal R, Jakubowski C, King J, et al. Outcome in patients on continuous ambulatory peritoneal dialysis and haemodialysis: 4-year analysis of a prospective multicenter study. Lancet 1987; ii:1105–1109.
4. Popovich RP, Moncrief JW, Decherd JF, Bomar JB, Pyle W. The definition of a novel portable/wearable equilibrium peritoneal dialysis technique. Trans Am Soc Artif Intern Organs 1976; 5:64. Abstract.
5. Oreopoulos DG, Robson M, Izatt S, Clayton S, de Veber GA. A simple and safe technique for continuous ambulatory peritoneal dialysis. Trans Am Soc Artif Inteen Organs 1978; 24:484–489.
6. Diaz-Buxo J, Walker P, Farmer C, Chandler J, Holt R. Continuous cyclic peritoneal dialysis—a preliminary report. Artif Organs 1981; 5:157–161.
7. Tenckhoff H, Schechter H. A bacteriologically safe peritoneal access device. Trans Am Soc Artif Intern Organs 1968; 14:181–187.
8. Fellin G, Gentile MG, Manna GM, Redaelli L, D'Amico G. Peritonitis prevention: a Y-connector and sodium hypochloride three years' experience. Report of the Italian CAPD study group. In: Khanna R, Nolph KD, Prowant B, Twardowski ZJ, Oreopoulo DG, eds. Advances in Continuous Peritoneal Dialysis. Toronto: Peritoneal Dialysis Bulletin, 1987:114–118.
9. Canadian CAPD Clinical Trials Group. Peritonitis in continuous ambulatory peritoneal dialysis. Randomized clinical trial comparing the Y connector disinfectant system to standard systems. Perit Dial Int 1989; 9:159–164.
10. Port FK, Held PJ, Nolph KD, Turenne MN, Wolfe RA. Risk of peritonitis and technique failure by CAPD connection technique: A national study. Kidney Int 1992; 42:867–974.
11. Golper TA, Geerlings W, Selwood NH, Brunner FP, Wing AJ. Peritoneal dialysis results in the EDTA registry. In: Nolph KD, ed. Peritoneal Dialysis. Dordrecht: Kluwer Academic, 1989:414–428.
12. Domrongkitchaiporn S, Karim M, Watson L, Moriarty M. The influence of continuous ambulatory peritoneal dialysis connection technique on peritonitis rate and technique survival. Am J Kidney Dis 1994; 24:50–58.

13. Dryden MS, McCann M, Wing AJ, Phillips I. Controlled trial of a Y-set dialysis delivery system to prevent peritonitis in patients receiving continuous ambulatory peritoneal dialysis. J Hosp Infect 1992; 20:185–192.
14. Holley JL, Bernardini J, Piraino B. Infecting organisms in continuous ambulatory peritoneal dialysis patients on the Y-set. Am J Kidney Dis 1994; 23:569–573.
15. Verbrugh HA. Organisms causing peritonitis. In: Coles G, Davies M, Williams JD, eds. CAPD: Host defence, nutrition and ultrafiltration. Contrib Nephrol 1990; 85: 39–48.
16. Lui SF, Cheng AB, Leung CB, Wong KC, Li PKT, Lai KN. Imipenem/cilastatin sodium in the treatment of continuous ambulatory peritoneal dialysis-associated peritonitis. Am J Nephrol 1994; 14:182–186.
17. Were AJ, Marsden A, Tooth A, Ramsden R, Mistry CD, Gokal R. Netilmicin and vancomycin in the treatment of peritonitis in CAPD patients. Clin Nephrol 1992; 37: 209–213.
18. Dryden MS, Wing AJ, Phillips I. Low dose intraperitoneal ciprofloxacin for the treatment of peritonitis in patients receiving continuous ambulatory peritoneal dialysis (CAPD). J Antimicrob Chemother 1991; 28:131–139.
19. Taylor PC. Routine laboratory diagnosis of continuous ambulatory peritoneal dialysis peritonitis using centrifugation/lysis and saponin-containing media. Eur J Clin Microbiol Infect Dis 1994; 13:249–252.
20. Ludlam HA. Infectious consequences of continuous ambulatory peritoneal dialysis. J Hosp Infect 1991; 18(suppl A):341–354.
21. Rotellar C, Black J, Winchester JF, et al. Ten years' experience with continuous ambulatory peritoneal dialysis. Am J Kidney Dis 1991; 17:158–164.
22. Wilcox MH, Finch RG, Burden RP, Morgan AG. Peritonitis complicating continuous ambulatory peritoneal dialysis in Nottingham 1983–1988. J Med Microbiol 1991; 34:137–141.
23. Dryden M, Eykyn SJ. Short-course gentamicin in gram-negative CAPD peritonitis. Lancet 1993; 341:497.
24. Viglino G, Cancarini C, Catizone L, et al. Ten years experience of CAPD in diabetics: comparison of results with non-diabetics. Nephrol Dial Transplant 1994; 9: 1443–1448.
25. Tebben JA, Rigsby MO, Selwyn PA, Brennon N, Kliger A, Finkelstein FO. Outcome of HIV-infected patients on continuous ambulatory peritoneal dialysis. Kidney Int 1993; 44:191–198.
26. Scalamogna A, Castelnouo C, De Vecchi A, Ponticelli C. Exit-site and tunnel infections in continuous ambulatory peritoneal dialysis patients. Am J Kidney Dis 1991; 18:674–677.
27. Luzar MA, Brown CB, Balf D, et al. Exit-site care and exit-site infection in continuous ambulatory peritoneal dialysis (CAPD): results of a randomized multicenter trial. Periton Dial Int 1990; 10:25–29.
28. Wood CJ, Fleming V, Turnidge J, Thompson N, Atkins RC. *Campylobacter* peritonitis in continuous ambulatory peritoneal dialysis: report of eight cases and a review of the literature. Am J Kidney Dis 1992; 19:257–263.

29. Muñoz P, Fernández-Baca V, Peláez T, Sánchez R, Rodriguez-Créixems M, Bouza E. Aeromonas peritonitis. Clin Infect Dis 1994; 18:32–37.
30. Steigbigel RT, Cross AS. Infections associated with haemodialysis and chronic peritoneal dialysis. In: Remington JS, Swartz MN, eds. Current Clinical Topics in Infectious Diseases. New York: McGraw-Hill, 1984:125–145.
31. Solary E, Cabanne JF, Tauter Y, Rifle G. Evidence for a role of plasticizers in "eosinophilic" peritonitis in continuous ambulatory peritoneal dialysis. Nephron 1986; 42:341–342.
32. Dratwa M, Glupczynski Y, Lameire N, et al. Treatment of gram-negative peritonitis with aztreonam in patients undergoing continuous ambulatory peritoneal dialysis. Rev Infect Dis 1991; 13(suppl 7):645–647.
33. Borra SI, Chaudarana J, Kleinfeld M. Fatal peritonitis due to group B β-hemolytic *Streptococcus* in a patient receiving chronic ambulatory peritoneal dialysis. Am J Kidney Dis 1992; 19:375–377.
34. Vas SI. Peritonitis. In: Nolph KD, ed. Peritoneal Dialysis, Dordrecht: Kluwer Academic, 1989:161–188.
35. Rubin J, Herrera GA, Collins D. An autopsy study of the peritoneal cavity from patients on continuous ambulatory peritoneal dialysis. Am J Kidney Dis 1991; 18: 97–102.
36. Schweinburg FB, Seligman AM, Fine J. Transmural migration of intestinal bacteria. N Engl J Med 1950; 242:747–751.
37. Wu G, Khanna R, Vas S, Oreopoulos DG. Is extensive diverticulosis of the colon a contra-indication to CAPD? Perit Dial Bull 1983; 3:180–183.
38. Fijen JW, Struyk DG, Krediet RT, Boeschoten EW, de Vries JP, Arisz L. Dialysate leukocytosis in CAPD patients without clinical infection. Neth J Med 1988; 33:270–280.
39. Van Bronswijk H. Microbial invasion and peritoneal defence in CAPD patients. PhD thesis, Free University of Amsterdam, Amsterdam, Netherlands, 1988.
40. Marrie TJ, Bobel MA, Costerton JW. Examination of the morphology of bacteria adhering to peritoneal dialysis catheters by scanning and transmission election microscopy. J Clin Microbiol 1983; 18:1388–1398.
41. Holmes CJ. Catheter-associated biofilm. In: Coles GA, Davies M, Williams JD, eds. CAPD: Host Defence, Nutrition and Ultrafiltration. Contrib Nephrol 1990; 85:49–56.
42. Gallimore B, Gagnon RF, Richards GK. Role of an intraperitoneal implant in the pathogenesis of experimental *Staphylococcus epidermidis* peritoneal infection in renal failure mice. Am J Nephrol 1988; 36:406–413.
43. Topley N, Williams JD. Role of the peritoneal membrane in the control of inflammation in the peritoneal cavity. Kidney Int 1994; 46(suppl 48):71–78.
44. Verbrugh HA, Keane WF, Conroy WE, Peterson PK. Bacterial growth and killing in chronic ambulatory peritoneal dialysis fluids. J Clin Microbiol 1984; 20:199–203.
45. Verbrugh HA, Keane WF, Hoidal JR, Freiberg MR, Elliott GR, Peterson PK. Peritoneal macrophages and opsonins: antibacterial defense in patients undergoing chronic peritoneal dialysis. J Infect Dis 1983; 147:1018–1029.
46. Dunn DL, Barke RA, Ahrenholtz DH, Humphrey EW, Simmons RL. The adjuvant

effect of peritoneal fluid in experimental peritonitis. Mechanisms and clinical implications. Ann Surg 1984; 199:37–43.

47. Zeillemaker AM, Mul FPJ, Hoynck van Papendrecht AAGM, et al. Polarized secretion of interleukin-8 by human mesothelial cells: a role in neutrophil migration. Immunol 1995; 84:227–232.

48. Betjes MGH, Tuk CW, Struijk DG, et al. Interleukin-8 production by human peritoneal mesothelial cells in response to tumor necrosis factor α, interleukin-1, and medium conditioned by macrophages co-cultured with *Staphylococcus epidermidis*. J Infect Dis 1993; 168:1202–1210.

49. Jonjic N, Peri G, Bernasconi S, et al. Expression of adhesion molecules and chemotactic cytokines in cultured human mesothelial cells. J Exp Med 1992; 176:1165–1174.

50. Duwe AK, Vas SI, Weatherhead JW. Effects of the composition of peritoneal dialysis fluid on chemiluminescence, phagocytosis and bacterial activity in vitro. Infect Immun 1981; 33:130–135.

51. Van Bronswijk H, Verbrugh HA, Bos HJ, et al. Cytotoxic effects of commercial continuous ambulatory peritoneal dialysis (CAPD) fluids and of bacterial exoproducts on human mesothelial cells in vitro. Perit Dial Int 1989; 9:197–202.

52. Keane WF, Comty CM, Verbrugh HA, Peterson PK. Opsonic deficiency of peritoneal dialysis effluent in continuous ambulatory peritoneal dialysis. Kidney Int 1984; 25:539–543.

53. Holmes CJ. Biocompatibility of peritoneal dialysis solutions. Perit Dial Int 1993; 13:88–94.

54. De Fijter CWH, Verbrugh HA, Heezius HCJM, et al. Effect of clindamycin on the intracellular bactericidal capacity of human peritoneal macrophages. J Antimicrob Chemother 1990; 26:525–532.

55. Khan GA, Bank N. An adult patient with hyperimmune globulinemia E (Job's) syndrome, end-stage renal disease and repeated episodes of peritonitis. Clin Nephrol 1994; 41:233–236.

56. Lewis SI, Young SA, Wood BJ, Morgan KS, Erickson DG, Holmes CJ. Relationship between frequent episodes of peritonitis and altered immune status. Am J Kidney Dis 1993; 22:456–461.

57. Holmes CJ. Peritoneal host defense mechanisms in peritoneal dialysis. Kidney Int 1994; 46(suppl 48):58–70.

58. Van Belkum A. DNA fingerprinting of medically important microorganisms by use of PCR. Clin Microbiol Rev 1994; 7:174–187.

59. Millikin SP, Matzke GR, Keane WF. Antimicrobial treatment of peritonitis associated with continuous ambulatory peritoneal dialysis. Perit Dial Int 1991; 11:252–260.

60. British Society for Antimicrobial Chemotherapy. Diagnosis and management of peritonitis in continuous ambulatory peritoneal dialysis. Lancet 1987; i:845–848.

61. Keane WF, Everett ED, Golper TA, et al. Peritoneal dialysis related peritonitis treatment recommendations; 1993 update. Perit Dial Int 1993; 13:14–28.

62. Bailie GR, Eisele G. Pharmacokinetic issues in the treatment of continuous ambulatory peritoneal dialysis-associated peritonitis. J Antimicrob Chemother 1995; 35:563–567.

63. Ludlam HA, Barton I, While L, McMullin C, King A, Phillips I. Intraperitoneal ciprofloxacin for the treatment of peritonitis in patients receiving continuous ambulatory peritoneal dialysis (CAPD). J Antimicrob Chemother 1990; 25:843–851.

64. Wilcox MH, Geary I, Spencer RC. In-vitro activity of imipenem, in comparison with cefuroxime and ciprofloxacin, against coagulase-negative staphylococci in broth and peritoneal dialysis fluid. J Antimicrob Chemother 1992; 29:49–55.

65. Zimmerman SW. Rifampin use in peritoneal dialysis. Perit Dial Int 1989; 9:241–243.

66. Innes A, Burden RP, Finch RG, Morgan AG. Treatment of resistant peritonitis in continuous ambulatory peritoneal dialysis with intraperitoneal urokinase: A double-blind clinical trial. Nephrol Dial Transplant 1994; 9:797–799.

67. Luzar MA, Coles GA, Faller B, et al. *Staphylococcus aureus* nasal carriage and infection in patients on continuous ambulatory peritoneal dialysis. N Engl J Med 1990; 322:505–509.

68. Faller B. European Multi Center Trial: results. Proceedings of the 15th Annual Conference on Peritoneal Dialysis, Baltimore, Feb. 12–14, 1995; 53–62.

69. Sanyal D, Williams AJ, Johnsons AP, Georgy RC. The emergence of vancomycin resistance in renal dialysis. J Hosp Infect 1993; 24:167–173.

70. Editorial. Prevention of peritonitis in CAPD. Lancet 1991; 337:22–23.

14

Infections Associated with Catheters Used for Hemodialysis and Hemodialysis Shunts

Verena A. Briner
Hospital of Lucerne, Lucerne, Switzerland

Andreas F. Widmer
University Hospital Basel, Basel, Switzerland

I. INTRODUCTION

In 1943 the first hemodialysis was performed by using simple glass cannulae. Blood samples were drawn from several subcutaneous veins. However, the dialyzed blood volume was small and loss of veins due to infection and thrombosis was significant. This renal replacement therapy was of low quality. Nearly 20 years later, the external arteriovenous Quinton-Scribner shunt (1) was developed (Fig. 1). Two Teflon-silastic cannulae were surgically inserted into a distal arm vein and artery. Continuous blood flow from the artery into the dialysis filter and from there to the vein increased the efficacy of therapy. After the dialysis procedure, the tip of the cannulae were bridged by a caoutchouc tube. Thus, it became possible to treat patients with renal failure for a prolonged time. Thrombosis and infections, however, were very frequent and limited their use (2,3). In 1966, the internal arteriovenous fistula (AVF) was developed by side-to-side and later also by side-to-end anastomosis of a superficial artery with an adjacent vein close to the wrist (Fig. 2). Blood flow was >200 ml/min through the dilated vein and made adequate dialysis possible. AVF soon became the first choice for vascular access and replaced external shunts (4). In the absence of appropriate vessels, particularly in diabetics, females, elderly patients, and patients with severe peripheral vascular disease, the AVF is created in the cubital fossa by interposition of bovine carotid artery, human umbilical vein, saphenous vein, and synthetic grafts (Fig. 3) to create a fistula, which, however, is named a shunt. It is rarely required to create femoral or transthoracic axilloaxillary shunts. Autologous veins or bovine arteries show shorter long-term survival (5) than the AVF (6). Improvement of the synthetic material for prosthetic vascular implants contributed to enhance shunt survival (7). Still, the main cause for the high revision rate and graft failure is outflow obstruction. Around the anastomosis intimal hyperplasia develops and may result in stenosis (8). Although revision is very frequent (>50%) (7,9) the 1-year patency rate of polytetrafluoroethylene grafts (50% to 75%) (9) is within the range of patency rates for AVF (55% to 65%) (9,10).

Patients with acute renal failure and those awaiting maturation of the AVF or synthetic graft require only transient vascular access for dialysis. In 1960 Shaldon et al. (11) positioned a single lumen catheter in the femoral vessels using the method of Seldinger which was suitable for adequate blood flow from the patient to the filter. Nowadays a similar method is still used. The patient donates and receives the blood intermittently by using a double pump dializing machine which passes the blood via the same catheter with a Y-shaped external tip representing venous and arterial access (Fig. 4). To prevent vascular access morbidity, patients with femoral catheters are confined to bed rest. In general, therefore, therapy is restricted to several days to a few weeks, until acute renal failure resolves. In 1967, the subclavian vein was used as vascular access. The mobility of patients with a catheter in the upper thoracic sites was less limited and therefore the catheter was also used for long-term treatment in chronic renal failure when AVF was not available. Modification of catheter design to include two lumina made it possible to have continuous blood flow from and to the patient using a single insertion site (Fig. 4). Adequate blood flow for dialysis (200 to 300 ml/min) requires rigid catheters which do not collapse during sucking. Stiff material such as Teflon and polypropylene tends to return to its basic linear shape and may favor kinking (12). High rates of stenosis and thrombosis of the subclavian vein and the risk for pneumothorax were reasons to switch to the internal jugular access site (13,14). The technique to insert a catheter percutaneously was modified in a way that subcutaneous tunnellization of the prethoracic part of the catheter should prevent dislocation. A Dacron cuff in the subcutaneous part allows fibroblasts to invade and stabilize catheter localization (15–17). Catheter survival now ranges between 50% and 74% at 1 year and between 30% to 43% at 2 years (10,16,18–21). Infection and thrombosis remain the major limiting factors. The incidence of infection seems less frequent with silicone and silicone-coated catheters than with polyurethane, Teflon, or polypropylene hemodialysis catheters (22–24).

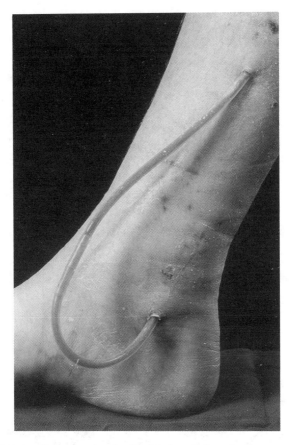

Figure 1   Quinton-Scribner shunt with the two Teflon-silastic cannulae that are bridged by a tube after dialysis.

II.   INFECTIONS IN HEMODIALYSIS PATIENTS

In hemodialysis patients, infections are the first cause of morbidity and the second cause of mortality in the U.S. (25) and Europe (26). An even greater mortality rate due to infection is found among diabetics on chronic hemodialysis (25). In the following section we focus on infections related to the vascular access site, which account for more than 70% of all infectious complications in hemodialysis patients (3,27).

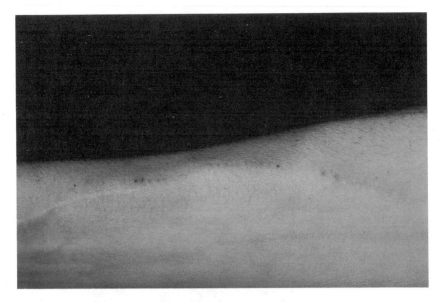

Figure 2   Arteriovenous fistula of a superficial artery and adjacent vein. Several puncture sites of the dilated vein are shown.

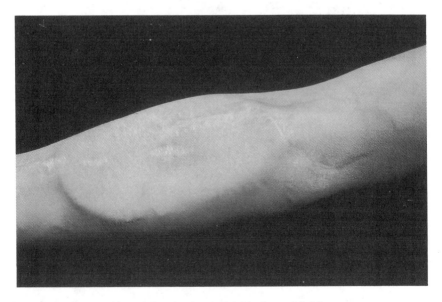

Figure 3   Interposition of Goretex loop distal to the cubital fossa.

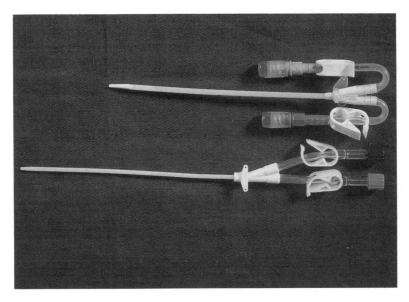

Figure 4   Top: single-lumen catheter. Bottom: double-lumen catheter.

A.   Infections Related to Arteriovenous Fistula and Shunt

The autologous AVF shows a high early failure rate (< 30 days) due to insufficient venous size and runoff (9). When these technical problems are overcome, a very low complication rate due to infection is demonstrated. Since vascular access site colonization and infection, bacteremia, and sepsis are not equally well defined in the various studies in the literature comparison of infection rates of different centers have to be done with caution. On average, the incidence of bacteremia and sepsis is lowest for AVF, five to 10 times increased for shunts and >10 times increased for subclavian catheters when appropriate study groups are compared (30). The incidence of bacteremia and sepsis per 100 access days ranges between <0.01 to 0.07 for patients with AVF (Table 1) (3,27–30). Episodes of bacteremia may be the result of access site infection. If local infection is severe enough to cause phlebitis, clotting may occur with attenuation of blood flow and loss of fistula (Fig. 5). Failure of prosthetic shunts usually result from thrombosis. The infection rate in synthetic grafts ranges from 0.03 to 0.11 per 100 access days (3,5,7,9,29). Bacteremia and sepsis related to localized vascular access site infection are caused in 60% to 100% by gram-positive organisms such as *Staphylococcus aureus* and coagulase-negative staphylococci (CoNS) (Table 2)

Table 1　Incidence of Bacteremia and Sepsis Associated With Vascular Access for Hemodialysis

	Reference	Total no. of patients	Incidence/100 access days
AV fistula	Higgins (30)	120	0.003
	Kaene et al. (3)	180	0.07
	Kaplowitz et al. (29)[a]	71	0.02
Shunt	Kaene et al. (3)	128	0.11
	Higgins (30)	55	0.03
Catheter			
V. subclavia	Cheesbrough et al. (39)[a]	53	0.77
	Dahlberg et al. (36)[a]	88	0.85
	Higgins (30)	50	0.63
	Sherertz et al. (35)[a]	27	0.77
	Uldall et al. (32)[a]	92	0.69
	Vanherweghem et al. (34)	148	0.6
	Vanholder et al. (33)	538	0.33
V. jugularis	Cappello et al. (20)	90	0.08
	Gibson et al. (19)	51	0.34
	Higgins (30)	9	0.2
	Moss et al. (23)	54	0.02
	Moss et al. (18)	131	0.01
	Shusterman et al. (21)	18	0.16
	Uldall et al. (15)	65	0.15

[a]Prospective study.

(3,27,29–31). The majority of infections in synthetic grafts occur within the first 3 to 4 months after surgery. This may suggest that incomplete neointimization of the graft favors local infection (5).

B.　Infections Related to Hemodialysis Catheters

The rate of hemodialysis catheter-related bacteremia and sepsis ranges from 1.5% to 35% of patients (12,16,21,22,32–36). Catheter-related infections are reported to be up to three times more frequent in diabetics than in nondiabetics (18,23,34). The incidence of bacteremia and sepsis associated with hemodialysis catheters is 0.01 to 0.85 infections per 100 access days (Table 1). To some extent the broad range may relate to patient selection, different assessment of infections (clinical or microbiological evaluation), the length of observation periods, and study design. The duration of catheter use varies from a few days (16,37) up to several

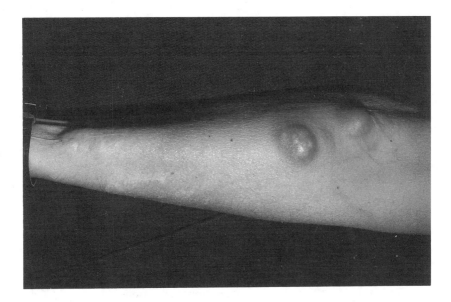

Figure 5   *S. aureus* abscess at the puncture sites of the shunt.

Table 2   Rates of Staphylococci as a Major Cause of Bacteremia and Sepsis in Hemodialysis Patients

Study	No. of catheters	No. of patients (with sepsis)	*S. aureus* (%)	CoNS (%)
Almirall et al. (38)	54	53 (9)	44.4	33.3
Bambauer et al. (12)	2626	1627 (296)	23	45.9
Cappello et al. (20)	107	90 (5)	80	0
Cheesbrough et al. (39)	64	53 (14)	42.9	35.7
Gibson et al. (19)	64	51 (18)	33.3	11.1
Higgins (30)	—	234 (16)	75.0	6.3
Levin et al. (17)	171	129 (12)	33.3	66.6
Shaffer et al. (22)	65	51 (14)	28.6	35.7
Vanherweghem et al. (34)	200	148 (17)	23.5	76.5

years (19). The incidence is clearly higher in studies done prospectively (32,35,36,38,39) and may roughly be 10- to 20-fold higher than for AVF. Exit site infection, defined as an infection that is limited to the cutaneous insertion site of the catheter, occurs in up to 40% of patients (16,35,36). More recent studies, however, reported a rather low incidence of infection associated with central venous dialysis catheters (15,18,20,22). These findings may relate partly to improvement of insertion technique and postinsertion care; this may also reflect shorter observation periods. Still, the infection rate tends to be lower in patients with internal jugular vein catheters than with subclavian catheters (Table 1). The infection risk per access day is constant, so infection rate increases linearly with the length of catheterization time (33–35,39). The effect of subcutaneous tunneling of catheters with and without cuff on infection rate is controversial. A similar rate of sepsis [3 of 21 (14%) patients without tunneled catheter vs. 2 of 19 (11%) patients with tunneled catheter] is reported by some authors (36). This contrasts to the significantly lower rate with tunnelization (9% without tunneled catheter and 5% with tunneled Hickman catheter) (20) and tunnelization with an additional Dacron cuff [four episodes of bacteremia in 112 noncuffed dialysis catheters (<4%) vs. no bacteremia in 80 patients with cuffed catheters such as Permcath and Hemocath] reported by others (16). The relationship between the rate of catheter infection and the number of lumina is still controversial (37,40).

Some infections may occur as a result of an inappropriate insertion technique or during usage of the catheter for dialysis. Each dialysis requires four connections to be made in the tubing, which offers ample opportunity for introducing microorganisms. In most cases, bacteria originate from the patients' skin (30,38,41). A potential source of intraluminal contamination, however, may also be the hands of medical staff manipulating the connections during hemodialysis. Colonization occurs most frequently through the catheter lumen (39). Catheters that are clinically uninfected at the time of removal have a 10% to 55% incidence of catheter colonization when routinely cultured (36,38,39). The majority of catheter-related infections are due to *S. aureus* and CoNS (12) (Table 2). Although CoNS most commonly colonize exit site and catheter, they account for fewer episodes of clinical sepsis than *S. aureus* (Table 3). This may reflect the low virulence of CoNS. In contrast, *S. aureus* colonization is frequently associated with sepsis and accounts for as much as 50% of all catheter-related bacteremias in hemodialysis patients (19,33,38,39). Other organisms than stapylococci, especially gram-negative bacteria such as *E. coli, Pseudomonas* spp., *Klebsiella* spp., *Proteus* spp., and *Serratia* spp. have been reported to cause vascular access-mediated infection (18,19,22). Hemodialysis catheter infection is rarely caused by fungi, although chronic hemodialysis and use of Hickman catheter have been shown to be risk factors for hospital-acquired candidemia (42).

III.   TREATMENT OF VASCULAR ACCESS SITE INFECTION IN HEMODIALYSIS

A.   Treatment of Arteriovenous Fistula- and Shunt-Related Infections

Native fistula infection is mainly limited to a needle site and resolves with local disinfection, oral antibiotic treatment for 1 to 3 weeks, and transient cessation of

Table 3   Gram-Positive Organisms Causing the Majority of Vascular Access Colonization, Bacteremia, and Sepsis in Hemodialysis Patients

Study	No. of catheters inserted	No. of patients	No. of catheters (Colon/BC +)[a]	S. aureus (Colon/BC +)[b] (%)	CoNS (Colon/ BC +)[b] (%)
Almirall et al. (38)	53	41	29/9	13.8/44.4	75.9/33.3
Cheesbrough et al. (39)	64	53	28/13	21.4/46.2	50.0/38.5
Kaene et al. (3)	728	445	590/73	30.8/47.9	33.8/27.4

[a]Number of catheters colonized/number of catheters associated with bacteremia (due to the same organism).
[b]Percent of catheters colonized with S. aureus or CoNS/% of catheters colonized with S. aureus or CoNS that are associated with sepsis.
Abbreviations: BC + = bacteremia and sepsis; Colon = colonization.

its use for hemodialysis (9,18,23). Selection of an appropriate antibiotic depends on the organisms isolated from the infection site. Empirical treatment should take into account that gram-positive cocci are preferentially causing these infections. If there is a low chance of methicillin-resistant S. aureus (MRSA) causing the infection in known S. aureus carriers, penicillinase-resistant synthetic penicillins may be administered. The infections in noncarriers are most often caused by CoNS, and a glycopeptid antibiotic should therefore be administered. Antibiotic therapy should be adjusted according to the culture results. When localized infection is not improving (especially in synthetic grafts) despite adequate therapy, surgical intervention such as drainage, excision, or bypassing of the lesion is required (5,9). Indications for excision and drainage (7) are (1) occluded grafts, (2) extended graft infections (Fig. 5), (3) infections with involvement of one anastomosis site, and (4) involvement of the entire subcutaneous tunnel with cellulitis. More than one-half of all grafts with severe and extended infection can be salvaged by these means. When infection persists, bleeding and pseudoaneurysm formation may occur (5).

B.   Treatment of Catheter-Related Infections

If the infection is limited to the cutaneous insertion site of the catheter, a swab is taken for microbiological analysis. Thereafter, the insertion site is disinfected with povidone-iodine (17) or chlorhexidine, and appropriate antibiotics (penicillinase-resistant penicillins such as nafcillin) are administered orally for 2 to 4 weeks (16,18,19,23). About 90% of exit site infections resolve with this regimen

(18). It has been reported that after an exit site infection has cleared, the catheter itself may become reinfected by the same organism unless it is replaced by a new one (15). However, less than 10% of exit site infections finally require another insertion site to cure the infection (16,23). When bacteremia or signs of systemic infection such as fever and chills are present, catheter removal is mandatory and parenteral antibiotics adapted to blood culture results should be administered. After catheter removal, sepsis most of the time resolves rapidly (12,17,22,30). However, complications such as endocarditis, osteomyelitis, and death are reported (3,16,34). Reimplantation of a new hemodialysis catheter should be delayed as long as possible. More recent reports demonstrate that prolonged intravenous treatment for several months with antibiotics may eradicate the infection in patients who for medical or personal reasons refuse to have their long-term catheters replaced (18,19,43–45). Bacteremia and sepsis may relapse when organisms other than CoNS, especially gram-negative bacteria, have caused the infection (18,19,22). Therefore, some authors recommend to change the catheter over a guide wire (15,45). In diabetics, access-related bacteremia resolves less frequently without catheter removal (18). It is common practice to administer antibiotics such as vancomycin, flucloxacillin, or gentamycin intravenously via the infected catheter (half of the dose through each lumen) and thereafter each catheter lumen is filled with antibiotics between two dialysis sessions (antibiotic lock) (46). At this time, proper studies supporting the beneficial effects of antibiotic lock are missing.

IV.   *S. AUREUS* COLONIZATION IN HEMODIALYSIS PATIENTS

A.   Nasal Carriage of *S. aureus* in Dialysis Patients

The bacterial flora of humans includes many organisms which under certain circumstances may cause diseases. *S. aureus* is a pathogen of major importance in hemodialysis patients, causing 30% to 80% of infections in these patients (27,30,47). The reservoir for *S. aureus* carriage has been shown to be the anterior nares (2,47). *S. aureus* nasal carriers tend to have persistent carriage. The prevalence of nasal carriage of *S. aureus* in hemodialysis patients is within the range of 30% to > 60% (17,31,47–49), compared to 21% of patients with chronic renal failure who are not on hemodialysis and 15% to 20% in the normal population (47). Regular needle puncture of the skin (insulin-requiring diabetics, drug users) increases selectively both the skin and nasal carrier rate of *S. aureus* (31) compared to healthy students. About 75% of nasal carriers on hemodialysis also have colonization of the shunt site with the same organism (2). On the other hand > 60% of patients with *S. aureus* shunt infection and > 70% with *S. aureus* bacteremia are nasal *S. aureus* carriers (27,31,47). Once established, *S. aureus* may colonize and invade skin lesions, especially if a foreign body is present, and may lead to local disease and dissemination. *S. aureus* carriers have a threefold higher risk of contracting catheter-related *S. aureus* sepsis compared to noncarriers (17). More than 90% of *S. aureus* infections in carriers are caused by the same phage type as that carried in the nares (47). However, persistent nasal carriage does not always lead to exit site infection.

B. Elimination of *S. aureus* in Nasal Carriers on Chronic Hemodialysis

In hemodialysis patients with vascular access infections, the number of hospital admissions is significantly greater than for patients whose vascular access remains uninfected (29). Furthermore, reduction of nasal *S. aureus* carriage results in a decrease of the yearly infection rate with *S. aureus* from 0.09 to 0.02 (50). These findings suggest that autoinfection is the mechanism of *S. aureus* infection, and an attempt to eradicate these organisms is therefore recommended. Several regimens of oral and local treatments have been effective in eradicating nasal *S. aureus* carriage in hemodialysis patients. Mupirocin ointment (2%) applied to the nose is very active against *S. aureus* including methicillin-resistant strains by inhibiting bacterial protein synthesis. After treating carriers two or three times a day for 5 to 7 days, eradication is achieved in about 80% to 100% (50–53). The rate of hand cultures positive for *S. aureus* is also reduced to 3%, compared to 58% in controls not treated with mupirocin (53). However, recolonization with the same phage type is noted in 20% to 75% 3 months after mupirocin treatment in dialysis patients (51,52) and up to 30% in healthy controls (53). In contrast, when daily therapy was followed by one application one to three times a week, recurrence of *S. aureus* was prevented in 95% of patients, and the yearly incidence of *S. aureus* bacteremia was reduced by 75% (50). Therefore, we recommend evaluation of chronic dialysis patients for their nasal carrier state. Demonstration of *S. aureus* in two subsequent nasal swabs (stable carriers) should give rise to routine treatment with the above regimen or 5 days treatment twice a day with mupirocin every 2 months. The development of resistance of *S. aureus* to mupirocin is uncommon (53). Microbiological analysis of nasal discharge is not required once stable carrier stage has been diagnosed. The intranasal application of mupirocin ointment is, compared with the application of systemic antimicrobials, relatively safe, well tolerated, and effective. Local application of mupirocin avoids a drug that may later be used for the treatment of systemic infections. Despite their effectiveness, oral regimens to eliminate nasal *S. aureus* (e.g., oral rifampin combined with various antibiotics such as cloxacillin, ciprofloxacin, or trimethoprim-sulfamethoxazole) are not recommended because systemic antibiotics may facilitate the development of resistant strains. Bacitracin, hexachlorophene, vancomycin, and penicillin failed to eradicate *S. aureus* carriage.

V.   PREVENTION OF VASCULAR ACCESS SITE INFECTION IN HEMODIALYSIS PATIENTS

The postinsertion catheter care remains the principal factor for preventing catheter-related infections (34,35). As many as 60% of dialysis patients are carriers of *S. aureus*, and *S. aureus* may cause 50% of catheter-related infections. Failure to comply with asepsis (poor hygiene, wet dressing) is a risk factor for vascular access site infection (29). The incidence of catheter-related infections can be reduced by meticulous aseptic care and elimination of nasal *S. aureus* in nasal carriers. Medical staff should disinfect their hands and wear gloves and masks when fistula, shunt, and catheter are manipulated for dialysis. Topical disinfection with povidone-iodine ointment applied to the exit site of hemodialysis catheters at each dressing change is superior to sterile gauze dressings alone in preventing infections at the catheter exit site, tip colonization, and sepsis (17). To prevent clotting, the catheters are filled with heparin at the end of dialysis and capped. Prophylactic antibiotics are not recommended (12). Recently, a lock with EDTA-minocyclin showed promising results. However, there are not sufficient data to promote this regimen at the time being. In between dialysis treatments the dressing should be kept dry. The access site should be swabbed with disinfecting solution before unlocking the catheter for the next dialysis.

Nurse training seems a key factor to prevent infections. Vanherweghem et al. (54) demonstrated during a period with a great number of untrained nurses working in the dialysis team that the incidence of sepsis was five times greater than before. The frequency of catheter manipulation correlates with endoluminal catheter colonization and thus with the risk of bacteremia and sepsis (39). Hemodialysis catheters therefore should be handled only by trained (dialysis) nurses, and the catheter should not be opened in between dialysis treatments.

REFERENCES

1. Quinton W, Dillard D, Scribner BH. Cannulation of blood vessels for prolonged haemodialysis. Trans Am Soc Artif Intern Organ 1960; 6:104–113.
2. Rebel MH, van Furth R, Stevens P, et al. The flora of renal haemodialysis shunt sites. J Clin Pathol 1975; 28:29–32.
3. Kaene WF, Shapiro FL, Raij L. Incidence and type of infections occurring in 445 chronic hemodialysis patients. Trans Am Soc Artif Intern Organs 1977; 23:41–46.
4. Brescia MJ, Cimino JE, Appel K, Hurwich EA. Chronic hemodialysis using vein-puncture and surgically created arteriovenous fistula. N Engl J Med 1966; 275:1089–1092.
5. Bhat DJ, Tellis VA, Kohlberg WI, et al. Management of sepsis involving expanded polytetrafluoroethylene grafts for hemodialysis access. Surgery 1980; 87:445–450.

6. Churchill DN, Taylor DW, Cook RJ, et al. Canadian hemodialysis morbidity study. Am J Kidney Dis 1992; 19:214–234.

7. Raju S. PTFE grafts for hemodialysis access. Ann Surg 1987; 206:666–673.

8. Hofstra L, Bergmans DCJJ, Hoek APG, et al. Mismatch in elastic properties around anastomoses of interposition grafts for hemodialysis access. J Am Soc Nephrol 1994; 5:1243–1250.

9. Palder SB, Kirkman RL, Whirremore AD, et al. Vascular access for hemodialysis. Ann Surg 1985; 202:235–239.

10. Mosquera DA, Gibson SP, Goldman MD. Vascular access surgery: a 2-year study and comparison with permcath. Nephrol Dial Transplant 1992; 7:1111–1115.

11. Shaldon S, Chiandussi L, Higgs B. Hemodialysis by percutaneous catheterisation of femoral artery and vein with regional heparinisation. Lancet 1961; II:857–859.

12. Bambauer R, Mestres P, Pirrung KJ. Frequency, therapy, and prevention of infections associated with large bore catheters. ASAIO J 1992; 38:96–101.

13. Clark DD, Albina JE, Chazan JA. Subclavian vein stenosis and thrombosisi: a potential serious complication in chronic hemodialysis patients. Am J Kidney Dis 1990; 15:265–268.

14. Swartz RD, Messana JM, Boyer CJ, et al. Successful use of cuffed central venous hemodialysis catheters inserted percutaneously. J Am Soc Nephrol 1994; 4:1719–1725.

15. Uldall R, De Bruyne M, Besley M, et al. A new vascular catheter for hemodialysis. Am J Kidney Dis 1993; 21:270–277.

16. Schwab SJ, Buller GL, McCann RL, et al. Prospective evaluation of a Dacron cuffed hemodialysis catheter for prolonged use. Am J Kidney Dis 1988; 11:166–169.

17. Levin A, Mason AJ, Jindal KK, et al. Prevention of hemodialysis subclavian vein catheter infections by topical povidone-iodine. Kidney Int 1991; 40:934–938.

18. Moss AH, Vasilakis C, Holley JL, et al. Use of silicone dual-lumen catheter with a Dacron cuff as a long-term vascular access for hemodialysis patients. Am J Kidney Dis 1990; 16:211–215.

19. Gibson SP, Mosquera D. Five years experience with the Quinton Permcath for vascular access. Nephrol Dial Transplant 1991; 6:269–274.

20. Cappello M, De Pauw L, Bastin G, et al. Central venous access for haemodialysis using the Hickman catheter. Nephrol Dial Transplant 1989; 4:988–992.

21. Shusterman NH, Kloss K, Mullen JL. Successful use of double-lumen, silicone rubber catheters for permanent hemodialysis access. Kidney Int 1989; 35:887–890.

22. Shaffer D, Madras PN, Williams ME, et al. Use of Dacron cuffed silicon catheters as long-term hemodialysis access. ASAIO J 1992; 38:55–58.

23. Moss AH, McLaughlin MM, Lempert KD, Holley JL. Use of a silicone catheter with a Dacron cuff for dialysis short-term vascular access. Am J Kidney Dis 1988; 12:492–498.

24. Harris JM, Martin LF. An in vitro study of the properties influencing *Staphylococcus epidermidis* adhesion to prosthetic vascular graft materials. Ann Surg 1987; 206:612–620.

25. 1994 Annual Data Report. United States Renal Data System. Washington: U.S. Department of Health and Human Services, 1995:95–105.

26. Jacobs J, Broyer M, Brunner FP, et al. Combined report on dialysis and transplantation in Europe. Proc Eur Dial Transplant Assoc 1981; 18:4–58.

27. Ralston AJ, Harlow GR, Jones DM, Davis P. Infections of Scribner and Brescia arteriovenous shunts. Br Med J 1971; 3:408–409.

28. Dobkin JF, Miller MH, Steigbigel NH. Septicemia in patients on chronic hemodialysis. Ann Intern Med 1978; 88:28–33.

29. Kaplowitz LG, Comstock JA, Landwehr DM, et al. A prospective study of infections in hemodialysis patients: patients hygiene and other risk factors for infection. Infect Control Hosp Epidemiol 1988; 9:534–541.

30. Higgins RM. Infection in a renal unit. Q J Med 1989; 261:41–51.

31. Kirmani N, Tuazon CU, Murray HW, et al. *Staphylococcus aureus* carriage rate of patients receiving long-term hemodialysis. Arch Intern Med 1978; 138:1657–1659.

32. Uldall PR, Merchant N, Woods F, et al. Changing subclavian hemodialysis cannulas to reduce infection. Lancet 1981; 1:1373.

33. Vanholder R, Hoenich N, Ringoir S. Morbidity and mortality of central venous catheter hemodialysis: a review of 10 years' experience. Nephron 1987; 47:274–279.

34. Vanherweghem JL, Cabolet P, Dhaene M, et al. Complications related to subclavian catheters for hemodialysis. Am J Nephrol 1986; 6:339–345.

35. Sherertz RJ, Falk RJJ, Huffman KA, et al. Infections associated with subclavian Uldall catheters. Arch Intern Med 1983; 143:52–56.

36. Dahlberg PJ, Yutuc WR, Newcomer KL. Subclavian hemodialysis catheter infections. Am J Kidney Dis 1986; 7:421–427.

37. Raja R, Kramer M, Alvis R, et al. Comparison of double lumen subclavian with single lumen catheter. Trans Am Soc Artif Intern Organs 1984; 30:508–509.

38. Almirall J, Gonzalez J, Rello J, et al. Infection of hemodialysis catheters: incidence and mechanisms. Am J Nephrol 1989; 9:454–459.

39. Cheesborough JS, Finch RG, Burden RP. A prospective study of the mechanism of infection associated with hemodialysis catheters. J Infect Dis 1986; 154:579–589.

40. Sariego J, Bootorabi B, Matsumoto T, Kerstein M. Major long-term complications in 1422 permanent venous access devices. Am J Surg 1993; 165:249–251.

41. Maki DG, Ringer M, Alvarado CJ. Prospective randomised trial of povidone-iodine, alcohol, and chlorhexidine for prevention of infection associated with central venous and arterial catheters. Lancet 1991; 338:339–343.

42. Wey SB, Mori M, Pfaller MA, et al. Risk factors for hospital-acquired candidemia. Arch Intern Med 1989; 149:2349–2353.

43. Rello J, Gatell JM, Almirall J, et al. Evaluation of culture techniques for identification of catheter-related infection in hemodialysis patients. Eur J Clin Microbiol Infect Dis 1989; 8:620–622.

44. Saltissi D, Macfarlane DJ. Successful treatment of *Pseudomonas paucimobilis* haemodialysis catheter-related sepsis without catheter removal. Postgrad Med J 1994; 70:47–48.

45. Carlisle EJ, Blake P, McCarthy F, et al. Septicemia in long-term jugular hemodialysis catheters; eradicating infection by changing the catheter over a guide wire. Int J Artif Organs 1991; 14:150–153.

46. Krzywda EA, Andris DA, Edmiston CE, et al. Treatment of Hickman catheter sepsis using the antibiotic lock technique. Infect Control Hosp Epidemiol 1995; 16:596.

47. Yu VL, Goetz A, Wagener M, et al. *Staphylococcus aureus* nasal carriage and infection in patients on hemodialysis. Efficacy of antibiotic prophylaxis. N Engl J Med 1986; 315:91–96.

48. Tuazon CU. Skin and skin structure infection in the patient at risk: carrier state of *Staphylococcus aureus*. Am J Med 1984; 76(suppl 51):166–171.

49. Goldblum SE, Ulrich JA, Reed WP. Nasal and cutaneous flora among hemodialysis patients and personnel: quantitative characterisation and pattern of staphylococcal carriage. Am J Kideny Dis 1982; 2:281–286.

50. Boelaert JR, Van Landyt HW, Godard CA, et al. Nasal mupirocin ointment decreases the incidence of *Staphylococcus aureus* bacteraemia in haemodialysis patients. Nephrol Dial Transplant 1993; 8:235–239.

51. Holton DL, Nicolle LE, Diley D, Bernstein K. Efficacy of mupirocin nasal ointment in eradicating *Staphylococcus aureus* nasal carriage in chronic haemodialysis patients. J Hosp Infect 1991; 17:133–137.

52. Watanakunokorn C, Brandt J, Durkin P, et al. The efficacy of mupirocin ointment and chlorhexidine body scrubs in the eradication of nasal carriage of *Staphylococcus aureus* among patients undergoing long-term hemodialysis. Am J Infect Control 1992; 20:138–141.

53. Reagan DR, Doebbeling BD, Pfaller MA, et al. Elimination of coincident *Staphylococcus aureus* nasal and hand carriage with intranasal application of mupirocin calcium ointment. Ann Intern Med 1991; 114:101–106.

54. Vanherweghem JL, Dhaene M, Goldman M, et al. Infections associated with subclavian dialysis catheters: the key role of nursing training. Nephron 1986; 42:116–119.

15

Catheter-Related Infections in Pediatric Patients

André Fleer, Tannette G. Krediet, Leo J. Gerards, and John J. Roord

University Hospital for Children and Youth "Het Wilhelmina Kinderziekenhuis," Utrecht, The Netherlands

I. INTRODUCTION

Central venous catheters (CVCs) have become a major asset in the treatment of infants and children with various forms of malignancy, nutritional disorders, and chronic debilitating diseases. Infection remains one of the most frequent and troublesome complications of CVCs in all categories of pediatric patients. In a large survey of nosocomial infections (NIs) with 4684 pediatric patients, it was found that the highest NI rate occurred in the neonatal intensive care unit (NICU) (14%), followed by neurosurgery (12%), hematology/oncology (12%), and neonatal surgery (9%) and the pediatric ICU (6%) (1). Both this last study and the National Nosocomial Infections Surveillance (NNIS) study in the U.S. (2–4) revealed that NIs in pediatric patients, particularly in the ICU and among neonatal and hematology/oncology patients, are primarily bloodstream infections which are intravascular device-related.

For this reason this chapter will be mainly confined to the epidemiology, host factors, and issues of management of CVC-related infections (CRI) in the most prominent categories of pediatric patients in which these infections occur—namely, intensive care patients, particularly premature newborns and neutropenic children—and to their predominant pathogen: coagulase-negative staphylococci (CoNS). A considerable experience has been gathered over the past 15 years with respect to CVC-related infections in infancy and childhood. The data published until 1988 were superbly reviewed by Decker and Edwards (5). Hence, 1988 will be used as starting point for the present review although some of the conclusions drawn by Decker and Edwards will inevitably be rehearsed here. Thus, the published data from 1988 onward together with some of our own observations will form the basis of the present review.

Since bacterial factors and pathogenetic mechanisms involved in these infections are dealt with in the various other chapters of this book, they will only be discussed here as far as they are relevant and specific for the pediatric situation.

II. DEFINITION AND DIAGNOSIS

Any review dealing with CRI is confronted not only with variations in patient populations and the way in which these infections are defined, but also with a variety of central venous access techniques used in the many studies that have appeared since the introduction of this approach in the 1970s. Moreover, the various types of CRI that are usually distinguished—i.e., exit site, tunnel, and septic infections—do overlap in clinical presentation since they not infrequently occur together.

A successful attempt to provide sharper definitions of the various types of CRI was recently published by Raad and Bodey (6). Apart from the more easily distinguished local CRI (exit site, tunnel segment), they defined catheter-related sepsis or septicemia (CRS) as probable when a positive blood culture (one or more) is accompanied by signs of sepsis (fever, chills, hypotension) and no source for the infection is apparent other than the catheter. It should be emphasized that catheter-related bacteremia (CRB) is often used as well for this type of infection, particularly in newborns. In the present paper catheter-related sepsis, septicemia, and bacteremia will mean the same condition and will be used synonymously— abbreviated as CRS or CRB, respectively. CRS or CRB is definite when there is clinical or microbiological evidence for the catheter as a source of infection. This evidence is based on either local signs of infection at the insertion site of the catheter, on a positive culture from the catheter (for which the catheter needs to be removed), or on quantitative blood cultures from CVC and a peripheral vein implicating the catheter as a source. In the latter case the diagnosis of CRS is supported by an at least 10-fold higher bacterial count in blood drawn through the CVC than in blood from a peripheral vein (7–9). The diagnostic value of CVC/peripheral vein blood count ratios is still not universally accepted, although in one of these studies (7), CVC bacterial counts were greatly higher than those of peripheral venous blood (ratios of up to 10^3 to 10^4 were found). In either case the organisms isolated from pus from the exit site, the catheter surface, or catheter blood sample should be identical to the peripheral blood isolate to substantiate the diagnosis of CRS.

A promising method to diagnose CRS is direct staining of blood collected through the catheter by acridine orange (10). This acridine orange leukocyte cytospin (AOLC) test requires only small amounts of blood and is therefore potentially useful in infants and small children. In infants and children suspected of CRS, the test proved to be both specific (94%) and reasonably sensitive (87%).

III. CATHETER-RELATED INFECTION IN THE NEONATAL ICU

A. Epidemiology

Nosocomial infection is an important cause of morbidity in neonatal intensive care units (NICUs) and is primarily device-related. The predominant manifestation in this setting is CVC-related bacteremia whose incidence varies from 5% to 25% (4,11–14) or 5 to 20 infections/1000 catheter-days. These variations can probably be explained by differences in definition and such variables as level and mode of care, length of stay, and degree of prematurity of hospitalized infants (4,11,12). Comparison of NICUs in the U.S. clearly demonstrated the influence of prematurity on CRB rates; infants of <1500 g birth weight were three times more likely to acquire a CVC-related bacteremia than infants of >1500 g (median infection rates of 14.6 and 5.1 bacteremias per 1000 catheter-days, respectively) (4). The possible influence of the mode of care was exemplified in our own study in which we observed a very sizable increase (4.5-fold) in the courses of intravenous therapy in 1977 and 1981, respectively (15). In 1981, total parenteral nutrition (TPN) was administered to 98.7% of infants hospitalized in our NICU for an average duration of 14.6 days. All infants had a CVC in place, either through an umbilical vein or inserted through a peripheral vein and passed into the right atrium. Clearly, increased instrumentation, particularly IV access through CVCs, may be in part responsible for the emergence of certain nosocomial pathogens, notably CoNS during the past decade.

Other factors, such as crowding, may also greatly influence the incidence rate of nosocomial infection in the NICU, as was demonstrated in the classic study of Goldmann et al. (12), in which a fivefold decrease in nosocomial infection rate was found after the NICU was moved to a new, more spacious facility.

The proportion of nosocomial infections that are CVC-related is evidently dependent on the extent to which CVCs are used in a particular NICU. As mentioned above, this rate is very high in the present-day intensive care nursery. As a result, CVC-related bacteremia features as one of the most important nosocomial infections in modern NICUs, with rates of up to 10% to 15%. This was exemplified in a nationwide survey conducted in the Netherlands on complications of parenteral nutrition in neonates involving seven NICUs, in which it was found that CRB was the most frequent complication, occurring in 11.7% of infants (16).

The results of the NNIS study which included NICUs (4) clearly showed that the use of devices characterized the NICU in terms of invasive practices as well as the average severity of illness of the infants. In addition, the NNIS study convincingly demonstrated that the utilization of devices was an important risk factor for the occurrence of nosocomial infections. Thus, the incidence of nosocomial bacteremia was found to be related mainly to the use of central or umbilical catheters.

However, it should be emphasized that other modes of care of hospitalized premature newborns may independently influence nosocomial infection rates. For example, lipid parenteral nutrition of the smallest infants, often necessitated by their poor condition, not only may promote CRI by specific agents such as the yeast *Malassezia furfur* (17,18) but also appears to be an independent risk factor for CoNS bacteremia (19,20) and candidemia (21,22).

In summary, it is evident from the large number of studies during the past 15 years that CVC-related bacteremia is an important nosocomial infection in premature infants hospitalized in the NICU and the CoNS dominate as causative agents (4,12,14,15,20,23–25). Other agents with varying incidence rates in this setting are *Staphylococcus aureus*, gram-negative bacilli, and *Candida* species, often depending on specific modalities of care, such as TPN.

B.   Causative Organisms

1.   Coagulase-Negative Staphylococci

CoNS have "invaded" and perhaps even surprised the medical world during the last decades as versatile pathogens in patients fitted with intravascular or prosthetic devices. A number of reviews has highlighted virtually all aspects of CoNS (26–31), among these two excellent reviews dealing with their exceptional significance as the foremost agents of CRI in the premature neonate (30,31).

In the beginning of the 1980s a number of NICUs noted an increase in bloodstream infections due to CoNS (15,20,23,26). It soon became evident that this phenomenon could no longer be discarded as contamination of blood culture bottles due to improper aseptic techniques. These latter studies clearly documented that CoNS bacteremia in the premature neonate is a separate disease entity which is almost exclusively intravascular device-related. In fact, CRB in prematures has become almost synonymous with CoNS bacteremia. Therefore, the following paragraphs, which discuss the epidemiology, risk factors, clinical findings, diagnosis, and management of CoNS bacteremia in the premature neonate, will deal with intravascular device-related infections due to these bacteria.

a.   Clinical Picture and Diagnosis

The clinical picture as well as the clinical setting in which these CoNS bacteremias occurred were identified and described in some detail in a number of studies (15,20,23–25). All studies mentioned the relatively indolent clinical presentation of CoNS bacteremia. A summary of clinical manifestations and labora-

Table 1 Signs and Symptoms and Laboratory Abnormalities in Infants With Coagulase-Negative Staphylococcal Bacteremia

Signs and symptoms
Recurrent bradycardia
Recurrent apneic attacks
Pallor and/or cyanosis
Fever or temperature instability
Increased oxygen requirement
Lethargy
Feeding intolerance
Laboratory abnormalities
Leukocytosis
Increased immature:total neutrophil ratio
Decreased platelet count
C-reactive protein increased

tory values most frequently found to be abnormal is presented in Table 1. It has to be realized that most of these signs and symptoms are rather unspecific.

These infections tend to occur during the second or third week of hospitalization, primarily in low-birth-weight, severely ill, premature infants with a CVC in situ (umbilical or inserted through a peripheral vein), being often on TPN and treated with broad-spectrum antibiotics. It should be mentioned that the data in all these studies were examined retrospectively, so conclusions are inevitably biased.

For this reason a more detailed analysis of clinical risk factors and manifestations was attempted in a few prospective studies. The essential findings of a prospective clinical study by Schmidt et al. (32) were that infants with CoNS bacteremia had temperature elevation, an increased oxygen requirement, lethargy, and feeding intolerance significantly more often than noninfected matched controls. The most frequently found laboratory abnormalities were an increased leukocyte count, particularly an increased Immature:Total Neutrophil (I:T) ratio, a decreased platelet count, and an elevated C-reactive protein (CRP). In addition, Schmidt et al. identified an elevated CRP as the best discriminating laboratory variable.

However, in a prospective study of the value of I:T ratio and CRP as diagnostic tools in early-onset and late-onset neonatal sepsis, including CoNS bacteremia, we could not confirm these results. We found the positive predictive value of both I:T ratio and CRP to be too low to be of any diagnostic value in both early-onset (41% and 36%, respectively) and late-onset neonatal sepsis (68% and

63%, respectively) (33). The negative predictive value of these parameters was found to be higher (90% to 98%), so their performance in excluding infection in the neonate appears to be better.

b.   Clinical and Host Risk Factors

A number of clinical risk factors for CoNS bacteremia in neonates have been identified and are summarized in Table 2. Obviously, one of the most important risk factors is an intravascular catheter, but very low birth weight, prematurity, endotracheal intubation, and TPN are also of significant importance (15,19,20,24,30,31). In an extensive case control study in two NICUs in the U.S., Freeman et al. (19) found that a CVC and TPN with lipid emulsions were the only risk factors out of 20 investigated to be causally related to CoNS bacteremia. Munson et al. (20) also noted a significant correlation among CoNS bacteremia, CVCs, and TPN.

In our study we identified a causal relationship between the occurrence of CoNS bacteremia and the previous administration of TPN fluids contaminated with CoNS (15). The incidence of CoNS bacteremia in infants who had received contaminated TPN fluids was 10 times higher than in those who had received sterile solutions. The disconcertingly high degree of contamination of TPN fluids by CoNS forced us to take strict hygienic precautions during preparation of these fluids. Laminar flow cabinet preparation of TPN fluids essentially eliminated contamination and led to a reduction in the incidence of CoNS bacteremia in our NICU from 12% to 4% in 1 year (34). Contamination of lipid TPN emulsions was also found to be the cause of *Klebsiella* and *Enterobacter* bacteremia in the NICU, with lethal consequences in two of five infants (35). Together, these data emphasize the need for rigorous control of sterility of TPN fluids, particularly for premature newborns.

An association between CoNS bacteremia and prematurity was noted in most studies. Munson et al. (20) found that 93% of cases occurred in infants of < 29

Table 2   Characteristic Features and Clinical Risk Factors of Coagulase-Negative Staphylococcal Bacteremia in Neonates

Onset ≥ 48 h after admission to neonatal intensive care unit
Occurrence primarily in premature infants of very low birth weight
Association with:
    Central venous catheters
    Total parenteral nutrition with lipid emulsions
    Contaminated parenteral fluids
    Antibiotic therapy

weeks' gestation. We observed that the attack rate of CoNS bacteremia in prematures was more than twice higher in those <28 weeks' gestation than in those >28 weeks (incidence rates of 20% and 9%, respectively) (15).

Finally, the site of insertion may also be a risk factor. We found by comparing CoNS bacteremia attack rates for umbilical CVCs and peripherally inserted CVCs that the incidence of bacteremia was significantly higher for peripheral CVCs (13.7 versus 7.4/1,000 CVC days, $P < 0.05$) (36). Conversely, a lower risk of infection for peripherally inserted CVCs (3.6% vs. 6.8%) was found in a French study (37). However, these authors did not mention the days in situ of peripherally and centrally inserted CVCs.

As cited above, there is a propensity for CoNS bacteremia to occur in the most premature infants. This is probably explained by the decline in host defenses, particularly opsonic defense, to CoNS with increasing prematurity (38,39). Opsonic defense to CoNS in premature infants proved to be exclusively dependent on complement activation (38), which is deficient itself in the premature infant (38,40–42). Moreover, CoNS strains from neonatal bacteremia may vary in their opsonic requirements (34,43,44). Particularly, some strongly hydrophobic CoNS strains proved to be almost opsonization-resistant in neonatal serum (34,45). Based on these findings it is not surprising that some of these CoNS strains cannot be cleared by premature newborns from their bloodstream. In addition, we found transplacental IgG to be opsonically deficient for CoNS, which adds to the neonate's host defense defects against these bacteria.

Together, these data may explain the premature newborn's exquisite susceptibility to infection with this otherwise harmless commensal microorganism.

c. Bacterial Factors and Epidemiological Characteristics

Apart from the bacterial properties discussed briefly in the previous paragraph, a number of other features of CoNS make this species particularly well equipped for causing infection in patients with CVCs and other prosthetic devices. These properties have been discussed in detail in the preceding chapters on pathogenesis and will not been reiterated here, as the pathogenic factors contributing to CoNS catheter-related infection are the same for adults and infants. However, the finding that slime production may characterize invasive CoNS isolates and may even be a risk factor for CoNS bacteremia in infants colonized with such strains (46,47) was not found in our study (48).

With the emergence of CoNS as important pathogens in certain hosts, typing becomes particularly important. An evaluation of CoNS typing methods was presented in an excellent and extensive review on the clinical significance of CoNS by Pfaller and Herwaldt (28), recently updated by Kloos and Bannerman (49). Phenotyping of CoNS strains from neonatal bacteremia by biochemical profile-based methods like API Staph-Ident has revealed that the majority of isolates belong to *S. epidermidis* (75% or more), the remainder to *S. haemolyticus, S.*

hominis, and *S. warneri* (15,46,47). However, a clear disadvantage of phenotype-based methods is their lack of discriminatory power in epidemiological studies (28,49).

For the latter purpose, molecular typing methods seem to be much better suited and have in the meantime proven to be an invaluable tool for epidemiological typing of CoNS isolates. For example, Bingen et al. (50) demonstrated that the random amplification of polymorphic DNA (RAPD) method provided a rapid differentiation of CoNS bacteremia isolates from a pediatric hospital. In addition, by using pulsed-field gel electrophoresis of chromosomal DNA from CoNS bloodstream isolates collected over 10 years in a neonatal unit, Huebner et al. (51) showed that certain CoNS strains can become endemic over long periods of time and can repeatedly cause bloodstream infections in neonates and even colonize personnel of the unit.

It is evident that nucleic acid-based methods have quickly become the gold standard of epidemiological typing of CoNS isolates, as is true for other pathogens.

d.   Management

CoNS are well known for their propensity to develop antibiotic resistance (28,49). This was experienced in an aminoglycoside resistance surveillance study conducted in our NICU (52). Within 1 year amikacin resistance from CoNS blood isolates increased from 6% to more than 40%. For fecal and respiratory CoNS isolates the pattern was similar, with resistance increasing from around 40% to more than 70%. For this reason it can be expected that CoNS from the NICU environment, in which antibiotics are extensively used, carry a high degree of antibiotic resistance. Indeed, most NICUs report widespread resistance of CoNS isolates to penicillin, methicillin, oxacillin, the cephalosporins, and gentamicin (30,31). However, isolates are still universally susceptible to vancomycin, and this is why this antibiotic is often recommended as the drug of choice for treating CoNS infections in the NICU.

Fortunately, vancomycin resistance among CoNS is still rare and appears to be confined to some strains of *S. haemolyticus* (28,49). It should be mentioned, however, that Herwaldt et al. (53) succeeded in generating vancomycin-resistant strains of both *S. haemolyticus* and *S. epidermidis* by serial passage in broth as well as on agar plates containing vancomycin. Decreased susceptibility to the other registered glycopeptide compound, teicoplanin, is more widespread than to vancomycin among CoNS isolates, notably *S. epidermidis* and *S. haemolyticus* (49).

Although catheter removal is often advocated, this is not necessary in our experience, since most infections quickly respond to appropriate antibiotic therapy without removal of the catheter. If infection persists despite adequate antibiotic treatment, the existence of focal infection, particularly endocarditis, should be considered (54). This is a potentially dangerous condition associated with an umbilical venous catheter placed in the right atrium. It is probably the only type of CoNS bacteremia in the newborn necessitating prompt removal of the catheter and antibiotic therapy.

Treatment with fresh plasma (fresh frozen plasma, FFP) is often recommended in cases of sepsis, among other things to increase opsonic activity. However, although we indeed found that FFP administration to neonates with CoNS bacteremia increased their opsonic activity in most cases, the effect was unpredictable (45). Thus, this mode of treatment in CoNS bacteremia in neonates cannot be recommended at present.

e. Prevention

Although the clinical picture of CVC-related CoNS bacteremia in neonates is relatively mild and the attributable mortality very low, probably less than 1% (30,31,55), the morbidity is extensive. Freeman et al. (55) found in a cohort study with matched controls that infants with CoNS bacteremia remained hospitalized an average of 19.8 days longer than matched controls without bacteremia. A similar analysis in our NICU revealed that CoNS bacteremia prolonged hospitalization for an average of 13.6 days. For this reason, prevention appears to be a worthwhile endeavor, particularly in view of the added hospital cost and possible discontinuation of essential treatment modes—e.g., TPN. Another incentive for prophylaxis is the possible eradication of CoNS strains prone to cause bacteremia (51).

The results of two prospective randomized trials of vancomycin prophylaxis in premature neonates have been recently reported and critically commented (56–58). Although the trials were successful in preventing CoNS bacteremia in this patient group, both in the reports and in the editorial comment, concern was expressed that widespread implementation of this kind of prophylaxis might induce development of vancomycin resistance among CoNS. However, vancomycin resistance among CoNS was detected in neither of the two studies. Despite this lack of resistance development, we concur with the recommendation that this approach should not be followed on a large scale until better data on the emergence of vancomycin-resistant CoNS are available.

Another approach to prevent CoNS bacteremia in the premature newborn is to boost antibacterial defenses. Considering the deficient host defenses against CoNS found in this population, particularly the low level of antibacterial IgG, which may, in addition, be opsonically deficient (38), prophylaxis with intravenous immunoglobulin (IVIG) is an apparently logical approach.

Hill summarized in a recent review (59) the data of 10 studies of IVIG prophylaxis in the neonatal ICU. He concluded that "prophylactic administration of IVIG to human neonates may never be shown to alter the overall instance of nosocomial infections, especially if catheter- and procedure-related infections are included." He added that this lack of efficacy of IVIG is probably explained by the fact that antibody alone may not play a major role against infections associated with indwelling devices. This notion is, however, not supported by experimental findings we obtained in a study of the opsonic requirements of surface-adherent CoNS that showed that IgG sufficed as an opsonin for efficient uptake by neutrophils (43). On the other hand, animal studies on the pathogenesis of device-related infection generally indicate that the host defense systems, particularly neutrophils are not very effective in clearing such infections once the organisms have settled themselves on the surface of the device, a situation likely to be the case in CVC-related infection. Slime production by CoNS interferes with neutrophil chemotaxis and phagocytosis (60), while in the vicinity of a foreign device neutrophils also manifest dysfunctions in bacterial killing and superoxide production (61).

2. Staphylococcus aureus

According to two large recent surveys *S. aureus* ranks second or third among nosocomial pathogens in pediatrics (1,62). CVC-related *S. aureus* bloodstream infections in the NICU present themselves in our experience in the same setting and in much the same way as CoNS infections. Management is similar to CoNS infections; i.e., antibiotic therapy without removal of the catheter is in our experience generally effective.

This is clearly different from the situation in adults, in which catheter removal appears to be warranted to prevent relapse and sepsis-related death (6). However, in the (premature) neonate it may also be prudent to remove the catheter, particularly in case of a CRI due to MRSA, as will be pointed out below.

The regimen of antimicrobial therapy, i.e., whether or not vancomycin should be the agent of choice, depends on the local susceptibility values. In our own NICU *S. aureus* is still oxacillin-sensitive, although MRSA may prevail in other units. Epidemics with MRSA in NICUs have occurred in various countries, if only sporadically (63–70). On the other hand, a nationwide survey of the prevalence of MRSA in children's hospitals in the U.S. revealed that the presence of a pediatric ICU or NICU was not a risk factor for MRSA (71). Apparently, in pediatric hospitals in the U.S. MRSA occurs just as likely in the ICU as in other departments. However, one should be aware that MRSA infection in the neonate may disseminate, particularly to the bone (72). The latter report also found that an intravascular device was the most frequent portal of entry of disseminated MRSA infection. Prompt treatment with vancomycin resulted in a good short-term response (95% cure rate) with minimal toxicity and no significant loss of function of the affected limb.

Together these data point out that it may be prudent to remove the catheter in all neonates with a CRI due to *S. aureus*, particularly when caused by MRSA, because of the potential danger of dissemination.

3. Gram-Negative Bacteria

CVC-related infections due to aerobic gram-negative bacteria (GNB) in the neonatal ICU have been reported in association with contaminated TPN infusion fluids (35). Contamination with *Klebsiella* and *Enterobacter* was traced to repeated entry of lipid emulsion bottles which had been extrinsically contaminated by hands of personnel. There was substantial morbidity and mortality: five of 20 infants developed a life-threatening illness, and two of these five died. This report underscores the need for rigorous hygienic measures when administering TPN to small infants, particularly hand hygiene during preparation of TPN fluids.

Apart from sporadic reports there is little information on the course and management of CVC-related GNB bacteremia in neonates and infants. There are no controlled studies about the optimal mode of therapy—for example, the need for catheter removal. In view of findings in older children and adults (6), however, it seems advisable to do so.

4. Yeasts

a. *Malassezia furfur*

CVC-related infection due to the lipophilic yeast *Malassezia furfur* has been observed in neonates and older infants receiving IV lipid emulsions (17,18,73). Most patients develop a mild to moderate infection with apneic and bradycardic attacks, low-grade fever, and respiratory symptoms. Patients promptly recover upon removal of the catheter. Antifungal therapy without removal of the catheter appears to be more problematic (73). Therefore, prompt removal of the catheter is recommended as the treatment of choice for CVC-related *Malassezia furfur* fungemia in infants.

b. *Candida* species

Candidemia is a much feared infection in the neonate, because of the mortality rate of up to 50% reported in earlier studies (74,75). However, the prognosis of CVC-related candidemia may be less terrifying. Two recent studies, both reporting on long-term experience, found mortality rates of CVC-related infection directly attributable to *Candida* of 20% and 12%, respectively (21,22). In the study with the highest mortality (five of 20 infants died), however, two of the infants died before initiation of treatment. Thus, in the treated infants therapy failed in three of 18, and in two of the three failures the clinical course was complicated by concomitant bacterial sepsis. Therefore, it appears that with prompt and adequate treatment the mortality rate of CVC-related candidemia is probably around 10%. The reason for this significantly better prognosis when compared to previous reports of neonatal candidemia (74,75) is probably an earlier awareness of candidemia in neonates with a CVC, less reluctance to discard *Candida* as a contaminant, and as a result prompt and aggressive antifungal therapy. In these earlier reports it was noted that rapid initiation of treatment with amphotericin B and 5-flucytosine resulted in a much better outcome than when there was a delay in diagnosis and initiation of therapy.

In fact, these earlier studies reported that as much as 20% to 30% of cases of neonatal systemic candidiasis may go undiagnosed during life and are only documented at autopsy. Both recent studies (21,22) clearly demonstrated that prolonged antibiotic therapy, hyperalimentation with lipid emulsions, and endotracheal intubation are major risk factors for CVC-related candidemia. Treatment with amphotericin B and 5-flucytosine with concurrent removal of the catheter is efficacious in most cases. In both reports it is emphasized that removal of the catheter is absolutely required to ensure effective management of neonatal CVC-related candidemia.

The value of the new antimycotic agents fluconazol and itraconazol in the treatment of neonatal candidiasis has still to be determined. Particularly, fluconazol seems promising because of its attractive pharmacokinetic properties in the neonate (76) and its proven efficacy in *Candida* infections in older children.

IV.   PEDIATRIC ICU

A number of large studies of nosocomial infection in pediatric ICU has revealed that, similar to the situation in the NICU, nosocomial infections are primarily device-related bacteremias (1,4,62). Gram-positive cocci are the major pathogens of these bacteremias, with CoNS predominating (1,62). According to one study (62), CRIs in the pediatric ICU peak after the fourth week of hospitalization. Arterial and central venous lines in place for more than 4 weeks had a cumulative chance of acquiring infection of 100% and 80%, respectively. Management of CRI in the pediatric ICU is identical to the approach outlined above for the neonatal ICU.

V.   CATHETER-RELATED INFECTIONS IN NEUTROPENIC CHILDREN

A.   Epidemiology and Risk Factors

Infection is one of the major complications of the use of long-term right atrial catheters of Hickman-Broviac type in patients with cancer (77–85). The incidence varies widely, from 0.68 to 6.8 episodes per 1000 catheter-days (Table 3). Catheter-related bacteremia, the most serious infectious complication of CVCs, occurs with a frequency of 0.52 to 6.8/1000 catheter-days (Table 3). As with CRI in neonates, the wide variation in incidence rates is probably explained by differences in patient populations and in definition of CRI.

Risk factors for the occurrence of CRI in pediatric oncology patients have been assessed in a number of studies, particularly the role of variables such as

Table 3   Incidence of Central Venous Catheter-Related Infections in Neutropenic Children[a]

	Incidence (rate/1000 catheter-days)	
Study	Local infection	Bacteremia
Darbyshire et al. (77)	N.S.[b]	6.8
Johnson et al. (78)	2.8	1.4
Hartman and Shochat (80)	2.5	2.1
Viscoli et al. (81)	0.16	0.52
van Hoff et al. (82)	0.54	2.3
Rizzari et al. (83)	0.15	4.4
Uderzo et al. (84)	2.5	0.58
Rikkonen et al. (85)	0.22	0.75

[a]Data compiled from eight studies, 1985–1993.
[b]N.S. = not stated.

neutropenia, chemotherapy, and age. Hartman and Shochat (80) found that neutropenia was associated with 70% of CRI but also that 75% of all other infections occurred during neutropenia. Thus, in this study neutropenia per se did not appear to increase the risk of CRI. However, insertion of a CVC during a neutropenic episode was associated with a more than twofold increased risk of bacteremia. In contrast, a large EORTC survey by Viscoli et al. (81) revealed that neutropenia did not impose an increased risk for CRI. This finding was confirmed in at least two other studies (86,87).

Contrary to these latter findings Hiemenz et al. (79) reported that from their experience with CVCs at the National Cancer Institute in Bethesda, MD, neutropenic patients had a fourfold increased risk of developing bacteremia if they had a CVC in place. Rizzari et al. also noted an increased risk of CRI during neutropenia (83).

Thus, the question whether neutropenia poses a risk factor for CRI in oncology patients appears to be unresolved. The only valid conclusion seems to be that placement of a catheter increases the risk of infection in both neutropenic and nonneutropenic oncological patients.

With respect to patient age in relation to the risk of CVC infection, Johnson et al. (78) clearly found an increased risk for young children. Toddlers (1 through 4 years of age) had a rate of 3.9 infections per 1000 catheter-days compared to rates of 2.7/1000 catheter-days for school children and 0.5/1000 catheter-days for adolescents. Similar observations were made by Mulloy et al. (88), who found that children <2 years of age were 2.6 times more likely to experience sepsis than older children.

The type of device also influences the rate of infection. A recent study from the Memorial Sloan-Kettering Cancer Center (89) reported that the rate of CRI in 1431 cancer patients was 10-fold lower in those with implanted ports (0.21/1000 catheter-days) than in those with Hickman-type silastic tunneled CVCs (2.77/1000 days). Similar findings were obtained by Rikkonen et al. (85), who observed that Hickman-Broviac type catheters carried a higher risk for bacteremia (0.75/1000 catheter-days) than implanted ports (0.14/1000 days). Moreover, these authors noted that CVCs in place for >300 days tended to be safer in this regard than those of shorter duration, although the difference was not statistically significant. It should be noted that patients with long infection-free intervals had leukocyte counts >1000 at the time of insertion of the CVC; thus, it is likely that their better host defenses contributed to the prevention of CRI, although the role of neutrophils is still uncertain (61). A possible explaration for this phenomenon is offered by the experimental studies by Sherertz et al. (90,91). These studies demonstrated both in a mouse and a rabbit model of subcutaneous catheter infection that catheters residing in the animal for 2 to 4 days before inoculation with microorganisms had up to a 40% lower infection rate than catheters challenged immediately after insertion. Presumably, if one allows an inflammatory reaction to be formed around the catheter, the likelihood of a subsequent CVC infection is less.

B.   Causative Organisms

In most studies gram-positive organisms constitute the majority of bloodstream isolates of CVC-related bacteremias, accounting for up to 78% of isolates (Table 4). In the previously cited studies (77–85) CoNS rank first among the gram-positive agents, comprising 13% to 51% of all agents, but 30% to almost 80% of gram-positive isolates (Table 4). Other causative agents include *Staphylococcus aureus*; viridans streptococci; enterococci; a variety of gram-negative bacilli, with *E. coli*, *Klebsiella/Enterobacter* and *Pseudomonas aeruginosa* as predominant isolates; and fungi and yeasts, primarily *Candida* species. More rare pathogens include *Bacillus* species (92) and *Mycobacterium chelonae/fortuitum* (93). Apart from the fact that these infections occurred in immunocompromised patients (mostly children treated for leukemia and lymphoma) and the obvious presence of a Hickman catheter, there were no predisposing factors to distinguish these cases.

C.   Clinical Findings and Diagnosis

Fever is a common event in neutropenic patients, often alerting the physician to an impending infection in a vulnerable patient. In the absence of signs of any

Table 4 Causative Agents of Central Venous Catheter-Related Infection in Neutropenic Children: Predominance of Gram-Positive Organisms[a]

Study	Gram-positive (%)	CoNS (%)
Darbyshire et al. (77)	67	51
Johnson et al. (78)	46	13.5
Hartman and Shochat (80)	46	19
Viscoli et al. (81)	78	30
van Hoff et al. (82)	59	30
Rizzari et al. (83)	56	43
Uderzo et al. (84)	75	50
Rikkonen et al. (85)	55	25

[a]Data compiled from eight studies, 1985–1993.

other site of infection, notably lungs, urinary tract, or gastrointestinal tract, an indwelling CVC is often suspected to be the source of infection, especially if the exit site and/or the tunnel tract of the CVC are inflamed. To substantiate the diagnosis of CVC-related infection one should obtain blood for culture from both the CVC and a peripheral vein simultaneously, in accordance with the diagnostic guidelines formulated in the beginning of this chapter (see section on Definition and Diagnosis). For rapid diagnosis, the AOLC test (10), also mentioned in the latter section, should be considered.

D. Management

Although removal of a foreign device is still the most effective way of treating a device-related infection, this is no longer considered to be necessary in the management of CVC-related infections in children, particularly in case of infection with CoNS. Numerous studies have clearly demonstrated that antibiotic treatment without removal of the catheter is highly successful in CVC-related bacteremia with eradication rates of more than 90% (Table 5). Treatment is usually started empirically with parenteral antibiotics and continued for 10 to 14 days, depending primarily on the patient's response. Apart from clinical signs, laboratory parameters such as C-reactive protein may be useful in determining the duration of therapy. Continuation of treatment beyond 2 weeks may be indicated if there is a slow but definite response (85). It should be remembered that CVCs are often a real "lifeline" in these patients, and sacrificing a CVC may be a much less attractive option than extending the antibiotic treatment course. The optimal choice of

Table 5   Central Venous Catheter-Related Infection in Neutropenic Children:
Response to Antibiotic Therapy Without Catheter Removal[a]

Study	Cure (%)	
	Local infection	Bacteremia
Darbyshire et al. (77)	N.S.[b]	38 (mult. isolates)
		88 (single isolates)
		72 (total)
Johnson et al. (78)	71	83
Hartman and Shochat (80)	N.S.[b]	93
Viscoli et al. (81)	0 (tunnel)	71
van Hoff et al. (82)	14	68
Rizzari et al. (83)	0 (tunnel)	90
Uderzo et al. (84)	72[c]	
Rikkonen et al. (85)	N.S.[b]	78

[a]Data compiled from eight studies, 1985–1993.
[b]N.S. = not stated.
[c]Response not specified separately for local and bacteremic infection.

empirical antibiotic therapy should be guided by the predominant isolates in a particular setting. As pointed out in the previous paragraph, these are usually CoNS, many of which are oxacillin- (methicillin-) resistant. Therefore, vancomycin is considered to be the antibiotic of choice for empiric treatment of CVC-related infections in neutropenic children. This choice is further supported by the excellent results that have been obtained with this drug in the treatment of CVC-related bacteremias.

When gram-negative bacilli are suspected, treatment should include an antipseudomonal beta-lactam agent such as ceftazidime or piperacillin. However, current data indicate that gram-negative CVC-related bacteremias, especially when due to *Pseudomonas*, are less successfully treated with antibiotics alone—i.e., without removal of the catheter (94). Similar considerations apply to CVC-related bacteremia due to more unusual pathogens, notably *Bacillus* species (92), *Mycobacterium chelonae* and *M. fortuitum* (93), and CVC-related candidemia (95,96). In these cases, catheter removal appears necessary to successfully treat CVC-related bloodstream infections. Also, with *S. aureus* as the pathogen, one should perhaps be more cautious about leaving the CVC in place (6).

Finally, catheter removal also seems the only effective treatment in 70% to 75% of tunnel infections, whereas exit site infections rarely necessitate catheter removal and can be treated by antibiotics alone in up to 80% of cases (78,94), with the exception of exit site and tunnel infections due to *M. chelonae* and *M. fortuitum*, which require surgical excision of the exit site or tunnel tract and surrounding tissues in addition to removal of the catheter (93).

E.   Prevention

CVC-related infections lead to extended hospital stay and increase hospital costs (55,97). Therefore, prevention is important for both medical and economical reasons. Because prophylaxis of CVC-related infections is discussed in more detail in Chapter 16, we will present only a brief account as far as it is relevant to the pediatric situation.

Prevention of CVC-related infection can be accomplished at three stages during the whole procedure of CVC placement and use. Obviously, the first point to be considered is the use of infection-resistant materials. There are some interesting developments in this field reviewed by Jansen (98).

Second, apart from the type of material of the device, the way in which the device is inserted may influence infection rates. As mentioned in the previous paragraph, totally implanted devices—i.e. without skin exit site, such as Port-a-caths—may have lower infection rates than Hickman-Broviac type CVCs (85, 89). Overall, tunneled catheters are less prone to catheter infection than nontunneled CVCs.

Third, prevention may be accomplished by the administration of antibiotics during CVC placement, e.g., by long-term administration of vancomycin. Although this regimen proved to be effective in preventing CVC-related CoNS bacteremia in newborns (56,57), the most obvious imminent danger is acquisition of resistance to vancomycin by gram-positive cocci, which would be a disastrous development. Thus, antibiotic prophylaxis during catheter insertion cannot be recommended at present.

A related approach is to flush the catheter with an antibiotic solution or to leave an antibiotic solution inside the catheter between uses. The first procedure was proven to be effective in preventing CVC-related bacteremia in oncological children (99). The second approach was used primarily to treat CVC-related sepsis without bacteremia, defined as positive cultures of blood drawn through the catheter but negative cultures of blood from a peripheral vein. Two studies (100,101) reported that this so-called antibiotic-lock technique (ALT) was effective in treating this type of CVC-related sepsis. We decided to use this approach as a preventive measure rather than for treatment and found ALT to be effective as a prophylactic regimen in patients on long-term TPN who had repeated CVC-related bacteremia and colonization of the CVC by the same organism. Although obviously successful, we do not strictly advocate this approach on a regular basis in all patients with long-term venous access, for similar reasons to those mentioned above for vancomycin prophylaxis in neonates.

VI. CONCLUSIONS

Central venous catheters are an integral part of modern medicine, especially in the care of ICU and oncological patients. This is true for both children and adults, although incidence rates of catheter-related infection in infants and children tend to be higher than in adults. In pediatrics, the highest incidence of CVC-related infection is observed in hospitalized premature newborns and neutropenic children. Coagulase-negative staphylococci are the predominant pathogens in both patient groups. Considering the fact that CVCs are here to stay, the main thrust of future studies should be to minimize the rate of infection. Although vancomycin prophylaxis is effective in both neonates and neutropenic children, the general consensus is that this is not the way in which this should be accomplished. The threat of vancomycin resistance among CoNS is sufficiently frightening to preclude this solution. Prophylaxis with IVIG in the premature neonate does not seem to be effective.

There are now sufficient data to conclude that CVC-related infection due to CoNS and *Staphylococcus aureus* can be treated by antibiotics alone although in selected cases in neonates and in neutropenic children one should possibly be more cautious of this approach if *S. aureus* is the pathogen. Treatment of a CVC-related infection due to gram-negative bacteria, *Bacillus* species, *M. fortuitum*, *M. chelonae*, *Candida* species, and *Malassezia furfur* requires removal of the catheter.

There is a continuous emergence of "new" pathogens associated with CVC-related infection (98,102); this is especially true for the immunocompromised host, which confronts the physician constantly with new treatment problems. These uncertainties and problems in management strongly emphasize the need for effective prevention, which becomes an issue of great importance. Besides, for other improvements in hygienic care of catheters, development of anti-infective biomaterials is of crucial significance. There are some promising developments in this field, pioneered by Jansen et al. (98) and Sherertz et al. (90,91), and these will be discussed in more detail in the next chapter.

REFERENCES

1. Ford-Jones EL, Mindorff CM, Langley JM, et al. Epidemiologic study of 4684 hospital-acquired infections in pediatric patients. Pediatr Infect Dis J 1989; 8:668–675.
2. Gaynes RP, Culver DH, Emori TG, et al. The national nosocomial infections surveillance system: plans for the 1990s and beyond. Am J Med 1991; 91(suppl 3B): 116S–120S.
3. Jarvis WR, Edwards JR, Culver DH, et al. Nosocomial infection rates in adult and pediatric intensive care units in the United States. Am J Med 1991; 91(suppl 3B): 185S–191S.

4. Gaynes RP, Martone WJ, Culver DH, et al. Comparison of rates of nosocomial infections in neonatal intensive care units in the United States. Am J Med 1991; 91(suppl 3B):192S–196S.

5. Decker MD, Edwards KM. Central venous catheter infections. Pediatr Clin North Am 1988; 35:579–612.

6. Raad II, Bodey GP. Infectious complications of indwelling vascular catheters. Clin Infect Dis 1992; 15:197–210.

7. Flynn PM, Shenep JI, Stokes DC, et al. In situ management of confirmed central venous catheter-related bacteremia. Pediatr Infect Dis J 1987; 6:729–734.

8. Flynn PM, Shenep JI, Barret FF. Differential quantitation with a commercial blood culture tube for diagnosis of catheter-related infection. J Clin Microbiol 1988; 26: 1045–1046.

9. Raucher HS, Hyatt AC, Barzilai A, et al. Quantitative blood cultures in the evaluation of septicemia in children with Broviac catheters. J Pediatr 1984; 104:29–33.

10. Rushforth JA, Hoy CM, Kite P, Puntis JWL. Rapid diagnosis of central venous catheter sepsis. Lancet 1993; 342:402–403.

11. Hemming VG, Overall JC, Britt MR. Nosocomial infections in a newborn intensive-care unit. Results of forty-one months of surveillance. N Engl J Med 1976; 294: 1310–1316.

12. Goldmann DA, Durbin WA Jr, Freeman J. Nosocomial infections in a neonatal intensive care unit. J Infect Dis 1981; 144:449–459.

13. Goldmann DA, Freeman J, Durbin WA Jr. Nosocomial infection and death in a neonatal intensive care unit. J Infect Dis 1983; 147:653–641.

14. Donowitz LG. Nosocomial infection in neonatal intensive care units. Am J Infect Control 1989; 17:250–257.

15. Fleer A, Senders RC, Visser MR, et al. Septicemia due to coagulase-negative staphylococci in a neonatal intensive care unit: clinical and bacteriological features and contaminated parenteral fluids as a source of sepsis. Pediatr Infect Dis 1983; 2:426–431.

16. Liem KD, van Lingen RA, Krediet TG. Complications of central venous catheters in neonates: a multicenter study. Abstracts of the 17th Annual Meeting of the Dutch Society for Pediatrics, Veldhoven, Netherlands, November 1–3, 1995. Abstract 156.

17. Powell DA, Aungst J, Snedden S, et al. Broviac catheter-related *Malassezia furfur* sepsis in five infants receiving intravenous fat emulsions. J Pediatr 1984; 105:987–990.

18. Azimi PH, Levernier K, Lefrak LM, et al. *Malassezia furfur:* a cause of occlusion of percutaneous central venous catheters in infants in the intensive care nursery. Pediatr Infect Dis J 1988; 7:100–103.

19. Freeman J, Goldmann DA, Smith NE, et al. Association of intravenous lipid emulsion and coagulase-negative staphylococcal bacteremia in neonatal intensive care units. N Engl J Med 1990; 323:301–308.

20. Munson DP, Thompson TR, Johnson DE, et al. Coagulase-negative staphylococcal septicemia: experience in a newborn intensive care unit. J Pediatr 1982; 101:602–605.

21. Weese-Mayer DE, Wheeler Fondriest D, Brouillette RT, et al. Risk factors associated with candidemia in the neonatal intensive care unit: a case control study. Pediatr Infect Dis J 1987; 6:190–196.

22. Leibovitz E, Iuster-Reicher A, Amitai M, et al. Systemic candidal infections associated with use of peripheral venous catheters in neonates: a 9-year experience. Clin Infect Dis 1992; 14:485–491.

23. Battisti O, Mitchison R, Davies P. Changing blood culture isolates in a referral neonatal intensive care unit. Arch Dis Child 1981; 56:775–778.

24. Baumgart S, Hall SE, Campos JM, et al. Sepsis with coagulase-negative staphylococci in critically ill newborns. Am J Dis Child 1983; 137:461–463.

25. La Gamma EF, Drusin LM, Mackles AW, et al. Neonatal infections. An important determinant of late NICU mortality in infants less than 1,000 g at birth. Am J Dis Child 1983; 137:838–841.

26. Lowy FD, Hammer SM. *Staphylococcus epidermidis* infections. Ann Intern Med 1983; 99:834–839.

27. Christensen GD. The confusing and tenacious coagulase-negative staphylococci. Adv Intern Med 1987; 32:177–192.

28. Pfaller MA, Herwaldt LA. Laboratory, clinical and epidemiological aspects of coagulase-negative staphylococci. Clin Microbiol Rev 1988; 1:281–299.

29. Patrick CC. Coagulase-negative staphylococci: pathogens with increasing clinical significance. J Pediatr 1990; 116:497–507.

30. Hall SL. Coagulase-negative staphylococcal infections in neonates. Pediatr Infect Dis J 1991; 10:57–67.

31. St. Geme JW, Harris MC. Coagulase-negative staphylococcal infection in the neonate. Clin Perinatol 1991; 18:281–302.

32. Schmidt BK, Kirpalani HM, Corey M, et al. Coagulase-negative staphylococci as true pathogens in newborn infants: a cohort study. Pediatr Infect Dis J 1987; 6:1026–1031.

33. Krediet T, Gerards LJ, Fleer A, et al. The predictive value of CRP and I/T ratio in neonatal infection. J Perinat Med 1992; 20:479–485.

34. Fleer A, Gerards LJ, Pascual A, et al. Coagulase-negative staphylococcal septicemia in premature neonates. Epidemiological features and the role of host defence and bacterial factors. In: Pulverer G, Quie PG, Peters G, eds. The Pathogenicity and Clinical Significance of Coagulase-Negative Staphylococci. Stuttgart: Gustav Fischer Verlag, 1987; 215–223.

35. Jarvis WR, Highsmith AK, Allen J, et al. Polymicrobial bacteremia associated with lipid emulsion in a neonatal intensive care unit. Pediatr Infect Dis 1983; 2:203–208.

36. Krediet TG, Heydendael VMR, Gerards LJ, et al. Infectious complications due to central venous catheters (CVC) in neonates. Program and Abstracts of 13th Meeting of the European Society for Paediatric Infectious Diseases, Birmingham, UK, April 19–21, 1995. Abstract 75.

37. Goutail-Flaud MF, Sfez M, Laguemie G, et al. Central venous catheter-related complications in newborns and infants: a 587-case survey. J Pediatr Surg 1991; 26:645–650.

38. Fleer A, Gerards LJ, Aerts P, et al. Opsonic defense to *Staphylococcus epidermidis* in the premature neonate. J Infect Dis 1985; 152:930–937.

39. Cates KL, Goetz C, Rosenberg N, et al. Longitudinal development of specific and functional antibody in very low birth weight premature infants. Pediatr Res 1988; 23:14–22.

40. Shaio M-F, Yang KD, Bohnsack JF, et al. Effect of immune globulin intravenous on opsonization of bacteria by classic and alternative complement pathways in premature serum. Pediatr Res 1989; 25:634–640.

41. Notarangelo LD, Chirico G, Chiara A, et al. Activity of classical and alternative pathways of complement in preterm and small for gestational age infants. Pediatr Res 1984; 18:281–285.

42. Geelen SPM, Fleer A, Bezemer AC, et al. Deficiencies in opsonic defense to pneumococci in the human newborn despite adequate levels of complement and specific IgG antibodies. Pediatr Res 1990; 27:514–518.

43. Pascual A, Fleer A, Westerdaal NAC, et al. Surface hydrophobicity and opsonic requirements of coagulase-negative staphylococci in suspension and adhering to a polymer substratum. Eur J Clin Microbiol Infect Dis 1988; 7:161–166.

44. van Bronswijk H, Verbrugh HA, Heezius CJM, et al. Heterogeneity in opsonic requirements of *Staphylococcus epidermidis:* relative importance of surface hydrophobicity, capsules and slime. Immunology 1989; 67:81–86.

45. Krediet TG, Gerards LJ, Beurskens F, Fleer A. Coagulase-negative staphylococcal (CONS) septicemia in premature neonates: effect of fresh frozen plasma on anti-CONS IgG and complement-dependent opsonisation. Program and Abstracts of the 6th International Congress for Infectious Diseases. Prague, April 26–30, 1994. Abstract 1155.

46. Hall RT, Hall SL, Barnes WG, et al. Characteristics of coagulase-negative staphylococci from infants with bacteremia. Pediatr Infect Dis J 1987; 6:377–383.

47. Hall SL, Hall RT, Barnes WG, et al. Colonization with slime-positive coagulase-negative staphylococci as a risk factor for invasive coagulase-negative staphylococci infections in neonates. J Perinatol 1988; 8:215–221.

48. Fleer A, Verhoef J. New aspects of staphylococcal infections: emergence of coagulase-negative staphylococci as pathogens. Antonie van Leeuwenhoek 1984; 50:729–744.

49. Kloos WE, Bannerman RL. Update on clinical significance of coagulase-negative staphylococci. Clin Microbiol Rev 1994; 7:117–140.

50. Bingen E, Barc M-C, Brahimi N, et al. Randomly amplified polymorphic DNA analysis provides rapid differentiation of methicillin-resistant coagulase-negative *Staphylococcus* bacteremia isolates in pediatric hospital. J Clin Microbiol 1995; 33:1657–1659.

51. Huebner J, Pier GB, Maslow JN, et al. Endemic nosocomial transmission of *Staphylococcus epidermidis* bacteremia isolates in a neonatal intensive care unit over 10 years. J Infect Dis 1994; 169:526–531.

52. Krediet TG, Fleer A, Gerards LJ. Development of resistance to aminoglycosides among coagulase-negative staphylococci and enterobacteriaceae in a neonatal intensive care unit. J Hosp Infect 1993; 24:39–46.

53. Herwald L, Boyken L, Pfaller M. In vitro selection of resistance to vancomycin in bloodstream isolates of *Staphylococcus haemolyticus* and *Staphylococcus epidermidis.* Eur J Clin Microbiol Infect Dis 1991; 10:1007–1012.

54. Noel GJ, O'Loughlin JE, Edelson PJ. Neonatal *Staphylococcus epidermidis* right-sided endocarditis: description of five catheterized infants. Pediatrics 1988; 82:234–239.

55. Freeman J, Epstein MF, Smith NE, et al. Extra hospital stay and antibiotic usage with nosocomial coagulase-negative staphylococcal bacteremia in two neonatal intensive care populations. Am J Dis Child 1990; 144:324–329.

56. Kacica MA, Horgan MJ, Ochoa L, et al. Prevention of gram-positive sepsis in neonates weighing less than 1500 grams. J Pediatr 1994; 125:253–285.

57. Spafford PS, Sinkin RA, Cox C, et al. Prevention of central venous catheter-related coagulase-negative staphylococcal sepsis in neonates. J Pediatr 1994; 125:259–263.

58. Barefield ES, Philips JB. Vancomycin prophylaxis for coagulase-negative staphylococcal bacteremia. J Pediatr 1994; 125:230–232.

59. Hill HR. Intravenous immunoglobulin use in the neonate: role in prophylaxis and therapy of infection. Pediatr Infect Dis J 1993; 12:549–559.

60. Johnson GM, Lee DA, Regelmann WE, et al. Interference with granulocyte function by *Staphylococcus epidermidis* slime. Infect Immun 1986; 54:13–20.

61. Zimmerli W, Lew PD, Waldvogel FA. Pathogenesis of foreign body infection: evidence for a local granulocyte defect. J Clin Invest 1984; 73:1191–1200.

62. Milliken J, Tait GA, Ford-Jones EL, et al. Nosocomial infections in a pediatric intensive care unit. Crit Care Med 1988; 16:233–237.

63. Graham DR, Correa-Villasenor A, Anderson RL et al. Epidemic neonatal gentamicin-methicillin-resistant *Staphylococcus aureus* infection associated with nonspecific topical use of gentamicin. J Pediatr 1980; 97:972–978.

64. Dunkle LM, Naqvi SH, MacCallum R, et al. Eradication of epidemic methicillin-gentamicin-resistant *Staphylococcus aureus* in an intensive care nursery. Am J Med 1981; 70:455–458.

65. Armington LA, Mooney BR. Early recognition and control of methicillin-resistant *Staphylococcus aureus* in a newborn ICU. Am J Infect Control 1986; 14:84.

66. Mulhern B, Griffin E. An epidemic of gentamicin/cloxacillin resistant staphylococcal infection in a neonatal unit. Irish Med J 1987; 74:228–229.

67. Price EH, Brain A, Dickson JAS. An outbreak of infection with a gentamicin and methacillin-resistant *Staphylococcus aureus* in a neonatal unit. J Hosp Infect 1980; 1:221–228.

68. Trallero EP, Arenzana JG, Castaneda AA et al. Unusual multiresistant *Staphylococcus aureus* in a newborn nursery. Am J Dis Child 1981; 135:689–692.

69. Gilbert GL, Asche V, Hewstone AS, et al. Methicillin-resistant *Staphylococcus aureus* in neonatal nurseries. Med J Aust 1982; 1:455–459.

70. Reboli AC, John JF, Levkoff AH. Epidemic methicillin-gentamicin-resistant *Staphylococcus aureus* in a neonatal intensive care unit. Am J Dis Child 1989; 143:34–39.

71. Jarvis WR, Thornsberry C, Boyce J, Hughes JM. Methicillin-resistant *Staphylococcus aureus* at children's hospitals in the United States. Pediatr Infect Dis 1985; 4:651–655.

72. Ish-Horowicz MR, McIntyre P, Nade S. Bone and joint infections caused by multiply resistant *Staphylococcus aureus* in a neonatal intensive care unit. Pediatr Infect Dis J 1992; 11:82–87.

73. Powell DA, Marcon MJ. Failure to eradicate *Malassezia furfur* Broviac catheter infection with antifungal therapy. Pediatr Infect Dis J 1987; 6:579–680.

74. Johnson DE, Thompson TR, Green TP, et al. Systemic candidiasis in very low-birthweight infants (<1,500 grams). Pediatrics 1984; 73:138–143.

75. Faix RG. Systemic *Candida* infections in infants in intensive care nurseries: high incidence of central nervous system involvement. J Pediatr 1984; 105:616–622.

76. van den Anker JN, van Popele NML, Sauer PJJ. Antifungal agents in neonatal systemic candidiasis. Antimicrob Agents Chemother 1995; 39:1391–1397.

77. Darbyshire PJ, Weightman NC, Speller DCE. Problems associated with indwelling central venous catheters. Arch Dis Child 1985; 60:129–134.

78. Johnson PR, Decker MD, Edwards KM, et al. Frequency of Broviac catheter infections in pediatric oncology patients. J Infect Dis 1986; 154:570–578.

79. Hiemenz J, Skelton J, Pizzo PA. Perspective on the management of catheter-related infections in cancer patients. Pediatr Infect Dis 1986; 5:6–11.

80. Hartman GE, Shochat SJ. Management of septic complications associated with Silastic® catheters in childhood malignancy. Pediatr Infect Dis J 1987; 6:1042–1047.

81. Viscoli C, Garaventa A, Boni L, et al. Role of Broviac catheters in infections in children with cancer. Pediatr Infect Dis J 1988; 7:556–560.

82. van Hoff J, Berg AT, Seashore JH. The effect of right atrial catheters on infectious complications of chemotherapy in children. J Clin Oncol 1990; 8:1255–1262.

83. Rizzari C, Palamone G, Corbetta A, et al. Central venous catheter-related infections in pediatric hematology-oncology patients: role of home and hospital management. Pediatr Hematol Oncol 1992; 6:115–123.

84. Uderzo C, D'Angelo P, Rizzari C, et al. Central venous catheter-related complications after bone marrow transplantation in children with hematological malignancies. Bone Marrow Transpl 1992; 9:113–117.

85. Rikkonen P, Saarinen UM, Lähteenoja K-M, et al. Management of indwelling central venous catheters in pediatric cancer patients with fever and neutropenia. Scand J Infect Dis 1993; 25:357–364.

86. Gorelick MH, Owen WC, Seibel NL, et al. Lack of association between neutropenia and the incidence of bacteremia associated with indwelling central venous catheters in febrile pediatric cancer patients. Pediatr Infect Dis J 1991; 10:506–510.

87. Gray JW, Pedler SJ, Craft AW, et al. Changing causes of septicemia in paediatric oncology patients: effect of imipenem use. Eur J Pediatr 1994; 153:84–89.

88. Mulloy RH, Jadavji T, Russell ML. Tunnelled central venous catheter sepsis: risk factors in a pediatric hospital. J Parenter Enter Nutr 1991; 15:460–463.

89. Groeger JS, Lucas AB, Thaler HT. Infectious morbidity associated with long-term use of venous access devices in patients with cancer. Ann Intern Med 1993; 119:1168–1174.

90. Sherertz RJ, Forman DM, Solomon DD. Efficacy of dicloxacillin-coated polyurethane catheters in preventing subcutaneous *Staphylococcus aureus* infection in mice. Antimicrob Agents Chemother 1989; 33:1174–1178.

91. Sherertz RJ, Carruth WA, Hampton AA, et al. Efficacy of antibiotic-coated catheters in preventing subcutaneous *Staphylococcus aureus* infection in rabbits. J Infect Dis 1993; 167:98–106.

92. Saleh RA, Schorin MA. *Bacillus* sp. sepsis associated with Hickman catheters in patients with neoplastic disease. Pediatr Infect Dis J 1987; 6:851–856.

93. Flynn PM, van Hooser B, Gigliotti F. Atypical mycobacterial infections of Hickman catheter exit sites. Pediatr Infect Dis J 1988; 7:510–513.

94. Benezra D, Kiehn TE, Gold JWM, et al. Prospective study of infections in indwell-

ing central venous catheters using quantitative blood cultures. Am J Med 1988; 85: 495–498.

95. Eppes SC, Troutman JL, Gutman LT. Outcome of treatment of candidemia in children whose central catheters were removed or retained. Pediatr Infect Dis J 1989; 8: 99–104.

96. Dato VM, Dajani AS. Candidemia in children with central venous catheters: role of catheter removal and amphotericin B therapy. Pediatr Infect Dis J 1990; 9:309–314.

97. Arnow PM, Quimosing EM, Beach M. Consequences of intravascular catheter sepsis. Clin Infect Dis 1993; 16:778–784.

98. Jansen B. Vascular catheter-related infection: aetiology and prevention. Curr Opin Infect Dis 1993; 6:526–531.

99. Schwartz C, Henrickson KJ, Roghmann K, et al. Prevention of bacteremia attributed to luminal colonization of tunneled central venous catheters with vancomycin-susceptible organisms. J Clin Oncol 1990; 8:1591–1597.

100. Messing B, Peitra-Cohen S, Debure A, et al. Antibiotic-lock technique: a new approach to optimal therapy for catheter-related sepsis in home-parenteral nutrition patients. J Parenter Enter Nutr 1988; 12:185–189.

101. Johnson DC, Johnson FL, Goldman S. Preliminary results treating persistent central venous catheter infections with the antibiotic lock technique in pediatric patients. Pediatr Infect Dis J 1994; 13:930–931.

102. Goldmann DA, Pier GB. Pathogenesis of infections related to intravascular catheterization. Clin Microbiol Rev 1993; 6:176–192.

16

Current Approaches to the Prevention of Catheter-Related Infections

Bernd Jansen
Johannes Gutenberg University, Mainz, Germany

I. INTRODUCTION

Since their introduction in 1945, polymeric catheters have gained widespread acceptance in all fields of medicine. Currently, they are used for various therapeutic and diagnostic purposes—e.g., infusion therapy, administration of blood products, or hemodynamic monitoring of ICU patients. Thus, they represent major progress in modern medicine.

It is estimated that more than half of all patients admitted to a hospital in the U.S., Europe, or elsewhere will receive an intravascular catheter. In the United States this would represent 15 million to 20 million patients, some of whom will be at high risk of catheter-related infection (CRI). The annual frequency of CRI in the U.S. is reported to be approximately 850,000 cases (1). Because CRIs are major causes of primary nosocomial bloodstream infection, they represent an important risk factor, influencing patient morbidity and mortality and also hospital economics. For example, CRIs lead to a cost increase of approximately $3000 to $6000 U.S. per each case, due to therapy and prolonged hospital stay (2,3).

Two further special features of CRIs contribute to their importance and enhance their impact on patient health and economics. First, the difficulties in finding an accurate diagnosis of CRI may lead to a considerable number of unnecessarily removed catheters with associated cost increase, whereas a failure in diagnosis may have severe consequences for the patient. Second, failure of antibiotic treatment in many cases of established CRI and the subsequent necessity for catheter removal again considerably contribute to morbidity and to cost increase. For all these reasons, effective prevention of CRI is of paramount importance. In the last 10 to 20 years, a large number of studies on various aspects of CRI such as epidemiology, pathogenesis, therapy, and prevention have been published and have substantially increased our knowledge about these unique infections. Surely, this also has inspired the development of preventive measures. The aim of this chapter is to give a comprehensive overview of current strategies in the prevention of CRI, by carefully considering their individual benefits and shortcomings. In the concluding remarks a list of selected recommendations for the prevention of CRI will be given.

II. BASIC CONSIDERATIONS

For effective prevention, a basic understanding of the underlying mechanisms leading to CRI is essential. These include the pathogenesis and epidemiology as well as patient risk factors and are intensively discussed in the respective chapters elsewhere in this book. In the following, certain aspects of these issues will be addressed that are relevant with regard to prevention of CRI.

A. Factors Contributing to the Establishment of CRI

A variety of different factors may contribute to the development and establishment of a CRI (Fig. 1), e.g., the nature and specific abilities of the pathogen involved are important. Gram-positive organisms like coagulase-negative staphylococci (CoNS) and *Staphylococcus aureus* are main causative organisms due to their occurrence on skin and mucous membranes and their adherence capability, but in recent years CRIs with gram-negative microorganisms are increasingly observed, especially in immunocompromised patients. Thus, modern preventive strategies must not only aim at gram-positive bacteria as the most frequent isolated organisms but also take into account gram-negative bacteria and fungi. Although CRIs occur in the immunocompromised as well as in the immunocompetent host, immunosuppression of a patient is an important risk factor for CRI regarding severity and outcome. Other patient risk factors include extremes of age, burns and other major traumas, major skin lesions, and severe underlying diseases. The catheter itself with its specific properties may also play a particular role in the generation of associated infection. Besides chemical composition, surface topography, and thrombogenicity of a specific material, the type of catheter and its particular application may display different risks (Table 1).

Further important factors that may influence the risk for CRI are insertion technique, location of catheter placement, hygienic care of catheters, frequency

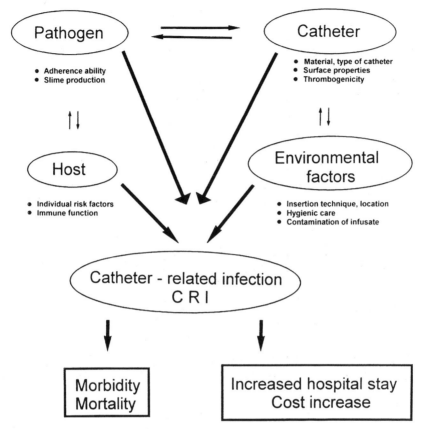

Figure 1   Factors contributing to catheter-related infections.

of manipulations at the catheter system, duration of catheterization, etc. Some of these factors may significantly contribute to CRI as has been pointed out by a variety of clinical studies and will be addressed more intensively in the next part of this chapter. A summary of the most important risk factors discussed so far is given in Table 2.

B.   Pathogenesis

There are three main routes by which microorganisms may adhere to and colonize an IV catheter (which are discussed in detail in the chapter by R. Sherertz, "Pathogenesis of Vascular Catheter-Related Infections"): (1) colonization by migration along the external catheter surface to the catheter tip; (2) colonization by contamination of the catheter hub or the infusate along the internal catheter

Table 1   Approximate Risks for Catheter-Related Septicemia Due to Various Types of Catheters

	Representative rate	Range
Short-term access[a]		
Steel needles	< 0.2	0–1
Peripheral IV catheters		
Percutaneously inserted	0.2	0–1
Cutdown	6	—
Arterial catheters	1	0–1
Central venous catheters		
All-purpose, multilumen	3	1–7
Swan-Ganz	1	0–5
Hemodialysis	10	3–18
Long-term access[b]		
Peripherally inserted CVC	0.20	—
Hickman, Broviac catheters	0.20	0.1–0.53
Central venous ports	0.04	0.00–0.1

[a]No. of septicemias per 100 devices.
[b]No. of septicemias per 100 device-days.
Source: Modified from Ref. 57.

Table 2   Risk Factors for Catheter-Related Infection

Patient factors	Extremes of age
	Burns, trauma
	Surgical patients, ICU patients
	Immunocompromised patients
	Severe skin lesions
	Severe underlying diseases
Catheter	Chemical composition (e.g., PVC)
	Surface topography
	Thrombogenicity
	Type (steel cannula, peripheral, central venous, etc.)
Catheterization and catheter care	Insertion technique
	Skill of medical personnel
	Access route
	Duration of placement
	Antiseptic measures (e.g., skin disinfection)
	Catheter dressing
	Interval of catheter and infusion system exchange
	Frequency of manipulations
	Kind of medicaments administered (e.g., parenteral alimentation)

surface; and (3) hematogenous spread of microorganisms from a distant site of infection (1).

Although the first pathway seems to be the most frequent in the pathogenesis of CRI, with regard to preventive measures the other two routes must also be considered. Figure 2 shows current prevention strategies aimed at the different pathways. Most of these are hygienic measures and will be discussed in detail later. Strategies aimed at the catheter material have been developed in recent years and require a basic understanding of the mechanisms by which microorganisms adhere to and colonize a catheter. Therefore, some of the principal adherence and colonization mechanisms will be discussed here.

There is evidence from many investigations that adherence to medical devices (in the majority, synthetic polymers) is the first and most important step in the pathogenesis of foreign-body-associated infection (4–6). This holds true also for CRI. Subsequent colonization, production of extracellular substances by microorganisms (slime, glycocalix), and involvement of host factors (e.g., blood and tissue proteins, platelets) lead to the formation of a compact matrix (biofilm)

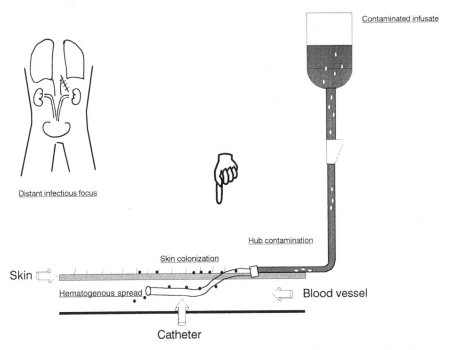

Figure 2 Strategies for prevention of CRI aimed at the different routes of catheter contamination.

on a device surface that is able to interfere with host defense mechanisms and antibiotic attack (6,7).

Principally, microbial interaction with synthetic surfaces can be divided in nonspecific and specific mechanisms (5). Nonspecific interactions can be assumed if microorganisms adhere to a native, uncoated catheter surface in the absence of specific host factors—e.g., adherence of *Staphylococcus epidermidis* to a pure polymer in a protein-free medium. These nonspecific mechanisms include van der Waals forces and electrostatic and hydrophobic interactions (Fig. 3), and have been extensively studied in a large number of investigations (for an overview see 4,5). Unspecific adherence can be described either using the DLVO-model or by a thermodynamical approach, provided that specific physico-chemical features of the microorganisms, the solid surface (medical device) and the surrounding medium are known or can be determined experimentally.

Regarding CRI, nonspecific adherence of skin microorganisms (e.g., *S. epidermidis*) to a native catheter surface may occur only very early at the time of insertion. However, virtually all foreign-body materials soon become coated by glycoproteins, derived from fluid or matrix phases containing fibrinogen, fibronectin, collagen, and other proteins (4,8), and lead to a fibrin sheath or, more generally, a biofilm around the catheter. It is well known that *S. aureus* binds to plastic surfaces via fibronectin as a mediator of adherence (9,10), but mediator-dependent adherence has been shown also for CoNS (11). Blood platelets seem to play another major role especially in the adherence of *S. aureus* (12,13). Further, specific factors on the bacterial surface of CoNS have been elucidated as

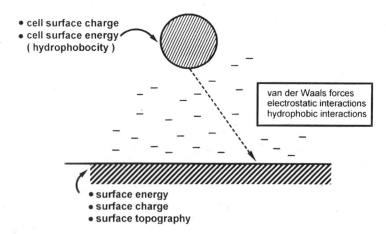

Figure 3   Unspecific adherence of a bacterial cell to a solid surface.

"adhesins" (14–18), so the overall adherence process appears to be very complex in nature (Fig. 4, Table 3)

C.   Basic Approaches to the Prevention of CRI

Regarding microbial adherence as an essential step in the pathogenesis of foreign-body infection and CRI, inhibition of adherence appears to be a very attractive approach for prevention. In Figure 5, important steps in the pathogenesis such as adhesion and colonization are schematically depicted by which way they could be inhibited. As long as there is no more detailed insight in the molecular pathogenesis of device-related infection, strategies directed against specific adherence mechanisms seem to be premature, especially because it is as yet unknown if a specific adhesin (e.g., protein, polysaccharide) is genus- or species-specific or merely strain-specific. Therefore, most of the recently developed strategies have focused on the modification of medical devices.

Alteration of the material surface (e.g., of a polymeric catheter) leads to a change in specific and nonspecific interactions with microorganisms. We could recently show for a large series of different modified polymers—each with unique physico-chemical properties—that nonspecific adherence of *S. epidermidis* KH6 could not be inhibited by surface modification, although this was thermodynamically predicted (19). We hypothesized that there must exist a certain "minimum of bacterial adherence" that cannot be remained under and which is independent of the nature of the device surface (19,20). Nevertheless, surface modification of polymeric medical devices may lead to a reduced microbial

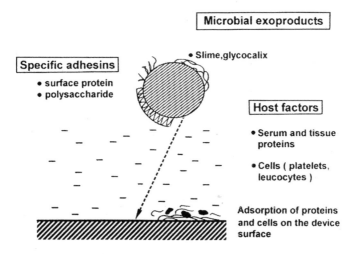

Figure 4   Factors involved in specific bacterial adherence to solid surfaces.

Table 3 Factors Involved in Specific Adherence of Staphylococci to Foreign Body Surfaces

	Specific factor determined	Species	Possible mode of action	Reference
Host factors	Fibronectin	*S. aureus*, CoNS	Adherence promotion	9–11
	Fibrinogen	*S. aureus*	Adherence promotion	9
	Thrombospondin	*S. aureus*	Adherence promotion	13
	Platelets	*S. aureus*, CoNS	Adherence promotion	12
Bacterial factors	Polysaccharide adhesin (PS/A)	*S. epidermidis*	Adhesin	14,15,18
	Surface protein	*S. epidermidis*	Adhesin	16
	Hemagglutinin	CoNS	Adhesin	17

adherence via altered interactions with proteins and platelets and will be discussed more detailed later on.

The development of so-called antimicrobial polymers aims predominantly at the prevention of microbial *colonization* rather than *adherence*. Catheters or parts of the catheter system containing antibiotics, disinfectants, or metals have been evaluated experimentally or in clinical trials, and are in part commercially available and already used in clinical applications. Prevention of biofilm formation by enzymatic destruction plus subsequent antibiotic therapy as well as the newly developed electrical enhancement of antibiotic penetration through biofilms are therapeutic strategies rather than preventive measures and will be discussed elsewhere in this book (21,22).

III. PREVENTION STRATEGIES AIMED AT CATHETERIZATION AND CATHETER CARE

As was pointed in the previous chapter, there are a variety of risk factors for CRI and, due to the particular pathogenesis, there exist several possible routes by which a catheter can become contaminated and thus infected (see Fig. 2). It is the goal of this chapter to review current prevention strategies which are directed against some of the most important risk factors and which are mainly based on

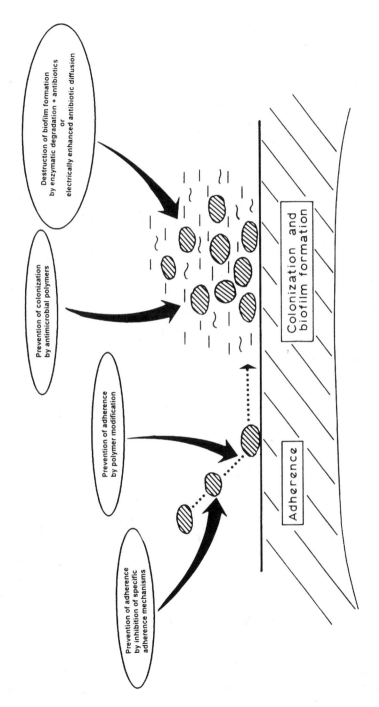

Figure 5   Current prevention strategies aimed at inhibition of bacterial adherence and/or colonization.

hygienic principles. A summary of these measures, which will be discussed in detail, is given in Table 4.

A. Catheter Insertion

1. Indication for Catheterization

A first important measure to avoid CRI is to question whether a patient needs an IV catheter at all and how long a catheter is really necessary. This appears rather trivial, but there are for sure many clinical situations in which a patient needs only short-term peripheral IV access, and, provided the patient offers no problems in venous puncture, IV access could be accomplished by the use of steel cannulae, which have a definitely lower risk than polymeric catheters (see Table 1). With a catheter in place—especially a central venous catheter—the indication to continue catheterization should be made daily, as it has been shown from various studies that the risk of CRI increases with prolonged catheterization (23–26). Thus, the effort to minimize the duration of catheterization is very important.

2. Catheter Material

It was emphasized that in an individual situation the choice of the catheter type may be of benefit in order to avoid CRI. Beside using steel cannulae, for short-term access rather than polymeric catheters, some recommendations for the choice of the appropriate catheter type can be given on the basis of several studies (27,28). Concerning the basic polymer material, it has been shown that polyvinylchloride (PVC) and even polyethylene are unsuitable due to their higher thrombogenicity and vulnerability for infection (29–33). Catheters made from silicone, polyurethane, or fluoropolymers are thus preferable (27). A recent study by Sherertz et al., however, demonstrated an increased risk for infection also for silicone catheters (34). The all-purpose, multilumen catheter is frequently used in many ICU units, although in a number of cases also single-lumen catheters could be used. It is unclear if there is a greater risk associated with multilumen catheters due to their bigger diameter (35–37), but, whenever possible, single-lumen catheters should be applied for longer periods, also for cost reasons. If it is anticipated that a catheter remains in place for more than 1 or 2 months, the implantation of a tunneled, cuffed catheter (Hickman or Broviac) or of a totally implantable catheter system (e.g., Port-a-Cath) should be considered. As was shown in Table 1, their use is associated with a significantly lower risk for CRI than with other CVCs.

3. Location of IV Access

Especially if a central venous or arterial catheter has to be inserted, the location of the IV access might be of concern regarding infections or mechanical compli-

Table 4 Currently Employed Strategies to
Avoid Catheter-Related Infection

Measures aimed at *catheter insertion*
  Handwashing
  Cutaneous antisepsis
  Barrier precautions
  IV teams
  Choice of location
  Choice of catheter type
  Antimicrobial prophylaxis[a]
Measures aimed at *catheter care*
  Use of dressings
  Minimizing manipulations
  Exchange protocols
  Topical antimicrobials[a]
Measures aimed at *administration set*
  In-line filters[a]
  Exchange protocols
Surveillance

---

[a]Currently not recommended.

cations. Whereas the jugular vein is supposed to be associated with a lower risk of mechanical complication but higher risk for infection, the opposite holds for the subclavian vein (38–40). Therefore, in ICU and highly immunocompromised patients, the subclavian route should be preferred due to its lower infectious complications. In patients in whom the jugular or subclavian site cannot be used the femoral vein access site can be an alternative (41,42).

4. Aseptic Measures and Barrier Precautions

With each IV catheterization the intact skin as an effective barrier against microorganisms is locally penetrated, and the catheter itself acts as a port of entry for microbes into the bloodstream. Thus, it is mandatory that strict aseptic conditions be followed during insertion of a catheter. This is valid for all types of catheters, but especially for arterial and central venous catheters. Hand washing with a disinfectant solution (e.g., chlorhexidin, alcohol) should precede each catheterization and is also of great importance for each later manipulation at the catheter or tubing system. Use of sterile gloves is strictly recommended in case of central venous and arterial catheters and should even taken into consideration during insertion of peripheral IV catheters in highly immunocompromised patients. The benefit of using maximal sterile barrier precautions to reduce the risk of CRI has been elucidated in two recent studies (43,44). In one study it was shown that the use of masks, caps, sterile gloves, gown, and a large drape during insertion of nontunneled, noncuffed central venous catheters leads to more than a sixfold reduction in catheter-related septicemia compared to a control group in which only sterile gloves and small sterile drapes were used (43). In another study on Swan-Ganz pulmonary artery catheters the application of such barrier precautions was associated with a twofold lower risk of infection (44). It is concluded that these measures are cost-effective, of benefit for the patient, and thus strongly recommended, at least for the insertion of central venous and arterial catheters.

5. IV Teams

Another important issue is the skill of the person or the team performing catheterization. A number of studies have shown that catheter insertion and catheter maintenance by a team of especially trained physicians, technicians, and nurses is associated with a lower risk of CRI and proves to be highly cost-effective (45–49). Thus, in a considerable number of hospitals in the United States such teams have been established whereas in most European countries IV teams are rarely instituted. In addition, the formulation of strict guidelines and protocols for catheter insertion and care as well as an intensive and repeated education of staff members is of paramount importance to reduce the incidence of infection.

6. Cutaneous Antisepsis

Due to the particular pathogenesis of CRI, skin disinfection at the insertion site is mandatory since contamination of a catheter during insertion by the patient's own microflora is supposed to be one of the commonest pathways of infection. However, even strict cutaneous antisepsis is not able to reduce all the resident flora, especially in deeper skin areas. Current protocols in the U.S. emphasize the use of chlorhexidine, while in European countries alcoholic disinfectants are more common (50,51). Although chlorhexidine seems to be slightly superior, alcohol is a reasonable and inexpensive alternative. As with every disinfectant, the recommended concentrations and duration of the application have to be carefully followed to obtain maximum success.

7. Antimicrobial Prophylaxis

A controversial issue is systemic (IV) antimicrobial prophylaxis during catheter insertion. In two trials, one randomized and one nonrandomized (52,53), a reduction of CRI has been demonstrated, whereas other controlled studies showed no benefit (54–56). At present, routine IV administration of antibiotics during catheter insertion cannot be recommended.

B.   Catheter Care

A general principle in catheter care is to restrict manipulations at the catheter or the administration system to a necessary minimum (1,57). Each healthcare worker managing patients with IV catheters (especially those on an ICU) should always be aware that the catheter is a conduit of the bloodstream to the environment with numerous risks of microbial contamination. Hand washing and wearing sterile gloves for each manipulation are essential, particularly in the case of central venous and arterial lines in high-risk patients.

1.   Catheter Site Dressings

To protect the insertion site of a catheter properly and to have an opportunity to inspect the site daily for suspicion of infection, transparent dressings have been introduced that are semipermeable, thus allowing no penetration of moisture from the outside and microbes but the evaporation of water vapor. There is up to now some controversy in the literature regarding the benefits and shortcomings of such dressings compared with sterile gauze (58–62). In a meta-analysis it was concluded that the risk of catheter tip infection is significantly increased by use of transparent rather than gauze dressings both for peripheral and central venous catheters (63). Accumulation of moisture under the polymeric dressing was associated with increased microbial contamination at the insertion site. Other studies, however, found no significant differences (61,62,64). The development of new dressings with high permeability and increased water vapor transmission rates will further minimize the risk of moisture buildup under the dressings (65).

There has been some concern about how frequently dressings should be changed. While with peripheral venous catheters no routine exchange is necessary (61), with CVCs, especially those used in ICUs, changing the dressings every other day is recommended (66). Another recent study comparing exchange intervals of dressings in hemato-oncological patients having a CVC concludes that a change twice a week can also be accepted (67). Dressings used for subcutaneously tunneled catheters (Hickman, Broviac) showed no increased risk of CRI; polyurethane dressings used for pulmonary artery catheters can probably be left in place for the duration of catheterization (≈4 days) without increased risks (68).

2.   Topical Antimicrobials

To minimize the risk of microbial ascension from the insertion site along the catheter surface, topical antimicrobials have been applied. A polyantibiotic ointment consisting of polymyxin, neomycin, and bacitracin has shown no benefit for site care of peripheral catheters, but it has been associated with an increased frequency of *Candida* infections (69). The use of topical polyvinylpyrrolidone-iodine (povidone-iodine) on the catheter site seems to be of benefit in patients with hemodialysis catheters, as a recently published study showed (70). Mupirocin, which is mainly applied for the eradication of (methicillin-resistant) *S. aureus* in nasal carriers, has also shown some success in the reduction of CRI, either used as local treatment or to decontaminate nasal staphylococcal carriage in hemodialysis patients (71,72). Although active only against gram-positive bacteria, topical application of mupirocin did not lead to a selection of fungi or gram-negative rods, so further clinical trials to evaluate its efficacy in reducing CRI are warranted.

3. Catheter Replacement

One of the key questions in catheter care and still a matter of controversy is how long a particular catheter can be left in place if no infection is suspected. It must again be emphasized that the responsible physician should assess daily whether a catheter is further needed. If a catheter is no longer necessary, it should be removed to avoid possible complications. There is no debate about that catheters inserted in emergency situations should be replaced as soon as possible. In case of peripheral IV (see also the chapter by G. Mayhall on Peripheral Venous Catheters) and pulmonary artery catheters, an exchange interval of 3 or 4 days is usually recommended. However, in one recently published prospective study it was shown that routine replacement of peripheral IV catheters seems to be not necessary (73). In case of central venous catheters, the most common practice is to keep a catheter as long as possible in place; guidelines for routine exchange are not given (74,75).

Another important factor—and this holds especially for short-term central venous lines—is by which way catheter replacement should be performed. It is common practice to change a central venous catheter over a guidewire by the Seldinger technique. The main purpose is to avoid complications associated with the new venous puncture, e.g., pneumothorax and other mechanical complications, and to have quickly a new catheter in place, especially in high-risk-patients with limited IV access. There have been a number of studies on the benefits and shortcomings of the Seldinger technique vs. new venous puncture (74–77), but up to now it has not been conclusively demonstrated if a guidewire exchange leads to increased infection rates. Thus, most authorities recommend the Seldinger technique for special situations, provided strict aseptic measures and the use of maximal sterile barrier precautions are applied. In case of an obvious infection at the exit site (purulent exudate) or if signs of septicemia occur, the new catheter should be inserted at a new site. In each case of guidewire exchange it is mandatory to culture the removed catheter, e.g., by the semiquantitative method, and to remove the newly inserted catheter immediately if the old catheter proves to be infected (75,76).

Concerning the exchange interval for infusion sets, in most hospitals in the U.S. a 72-hour interval is recommended, based on controlled studies (78,79) and contrary to the CDC Guidelines for Prevention of Intravascular Infections published in 1981 (80). Exceptions are the administration of blood products, lipid emulsions, and total parenteral nutrition (81–83). In those cases the administration systems should be replaced according to a 24-hour or 48-hour interval, respectively.

To minimize the risk of CRI due to extrinsic contamination by the infusate, in-line filters are frequently used with a pore size of 0.22 to 0.45 μm to retain bacteria and endotoxins (84–87). However, most of them are not able to prevent the passage of endotoxins; they frequently have to be exchanged and may become blocked with an ever higher risk of contamination. Regarding the relatively high costs associated with their use along with a doubtful benefit for minimizing CRI, they cannot be recommended for routine use at present (57).

C. Surveillance

Because skin colonization is thought to be an important risk factor for CRI, a few studies have dealt with surveillance cultures of skin and hub to find correlations between the extent of contamination and the development of CRI (88–90). However, despite a sensitivity of approximately 80%, the positive predictive value was only 44% in one study (89). Further studies are needed to evaluate the significance of surveillance cultures in the diagnosis and prevention of CRI.

Maki suggested surveillance of intravascular device-related bacteremias as a valuable tool in infection control, provided all blood isolates—especially CoNS—are identified to species level, the antibiotic phenotype is determined by standardized methods, and bloodstream isolates are saved for 2 years to enable performance of future epidemiological studies (91).

IV. MODIFICATION OF CATHETERS FOR THE PREVENTION OF CRI

In Section II of this chapter, the basic considerations regarding prevention of CRI by developing innovative catheter systems were discussed. It seems obvious that, due to the particular pathogenesis of CRI, approaches that are directed against bacterial contamination of a device are most promising. Catheters made out of a material that is antiadhesive or at least colonization-resistant in vivo would be the most suitable candidates to avoid associated infection and thus increase the lifetime of a catheter considerably. In the last 10 or 15 years there has been a large number of studies dealing with this problem, in part using different strategies. A general overview is given in Table 5. Most of the studies have been performed with intravascular catheters. A few studies have dealt with the development of infection-resistant CAPD and ventricular or urinary catheters, which will be discussed at the end of this section.

A. Antiadhesive Polymer Materials

The most attractive approach to obviate foreign-body-associated infections—in particular, CRIs—would be to develop a medical material which proves to be resistant against microbial adherence, even after insertion into the bloodstream and despite the ever occurring interactions of the device surface with host factors like proteins and cells. We have recently demonstrated that it seems to be impossible to create a polymeric surface which shows an absolute bacterial zero adherence in vitro (19,20). Hence, it seems not possible to design an absolute antiadhesive material which retains its properties even in the more complex, in vivo situation. However, there is some evidence that intrinsic properties of a material might be of advantage regarding resistance to infection. These are: (1) surfaces that are coated with albumin or preferentially absorb albumin; (2) hydrophilic, smooth surfaces; and (3) antithrombogenic materials. Thus, improvement of the surface texture, tailoring the protein adsorption characteristics, and improving the antithrombogenicity of a given material are key features in the development of innovative, infection-resistant materials. However, this goal has not been reached satisfactorily.

Several research groups have tried to develop polymers with new surface properties leading to a reduction of bacterial adhesion. Bridgett et al. studied the adherence of three isolates of *S. epidermidis* to polystyrene surfaces which were modified with a copolymer of poly(ethylene oxide) and poly(propylene oxide) (92). In vitro, a substantial reduction in bacterial adhesion was achieved with all surfactants tested. Similar results were found by Desai et al., who investigated the adhesion of *S. epidermidis*, *S. aureus*, and *Pseudomonas aeruginosa* to polymers that were surface-modified with poly(ethylene oxide) (93). They observed reductions in adherent bacteria between 70% and 95%, compared to the untreated poly-

Table 5 Prevention Strategies Aimed at the Modification of Catheters

Modified devices	Type of modification
Intravascular catheters Urinary catheters CAPD catheters	Modification of basic polymers (antiadhesive polymers)
Ventricular catheters	Incorporation or superficial bonding of antimicrobial substances
Catheter hub	Antibiotics
Cuffs	Antiseptics
Tubing systems	Metals with antimicrobial activity

mer. A photochemical coating of polymers was used by Dunkirk et al., demonstrating that the coating reduced adhesion of a variety of bacterial strains (94). Tebbs et al. compared the adherence of five *S. epidermidis* strains to a polyurethane catheter and to a commercial hydrophilic, coated polyurethane catheter (Hydrocath) (95). Adhesion of three strains to the coated catheters was considerably reduced. Bacterial colonization was further reduced by the addition of benzalkonium chloride to a hydrophilic polyurethane (Hydrocath) catheter (96). Our own approaches to develop antiinfective materials comprised the modification of polymer surfaces by radiation or glow discharge techniques; e.g., 2-hydroxymethylmethacrylate (HEMA) was covalently bonded to a polyurethane surface by means of radiation grafting, leading to a reduced in vitro adhesion of *S. epidermidis* (97,98).

So far none of the modified polymers have been used in clinical applications with the exception of the hydrophilic, polyvinylpyrrolidone-coated Hydrocath catheter based on polyurethane. Its relatively low thrombogenicity and low in vitro bacterial adherence should also be of benefit regarding infection resistance; however, this has as yet not been demonstrated in a clinical trial.

B.   Incorporation of Antimicrobial Agents Into Catheters

The loading of medical polymers with antimicrobial substances either for therapeutic or preventive purposes has a long tradition. The best-known anti-infective polymeric drug delivery systems are the polymethylmethacrylate (PMMA)-gentamicin bone cement and the PMMA-gentamicin beads (Septopal) used for treatment of bone and soft-tissue infections (99,100). Vascular prostheses from Dacron have been treated with various antibiotic substances to create infection-resistant grafts, but without routine clinical application up to now (101–103). In recent years, catheters or parts of the catheter system have been coated with antimicrobial drugs, and some of these antimicrobial devices are commercially available. The main principle of such devices is that an antimicrobial drug (an antibiotic, disinfectant, or metal) is bound superficially to a catheter—either directly or by means of a carrier—or incorporated into the interior of the polymer. If such a device comes into contact with an aqueous environment, release of the drug into the near vicinity occurs. Most such materials exhibit a release pattern according to first-order kinetics with an initially high drug release and, afterward, exponential decrease of the released drug. The amount of the antimicrobial substance released is influenced by the processing parameters, loading dose, applied technique, molecular size of the drug, and the physico-chemical properties of the polymeric device. A high antimicrobial concentration is reached (at least initially) in the very near vicinity of the device surface, mostly exceeding the MIC and MBC of susceptible organisms. It is as yet unclear whether such a device is capable of inhibition of microbial adherence per se, but at least a rapid elimination of already adherent microorganisms can be achieved. Thus, such materials are especially suitable to prevent "early-onset" CRIs, which originate from contamination during the insertion or shortly thereafter.

1. Development of Antimicrobial Catheters

There is a large number of studies on the bonding of antibiotics to biomaterials (Table 6). Solovskj et al. prepared polymers to which ampicillin and 6-aminopenicillanic acid were covalently bonded and which inhibited the in vitro growth of *S. aureus* (104). However, most studies have focused on the incorporation or superficial coating of antimicrobials rather than on covalent bonding by chemical reaction; e.g., Sherertz et al. used a rabbit model to investigate intravascular catheters coated with several antimicrobial compounds (dicloxacillin, clindamycin, fusidic acid, and chlorhexidine) (105). The frequency of catheter infections was significantly reduced compared with the control group when the dicloxacillin-coated catheter was used. We have investigated the incorporation of flucloxacillin, clindamycin, and ciprofloxacin into polyurethane polymers and demonstrated a considerable reduction of the in vitro adherence of *S. epidermidis*

Table 6 Bonding of Antibiotics to Polymers for the Prevention of Catheter-Related Infection

Polymer	Antibiotic	Determination of antimicrobial activity	Reference
Copolymers of methacrylamide with methacryloylated peptides	Ampicillin 6 Amino-penicillanic acid	In vitro inhibition of bacterial growth	Solovskj et al. (104)
Polyurethane catheter	Dicloxacillin Clindamycin Fusidic acid Ciprofloxacin Cefuroxime Cefotaxime	Mouse model Rabbit model	Sherertz et al. (164) Sherertz et al. (105)
Silicone catheter	Vancomycin Teicoplanin	In vitro colonization	Wilcox et al. (165)
Polyurethane catheter	Clindamycin Flucloxacillin Vancomycin Ciprofloxacin	In vitro colonization	Jansen et al. (97)
Polyrethane catheter (Hydrocath)	Teicoplanin	In vitro colonization Mouse model	Jansen et al. (107) Romano et al. (108)

(97,106). As a more recent development, a commercially available central venous catheter (Hydrocath) was loaded with the glycopeptide teicoplanin (107,169). In in vitro studies as well as in a mouse model the capability of this catheter to prevent colonization with *S. epidermidis* and *S. aureus*, respectively, for a period of at least 48 hours was proven, rendering the catheter suitable to prevent early-onset infection (107,108). In a clinical pilot trial with 60 patients undergoing cardiac surgery in which the Hydrocath catheters were loaded over 15 min with teicoplanin before insertion into the jugular vein, it was demonstrated that the catheters were well tolerated by the patients; no infections occurred, but the mean duration of catheterization was only 5 days (169). To extend the antimicrobial spectrum of such a catheter to include gram-negative bacteria and fungi, a combination of teicoplanin with silver was incorporated into Hydrocath catheters, exhibiting considerable activity against *S. epidermidis*, *Escherichia coli*, and *Candida albicans* (109).

Also, antimicrobial substances different from antibiotics like antiseptics have been used to develop new catheter materials (Table 7); e.g., the disinfectant

Table 7 Bonding of Antiseptics or Metals to Polymers for the Prevention of Catheter-Related Infection

Polymer	Antiseptic/metal	Determination of antimicrobial effect	Reference
Ethylvinylacetate Polyethylene Polypropylene Poly-(4-methyl-1-pentane)	Irgasan	Rabbit model	Kingston et al. (110)
Polyurethane catheter		Baboon model	Kingston et al. (166)
Polyurethane catheter (Hydrocath)	Iodine	In vitro colonization	Jansen et al. (111)
Polyurethane catheter	Chlorhexidine + silver sulfadiazine	Rat model	Bach et al. (167)
Silicone catheter	Silver	In vitro colonization	Sioshansi et al. (112)
Silicone PVC Teflon Butyl rubber	Silver, copper	In vitro colonization	Mc Lean et al. (113)
Polyurethane catheter	Silver	In vitro colonization	Jansen et al. (168)

Irgasan was incorporated into several polymer catheters showing a reduction of infections in rabbits (110). We used the hydrophilic Hydrocath catheter to incorporate iodine, leading to a polyvinylpyrrolidone-iodine complex on the inner and outer catheter surface (111). In vitro adherence of various microorganisms (*Staphylococcus* spp., *Escherichia coli*, *Candida* sp., *Pseudomonas* sp.) was completely inhibited for the time of iodine release. After iodine exhaustion, reloading of the catheter was possible. Tebbs and Elliot incorporated benzalkonium chloride into triple-lumen Hydrocath catheters and demonstrated a long-lasting antimicrobial activity of the catheters against staphylococci and a somewhat lesser activity against gram-negative bacteria and *C. albicans* (96).

Among metals with antimicrobial activity, silver has raised the interest of many investigators because of its good antimicrobial action and low toxicity. Sioshansi et al. used ion implantation to deposite silver-based coatings on a silicone rubber, which thereafter demonstrated antimicrobial activity (112). Also silver-copper surface films, sputter-coated onto catheter materials, showed antibacterial activity against *P. aeruginosa* biofilm formation (113). Silver has also been used extensively for the development of infection-resistant urinary catheters (see Section IV.C).

2. Clinical Studies

As silver has a broad-spectrum antimicrobial activity, is of minor toxicity, and lacks cross-resistance to classical antibiotics, it appears to be an attractive agent for antimicrobial biomedical devices. This is reflected by a few clinical studies that have been performed with silver-containing intravascular catheters. A novel catheter containing silver-sulfadiazine and chlorhexidine was evaluated in a randomized, comparative trial in 402 patients in a surgical ICU and proved to bear a fourfold reduced risk to produce bacteremia (114,115). Other trials have also demonstrated the clinical usefulness of this catheter, which is already commercially available (Arrowgard; Arrow International, U.S.) (116–118). In another randomized prospective study in hemato-oncological patients a novel silver sulfate-polyurethane catheter (Fresenius AG, Germany) was associated with a significantly lower rate of bacteremia (10,2%) than in the control group (22.5%) (119).

Only a few other clinical trials have been performed with antimicrobial IV catheters. Kamal et al. have evaluated the efficacy of a cefazolin-containing catheter in a prospective, randomized trial (120). There was a significant decrease in catheter infection as determined by the semiquantitative method of Maki (121). In a more recent study involving over 800 patients in each group, a twofold reduction in CRI was observed for the cefazolin-bonded catheter. Raad et al. recently reported about the clinical efficacy of a central venous catheter coated with minocycline and rifampicin to prevent catheter-related bacteremia in immunosuppressed patients (123).

A summary of the clinical studies performed so far with antimicrobial IV catheters is given in Table 8.

3. Modified Cuffs

As an alternative approach, protective cuffs have been developed for central venous catheters. These cuffs were coated with silver compounds to increase the anti-infective effect and, attached to the catheter prior to insertion, to act as a tissue interface barrier and thus to inhibit bacterial migration from the skin along the catheter; e.g., the Vita Cuff (Vita fore Corporation, San Carlos, U.S.) consists of a detachable cuff made of biodegrable collagen to which silver ions are chelated. In a prospective, randomized multicenter trial it was found that catheters inserted with the cuff were three times less likely to be colonized on removal than were control catheters, and nearly four times less likely to produce bacteremia (124). Similar results were observed in another study (125), whereas Groeger et al. found no difference in the frequency of colonized catheters between the test and control group (126). A reason for the controversial results might be that Groeger et al. used the cuff in patients with long-term catheterization in whom hub colonization may be a more important factor for CRI than extraluminal contamination against which the cuff confers protection. Based on their own results from a recently published study, Smith et al. recommended to use the Vita Cuff in patients requiring prolonged central venous catheterization (127).

C. Other Anti-Infective Catheters

Another interesting phenomen was detected in a meta-analysis of prospective studies of Swan-Ganz pulmonary artery catheters (128). Heparin is now commonly bonded to the external surface of Swan-Ganz catheters to enhance their antithrombogenicity (129), and heparin-bonded catheters obviously showed a lower frequency of CRI. In in vitro studies it has been demonstrated that a coating with heparin reduces bacterial adherence, but it is speculated that benzalkonium chloride to which heparin is bonded is mainly responsible for the anti-infective properties of these Swan-Ganz catheters.

A number of studies have been published on anti-infective urinary catheters. Aminoglycosides like dibekacin sulfate or kanamycin as well as cephalotin or cefoxitin have been bonded to hydrophilic polymers, polyethylene, and silicone rubber catheters and evaluated experimentally or in part in clinical studies, showing some effectiveness in the prevention of urinary catheter-associated infection. Most studies have dealt with the development of silver-containing catheters; e.g., Liedberg et al. investigated the interaction between silver alloy-coated urinary catheters and *P. aeruginosa* and demonstrated suppression of in vitro biofilm formation (130). In a randomized clinical trial, the incidence of catheter-associated urinary tract infection was reduced (131). In another prospective study involving

Table 8 Clinical Studies Performed With Antimicrobial Catheters

Type of catheter	Number of patients		Percentage of infections[a]		Significance	Reference
	Study	Control	Study	Control		
Polyurethane, chlorhexidine/silver sulfadiazine (Arrowgard)	—	—	13.6 (I)	24.6 (I)	$P = 0.003$	Maki et al. (114)
			1.0 (B)	4.7 (B)	$P = 0.02$	
	—	—	4.83 bacteremias/1000 catheter days	8.66 bacteremias/1000 catheter days	—	Clemence et al. (117)
	12	14	0 (I)	15.4 (I)	$P = 0.04$	Bach et al. (116)
	19	189	33 (C)	45 (C)	$P < 0.05$	Ramsay et al. (118)
			0.5 (B)	2 (B)	$P = 0.08$	
Polyurethane-cefazoline	97	81	2 (I)	14 (I)	$P = 0.004$	Kamal et al. (120)
	811	890	5.39 infections/1000 patient days	10.46 infections/1000 patient days	$P = 0.005$	Kamal et al. (122)
Polyurethane-silver	120	113	10.2 (I)	21.2 (I)	$P = 0.011$	Goldschmidt et al (19)
Polyurethane-minocycline/rifampicin	117	117	9 (C)	30 (C)	$P < 0.001$	Raad et al. (123)
			0 (B)	6 (B)	$P = 0.01$	

[a]C = colonization; I = infection; B = bacteremia.

482 hospitalized patients, Johnson et al. observed a similar rate of catheter-associated urinary tract infections in patients with a silver oxide urinary catheter compared to patients with normal catheters (132).

Trooskin et al. developed an infection-resistant continuous ambulatory peritoneal dialysis (CAPD) catheter by binding of penicillin via the cationic surfactant tridodecylmethylammonium chloride (TDMAC) to the silicone elastomer. In in vivo studies with rats, the antibiotic-bonded catheters were more resistant to colonization after exit site and intraluminal bacterial challenges (133).

Infection of central nervous systems (hydrocephalus) shunts is a major problem in patients with ventricular drainage. Therefore, efforts have been made to develop infection-resistant hydrocephalus shunts or other neurological prostheses. Bayston et al. have published a considerable number of experimental work on impregnation of silicone shunt catheters with various antimicrobials (134–137). Bridgett et al. reported on the reduced staphylococcal adherence to Hydromer-coated and thus hydrophilic cerebrospinal fluid shunts; however, there were technical difficulties in achieving a uniform Hydromer layer on the silicone rubber (138).

We have recently developed an incorporation method for rifampicin and other hydrophobic antibiotics into silicone ventricular catheters (139)—e.g., a rifampicin-loaded catheter is capable of inhibiting in vitro adherence of staphylococci. In an animal model using New Zealand white rabbits, catheters were implanted into the ventricular space and infection was induced by inoculation of certain dosages of *S. epidermidis* or *S. aureus* (140). None of the animals having received the rifampicin-loaded catheter showed clinical signs of infection, and the infecting strain could not be recovered from the catheter, brain tissue, or cerebrospinal fluid. In contrast, all animals with the uncoated catheters showed signs of severe meningitis or ventriculitis, and the infecting strains were cultivated in each case from the catheter and from surrounding tissue. A silicone catheter containing a combination of rifampicin and another hydrophobic antimicrobial agent is now under development to minimize the risk of rifampicin resistance.

V.   OTHER APPROACHES TO THE PREVENTION OF CRI

Stotter et al. developed a novel catheter hub to reduce the risk of hub contamination. It could be demonstrated that the rate of catheter-related bacteremia was significantly reduced (141). Segura et al. also have developed a contamination-resistant hub and have recently evaluated its efficacy to reduce catheter-related bloodstream infection in a clinical trial (142–144). A novel catheter system, equipped with a diaphragm instead of a stopcock for drawing blood specimen from arterial lines, proved to be associated with a sixfold lower rate of fluid contamination than a system using standard stopcocks (145).

An approach to reduce the risk of transmission of bloodborne infections to healthcare workers led to the design and introduction of needleless devices (146–149). At present, there are few data available on the benefit of such systems, but it seems that technical problems arise with the use of such systems which have to be solved before these devices should be evaluated in longer trials. Further, the use of nontoxic, biodegradable antiseptics to IV fluids as a measure to avoid fluid contamination and thereby to minimize the risk of hub contamination was proposed (150). Replacement of heparin in flush solutions by substances with intrinsic antimicrobial activity like EDTA might be of further benefit in reducing the risk of catheter-related bacteremia (151). The risk of phlebitis due to the administration of certain drugs (e.g., potassium chloride, lidocaine, antimicrobials) may be reduced by using intravenous additives, such as hydrocortisone (152,153). The topical application of glycerol trinitrate, or anti-inflammatory agents like cortisone near the catheter site, has effectively reduced the incidence of infusion-related thrombophlebitis and thus increased the lifespan of the catheters (154–156).

A very interesting approach to prevent biofilm formation has been suggested by Costerton et al. (22). They found that by application of an electric field together with antibiotics the killing of biofilm-embedded bacteria is dramatically enhanced (e.g., killing of *P. aeruginosa* by tobramycin). Although being more a therapeutical strategy than a preventive measure, the use of electric current might be useful for the prevention of CRI, as was already proposed in a previous study (157).

There are only very limited studies on innovative approaches for the prevention of foreign-body infection and CRI which do not aim at the medical device (implant or catheter). Tojo et al. isolated a polysaccharide from a *S. epidermidis* strain that appears to be involved in adhesion to synthetic polymers such as silicone (14,15). Active immunization of rabbits with this polysaccharide-adhesin (PS/A) factor led to reduced bacteremia caused by catheters contaminated with the specific *S. epidermidis* strain (158). In a further study, *S. epidermidis* prosthetic valve endocarditis was successfully prevented by active and passive immunization of the rabbits (159).

In a multicenter trial on the efficacy of a vaccination with staphylococcal toxoid in patients with CAPD catheters, no increase of the intraperitoneal bactericidal activity and no reduction of catheter-associated peritonitis or exit-site infection was observed (160). Finally, it has been proposed to develop monoclonal antibodies against fibronectin and other mediators of bacterial (staphylococcal adherence) to inhibit the specific adherence process (161). Whether such approaches—immunization with staphylococcal vaccines or blocking of specific adherence mechanisms—may be of general value for the prevention of CRI has yet to be determined.

Table 9   Selected Recommendations for the Prevention of CRI

	General recommendations	Specific recommendations
Strongly recommended	Healthcare worker education and training Daily inspection of catheter site Hand washing before handling catheters Barrier precautions during catheter insertion and care Catheter site care (appropriate cutaneous antisepsis, use of sterile gauze or transparent dressing) Removal of a catheter that is no longer needed Change of intravenous tubing no more frequently than at 72-hour intervals (except for the administration of blood and blood products: 24–48 h interval)	Use of Teflon and polyurethane catheters, or steel needles, for peripheral catheterization[a] Change of peripheral venous catheters every 48–72 h[a] Use of single-lumen rather than multilumen catheters[b] Use of tunnelled, cuffed, or totally implantable vascular access devices, if catheterization > 30 days is anticipated[b] Use of subclavian rather than jugular or femoral vein for vascular access[b] Change peripherally inserted CVC at least every 6 weeks[b] Change pulmonary artery catheters at least every 5 days[b] Do not change routinely percutaneously inserted central venous catheters[b]
Suggested for implementation	Surveillance for device-related infections	Use of antimicrobial central venous catheters in adult patients at high risk for CRI[b]
No recommendation	Use of in-line filters Use of needleless intravascular devices Antimicrobial prophylaxis	Use of antimicrobial peripheral venous catheters[b] Routine changes of CVC dressings and of totally implantable devices[b] Guidewire-assisted catheter exchange in case of documented CRI[b]

[a]Peripheral catheters.
[b]Central venous or arterial catheters.
Source: Adapted from Ref. 163.

VI. CONCLUDING REMARKS

Due to the difficulties in treatment of CRI and because of their impact on morbidity and (sometimes) mortality as well as cost increase, prevention of CRI
remains a major goal in modern medicine. In the preceding sections of this chapter we have tried to highlight modern preventive strategies, based on advances in
catheterization technique and care, and on innovative technology. Since the first
CDC guidelines for prevention of intravascular infection appeared in 1981, we
have learned much more about different aspects of CRI, and a considerable number of well-performed, controlled clinical studies have contributed to our actual
practice in intravascular catheterization. The development of new catheters, based
on modified materials, and other innovative approaches in this field will surely
lead to a further reduction in the incidence of CRI. It would be beyond the scope
of this chapter to give detailed guidelines for the daily management of catheters
and prevention of CRI, and the reader is referred to recently published or proposed guidelines (162,163). However, some concluding recommendations will be
given here, according to the proposal for the revised CDC guidelines (163). These
are summarized in Table 9.

REFERENCES

1. Widmer AF. IV-related Infections. In: Wenzel RP, ed. Prevention and Control of
    Nosocomial Infection. 2nd ed. Baltimore: Williams and Wilkins, 1993:556–579.
2. Arnow PM, Quimosing EM, Beach M. Consequences of intravascular catheter infec-
    tion. Clin Infect Dis 1993; 16:778–784.
3. Maki DG. Nosocomial bacteremia. An epidemiologic overview. Am J Med 1981;
    70:719–732.
4. Dankert J, Host AH, Feijen J. Biomedical polymers: bacterial adhesion, colonization
    and infection. In: Williams DF, ed. Critical Reviews in Biocompatibility. Boca
    Raton, FL; CRC Press, 1986; 2(3):219–301.
5. Jansen B, Peters G, Pulverer G. Mechanisms and clinical relevance of bacterial adhe-
    sion to polymers. J Biomat Appl 1988; 2:520–543.
6. Jansen B, Schumacher-Perdreau F, Peters G, Pulverer G. New aspects in the patho-
    genesis and prevention of polymer-associated foreign body infections caused by
    coagulase negative staphylococci. J Investig Surg 1989; 2:361–380.
7. Peters G, Schumacher-Perdreau F, Jansen B, Bey M, Pulverer G. Biology of *S. epi-
    dermidis* slime. In: Pulverer G, Quie P, Peters G, eds. Clinical Significance and Path-
    ogenicity of Coagulase-Negative Staphylococci. Stuttgart: Gustav Fischer Verlag,
    1987:15–32.
8. Gristina AG. Biomaterial-centered infection: microbial adhesion versus tissue inte-
    gration. Science 1987; 237:1588–1595.
9. Herrmann M, Vaudaux PE, Pittet D, et al. Fibronectin, fibrinogen, and laminin act as

mediators of adherence of clinical staphylococcal isolates to foreign material. J Infect Dis 1988; 158:693–701.

10. Vaudaux P, Suzuki R, Waldvogel FA, Morgenthaler JJ, Nydegger UE. Foreign body infection: role of fibronectin as a ligand for the adherence of *Staphylococcus aureus*. J Infect Dis 1984; 150:546–553.

12. Herrmann M, Lai QJ, Albrecht RM, Mosher DF, Proctor RA. Adhesion of *Staphylococcus aureus* to surface-bound platelets: role of fibrinogen/fibrin and platelet integrins. J Infect Dis 1993; 167:312–322.

13. Herrmann M, Suchard SJ, Boxer LA, Waldvogel FA, Lew PD. Thrombospondin binds to *Staphylococcus aureus* and promotes staphylococcal adherence to surfaces. Infect Immun 1991; 59:279–288.

14. Muller E, Hübner J, Gutierrez N, Takeda S, Goldmann DA, Pier GB. Isolation and characterization of transposon mutants of *Staphylococcus epidermidis* deficient in capsular polysaccharide/adhesin and slime. Infect Immun 1993; 61:551–558.

15. Tojo M, Yamashita N, Goldmann DA, Pier GB. Isolation and characterization of a capsular polysaccharide adhesin from *Staphylococcus epidermidis*. J Infect Dis 1988; 157:713–730.

16. Timmermann CP, Fleer A, Besnier JM, DeGraaf L, Cremers F, Verhoef J. Characterization of a proteinaceous adhesin of *Staphylococcus epidermidis* which mediates attachment to polystyrene. Infect Immun 1991; 59:4187–4192.

17. Rupp ME, Archer GL. Hemagglutination and adherence to plastic by *Staphylococcus epidermidis*. Infect Immun 1992; 60:4322–4327.

18. Mack D, Siemssen N, Laufs R. Parallel induction by glucose of adherence and a polysaccharide antigen specific for plastic-adherent *Staphylococcus epidermidis:* evidence for functional relation to intercellular adhesion. Infect Immun 1992; 60: 2048–2057.

19. Kohnen W, Ruiten D, Jansen B. Correlation between free energy for adhesion and bacterial adhesion to polymers—the minimum adherence hypothesis. American Society for Microbiology, 93th Meeting, Las Vegas, 1994. Abstract L35.

20. Jansen B, Kohnen W. Prevention of biofilm formation by polymer modification. J Industr Microbiol 1995; 15:391–396.

21. Ascher DP, Shoupe BA, Maybee D, Fischer GW. Persistent catheter-related bacteremia: clearance with antibiotics and urokinase. J Ped Surg 1993; 28:627–629.

22. Khoury AE, Lam K, Ellis B, Costerton JW. Prevention and control of bacterial infections associated with medical devices. ASAIO J 1992; 38(3):174–178.

23. Gil RT, Kruse JA, Thill-Baharozian MC, Carlson RW. Triple vs single-lumen central venous catheters. A prospective study in a critically ill population. Arch Intern Med 1989; 149:1139–1143.

24. Richet H, Hubert B, Nitemberg G, et al. Prospective multicenter study of vascular catheter-related complications and risk factors for positive central-catheter cultures in intensive care unit patients. J Clin Microb 1990; 28:2520–2525.

25. Miller JJ, Bahman V, Mathru M. Comparison of the sterility of long-term central venous catheterization using single-lumen, triple-lumen, and pulmonary artery catheters. Crit Care Med 1984; 12:634–637.

26. Ullman RF, Gurevich I, Schoch PE, Cunha BA. Colonization and bacteremia relat-

ed to duration of triple-lumen intravascular catheter placement. Infect Control 1990; 18:201–207.

27. Band JD, Maki DG. Steel needles used for intravenous therapy. Morbidity in patients with hematologic malignancy. Arch Intern Med 1980; 140:31–34.

28. Tully JL, Friedland GH, Baldini LM, Goldmann DA, Complications of intravenous therapy with steel needles and Teflon catheters. A comparative study. Am J Med 1981; 70:702–706.

29. Maki DG, Ringer M. Risk factors for infusion-related phlebitis with small peripheral venous catheters. A randomized controlled trial. Ann Intern Med 1991; 114:845–854.

30. Sheth NK, Rose HD, Franson TR, et al. In vitro quantitative adherence of bacteria on polyvinyl chloride and teflon catheters in hospitalized patients. J Clin Microb 1983; 18:1061–1063.

31. Collins RN, Braun PA, Zinner SH, Kass EH. Risk of local and systemic infection with polyurethane intravenous catheters. N Engl J Med 1968; 279:340–343.

32. Maki DG, Goldmann DA, Rhame FS. Infection control in intravenous therapy. Ann Intern Med. 1973; 79:867–887.

33. Mitchell, A, Atkins S, Royle GT, Kettlewell MGW. Reduced catheter sepsis and prolonged catheter life using a tunneled silicone rubber catheter for total parenteral nutrition. Br J Surg 1982; 69:420–422.

34. Sherertz RJ, Carruth WA, Marosok RD, Espeland MA, Johnson RA, Solomon DD. Contribution of vascular catheter material to the pathogenesis of infection: the enhanced risk of silicon in vivo. J Biomed Mater Res 1995; 29(5):635–645.

35. Yeung C, May J, Hughes R. Infection rate for single-lumen vs. triple-lumen subclavian catheters. Infect Control Hosp Epidemiol 1988; 9:154–158.

36. McCarthy MC, Shives JK, Robinson RJ, Broadie TA. Prospective evaluation of single- and triple-lumen catheters in total parenteral nutrition. J Parenter Enter Nutr 1987; 11:259–262.

37. Clark-Christoff N, Watters VA, Sparks W, Snyder P, Grant JP. Use of triple-lumen subclavian catheters for administration of total parenteral nutrition. J Parenter Enter Nutr 1992; 16:403–407.

38. Collignon P, Soni N, Pearson I, Sorrell T, Woods P. Sepsis associated with central vein catheters in critically ill patients. Intens Care Med 1988; 14:227–231.

39. Horowitz HW, Dworkin BM, Savino JA, et al. Central catheter-related infections: comparison of pulmonary artery catheters and triple lumen catheters for the delivery of hyperalimentation in a critical care setting. J Parenter Enter Nutr 1990; 14:558–592.

40. Pinilla JC, Ross DF, Martin T, Crump H. Study of the incidence of intravascular catheter infection and associated septicemia in critically ill patients. Crit Care Med 1983; 11:21–25.

41. Lazarus HM, Creger RJ, Bloom AD, Shenk R. Percutaneous placement of femoral central venous catheter in patients undergoing transplantation of bone marrow. Surg Gynecol Obstet 1990; 170:403–406.

42. Williams JF, Seneff MG, Friedman BC, et al. Use of femoral venous catheters in critically ill adults: prospective study. Crit Care Med 1991; 19:550–553.

43. Raad, II, Hohn DC, Gilbreath BJ, et al. Prevention of central venous catheter-relat-

ed infections by using maximal sterile barrier precautions during insertion. Infect Control Hosp Epidemiol 1994; 15:231–238.

44. Mermel LA, McCormick RD, Springman SR, Maki DG. The pathogenesis and epidemiology of catheter-related infection with pulmonary artery Swan-Ganz catheters: a prospective study utilizing molecular subtyping. Am J Med 1991; 91:197–205.

45. Faubion WC, Wesley JR, Khalidi N, Silvia T. Total parenteral nutrition catheter sepsis: impact of the team approach. J Parenter Enter Nutr 1986; 10(6):642.

46. Keohane PP, Jones BJ, Attrill H, et al. Effect of catheter tunnelling and a nutrition nurse on catheter sepsis during parenteral nutrition. A controlled trial. Lancet 1983; 2:1388–1390.

47. Nelson DB, Kein CL, Mohr B, Frank S, Davis SD. Dressing changes by specialized personnel reduce infection rates in patients receiving central venous parenteral nutrition. J Parenter Enter Nutr 1986; 10(2):220.

48. Tomford JW, Hershey CO, McLaren CJE, Porter DK, Cohen DI. Intravenous therapy team and peripheral venous catheter-associated complications. A prospective controlled study. Arch Intern Med 1984; 144:1191.

49. Tomford JW, Hershey CO. The I.V. therapy team. Impact on patient care and costs of hospitalization. NITA 1985; 8:387.

50. Henderson DK. Bacteremia due to percutaneous intravascular devices. In: Mandell GL, Douglas RG, Bennet JE, eds. Principles and Practice of Infectious Diseases. 3rd ed. New York: Churchill Livingstone, 1990:2189–2199.

51. Rutala WA. APIC guideline for selection and use of disinfectants. Am J Infect Control 1990; 18:99–117.

52. Bock SN, Lee RE, Fischer B, et al. A prospective randomized trial evaluating prophylactic antibiotics to prevent triple-lumen catheter-related sepsis in patients treated with immunotherapy. J Clin Oncol 1990; 8(1):161–169.

53. Al-Sibai MB, The value of prophylactic antibiotics during insertion of long-term indwelling silastic right arial catheters in cancer patients. Cancer 1987; 60:1891–1895.

54. McKee R. Does antibiotic prophylaxis at the time of catheter insertion reduce the incidence of catheter related sepsis in intravenous nutrition? J Hosp Infect 1985; 6:419–425.

55. Ranson MR, Oppenheim BA, Jackson A, Kamthan AG, Scarffe JH. Double-blind placebo controlled study of vancomycin prophylaxis for central venous catheter insertion in cancer patients. J Hosp Infect 1990; 15:95–102.

56. Rackoff WR, Weiman M, Jakobowski D, et al. A randomized, controlled trial of the efficacy of a heparin and vancomycin solution in preventing central venous catheter infections in children. J Pediatr 1995; 127(1):147–151.

57. Maki DG. Infections due to infusion therapy. In: Bennett JV, Brachman PS, eds. Hospital Infections. 3rd ed. Boston: Little, Brown, 1994:849–898.

58. Craven DE, Lichtenberg A, Kunches LM, et al. A randomized study comparing a transparent polyurethane dressing to a dry gauze dressing for peripheral intravenous catheter sites. Infect Control 1985; 361–366.

59. Dickerson N, Horton P, Smith S, Rose RC III. Clinically significant central venous catheter infections in a community hospital: association with type of dressing. J Infect Dis 1989; 160:720–721.

60. Conly JM, Grieves K, Peters B. A prospective, randomized study comparing transparent and dry gauze dressings for central venous catheters. J Infect Dis 1989; 159: 310–319.

61. Maki DG, Ringer M. Evaluation of dressing regimes for prevention of infection with peripheral intravenous catheters. Gauze, a transparent polyurethane dressing, and an iodophor-transparent dressing. JAMA 1987; 258:2396–2403.

62. Ricard P, Martin R, Marcoux JA. Protection of indwelling vascular catheters: incidence of bacterial contamination and catheter-related sepsis. Crit Care Med 1985; 13:541–543.

63. Hoffmann KK, Weber DJ, Samsa GP, Rutala WA. Transparent polyurethane film as an intravenous catheter dressing: a meta-analysis of the infection risks. JAMA 1992; 267:2072–2076.

64. Hoffmann KK, Western S, Groschel DHM, et al. Bacterial colonization and phlebitis-associated risk with transparent polyurethane film for peripheral intravenous site dressings. Am J Clin Pathol 1988; 16:101–106.

65. Thomas S, Loveless P, Hay NP. Comparative review of the properties of six semipermeable film dressings. Pharm J 1988; 241:785.

66. Gantz NM, Presswood GM, Goldberg R, Doern G. Effects of dressing type and change interval on intravenous therapy complications rates. Diagn Microbiol Infect Dis 1984; 2:325–332.

67. Engervall P, Ringertz S, Hagman E, Skogman K, Björkholm M. Change of central venous catheter dressings twice a week is superior to once a week in patients with hematological malignancies. J Hosp Infect 1995; 29:275–286.

68. Maki DG, Stolz SS, Wheeler S, Mermel LA. A prospective randomized trial of gauze and two polyurethane dressings for site care of pulmonary artery catheters: implications for catheter management. Crit Care Med 1994; 22(11):1729–1737.

69. Maki DG, Band JD. A comparative study of polyantibiotic and iodophor ointment in prevention of vascular catheter-related infection. Am J Med 1981; 70:739–744.

70. Fong IW. Prevention of haemodialysis and peritoneal dialysis catheter related infection by topical povidone-iodine. Postgrad Med J 1993; 69(3):15–17.

71. Hill RLR, Casewell MW. Reduction in the colonization of central venous cannulae by mupirocin. J Hosp Infect 1991; 19(B):47–57.

72. Boelart JR, De Baere YA, Gernaert MA, Godard CA, van Landuyt HW. The role of nasal mupirocin ointment to prevent Staphylococcus aureus bacteremias in hemodialysis patients: an analysis of cost-effectiveness. J Hosp Infect 1991; 19(B):41–46.

73. Bregenzer T, Conen D, Widmer AF. Routine replacement of peripheral IV-catheters is not necessary: A prospective study. Can J Infect Dis 1995; 6(C):247C.

74. Cobb DK, High KP, Sawyer RG, et al. A controlled trial of scheduled replacement of central venous and pulmonary artery catheters. N Engl J Med 1992; 327(15): 1062–1068.

75. Eyer S, Brummitt C, Crossley K, et al. Catheter-related sepsis: prospective, randomized study of three different methods of long-term catheter maintenance. Crit Care Med 1990; 18:1073–1079.

76. Amstrong CW, Mayhall CG, Miller KB, et al. Prospective study of catheter replacement and other risk factors for infection of hyperalimentation catheters. J Infect Dis 1986; 154:808–816.

77. Snyder RH, Archer FJ, Endy T, et al. Catheter infection: a comparison of two catheter maintenance techniques. Ann Surg 1988; 208:651–653.

78. Josephson A, Gombert ME, Sierra MF, Karanfil LV, Tansino GF. The relationship between intravenous fluid contamination and the frequency of tubing replacement. Infect Control 1985; 6:367–370.

79. Maki DG, Botticelli JT, LeRoy ML, Thielke TS. Prospective study of replacing administration sets for intravenous therapy at 48 vs 72-hour intervals: 72 hours is safe and cost-effective. JAMA 1987; 258:1777–1781.

80. Simmons BP: Guideline for prevention of intravascular infections (CDC guidelines). Am J Infect Control 1981; 183–199.

81. McKee KT, Melly MA, Greene HL. Gram-negative bacillary sepsis associated with use of lipid emulsion in parenteral nutrition. Am J Dis Child 1979; 133:649–650.

82. Jarvis WR, Highsmith AK, Allen JR, Haley RW. Polymicrobial bacteremia associated with lipid emulsion in neonatal intensive care unit. Pediatr Infect Dis 1983; 2: 203–208.

83. Crocker KS, Noga R, Filibeck DJ, et al. Microbial growth comparisons of five commercial parenteral lipid emulsions. J Parenter Enter Nutr 1984; 8:391–395.

84. Falchuk KH, Peterson L, McNeil BJ. Microparticulate-induced phlebitis: its prevention by in-line filtration. N Engl J Med 1985; 312:78–82.

85. Maddox RR, John JF Jr, Brown LL, Smith CE. Effect of in-line filtration on postinfusion phlebitis. Clin Pharm 1983; 2:58–61.

86. Baumgartner TG, Schmidt GL, Thakker KM, et al. Bacterial endotoxin retention by in-line intravenous filters. Am J Hosp Pharm 1986; 43:681–684.

87. Freeman JB, Litton AA. Preponderance of gram-positive infections during parenteral alimentation. Surg Gynecol Obstet 1974; 139:905–908.

88. Guidet B, Nicola I, Barakett JM, et al. Skin versus hub cultures to predict colonization and infection of central venous catheter in intensive care patients. Infection 1994; 22(1):43–48.

89. Fan ST, Teoh CC, Lau KF: Evaluation of central venous catheter sepsis by differential quantitative blood culture. Eur J Clin Microbiol Infect Dis 1989; 8:142–144.

90. Raad II, Baba M, Bodey GP. Diagnosis of catheter-related infections: The role of surveillance and targeted quantitative skin cultures. Clin Infect Dis 1995; 20:593–597.

91. Maki DG. Infections caused by intravascular devices used for infusion therapy: pathogenesis, prevention and management. In: Bisno AL, Waldvogel FA, eds. Infections Associated With Indwelling Medical Devices. 2nd ed. Washington D.C.; ASM Press, 1994:155–212.

92. Bridgett MJ, Davies MC, Deneyer SP. Control of staphylococcal adhesion to polystyrene surfaces by polymer surface modification with surfactants. Biomaterials 1992; 13:411–416.

93. Desai NP, Hossainy SF, Hubbell JA. Surface-immobilized polyethylene oxide for bacterial repellence. Biomaterials 1992; 13:417–420.

94. Dunkirk SG, Gregg SL, Duran LW, et al. Photochemical coatings for the prevention of bacterial colonization. J Biomat App 1991; 6:131–155.

95. Tebbs SE, Sawyer A, Elliott TS. Influence of surface morphology on in vitro bacterial adherence to central venous catheters. Br J Anaesth 1994; 72:587–591.

96. Tebbs SE, Elliott TS. Modification of central venous catheter polymers to prevent in vitro microbial colonisation. Eur J Clin Microbiol Infect Dis 1994; 13:111–117.

97. Jansen B, Schareina S, Steinhauser H, Peters G, Schumacher-Perdreau F, Pulverer G. Development of polymers with antiinfective properties. Polym Mater Sci Eng 1987; 57:43–46.

98. Jansen B. New concepts in the prevention of polymer associated foreign body infections. Zbl Bakt 1990; 272:401–410.

99. Marcinko DE. Gentamicin-impregnated PMMA beads: an introduction and review. J Foot Surg 195; 24(2):116–121.

100. Welch AG. Antibiotics in acrylic bone cement. J Biomed Mater Res 1978; 12:679.

101. Moore WA, Chrapil M, Seiffert G, Keown K. Development of an infection-resistant vascular prosthesis. Arch Surg 1981; 116:1403.

102. Powell TW, Bernham SJ, Johnson G. A passive system using rifampicin to create an infection-resistant vascular prosthesis. Surgery 1983; 945:765–769.

103. McDougal EG, Burnham SJ, Johnson G. Rifampicin protection against experimental graft sepsis. Vasc Surg 1986; 4(1):5.

104. Solovskj MV, Ulbrich K, Kopecek J. Synthesis of N-(2-hydroxypropyl)methacrylamide copolymers with antimicrobial activity. Biomaterials 1993; 4:44–48.

105. Sherertz RJ, Carruth WA, Hampton AA, Byron MP, Solomon DD. Efficacy of antibiotic-coated catheters in preventing subcutaneous *Staphylococcus aureus* infection in rabbits. J Infect Dis 1993; 167:98–106.

106. Jansen B, Peters G. Modern strategies in the prevention of polymer-associated infections. J Hosp Infect 1991; 19:83–88.

107. Jansen B, Jansen S, Peters G, Pulverer G. In-vitro efficacy of a central venous catheter ("Hydrocath") loaded with teicoplanin to prevent bacterial colonization. J Hosp Infect 1992; 22:93–107.

108. Romano E, Berti M, Goldstein BP, Borghi A. Efficacy of a central venous catheter (Hydrocath) loaded with teicoplanin in preventing subcutaneous staphylococcal infections in mouse. Zbl Bakt 1993; 279:426–433.

109. Jansen B, Ruiten D, Pulverer G. In-vitro activity of a catheter loaded with silver and teicoplanin to prevent bacterial and fungal colonization. J Hosp Infect 1995; 31:238–241.

110. Kingston D, Seal DV, Hill ID. Self-disinfecting plastics for intravenous catheters and prosthetic inserts. J Hyg Lond 1986; 98(2):185–198.

111. Jansen B, Kristinsson KG, Jansen S, Peters G, Pulverer G. In-vitro efficacy of a central venous catheter complexed with iodine to prevent bacterial colonization. J Antimicrob Chemother 1992; 30:135–139.

112. Sioshansi P. New processes for surface treatment of catheters. Artif Organs 1994; 18:266–272.

113. McLean RJ, Hussain AA, Sayer M, Vincent PJ, Hughes DJ, Smith TJ. Antibacterial activity of multilayer silver-copper surface films on catheter material. Can J Microbiol 1993; 39:895–899.

114. Maki DG, Wheeler SJ, Stolz SM, Mermel LA. Clinical trial of a novel antiseptic central venous catheter. In: Program and Abstracts of the 31st Interscience Conference on Antimicrobial Agents and Chemotherapy. Chicago: American Society for Microbiology, 1991. Abstract 461.

115. Maki DG, Wheeler SJ, Stolz SM. Study of a novel antiseptic-coated central venous catheter. Crit Care Med 1991; 19(suppl):99.

116. Bach A, Böhrer H, Böttiger BW, Motsch J, Martin E. Reduction of bacterial colonization of triple-lumen catheters with antiseptic bonding in septic patients. Anaesthesiology 1994; 81(A):261.

117. Clemence MA, Anglim AM, Jernigan JA, et al. A study of prevention of catheter related bloodstream infection with an antiseptic impregnated catheter. In: Program and Abstracts of the 34th Interscience Conference on Antimicrobial Agents and Chemotherapy, New Orleans, 1994. Abstract J199.

118. Ramsay J, Nolte F, Schwarzmann S. Incidence of catheter colonization and catheter related infections with an antiseptic impregnated triple lumen catheter. Crit Care Med 1994; 22:A115.

119. Goldschmidt H, Hahn U, Salwender HJ, et al. Prevention of catheter-related infections by silver coated central venous catheters in oncological patients. Zbl Bakt 1995; 283:215–223.

120. Kamal GD, Pfaller MA, Rempe LE, Jebson PJ. Reduced intravascular catheter infection by antibiotic bonding. A prospective, randomized, controlled trial. JAMA 1991; 265:2364–2368.

121. Maki DG, Weise CE, Sarafin HW. A semiquantitative culture method for identifying intravenous catheter-related infection. N Engl J Med 1977; 296:1305–1309.

122. Kamal GD, Divishek D, Adams J, Jebson P, Tatman D. Reduced intravascular catheter infection by routine use of antibiotic bonded catheters. Crit Care Med 1994; 22: A115.

123. Raad I, Darouiche R. Central venous catheters (CVC) coated with minocycline and rifampicin (M/R) for the prevention of catheter-related bacteremia (CRB). In: Program and Abstracts of the 35th Interscience Conference on Antimicrobial Agents and Chemotherapy, San Francisco, 1995. Abstract J7, 258.

124. Maki DG, Cobb L, Garman JK, Shapiro JM, Ringer M, Helgerson RB. An attachable silver-impregnated cuff for prevention of infection with central venous catheters. A prospective randomized multi-center trial. Am J Med 1988; 85:307–314.

125. Flowers R, Schwenzer KJ, Kopel RF, Fisch MJ, Tucker SI, Farr BM. Efficacy of an attachable subcutaneous cuff for the prevention of intravascular catheter-related infection. A randomized, controlled trial. JAMA 1989; 261:878–883.

126. Groeger JS, Lucas AB, Coit D, et al. A prospective, randomized evaluation of the effect of silver impregnated subcutaneous cuffs for preventing tunneled chronic venous access catheter infection in cancer patients. Ann Surg 1993; 218:206–210.

127. Smith HO, DeVictoria CL, Garfinkel D, et al. A prospective randomized comparison of an attached silver-impregnated cuff to prevent central venous catheter-associated infection. Gynecol Oncol 1995; 58(1):92–100.

128. Mermel LA, Stolz SM, Maki DG. Surface antimicrobial activity of heparin-bonded and antiseptic-impregnated vascular catheters. J Infect Dis 1993; 167:920–924.

129. Hoar PF, Wilson RM, Mangano DT, Avery GJ, Szarnicki RJ, Hill JD. Heparin bonding reduces thrombogenicity of pulmonary artery catheters. N Engl J Med 1981; 305:993–995.

130. Liedberg H, Ekman P, Lundeberg T. Pseudomonas aeruginosa: adherence to and growth on different urinary catheter coatings. Int Urol Nephrol 1990; 22:487–492.

131. Liedberg H, Lundeberg T. Silver alloy coated catheters reduce catheter-associated bacteriuria. Br J Urol 1990; 65:379–381.

132. Johnson JR, Roberts PL, Olson RJ, Moyer KA, Stamm WE. Prevention of urinary tract infection with a silver oxide-coated urinary catheter: clinical and microbiologic correlates. J Infect Dis 1990; 162:1145–1150.

133. Trooskin SZ, Donetz AP, Baxter J, Harvey RA, Greco RS. Infection-resistant continuous peritoneal dialysis catheters. Nephron 1987; 46:263–267.

134. Bayston R, Millner RDG. Antimicrobial activity of silicone rubber used in hydrocephalus shunts, after impregnation with antimicrobial substances. J Clin Pathol 1981; 34:1057–1062.

135. Bayston R, Adroyewski V, Barsham S. Use of an in vitro model to study eradication of catheter colonization by *Staphylococcus epidermidis*. J Infect 1988; 16:141–146.

136. Bayston R, Barsham C. Catheter colonization: a laboratory model suitable for aetiological, therapeutic and preventive studies. Med Lab Sci 1988; 45:235–239.

137. Bayston R, Grove N, Siegel J, et al. Prevention of hydrocephalus shunt catheter colonisation in vitro by impregnation with antimicrobials. J Neurosurg 1989; 52: 605–609.

138. Bridgett MJ, Davies MC, Denyer SP, Eldridge PR. In vitro assessment of bacterial adhesion to Hydromer-coated cerebrospinal fluid shunts. Biomat 1993; 14(3):184–188.

139. Schierholz J, Jansen B, Jaenicke L, Pulverer G. In-vitro efficacy of an antibiotic releasing silicone ventricle catheter to prevent shunt infection. Biomaterials 1994; 15(12):996–1000.

140. Hampl J, Schierholz J, Jansen B, Aschoff A. In vitro and in vivo efficacy of a rifampicin-loaded silicone catheter for the prevention of CSF shunt infections. Acta Neurochir 1995; 133:147–152.

141. Stotter AT, Ward H, Waterfield AH, Sim AJW. Junctional care: the key to prevention of catheter sepsis in intravenous feeding. J Parenter Enter Nutr 1987; 11:159.

142. Segura M, Alia C, Valverde J, Franch G, Torres-Rodriguez JM, Sitges-Serra A. Assessment of a new hub design and the semiquantitative catheter culture method using an in vivo experimental model of catheter sepsis. J Clin Microbiol 1990; 28(11):2551.

143. Segura M, Alia C, Oms L, Sanco JJ, Torres-Rodriguez JM, Sitges-Serra A. In vitro bacteriological study of a new hub model for intravascular catheters and infusion equipment. J Clin Microbiol 1989; 27(12):2656.

144. Segura M, Alvarez F, Lerma JM, et al. Clinical trial of the effect of new catheter hub on the prevention of central venous catheter-related sepsis. In: Program and Abstracts of the 35th Interscience Conference on Antimicrobial Agents and Chemotherapy. San Francisco, 1995. Abstract J10, 258.

145. Crow S, Conrad SA, Chaney-Rowell K, King JW. Microbial contamination of arterial infusions used for hemodynamic monitoring: A randomized trial of contamination with sampling through conventional stopcocks versus a novel closed system. Infect Control Hosp Epidemiol 1989; 10:557.

146. Adams KS, Zehrer CL, Thomas W. Comparison of a needleless system with conventional heparin locks. Infect Control Hosp Epidemiol 1993; 21:263–269.

147. Danzig LE, Short L, Collins K, et al. Bloodstream infections associated with a

needleless intravenous infusion system and total parenteral nutrition. Infect Control Hosp Epidemiol 1995; 16(pt 2):22.

148. Kellermann S, Shay D, Howard J, Feusner J, Goes C, Jarvis W. Bloodstream infections associated with needleless devices used for central venous catheter access in children receiving home health care. In: Program and Abstracts of the 35th Interscience Conference on Antimicrobial Agents and Chemotherapy, San Francisco 1995: abstr. J11, 258.

149. Vassallo D, Blanc-Jouvan M, Bret M, et al. *Staphylococcus aureus* septicemia and a needleless system of infusion. In: Program and Abstracts of the 35th Interscience Conference on Antimicrobial Agents and Chemotherapy, San Francisco, 1995. Abstract J12, 259.

150. Freeman R. Addition of sodium metabisulfite to left atrial catheter infusate as a means of preventing bacterial colonization of the catheter tip. Thorax 1982; 37:142.

151. Root JL. Inhibitory effect of disodium EDTA upon the growth of *Staphylococcus epidermidis* in vitro; relation to infection prophylaxis of Hickman catheters. Antimicrob Agents Chemother 1988; 32:1627–1631.

152. Sketch MH. Use of percutaneously inserted venous catheters in coronary care units. Chest 1972; 62:684–689.

153. Bassan MM. Prevention of lidocaine-infusion phlebitis by heparin and hydrocortisone. Chest 1983; 84:439–441.

154. Wright A. Use of transdermal glyceryl trinitate to reduce failure of intravenous infusion due to phlebitis and extravasation. Lancet 1985; 2:1148–1150.

155. Woodhouse CR. Movelat in the prevention of infusion thrombophlebitis. Br Med J 1979; 1:454–455.

156. O'Brien BJ, Buxton MJ, Khawaja HT. An economic evaluation of transdermal glyceryl trinitrate in the prevention of intravenous infusion failure. J Clin Epidemiol 1990; 43:757–763.

157. Crocker IC, Liu WK, Byrne PO, Elliott TSJ. A novel electrical method for the prevention of microbial colonization of intravascular cannulae. J Hosp Infect 1992; 22: 7–17.

158. Kojima Y, Tojo M, Goldmann DA, Tosteson TD, Pier GB. Antibody to the capsular polysaccharide/adhesin protects rabbits against catheter-related bacteremia due to coagulase-negative staphylococci. J Infect Dis 1990; 162:435–441.

159. Takeda S, Pier GB, Kojima Y, et al. Protection against endocarditis due to *Staphylococcus epidermidis* by immunization with capsular polysaccharide/adhesin. Circulation 1991; 84:2539–2546.

160. Poole-Warren LA, Hallett MD, Hone PW, Burden SH, Farrell PC. Vaccination for prevention of CAPD associated staphylococcal infection: results of a prospective multicentre clinical trial. Clin Nephrol 1991; 35:198–206.

161. Vaudaux P, Yasuda H, Velazco MI, et al. Role of host and bacterial factors in modulating staphylococcal adhesion to implanted polymer surfaces. J Biomat Appl 1990; 5(2):134–153.

162. Elliott TSF, Faroqui MH, Armstrong RF, Hanson GC. Guidelines for good practice in central venous catheterization. J Hosp Infect 1994; 28(3):163–176.

163. Draft guidelines for prevention of intravascular device-related infections. Fed Reg 1995; 60:49978–50006.

164. Sherertz RJ, Forman DM, Solomon DD. Efficacy of dicloxacillin-coated polyurethane catheters in preventing subcutaneous *Staphylococcus aureus* infection in mice. Antimicrob Agents Chemother 1989; 33:1174–1178.
165. Wilcox MH, Winstanley TG, Spencer RC. Binding of teicoplanin and vancomycin to polymer surfaces. J Antimicrob Chemother 1994; 33:431–441.
166. Kingston D, Birnie EDC, Martin J, Pearce PC, Manek S, Quinn CM. Experimental pathology of intravenous polyurethane cannulae containing disinfectant. J Hosp Infect 1992; 20:257–270.
167. Bach A, Böhrer H, Martin E, Geiss HK, Sonntag HG. Prevention of catheter-related infections by antiseptic surface bonding. J Surg Res 1993; 55:640–646.
168. Jansen B, Rinck M, Wolbring P, Strohmeier A, Jahns T. In vitro evaluation of the antimicrobial efficacy and biocompatibility of a silver-coated central venous catheter. J Biomat Appl 1994; 9(1):55–70.
169. Jansen B. Beschichtung von Kathetern und Implantaten mit Teicoplanin zur Prävention von Fremdkörperinfektionen. Chemotherapie Journal 1996; 11(suppl):42–44.

Index

About the Editors

HARALD SEIFERT is an Assistant Professor at the Institute of Medical Microbiology, University of Cologne, Germany. The author or coauthor of numerous journal publications and book chapters, he is a member of the American Society of Microbiology and the German Infectious Disease Society, among others. Dr. Seifert received the M.D. degree (1981) from the University of Bonn, Germany.

BERND JANSEN is a Professor of Medical Microbiology and Hygiene and the Head of the Department of Hygiene and Environmental Medicine, Johannes Gutenberg University, Mainz, Germany. The author or coauthor of over 100 publications, he is a member of the American Society of Microbiology, the Society of Healthcare Epidemiology of America, and the American Chemical Society, among others. Dr. Jansen received the Ph.D. degree (1980) in chemistry and the M.D. degree (1987) from the University of Cologne, Germany.

BARRY M. FARR is the Hospital Epidemiologist and the William S. Jordan Jr. Professor in the Department of Internal Medicine, University of Virginia, Charlottesville. One of the consultants to the Centers for Disease Control for their 1996 *Guidelines for Prevention of Intravascular Device-Related Infections*, he was also a member of a task force convened by the Food and Drug Administration that developed a 1994 guideline for preventing central venous catheter complications. Dr. Farr is the author or coauthor of over 180 publications, a Fellow of the American College of Physicians as well as the Infectious Diseases Society of America, and a member of the American Epidemiological Society, among others. He received the M.D. degree (1978) from Washington University, St. Louis, Missouri, and the M.Sc. degree (1984) in epidemiology from the London School of Hygiene and Tropical Medicine, London, England.